Current Trends in the Diagnosis and Management of Metabolic Disorders

This volume provides an overview of the biochemical basis of metabolic diseases and the molecular basis of chemical pathologies. Metabolic disorders occur when metabolic processes in the body are disrupted. They contribute a significant burden to human health globally. They can be congenital or acquired, for example, diabetes mellitus, obesity, metabolic syndrome, osteoporosis, osteopenia, mild-moderate hypovitaminosis D, erectile dysfunction, dyslipidemia, and thyroiditis. Metabolic disorders have gained significant importance due to the exponential increase in obesity worldwide. Early diagnosis of metabolic disorders is important in order to employ lifestyle and risk factor modification.

Features:

- An overview of the biochemical basis of metabolic diseases and the molecular basis of chemical pathologies.

- Describes recent trends in the diagnosis of metabolic disorders.

- Discusses management and treatment of metabolic diseases.

- Allows quick identification and retrieval of material by researchers learning the efficacy, associated dosage, and toxicity of each of the classes of drugs.

- Suitable globally for graduate and postgraduate students studying metabolic diseases.

Current Trends in the Diagnosis and Management of Metabolic Disorders

Edited By

Seth Kwabena Amponsah

Emmanuel Kwaku Ofori

Yashwant V. Pathak

CRC Press
Taylor & Francis Group
Boca Raton London New York

CRC Press is an imprint of the
Taylor & Francis Group, an **informa** business

First edition published 2024
by CRC Press
2385 Executive Center Drive, Suite 320, Boca Raton, FL 33431

and by CRC Press
4 Park Square, Milton Park, Abingdon, Oxon, OX14 4RN

Library of Congress Cataloging-in-Publication Data

Names: Amponsah, Seth Kwabena, editor. | Ofori, Emmanuel Kwaku, editor. |
Pathak, Yashwant, editor.
Title: Current trends in the diagnosis and management of metabolic disorders / edited by
Seth Kwabena Amponsah, PhD, Department of Medical Pharmacology, University of Ghana Medical
School, Accra, Ghana, Emmanuel Kwaku Ofori, PhD, Department of Chemical Pathology, University of
Ghana Medical School, Accra, Ghana, Yashwant V. Pathak, PhD, FAAAS, USF Health Taneja College of
Pharmacy, University of South Florida, Tampa FL, USA & Faculty of Pharmacy, Airlangga University,
Surabaya, Indonesia.
Description: First edition. | Boca Raton : CRC Press, 2024. | Includes bibliographical
references and index.
Identifiers: LCCN 2023030934 (print) | LCCN 2023030935 (ebook) |
ISBN 9781032469676 (hbk) | ISBN 9781032471600 (pbk) | ISBN 9781003384823 (ebk)
Subjects: LCSH: Metabolism--Disorders. | Metabolism--Disorders--Diagnosis. |
Metabolism--Disorders--Treatment.
Classification: LCC RC627.54 .C87 2024 (print) | LCC RC627.54 (ebook) |
DDC 616.3/9--dc23/eng/20231002
LC record available at https://lccn.loc.gov/2023030934
LC ebook record available at https://lccn.loc.gov/2023030935

ISBN: 978-1-032-46967-6 (hbk)
ISBN: 978-1-032-47160-0 (pbk)
ISBN: 978-1-003-38482-3 (ebk)

DOI: 10.1201/9781003384823

Typeset in Palatino
by Deanta Global Publishing Services, Chennai, India

Dedication

I dedicate this book to my wife Adwoa and my children (Ethan and Elyse), who continuously motivate me. I am also indebted to my mother, Comfort Aboagye-Adu, my sister Adwoa Kyerewa Akoto, and my brother-in-law Odeneho Kwafo Akoto III.

I also dedicate this book to a very good friend who keeps encouraging me to write more books, Kwame Sam Biney, and to his brother, George Biney, of blessed memory. I cannot forget "The Body", a group of close friends who have become like family.

Seth K. Amponsah

I dedicate this book to the loving memory of my dad, Emmanuel Addae Ofori, who I know would be pleased with what I have accomplished. I also dedicate it to my mother, Mabel Ofori, who, from the very beginning, instilled in me the values of resiliency and perseverance.

To my wife Irene, and three wonderful children, Michelle, Janelle, and Kwabena, you are my source of strength and inspiration.

Emmanuel K. Ofori

To the loving memories of my parents and Dr Keshav Baliram Hedgewar, founder of Rashrtriya Swayamsevak Sangh (RSS) in Bharat, who gave proper direction to my life, to my beloved wife Seema, who gave positive meaning, and my son Sarvadaman, who gave a golden lining to my life.

I would like to dedicate this book to Prof. Ved Nanda, Prof. Radheshyam Dwivedi, Prof. Manohar Shinde and Shri Baburam Guptajee, who were my mentors and role models; I learned a lot from them.

Yashwant V. Pathak

Table of Contents

Preface

Metabolic disorders occur when metabolic processes in the body are disrupted. Metabolic diseases contribute a significant burden to human health throughout the world. These disorders can be congenital or acquired, for example, diabetes mellitus, obesity, metabolic syndrome, osteoporosis, osteopenia, mild-moderate hypovitaminosis D, erectile dysfunction, dyslipidemia, and thyroiditis. Metabolic disorders have gained significant importance due to the exponential increase in obesity worldwide. Early diagnosis of metabolic disorders is important in order to employ lifestyle and risk factor modification.

Over the years, there has been growing interest in the field of metabolic disorders; however, there appears to be few books that address recent trends. After carefully studying the literature, we found that there are few books available on the market that compile the various biomedical aspects of metabolic diseases/disorders; hence, this book will be a great resource for clinicians, scientists, researchers, and students.

Due to the fact that medicine is a fast-evolving field, it is important that information on current trends is documented. This book offers details of many aspects of metabolic disorders (diabetes mellitus, obesity, etc.). We believe that this book is timely and will be in high demand among primary audiences (health care professionals, academicians and scientist/researchers in the field of endocrinology, chemical pathology, medical biochemistry, and pharmacology) as well as secondary audiences (graduate students, young researchers, and young investigators). Due to high priority given to the treatment of metabolic disorders, the needs of both primary and secondary audiences will be met by this book. The book contains 20 chapters with rich content, presenting fundamental facts, as well as practical and clinically related data. The book has the following key features:

- Molecular basis of chemical pathologies

- Recent trends in the diagnosis of metabolic disorders

- Management and treatment of metabolic diseases

The editors are grateful to all contributing authors, who continue to have a positive influence in their roles as researchers and academicians. The editors also thank CRC Press (Taylor & Francis Group) for facilitating all the processes involved in the production and publishing of this book.

Seth K. Amponsah
Emmanuel K. Ofori
Yashwant V. Pathak

Foreword

In this current era, many more people suffer from metabolic disorders such as diabetes mellitus, dyslipidemia, and cardiovascular diseases. Indeed, these conditions have become more widespread even in developing countries. Although there has been significant progress made in the diagnosis and management of diseases associated with metabolic disorders, it could be argued that there are still many unanswered questions regarding their etiology and management modalities. Metabolic disorders pose a multi-faceted (health, economic, emotional, and social) burden on individuals, families, and public health systems. Often, the costs associated with diagnosis, treatment, and management of metabolic disorders can be high, and thus, there is the need for patients to make lifestyle changes, adhere to drug treatment regimens, and constantly monitor metabolic biomarkers. Considering the burden that these diseases pose to humans, it is important to review current literature and document novel approaches used to mitigate the development and progression of these disorders.

The current book provides an overview of a number of metabolic disorders, including their etiology, diagnosis, current trends in their management, and future directives. The book has 20 individual chapters that are devoted to important topics such as biochemical and nutritional aspects of metabolic disorders, artificial intelligence use in metabolic disorders, and the clinical management of renal, neurological, bone, and cardiovascular disorders.

I can attest to the fact that the chapters found in this book are well written, and the text integration is outstanding. The themes for the chapters are clear, concise, and easy-to-understand.

Students, researchers, and professionals working in the fields of laboratory medicine, clinical sciences, and allied health sciences will find this book valuable. In my capacity as a clinician and consultant, I highly recommend this book to all healthcare professionals who wish to stay abreast with the current trends in the management and diagnosis of metabolic diseases. I also wish to congratulate the editors, Seth K. Amponsah, Emmanuel K. Ofori, and Yashwant V. Pathak, and all contributors for this remarkable resource.

Prof. Enyonam Yao Kwawukume
President
Family Health Medical School, Family Health University College, Ghana

Editors

Seth Kwabena Amponsah (PhD) is a Senior Lecturer and Head of the Department of Medical Pharmacology, University of Ghana Medical School. He has an MPhil and PhD in Pharmacology. He has had post-doctoral fellowships under BANGA-Africa Project and BSU III (DANIDA – Denmark). He has over 12 years of experience in teaching and research. His research focus includes clinical pharmacology (infectious disease and antimicrobial stewardship): the prudent use of antimicrobials, antimicrobial level monitoring, and the efficacy of antimicrobials in patients. He also has experience in population pharmacokinetic modeling; non-compartment pharmacokinetic estimation; and pharmacokinetic evaluation of new drug formulations. He has published over 50 research articles, 1 book, 10 book chapters, and several conference abstracts. He is an Academic Editor for *PLoS ONE* and an Associate Editor for *Pan African Medical Journal*.

Emmanuel Kwaku Ofori (PhD) is currently a Senior Lecturer and Head of the Department of Chemical Pathology, University of Ghana Medical School. He earned his PhD in July 2018 from the University of Lausanne, Switzerland. He teaches several disciplines in the health sciences (medical, nursing, veterinary, and laboratory sciences, among others). He has supervised and mentored many undergraduate and postgraduate students. His research focuses on lipidomics, metabolic medicine, and steroidal adaptations to diet and exercise. He aims to become an international expert on translational research into metabolic diseases. He has about 22 publications to his name in top-ranked peer-reviewed journals. He has also presented several abstracts at international conferences.

Yashwant V. Pathak (PhD) has over 15 years of experience as Dean in an institution of higher education and over 30 years as faculty and as a researcher in higher education following his PhD. Presently he is Associate Dean for Faculty Affairs and Tenured Professor of Pharmaceutical Sciences. He is an internationally recognized scholar, researcher, and educator in the areas of healthcare education, nanotechnology, drug delivery systems, and nutraceuticals. Professor Pathak is an Adjunct Professor at Faculty of Pharmacy, Airlangga University, Surabaya, Indonesia. He has received many international and national awards, including four Fulbright Fellowships, an Endeavour Executive Fellowship from Australian government, four outstanding faculty awards, and he was selected as Fellow of American Association for Advancement of Science (AAAS) in 2021 for his contribution to the advancement of science. He has published over 350 research publications, reviews, and chapters in various books. He has edited over 60 books in various fields, including nanotechnology, nutraceuticals, conflict management, and cultural studies. He is also actively involved in many non-profit organizations, including Hindu Swayamsevak Sangh, USA, Sewa International USA, International Accreditation Council for Dharma Schools and Colleges, the International Commission for Human Rights and Religious Freedom, and the Uberoi Foundation for Religious Studies, among others.

List of Contributors

Mohit Agrawal
School of Medical and Allied Sciences, K.R. Mangalam University, Gurugram Pin 122103 Haryana, India

Aparna Anandan
Translational Research Laboratory, Department of Biotechnology, Bharathiar University, Coimbatore – 641 046, Tamil Nadu, India

Unais AK
Translational Research Laboratory, Department of Biotechnology, Bharathiar University, Coimbatore – 641 046, Tamil Nadu, India

Seth Kwabena Amponsah
Department of Medical Pharmacology, University of Ghana Medical School, Accra, Ghana

Michael Amponsah-Offeh
Department of Cardiovascular Research, European Center for Angioscience (ECAS), Medical Faculty Mannheim, Heidelberg University, 6 8167 Mannheim, Germany

Abigail Aning
Department of Clinical Pathology, Noguchi Memorial Institute for Medical Research, University of Ghana, Ghana

Niyati Acharya
Institute of Pharmacy, Nirma University, Ahmedabad, India

Sanjeev Acharya
SSR College of Pharmacy, Sayli – Silvassa Road, Sayli, Silvassa – 396 230, Union Territory of Dadra and Nagar Haveli and Daman and Diu, India

Vishnu Prabhu Athilingam
Translational Research Laboratory, Department of Biotechnology, Bharathiar University, Coimbatore – 641 046, Tamil Nadu, India

Rajashri Bezbaruah
Institute of Pharmacy, Assam Medical College and Hospital, Dibrugarh – 786002, Assam, India

Raktim Borgohain
Department of Pharmacology, Lakhimpur Medical College and Hospital, Assam, India

Kwasi Agyei Bugyei
Department of Medical Pharmacology, University of Ghana Medical School, Accra, Ghana

Hema Chaudhary
School of Medical and Allied Sciences, K.R. Mangalam University, Gurugram Pin 122103 Haryana, India

Jitu Das
Department of Community Medicine, Lakhimpur Medical College and Hospital, North Lakhimpur, India

Paige DeBlieux
University of South Florida Morsani College of Medicine, MD Program, Tampa, Florida, USA

Chinmoyee Deori
Department of Pharmacology, Lakhimpur Medical College and Hospital, North Lakhimpur, India

Rumi Deori
Department of Biochemistry, Lakhimpur Medical College and Hospital, North Lakhimpur, India

Migom Doley
Department of Community Medicine, Lakhimpur Medical College and Hospital, Assam, India

Partha P Kalita
Program of Biotechnology, Assam Down Town University, Panikhaiti, Guwahati – 781026, Assam, India

Shradha Devi Dwivedi
University Institute of Pharmacy, Pt. Ravishankar Shukla University, Raipur (C.G.), India

Andrew A. Dwyer
Boston College, William F. Connell School of Nursing, Chestnut Hill, MA, USA

Jenifer L. Ferreir
SSR College of Pharmacy, Sayli – Silvassa Road, Sayli, Silvassa – 396 230, Union Territory of Dadra and Nagar Haveli and Daman and Diu, India

Gaurab Kumar Gogoi
Department of Pharmacology, Lakhimpur
   Medical College and Hospital, Assam,
   India

Madhusmita Gogoi
Faculty of Science and Engineering,
   Department of Pharmaceutical Sciences,
   Dibrugarh University, Dibrugarh, Assam,
   India

Nilayan Guha
Faculty of Science and Engineering,
   Department of Pharmaceutical Sciences,
   Dibrugarh University, Dibrugarh, Assam,
   India

Shivani Jani
Department of Pharmaceutical Quality
   Assurance, SMT. S.M. Shah Pharmacy
   College, Gujarat Technological University,
   Amsaran 387130, Gujarat, India

Yash Jasoria
School of Medical and Allied Sciences, K.R.
   Mangalam University, Gurugram Pin 122103
   Haryana, India

Bibhuti Bhusan Kakoti
Department of Pharmaceutical Sciences,
   Faculty of Science and Engineering,
   Dibrugarh University, Dibrugarh – 786004,
   Assam, India

Richard Kang
University of South Florida Morsani College
   of Medicine, MD Program, Tampa, Florida,
   USA

Hitesh Katariya
Department of Pharmaceutics, SMT. S. M.
   Shah Pharmacy College, Gujarat
   Technological University, Amsaran 387130,
   Gujarat, India

Jordan Keels
Boston College, William F. Connell School of
   Nursing, Chestnut Hill, MA, USA

Elikem Kwami Kumahor
Laboratory Sub-BMC, Korle-Bu Teaching
   Hospital, Accra, Ghana

Santhana Kumar
SSR College of Pharmacy, Sayli – Silvassa Road,
   Sayli, Silvassa – 396 230, Union Territory of
   Dadra and Nagar Haveli and Daman and
   Diu, India

Tridip Kutum
Department of Biochemistry, Lakhimpur
   Medical College and Hospital, North
   Lakhimpur, India

Patrick Diaba-Nuhoho
Division of Vascular Endothelium and
   Microcirculation, Department of Medicine III,
   University Hospital and Faculty of Medicine
   Carl Gustav Carus, Technische Universität
   Dresden, 01307 Dresden, Germany

Emmanuel Kwaku Ofori
Department of Chemical Pathology, University
   of Ghana Medical School, Accra, Ghana

V. Vijaya Padma
Translational Research Laboratory, Department
   of Biotechnology, Bharathiar University,
   Coimbatore – 641 046, Tamil Nadu, India

Riya Patel
SSR College of Pharmacy, Sayli – Silvassa Road,
   Sayli, Silvassa – 396 230, Union Territory of
   Dadra and Nagar Haveli and Daman and
   Diu, India

Yashwant V. Pathak
USF Health Taneja College of Pharmacy,
   University of South Florida, Tampa, Florida,
   USA
and the Faculty of Pharmacy, Airlangga
   University, Surabaya, Indonesia

Pompy Patowary
Faculty of Science and Engineering,
   Department of Pharmaceutical Sciences,
   Dibrugarh University, Dibrugarh, Assam,
   India

Arpita Paul
Faculty of Science and Engineering,
   Department of Pharmaceutical Sciences,
   Dibrugarh University, Dibrugarh, Assam,
   India

Bhupendra Prajapati
Department of Pharmaceutics and
   Pharmaceutical Technology, Shree S.K.
   Patel College of Pharmaceutical Education
   and Research, Ganpat University, Mehsana
   384012, Gujarat, India

Charles Preuss
University of South Florida Morsani College
   of Medicine, Department of Molecular
   Pharmacology and Physiology, Tampa,
   Florida, USA

Lokendra Singh Rathor
University Institute of Pharmacy, Pt.
Ravishankar Shukla University, Raipur
(C.G.), India

Nensi Raytthatha
Sigma Institute of Pharmacy, Vadodara,
Gujarat, India

Dhritiman Roy
Department of Pharmaceutical Sciences,
Faculty of Science and Engineering,
Dibrugarh University, Dibrugarh – 786004,
Assam, India

Divya Sahu
University Institute of Pharmacy, Pt.
Ravishankar Shukla University, Raipur
(C.G.), India

Surovi Saikia
Translational Research Laboratory, Department
of Biotechnology, Bharathiar University,
Coimbatore – 641 046, Tamil Nadu, India

Ngurzampuii Sailo
Department of Pharmaceutical Sciences, Faculty
of Science and Engineering, Dibrugarh
University, Dibrugarh – 786004, Assam, India

Sheila A. Santa
Department of Medical Laboratory Sciences,
School of Biomedical and Allied Health
Sciences, University of Ghana, Accra Ghana

Zakaria Seidu
Department of Biochemistry and Molecular
Biology, Faculty of Biosciences, University
for Development Studies, Ghana

Deependra Singh
University Institute of Pharmacy, Pt.
Ravishankar Shukla University, Raipur
(C.G.), India

Manju Rawat Singh
University Institute of Pharmacy, Pt.
Ravishankar Shukla University, Raipur
(C.G.), India

Manmohan Singhal
Faculty of Pharmacy, DIT University,
Dehradun, Uttrakhand, India

Arun Soni
SSR College of Pharmacy, Sayli – Silvassa Road,
Sayli, Silvassa – 396 230, Union Territory of
Dadra and Nagar Haveli and Daman and
Diu, India

Monica Stevens
University of South Florida Morsani College
of Medicine, MD Program, Tampa, Florida,
USA

Jennifer Suurbaar
Department of Biochemistry and Molecular
Medicine, School of Medicine, University for
Development Studies, Ghana

Emmanuel A. Tagoe
Department of Medical Laboratory Sciences,
School of Biomedical and Allied Health
Sciences, University of Ghana, Accra,
Ghana

Patricia Underwood
Boston College, William F. Connell School of
Nursing, Chestnut Hill, MA, USA

Jigar Vyas
Sigma Institute of Pharmacy, Vadodara,
Gujarat, India

Kamaruz Zaman
Faculty of Science and Engineering,
Department of Pharmaceutical Sciences,
Dibrugarh University, Dibrugarh, Assam,
India

1 Overview
Biochemical Basis of Metabolic Diseases

Emmanuel Kwaku Ofori, Seth Kwabena Amponsah, and Yashwant V. Pathak

1.1 INTRODUCTION

Metabolism refers to a set of chemical events that take place within the cells of living organisms to maintain life. The process of metabolism is comprised of a plethora of interrelated metabolic pathways, all of which work together to ultimately supply cells with the energy that is necessary for them to perform their function [1]. The development of metabolic disease is caused by errors that disrupt the metabolic processes. These metabolic inconsistencies are typically the result of either an excess or a deficiency in the production of vital compounds that are required by the organism. Some of them affect the breakdown of lipids, amino acids, or carbohydrates [2]. Mitochondrial illnesses are another group that damages the components of the cell that are responsible for producing energy. There is a substantial amount of room for error within the system; hence, the presence of a mutation in a single enzyme does not necessarily indicate that an individual will be afflicted with a disease [3]. There may be more than one way to accomplish the same goal for several different metabolic intermediates, and multiple enzymes may compete with one another to change the same molecule. In this chapter, some metabolic illnesses are highlighted.

1.2 DIABETES MELLITUS

Diabetes mellitus (DM) is a metabolic illness that is characterized by hyperglycaemia due to abnormalities in insulin secretion, insulin action, or both [4]. DM manifests itself in abnormalities in insulin synthesis, insulin action, or both. Other variables may also be implicated. Over 1.6 million people across the world have lost their lives as a direct or indirect result of DM [5, 6]. As a result of the osmotic influence of high glucose in the blood and urine, there is frequent urination, loss of fluids, and thirst.

DM can lead to long-term complications such as cardiovascular disease (including atherosclerosis and stroke), as well as damage to nerves, the kidneys, and the eyes [7]. DM can be classified into several subtypes, the most common of which are type 1 (T1DM), type 2 (T2DM), maturity-onset diabetes of the young (MODY), gestational diabetes (GD), and neonatal diabetes (ND), as well as secondary causes such as endocrinopathies and steroid use, etc. [8, 9], summarized in Table 1.1.

1.2.1 Insulin and Normal Physiology of Food Metabolism

Several different enzymes and processes are responsible for the digestion of ingested food and its absorption from the intestinal tract into the bloodstream. Triglycerides are stored in fat cells, whereas carbohydrates are stored as glycogen in the liver and muscle cells for future use as fuel. This is especially important for the functioning of the brain, which is wholly reliant on glucose for its processes [10, 11].

The pace at which glucose enters the blood and the rate at which it is utilized (that is, used up by cells) both contribute to the overall concentration of glucose in the blood. A normal person's levels are strictly managed, and as a result, they rarely go below 2.5 mmol/L or above 8.0 mmol/L after a meal at any point in time, or above 6.0 mmol/L after an overnight fast. Under the influence of blood glucose levels that are greater than 5.0 mmol/L, the beta (β) cells in the islets of Langerhans of the pancreas secrete insulin into the bloodstream [12, 13]. Insulin is a protein hormone required for glucose to be transported into the cells, where it can either be used as fuel or stored. In addition to this, it makes it easier for fat cells to take in fatty acids and store them, as well as for all cells to take in amino acids [14, 15]. Insulin functions on its three primary target tissues: the liver, which is where it reduces hepatic glucose output, the muscle, which is where it stimulates glucose disposal, and the adipocyte, which is where it decreases lipolysis and enhances lipogenesis [16]. A lack of insulin, on the other hand, causes the opposite of these processes to occur, which ultimately leads to a condition that is analogous to famine. Insulin can communicate with cells through its interaction with a protein on the cell surface known as an insulin receptor. This connection activates a cascade of intracellular processes, each of which is catalyzed by a separate enzyme, which finally culminates in the synthesis of another protein that is known as glucose transporter (GLUT 1-5) that is responsible for transporting glucose molecules across the cell membranes (Figure 1.1). On

DOI: 10.1201/9781003384823-1

Table 1.1   General classification of diabetes mellitus

Type 1 (*β cell destruction usually leading to absolute insulin deficiency*)

    A. Immune-mediated: formerly known as IDDM or juvenile-onset diabetes, this kind of diabetes is caused by cellular (T-cell) mediated autoimmune destruction of the beta cells of the pancreas and results in type 1 diabetes

    B. Environmental factors (such as viral infection, diet, etc.)

    C. Idiopathic – no known aetiologies

Type 2 (*characterized by insulin resistance, which is a deficiency in the body tissues' ability to respond normally to insulin*)

    • Although the exact causes of the disease are unknown, it is known that several lifestyle factors, such as being overweight, having a poor diet, not getting enough exercise, and being stressed, play a significant role in its progression

Gestational DM (*any degree of glucose intolerance that begins during pregnancy or is recognized for the first time during pregnancy*)

Other types

    The genetic defect of β cell function – chromosomal

    Disease of the pancreas (pancreatitis, cancer)

    Endocrinopathies (Cushing's syndrome, acromegaly, glucagonoma, etc.)

    Drug or chemical-induced (Corticosteroids, thiazide, beta-blockers, diuretics, etc.)

    Infections (viral, etc.)

Note: DM is diabetes mellitus, IDDM is insulin-dependent diabetes mellitus

the other hand, glucagon and other antagonistic hormones (such as cortisol, growth hormone, somatostatin, thyroid hormones, and so on) raise blood glucose levels by increasing the rate at which glycogen, fat, and protein are broken down [17, 18]. This is achieved by the operation of a convoluted process that requires cooperation with several other systems.

1.2.2 Type 1 Diabetes Mellitus, Complications, and Ketoacidosis

Type 1 diabetes mellitus (T1DM) is primarily associated with two HLA class 2 haplotypes that play a role in antigen presentation [19]. The autoimmune-mediated death of pancreatic beta cells is what characterizes T1DM. There is a specific band on the short arm of chromosome 6 that carries the genes responsible for this disease. The major histocompatibility complex is a group of genes located in this region that are responsible for controlling the immune system. The ability of the immune system to recognize itself can be hindered when some genes in this complex fail to function properly or are aberrant [20]. There is more to the story than just genetics, as not everyone who carries these genes will eventually get the disease. About half of all sets of identical twins

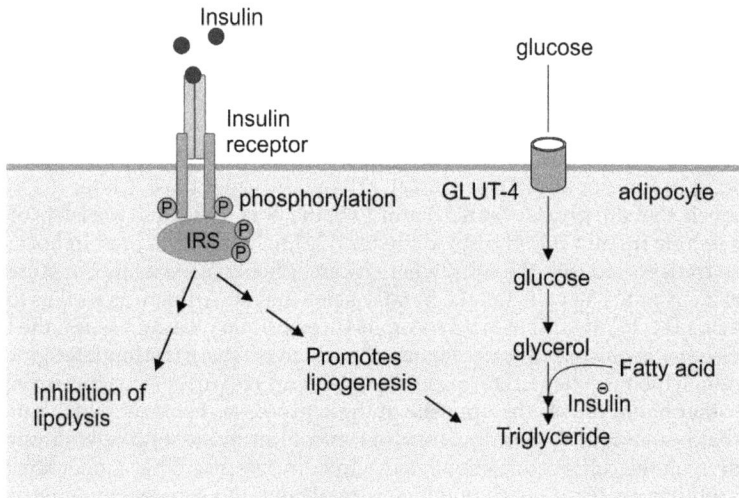

Figure 1.1   Insulin signalling in an adipocyte

with these genes will develop the disease [21]. Increased or aberrant gastric emptying after a meal, uncontrolled hepatic glucose synthesis, and impaired glucose disposal in the presence of insulin all contribute to elevated glucose levels in the blood after a meal [22].

Environmental factors almost certainly play a role in the onset of islet autoimmunity, which leads to the destruction of beta cells in the pancreas and a subsequent lack of insulin. This is demonstrated by the rise in the number of people who have been diagnosed with T1DM after migrating from areas with a lower incidence of the disease to areas with a higher incidence of the disease [23]. Some risk factors have been linked to the development of T1DM, including food, vitamin D consumption, infections, and the microbiota in the gut, according to both experimental and epidemiological research [24]. It has been hypothesized that all of these factors could, collectively, alter gene expression via epigenetic pathways, thereby generating an abnormal immune response and islet autoimmunity [25]. It has also been suggested that eating certain foods, such as gluten, during the first year of a person's life may increase their risk of developing T1DM [26, 27]. Infections with viruses belonging to the *Herpesviridae* and *Parvoviridae* families of DNA viruses, as well as the *Togaviridae, Paramyxoviridae, Retroviridae,* and *Picornaviridae* families of RNA viruses, have further been linked to type 1 DM [28]. Both newborn formulae made with cow milk and the use of cow milk during infancy have additionally been hypothesized to contribute to the development of T1DM [29].

More than 90% of children who are diagnosed with type 1 DM have one of these three types of anti-islet autoantibodies: autoantibodies that react with insulin (IAA), an islet enzyme called glutamic acid decarboxylase 65 (GAD 65), or a molecule of uncertain function called islet antigen 2 (IA-2) [30].

Based on the degree of hyperglycaemia, ketosis, and age at presentation as well as the rate of disease progression, type 1 DM can be broken down into three subtypes namely acute-onset type 1 diabetes (AT1DM), slowly progressive type 1 diabetes (SP1DM), and fulminant type 1 diabetes (FT1DM) [31]. AT1DM is known as the "typical" TIDM since it is characterized by decreased endogenous insulin production and positive islet-related autoantibodies [32]. SP1DM, also known as latent-onset autoimmune diabetes in adults (LADA), is a type of autoimmune diabetes that is characterized by maintained pancreatic beta-cell activity at the outset and positive islet-related autoantibodies. This kind of T1DM is considered to be on the milder end of the autoimmune diabetes spectrum [33]. SP1DM can be distinguished from T2DM by the presence and persistence of pancreatic autoantibodies, particularly an autoantibody called glutamic acid decarboxylase (GAD), which is also an excellent predictor of future T1DM. Because of the quick onset of the condition, patients with FT1DM have a comparatively low level of glycated haemoglobin levels (HbA1c of less than 8.7%). Secretion of endogenous insulin is significantly reduced in patients with FT1DM, and the majority of islet-related autoantibodies are negative [34]. In all cases of T1DM, the T lymphocytes of the immune system are responsible for the destruction of beta cell populations in the pancreas, which results in a cessation of insulin production and the insulin deficit that develops is both permanent and severe.

An absolute lack of insulin results in the failure of anabolic processes. Due to a barrier that prevents glucose from entering cells, it builds up in the blood. As a consequence of hyperglycaemia, the individual experiences excessive urination (known medically as polyuria), followed by excessive thirst (known medically as polydipsia) to make up for the loss of water, and finally, excessive hunger (known medically as polyphagia) since the cells do not have enough fuel. In addition, there is a loss of weight, as well as cell death and loss. Dehydration and a lack of electrolytes can set in when the body's intake of fluids and food is unable to keep up with its output of fluids and food. When fat is broken down, free fatty acids, also known as FFAs, are released from the cells that store fat. FFAs are transported to the liver, where they undergo a metabolic process that results in the production of ketone bodies, which include acetone, acetoacetic acid, and beta-hydroxybutyric acid. The presence of acidosis is directly proportional to the amount of ketone bodies that have been produced. The consequence of this is ketoacidosis, which, if left untreated, can lead to unconsciousness and ultimately death [35, 36].

1.2.3 Type 2 Diabetes Mellitus (T2DM) and Acute Complications

Insufficient insulin secretion from pancreatic islet β-cells, insulin resistance (IR), and an insufficient compensatory insulin secretory response characterize T2DM [37]. T2DM is a complex disease caused by environmental and genetic factors [38]. Getting older, leading a sedentary lifestyle, and being overweight are all environmental factors. The action of insulin can be affected by a deficiency in genes that control the creation of certain enzymes that regulate multiple chemical processes in the functioning of beta cells, insulin secretion, insulin action at the cellular level, insulin receptor development by the cell, and insulin action inside the cell. This decrease in insulin activity can interfere with the cell's ability to take in glucose, create an increase in the creation of glucose by the liver, hinder the uptake of glucose and fatty acids by fat cells, lead to an increase in the breakdown of triglycerides, and cause a variety of other metabolic abnormalities [39]. Insulin resistance (IR) is probably the first problem that develops in T2DM. It starts several years before the emergence of symptoms or the development of a blood glucose level that is high enough to diagnose the condition. The peripheral cells (mainly muscle and fat cells) of the body, as well as the liver, are where IR manifests itself. When IR develops, beta cells in the pancreas produce more insulin to compensate and keep blood glucose levels within the narrow range that is necessary for normal bodily function. It is hypothesized that IR manifests itself at the cellular level in the majority of instances due to post-receptor abnormalities in insulin signalling [40, 41]. Down-regulation, inadequacies, or genetic polymorphisms of tyrosine phosphorylation of the insulin receptor, IRS proteins, or PIP-3 kinase are all examples of possible pathways [42]. Abnormalities of GLUT 4 function may also play a role in this condition [41]. If IR continues or worsens over time (usually years), beta cells will begin to fail as a result of a genetic defect, toxicity caused by glucose and/or fat, or exhaustion. This can happen for several reasons.

There is a degree of IR and compensatory hyperinsulinaemia in obese people, although not all of these people will develop DM, and the exact mechanism by which obesity produces IR is not understood [43]. Obese people have compensatory hyperinsulinaemia. As more and more fatty tissue is accumulated, it is common knowledge that the tissue becomes increasingly resistant to the effects of insulin. This is especially true of abdominal fat. Muscle tissue that is not used regularly also develops IR [44]. These processes are reversible through the use of medications that increase insulin sensitivity (IS), as well as by the reduction of calories in one's diet and increased metabolic function through exercise. Diabetic ketoacidosis (DKA) (see section 2.2), hyperosmolar non-ketotic (HONK) syndrome/coma, and hypoglycaemia are the most common severe acute consequences of DM.

In people who have T2DM, HONK is the most serious acute hyperglycaemic emergency that can occur [45]. It is distinguished from ketoacidosis by extreme hyperglycaemia (more than 50 mmol/L), hyperosmolality, and severe dehydration [46]. Ketoacidosis is not present. The severity of dehydration, the degree of water and electrolyte depletion, the existence of comorbidities, and advanced age are the factors that define the prognosis. In addition to addressing hyperosmolality, hyperglycaemia, and electrolyte abnormalities, treatment focuses on managing the underlying condition that led to metabolic derailment (rehydrating the patient and giving them insulin) [47]. This is done by replenishing the volume that was lost and correcting hyperosmolality and hyperglycaemia.

Plasma glucose values that are lower than 2.2 mmol/L are the diagnostic threshold for hypoglycaemia. Both T1DM and T2DM can be made more difficult to treat if hypoglycaemia occurs. The beginning of symptoms and the glucose concentration both play a role in how symptoms manifest. Gastric hyperactivity, feelings of hunger, and irritation are examples of mild symptoms. In severe cases, patients may exhibit symptoms such as mental disorientation, thick speech, intoxication, convulsions, or coma. Children who have untreated chronic hypoglycaemia run the risk of developing mental impairment [48, 49].

1.2.3.1 *Macrovascular Complications*

The large blood vessels of the heart, brain, and legs are together referred to as the macrovascular system [50]. Alterations in lipid metabolism are a contributing factor in the development of abnormalities in the bigger arteries. Coronary artery, cerebrovascular, or peripheral vascular insufficiency are all possible manifestations of this condition [51]. People who have T2DM are more likely to suffer from atherosclerosis of the coronary arteries, which is also the leading cause of death among those who have this condition [52, 53]. At any level of risk factors, such as cholesterol, smoking, leading a sedentary lifestyle, being overweight, having hypertension, etc., there is an increased likelihood of coronary artery disease and its associated complications. It is also common knowledge that excessive levels of glucose in the blood can harm platelets, fibrin, and the mechanism responsible for blood clotting. Therefore, having high glucose levels can both increase the risk of thrombosis and delay the removal of fibrin, both of which are important factors in coronary thrombosis [54, 55].

1.2.3.2 Microvascular Complications

Because microvascular diseases affect capillaries located throughout the body, the symptoms of the disease can be spread out in a variety of locations. The kidneys, the optic nerves, and the nervous system are the organs that are affected the most. Both diabetic retinopathy and diabetic nephropathy are serious complications of diabetes. Diabetic retinopathy is the leading cause of blindness in adults, and diabetic nephropathy affects more than half of those who require dialysis or a kidney transplant [56, 57]. The polyol route, enzymatic glycosylation, and non-enzymatic glycosylation are the three primary pathways that contribute to the development of microvascular illness [58].

Prolonged exposure to high glucose concentrations leads to the creation of sorbitol (alcohol generated from glucose) by the activity of aldose reductase. The accumulation of sorbitol in the cells causes osmotic damage, leading to the narrowing of the lumens of small blood arteries [59]. When glucose builds up as a result of a blockage in the normal pathways of glucose metabolism, an alternative pathway of glucose metabolism known as the polyol pathway can help clear it out. Glucose is converted into an alcohol form known as sorbitol when an enzyme known as aldose reductase is present. This enzyme is found in most tissues, including nerve tissue, and it is responsible for the transformation. Sorbitol gradually builds up in the cells. By acting as a competitive inhibitor, sorbitol hinders the absorption of myoinositol from meals when it builds up inside the cells and accumulates to high levels [60]. A myoinositol deficit causes oxidative stress and cellular damage by inhibiting the scavenging of free radicals, which can occur when there is not enough of the nutrient [61]. This is most likely the principal mechanism responsible for the nerve damage seen in diabetic neuropathy.

Aberrations of lipids, specifically glycation, and the oxidation of lipoproteins also contribute to build-up, as well as alterations in lipoprotein metabolism. The hexosamine pathway is a subsidiary branch of the glycolytic system, contributing less than three 3% of glucose to the final product. Glucose/glycosyl side chains are provided for proteins and lipids by the conversion of fructose-6-phosphate to glucosamine-6-phosphate, which is catalyzed by the first and rate-limiting enzyme, glutamine:fructose-6-phosphate amidotransferase (GFAT). There is a greater preference for this pathway in DM, which ultimately results in an increased number of alterations [60]. Recent research has shown that activation of protein kinase C (PKC) plays a significant part in atherosclerosis brought on by hyperglycaemia. The activation of PKC has a role in a variety of cellular responses, including the expression of many different growth factors, the activation of signalling pathways, and the amplification of oxidative stress in hyperglycaemia. PKC is involved in the modulation of cholesterol efflux, monocyte recruitment, macrophage infiltration, and lipid content in diabetic plaque, all of which are factors that contribute to diabetes-induced inflammation [62, 63]. To prevent this damage, the levels of glucose in the blood must be maintained within the normal range the majority of the time. When there is a high concentration of glucose in these cells, the glucose must be removed through some process. These waste removal processes are essential, but they do have side effects. The repercussions have the potential to inflict damage on the nerves and blood vessels, as well as the organs that these structures support.

The nonenzymatic glycosylation process is the third way in which vascular injury can occur. Glucose can undergo cross-linking with proteins and accumulate in vessel walls and tissues, which can lead to structural and functional damage [58]. Both a lack of insulin and an abundance of glucose are responsible for the enzymatic process of glycosylation. Proteinuria is the first symptom that one may notice when diabetic nephropathy has begun to develop. The same process can be identified through fluorescein leaking into the retina and albumen leaking into peripheral tissues. A thickening of the basement membrane can also reduce the diameter of the blood vessel, which in turn reduces the amount of blood that can flow through the channel and raises the intravascular pressure. Nonenzymatic glycosylation is completely determined by the glucose concentration in the blood and can take place in virtually every protein found in the body. The production of glycated haemoglobin (also known as HbA1c) is arguably the greatest example of the chemical reaction that occurs during this process. Red blood cells (RBCs) are home to the oxygen-carrying protein known as haemoglobin, which is found throughout the blood. RBCs are also known as erythrocytes. Glucose can pass through the membrane of red blood cells, and once inside, it binds to the terminal amino acid of the chain of haemoglobin, where it becomes permanently connected to the protein. It stays on the haemoglobin until the RBCs are no longer present in the blood, after about 120 days. When a protein molecule in the body is subjected to high quantities of glucose, the same reaction can take place in virtually every protein molecule. In other proteins, including collagen, elastic tissue, immunoglobulins, and so on, the amino acid-glucose molecule goes through a further chemical transformation to generate what is known as an Advanced Glycosylation End product, or AGE [64]. This can result in the tissue losing its elasticity and becoming rigid. People who have DM tend to have blood vessels with stiff walls, which is a contributing factor in the development of systolic hypertension. AGE products have been shown to form links with cholesterol that is already present in the walls of blood arteries, which can initiate the process of atherosclerosis [65]. Glycosylation of serum proteins such as immunoglobulins can render these proteins inactive and harm the body's ability to fight infection. Postoperative blood glucose control must take this into consideration. Physiologic control of blood glucose levels (HbA1c 6.5%), blood pressure control (130/80), and cholesterol control (LDL 100mg/dL) are all necessary for preventing the chronic consequences of diabetes, both macrovascular and microvascular [66].

1.3 OBESITY

The prevalence of obesity in several regions of the world has now reached epidemic levels. The percentage of adults who are obese has nearly doubled over the past four decades [67]. Almost 40% of the population of the world is considered to be overweight, and the number of children and adolescents who are obese is also on the rise [68]. An individual is considered to be overweight or obese when they have a body weight that is disproportionate to their height. It is generally accepted that the body mass index (BMI), which is derived from the ratio of a person's body mass in kilograms to their height in metres squared, although useful in large epidemiological studies, is an imprecise method of determining whether or not a person is overweight or obese. According to the World Health Organization (WHO) classification, normal values for BMI range from 18.5 to 24.9 kg/m^2; overweight is defined as 25–29.9 kg/m^2; and obesity is defined as 30 kg/m^2. The intricate interplay of energy intake and expenditure, psychosocial factors, genetic factors, and the body's neurological and endocrine systems all have a role in determining an individual's body weight, and subsequently, their likelihood of being obese [69, 70]. This was once believed to be a concern of the industrialized world, but it is becoming increasingly prevalent in low- and middle-income nations. The risk of developing metabolic disorders and ailments including T2DM, cardiovascular disorders, metabolic syndrome, chronic kidney disease (CKD), non-alcoholic fatty liver disease (NAFLD), osteoarthritis, and certain kinds of cancer is raised when a person is obese [71].

Several different pathways could ultimately lead to obesity. The conventional view and primary explanation is that obesity is the result of the body amassing a sizeable amount of extra energy in in excess of the amount of energy it has spent. The extra energy is deposited in the body's fat cells, which leads to the pathology that is characteristic of obesity. The nutritional signals that are responsible for obesity are changed as a result of the pathological growth of fat cells [72]. Additional aetiologies or defects that lead to obesity can be identified under the categories of genetic factors, epigenetic factors, and environmental factors [73, 74].

Numerous gene variants linked to obesity through physiological processes like the control of appetite and energy metabolism have been discovered as a result of studies looking at the genetic basis of obesity in the general population. This suggests that obesity is a polygenic disorder that is influenced by multiple genes, along with lifestyle and environmental factors [75]. In recent years, there has been a great deal of interest in the gut microbiota (also known as the microorganisms that are native to the gut) and its links to obesity. Researchers have found that persons with obesity have a microbiome that is more varied than that of individuals who have a normal weight [76]. Also, studies of the microbiota of twins who are discordant for obesity have demonstrated that the metabolic phenotype (that is, normal or obese) can be transmitted to germ-free mice by transplanting the human faecal microbiota [77]. It is not known what basis there is for the various impacts that microbiota have on body weight; nevertheless, it may be related to variances in the metabolic processes that microbes use to process fibre or other nutrients.

1.3.1 Therapeutics of Obesity

Given the lack of targeted pharmaceutical interventions, the lack of clear guidelines, and the wide range of possible adverse effects, adjusting one's way of life remains the most important component of obesity management. It is recommended that people who are overweight lose at least 10% of their body weight through a combination of dietary changes, increased physical activity, and behavioural therapy [78, 79]. Diets that restrict portion sizes can result in a significant amount of weight loss in a relatively short period. Maintaining long-term control of one's weight can be accomplished by also engaging in high volumes of physical exercise and maintaining communication with one's healthcare practitioner. In many instances, making changes to one's lifestyle leads to a substantial reduction in total body weight, which in turn results in a considerable reduction in the risk of developing cardiovascular disease [80]. Because people's food choices are largely influenced by their environments, governments need to take steps to improve both their policies and the environment to reduce the availability of foods that are bad for people's health and increase the accessibility of foods that are healthy for them. Obesity can be mitigated through a combination of preventative measures (such as health promotion, nutrition education, incentives for healthy living, a sugar-sweetened beverage tax, and social marketing) and corrective measures (such as policy changes, regulations, and laws). Modifying eating behaviours also requires adhering to certain guidelines. Purchase foods that are low in fat. Current food guidelines should be revised to encourage the production of foods that are lower in sugar, fat, and salt; at the same time, the availability of foods that promote childhood obesity should be limited. Create a shopping list, and then do your best to stick to it. Never go shopping while you are feeling hungry. Determine the situations in which you indulge in unnecessary eating, such as when you are with other people who are eating or when you are unable to stomach the thought of throwing food away. Maintain a constant supply of a variety of low-calorie snacks, such as raw vegetables, for example. Find people to assist you, such as members of your family, your circle of friends, your coworkers, or "weight-watchers". Eat more slowly and make your portions look bigger to trick yourself into thinking you are getting more food. Take preventative measures against hunger by avoiding feelings of isolation, melancholy, boredom, anger, and exhaustion. Engage in regular physical activity.

Those who have a body mass index (BMI) of 30 kg/m² or more and who have failed to lose weight through diet and exercise alone might consider pharmacotherapy [81]. Only people with extreme obesity who struggle with hunger when on a reduced-calorie diet may benefit from supportive medication therapy. Its use is restricted to supervised behavioural modification therapy for short periods and under strict medical supervision.

Bariatric surgery is an additional treatment option for those who have a BMI that is greater than 35 kg/m² and who are unable to reduce their weight through changes in lifestyle or medication. According to some studies, the benefits of bariatric surgery extend far beyond the straightforward prospect of weight loss. It has been shown that bariatric surgery can bring about a reduction in the chronic inflammation that is associated with obesity, as well as changes in metabolic biomarkers, the gut microbiome, and long-term remission from type 2 diabetes [82, 83]. For instance, following Roux-en-Y gastric bypass (RYGB) surgery, the total richness of gut microbes was shown to have increased in human participants [84]. Further investigation demonstrated that RYGB was responsible for the overexpression of genes that are key to the transforming growth factor-β signalling pathway, the dramatic downregulation of genes that are involved in metabolic pathways and inflammatory responses, and the rise in the expression of certain genes that are found in white adipose tissue [85]. The typical outcome of bariatric surgery is a reduction in blood leptin levels, which is correlated with a lower BMI [86].

1.3.2 Adipose Tissue Physiology

As a huge endocrine organ, adipose tissue (AT) is responsible for the release of a wide variety of proteins and hormones. It is also involved in the storage of triglycerides (TG). This endocrine system is responsible for detecting the amount of stored energy and secreting hormones like leptin and adiponectin. Adiponectin increases insulin sensitivity, which promotes glucose uptake and, eventually, fat accumulation when there is increased storage capacity [87]. Leptin decreases food intake and activates pathways that cause lipolysis [88]. Adipocytes expand in size and number in response to an increase in the demand for fat storage during times of overnutrition; nevertheless, at a certain point, the maximum capacity is reached, and the stressed or damaged adipocytes initiate an inflammatory process that contributes to the health problems associated with obesity. The deposits of AT can be found either subcutaneously in the buttocks and thighs, as is commonly seen in obese males, or they can be found in the abdominal region. Not all AT depots pose the same metabolic hazards, despite this being a widely held belief. For instance, having excess fat in the abdomen region is known to play a significant role in IR [89]. There are two primary depots of fat in the abdominal region: subcutaneous and visceral fat. The layer of AT that lies between the dermis and the fascia is known as abdominal subcutaneous adipose tissue (ASAT). When there is a low level of energy expenditure but a high level of energy intake, ASAT acts as a physiological buffer for the extra energy [90]. Subcutaneous adipose tissue accounts for around 80% of total body fat. When the capacity of the body's subcutaneous fat depots to operate normally is exceeded, this leads to the accumulation of TGs in visceral fat, also known as VAT. In men, VAT makes up around 10–20% of total fat, while in women it makes up about 5–8% of total fat [91]. The build-up of VAT leads to an increase in IR in both hepatic and fat tissues, in addition to other metabolic abnormalities (such as glucose intolerance, increased triglycerides, and hypertension) [92]. At the moment, the full significance of this relationship is not fully known. There is a theory that visceral adipocytes are more lipid active than other types of adipocytes, which causes a significant increase in the amount of free fatty acids (FFA) that enter the portal circulation and are transported to the liver. It is thought that high FFA concentrations can cause lipotoxicity, which is defined as the ectopic deposition of lipids in various tissues of the body [93, 94]. It is important to note that not all of the fat that accumulates in the thighs is subcutaneous. Intermuscular adipose tissue (IMAT) is a type of fat that may be found both underneath the fascia and within the muscle itself. This fat has been linked to poor metabolic health in some studies [95–97]. In addition, the distribution of body fat in men and women differs significantly. Women typically have a higher SAT and overall body fat mass than males with the same waist circumference. When compared to women, men have a significantly higher percentage of VAT since they tend to accumulate fat in the abdominal or android region first which contributes to an increased risk of metabolic disease and IR. On the other hand, premenopausal women tend to store fat in their hips, thighs, and buttocks, which results in a gluteal-femoral adipose tissue distribution pattern (also known as gynoid or "pear shape"). After menopause, an increase in VAT accrual can be expected. This change is accompanied by an increase in metabolic risk parallel to that reported in men [98].

The inflammatory response in adipose tissue that causes an increase in the production of the pro-inflammatory cytokines tumour necrosis factor-alpha (TNF-α) and interleukin 6 (IL-6) has been linked to several different metabolic derailment processes. Some of the factors that contribute to this include a lack of oxygen supply to the adipose tissue (hypoxia), death of the stressed adipocytes leading to an influx of monocytes that are transformed into resident macrophages that secrete the inflammatory cytokines, and mechanical stresses caused by the interaction of the adipocytes with the dense extracellular matrix in which they are embedded [92, 99].

1.4 ATHEROSCLEROSIS

The word "atherosclerosis" is Greek in origin. "Atherosis", which is a build-up of fat accompanied by many macrophages, and "sclerosis", which is a fibrosis layer made up of smooth muscle cells, leukocytes, and connective tissue, are the two components of the word [100]. The accumulation of cholesterol crystals in the intima and the smooth muscle that lies underneath it is the first step in the process that leads to the creation of these plaques. The plaques then expand inside the arteries as a result of the expansion of fibrous tissues and the surrounding smooth muscle, which causes the blood flow to be reduced. Sclerosis, also known as the hardening of the arteries, is caused by the formation of connective tissue by fibroblasts and the accumulation of calcium in the lesion. Last but not least, the uneven surface of the arteries causes clot development and thrombosis, which in turn causes an abrupt restriction in the flow of blood [101].

Atherosclerosis begins at the molecular level when injured endothelial cells start to increase their expression of adhesion molecules such as E-selectin, vascular cell adhesion molecule-1 (VCAM-1), and intercellular adhesion molecule-1 (ICAM-1) [102]. These adhesion molecules facilitate the progression of leukocyte adhesion to the endothelium and migration to the subendothelial area, which ultimately results in atherosclerosis in its advanced stage. Atherosclerosis is a complicated disease that is brought on by several different genetic and environmental factors, as well as intricate interactions between genes and their environments [103, 104]. Clinically evident atherosclerosis begins with endothelial activation and inflammation, the encouragement of intimal lipoprotein deposition, retention, modification, and foam cell formation, the progression of complex plaques by plaque growth, enlargement of the necrotic core, fibrosis, thrombosis, and remodelling, and the triggering of acute events.

1.5 CANCER

Cancer is typified by uncontrolled cell development, which results in tissue invasion and subsequent metastasis [105]. The abnormal growth, also known as a tumour, can be generally categorized as either benign (meaning it grows locally without invading neighbouring tissues) or malignant (meaning it invades neighbouring tissues and can spread to other parts of the body). Although the vast majority of tumours found in humans are noncancerous and do not pose a threat to the health of their host, certain types of tumours can be fatal due to their proximity to vital organs (as in the case of a brain tumour), or the hormones that they secrete (in the case of thyroid adenomas). The majority of deaths from cancer are caused by malignant tumours, more specifically the metastases that develop [106]. Cancers are most commonly classified according to the place in the body where they first appeared. To date, over 200 distinct forms of cancer have been identified [107]. Many of these cancers occur with wildly varying frequencies in certain population groups or geographical areas. In general, lung, liver, stomach, and breast cancer account for the majority of fatalities caused by the disease [108, 109].

It is generally accepted that genetic mutations that occur on a cellular level are the root cause of cancer. Both biochemical and genomic evidence suggests that tumours originate from a single ancestral cell, giving rise to the term "clonal" to describe these disorders. The reasons are complex, involving a combination of individual genetic predispositions and environmental variables [110]. As a result of a breakdown in cellular DNA damage repair or recognition mechanisms, genetic aberrations (also known as single-point mutations, large chromosomal deletions, amplifications, or translocations in DNA) may arise spontaneously during the massive amount of cell turnover in the body throughout a human lifetime. These mutations are known as somatic mutations [111]. Alternatively, mutations can result from inherited genetic issues (known as germline mutations) or environmental influences (such as chemical carcinogens, UV exposure, or infectious agents). The most frequently impacted genes are those that play a role in maintaining proliferative signalling, dodging growth inhibitors, triggering invasion and metastasis, enabling replicative immortality, inducing angiogenesis, and resisting cell death [105, 112].

1.6 ALCOHOLIC LIVER DISEASE

Alcohol is converted to acetaldehyde in the liver by the enzyme alcohol dehydrogenase, which is then converted to acetate in the bloodstream by aldehyde dehydrogenase [113]. Both reactions require nicotinamide adenine dinucleotide (NAD+) as a cofactor, which results in the production of reduced nicotinamide adenine dinucleotide (NADH).

Consuming an excessive amount of alcohol is one of the most prevalent causes of liver illness, and it is also related to an increased risk of cancer and cardiovascular disease [114, 115]. Because it is the primary site of alcohol metabolism, the liver takes the brunt of the damage done to the body's tissues by alcohol consumption. Because the liver can regenerate itself, symptoms of liver damage might not present themselves until the damage has become quite severe. Damage to the liver caused by alcohol can be categorized into fatty liver disease caused by alcohol consumption, alcoholic hepatitis, and cirrhosis caused by alcohol consumption [116].

The first category, a build-up of fat in the liver, is something that occurs in practically all heavy drinkers and can even develop after just one session of drinking. It is normally reversible if drinking is stopped, and there are rarely any symptoms that last for an extended period. The second type, known as alcoholic hepatitis, is separate from infectious hepatitis and most frequently affects those who have engaged in heavy drinking for a significant amount of time. Inflammation of the liver leads to the death of liver cells and the gradual replacement of some healthy tissue with scar tissue (also known as a fibrosis); these are the defining characteristics of this condition [117]. Symptoms include jaundice, nausea and vomiting, weight loss, and exhaustion.

The most severe stage of the disease, known as cirrhosis, is characterized by significant fibrosis, which, in turn, causes liver failure and frequently results in death [118]. This causes the blood arteries to become rigid and affects the interior structure of the liver, which ultimately results in serious problems and the liver's failure to function. In addition to the liver, drinking alcohol while pregnant can have negative consequences on the growing foetus. These effects are referred to as foetal alcohol syndrome, and they include growth retardation, mental retardation, and facial deformities [119].

1.7 CONCLUSION

The prevalence of metabolic illnesses is unquestionably an increasing public health concern, and these conditions have a significant and detrimental effect on an individual's quality of life. These modifications may cause a disruption in the normal regulation of energy levels, hamper the production of energy by cells, or interfere with the effective breakdown of large molecules for energy. The improper management of one's energy consumption is one of the primary factors leading to the development of metabolic diseases and obesity. Therefore, it is essential to have a thorough understanding of the metabolic risk and conduct an evaluation of that risk to give patients with such illnesses the right comprehensive care in order to lower the risk of morbidity and mortality.

REFERENCES

1. Huang, C., K. Deng, and M. Wu, Mitochondrial cristae in health and disease. *International Journal of Biological Macromolecules*, 2023: p. 123755.

2. Kaenkumchorn, T.K., et al., Dietary Management of Metabolic Liver Disease. *Current Hepatology Reports*, 2023. **22**(1): pp. 24–32.

3. Mak, C.M., et al., Inborn errors of metabolism and expanded newborn screening: Review and update. *Critical Reviews in Clinical Laboratory Sciences*, 2013. **50**(6): pp. 142–162.

4. Alam, U., et al., General aspects of diabetes mellitus. *Handbook of Clinical Neurology*, 2014. **126**: pp. 211–222.

5. Lin, X., et al., Global, regional, and national burden and trend of diabetes in 195 countries and territories: An analysis from 1990 to 2025. *Scientific Reports*, 2020. **10**(1): pp. 1–11.

6. Ofori, E.K., et al., Dyslipidaemia is common among patients with type 2 diabetes: A cross-sectional study at Tema Port Clinic. *BMC Research Notes*, 2019. **12**(1): pp. 1–5.

7. Papatheodorou, K., et al., *Complications of Diabetes 2017*, 2018, Hindawi.

8. Baynes, H.W., Classification, pathophysiology, diagnosis and management of diabetes mellitus. *Journal of Diabetes & Metabolism*, 2015. **6**(5): pp. 1–9.

9. Banday, M.Z., A.S. Sameer, and S. Nissar, Pathophysiology of diabetes: An overview. *Avicenna Journal of Medicine*, 2020. **10**(04): pp. 174–188.

10. Courchesne-Loyer, A., et al., Emulsification increases the acute ketogenic effect and bioavailability of medium-chain triglycerides in humans: Protein, carbohydrate, and fat metabolism. *Current Developments in Nutrition*, 2017. **1**(7): p. e000851.

11. Vandenberghe, C., et al., Medium chain triglycerides modulate the ketogenic effect of a metabolic switch. *Frontiers in Nutrition*, 2020. **7**: p. 3.

12. Eberhard, D. and E. Lammert, The pancreatic β-cell in the islet and organ community. *Current Opinion in Genetics & Development*, 2009. **19**(5): pp. 469–475.

13. Da Silva Xavier, G., The cells of the islets of langerhans. *Journal of Clinical Medicine*, 2018. 7(3): p. 54.

14. Bano, G., Glucose homeostasis, obesity and diabetes. *Best Practice & Research Clinical Obstetrics & Gynaecology*, 2013. **27**(5): pp. 715–726.

15. Sonksen, P. and J. Sonksen, Insulin: Understanding its action in health and disease. *British Journal of Anaesthesia*, 2000. **85**(1): pp. 69–79.

16. Czech, M.P., Mechanisms of insulin resistance related to white, beige, and brown adipocytes. *Molecular Metabolism*, 2020. **34**: pp. 27–42.

17. Maughan, R., Carbohydrate metabolism. *Surgery (Oxford)*, 2009. **27**(1): pp. 6–10.

18. Møller, N. and J.O.L. Jørgensen, Effects of growth hormone on glucose, lipid, and protein metabolism in human subjects. *Endocrine Reviews*, 2009. **30**(2): pp. 152–177.

19. Saberzadeh-Ardestani, B., et al., Type 1 diabetes mellitus: Cellular and molecular pathophysiology at a glance. *Cell Journal (Yakhteh)*, 2018. **20**(3): p. 294.

20. Nicholson, L.B., The immune system. *Essays in Biochemistry*, 2016. **60**(3): pp. 275–301.

21. Noble, J.A. and A.M. Valdes, Genetics of the HLA region in the prediction of type 1 diabetes. *Current Diabetes Reports*, 2011. **11**: pp. 533–542.

22. Boland, B.B., C.J. Rhodes, and J.S. Grimsby, The dynamic plasticity of insulin production in β-cells. *Molecular Metabolism*, 2017. **6**(9): pp. 958–973.

23. Rewers, M. and J. Ludvigsson, Environmental risk factors for type 1 diabetes. *The Lancet*, 2016. **387**(10035): pp. 2340–2348.

24. Butalia, S., et al., Environmental risk factors and type 1 diabetes: past, present, and future. *Canadian Journal of Diabetes*, 2016. **40**(6): pp. 586–593.

25. Pociot, F. and Å. Lernmark, Genetic risk factors for type 1 diabetes. *The Lancet*, 2016. **387**(10035): pp. 2331–2339.

26. Antvorskov, J.C., et al., Association between maternal gluten intake and type 1 diabetes in offspring: National prospective cohort study in Denmark. *BMJ*, 2018. **362**: p. k3547.

27. Antvorskov, J.C., et al., Dietary gluten and the development of type 1 diabetes. *Diabetologia*, 2014. **57**: pp. 1770–1780.

28. Precechtelova, J., et al., Type I diabetes mellitus: Genetic factors and presumptive enteroviral etiology or protection. *Journal of Pathogens*, 2014. **2014**: p. 738512.

29. Lamminsalo, A., et al., Cow's milk allergy in infancy and later development of type 1 diabetes–nationwide case-cohort study. *Pediatric Diabetes*, 2021. **22**(3): pp. 400–406.

30. Pietropaolo, M., R. Towns, and G.S. Eisenbarth, Humoral autoimmunity in type 1 diabetes: Prediction, significance, and detection of distinct disease subtypes. *Cold Spring Harbor Perspectives in Medicine*, 2012. **2**(10): p. a012831.

31. Nishimura, A., et al., Slowly progressive type 1 diabetes mellitus: Current knowledge and future perspectives. *Diabetes, Metabolic Syndrome and Obesity: Targets and Therapy*, 2019. **12**: pp. 2461–2477.

32. Kawasaki, E., et al., Diagnostic criteria for acute-onset type 1 diabetes mellitus (2012) Report of the Committee of Japan Diabetes Society on the Research of Fulminant and Acute-onset Type 1 Diabetes Mellitus. *Diabetology International*, 2013. **4**: pp. 221–225.

33. Kobayashi, T., et al., Pathological changes in the pancreas of fulminant type 1 diabetes and slowly progressive insulin-dependent diabetes mellitus (SPIDDM): Innate immunity in fulminant type 1 diabetes and SPIDDM. *Diabetes/Metabolism Research and Reviews*, 2011. **27**(8): pp. 965–970.

34. Imagawa, A. and T. Hanafusa, Pathogenesis of fulminant type 1 diabetes. *The Review of Diabetic Studies*, 2006. **3**(4): p. 169.

35. Dhatariya, K.K., et al., Diabetic ketoacidosis. *Nature Reviews Disease Primers*, 2020. **6**(1): p. 40.

36. Evans, K., Diabetic ketoacidosis: Update on management. *Clinical Medicine*, 2019. **19**(5): p. 396.

37. Rachdaoui, N., Insulin: The friend and the foe in the development of type 2 diabetes mellitus. *International Journal of Molecular Sciences*, 2020. **21**(5): p. 1770.

38. Kido, Y., Gene–environment interaction in type 2 diabetes. *Diabetology International*, 2017. **8**: pp. 7–13.

39. Rathmann, W., B. Kowall, and G. Giani, Type 2 diabetes: Unravelling the interaction between genetic predisposition and lifestyle. *Diabetologia*, 2011. **54**: pp. 2217–2219.

40. Mlinar, B., et al., Molecular mechanisms of insulin resistance and associated diseases. *Clinica Chimica Acta*, 2007. **375**(1–2): pp. 20–35.

41. Wilcox, G., Insulin and insulin resistance. *Clinical Biochemist Reviews*, 2005. **26**(2): p. 19.

42. Guo, Y., et al., The role of nutrition in the prevention and intervention of type 2 diabetes. *Frontiers in Bioengineering and Biotechnology*, 2020. **8**: p. 575442.

43. Gbadegesin, R.A., M.P. Winn, and W.E. Smoyer, Genetic testing in nephrotic syndrome—Challenges and opportunities. *Nature Reviews Nephrology*, 2013. **9**(3): pp. 179–184.

44. Turcotte, L.P. and J.S. Fisher, Skeletal muscle insulin resistance: Roles of fatty acid metabolism and exercise. *Physical Therapy*, 2008. **88**(11): pp. 1279–1296.

45. Dhatariya, K., Diabetic ketoacidosis and hyperosmolar crisis in adults. *Medicine*, 2014. **42**(12): pp. 723–726.

46. Kalra, S. and S. K. Sharma, Diabetes in the elderly. *Diabetes Therapy*, 2018. **9**(2): pp. 493–500.

47. Mustafa, O.G., et al., Management of Hyperosmolar Hyperglycaemic State (HHS) in Adults: An updated guideline from the Joint British Diabetes Societies (JBDS) for Inpatient Care Group. *Diabetic Medicine*, 2023. **40**(3): p. e15005.

48. Morales, J. and D. Schneider, Hypoglycemia. *The American Journal of Medicine*, 2014. **127**(10): pp. S17–S24.

49. Yale, J.-F., et al., Hypoglycemia. *Canadian Journal of Diabetes*, 2018. **42**(Supplement 1): pp. S104–S108.

50. Chawla, A., R. Chawla, and S. Jaggi, Microvasular and macrovascular complications in diabetes mellitus: Distinct or continuum? *Indian Journal of Endocrinology and Metabolism*, 2016. **20**(4): p. 546.

51. Climie, R.E., et al., Macrovasculature and microvasculature at the crossroads between type 2 diabetes mellitus and hypertension. *Hypertension*, 2019. **73**(6): pp. 1138–1149.

52. Mazzone, T., A. Chait, and J. Plutzky, Cardiovascular disease risk in type 2 diabetes mellitus: Insights from mechanistic studies. *The Lancet*, 2008. **371**(9626): pp. 1800–1809.

53. Einarson, T.R., et al., Prevalence of cardiovascular disease in type 2 diabetes: A systematic literature review of scientific evidence from across the world in 2007–2017. *Cardiovascular Diabetology*, 2018. **17**(1): pp. 1–19.

54. La Corte, A.L.C., H. Philippou, and R.A. Ariëns, Role of fibrin structure in thrombosis and vascular disease. *Advances in Protein Chemistry and Structural Biology*, 2011. **83**: pp. 75–127.

55. Sobczak, A.I. and A.J. Stewart, Coagulatory defects in type-1 and type-2 diabetes. *International Journal of Molecular Sciences*, 2019. **20**(24): p. 6345.

56. Kropp, M., et al., Diabetic retinopathy as the leading cause of blindness and early predictor of cascading complications—Risks and mitigation. *EPMA Journal*, 2023: pp. 1–22.

57. Shahbazian, H. and I. Rezaii, Diabetic kidney disease; review of the current knowledge. *Journal of Renal Injury Prevention*, 2013. **2**(2): p. 73.

58. Chilelli, N., S. Burlina, and A. Lapolla, AGEs, rather than hyperglycemia, are responsible for microvascular complications in diabetes: A "glycoxidation-centric" point of view. *Nutrition, Metabolism and Cardiovascular Diseases*, 2013. **23**(10): pp. 913–919.

59. Reddy, G.B., et al., Erythrocyte aldose reductase activity and sorbitol levels in diabetic retinopathy. *Molecular Vision*, 2008. **14**: p. 593.

60. Forbes, J.M. and M.E. Cooper, Mechanisms of diabetic complications. *Physiological Reviews*, 2013. **93**(1): pp. 137–188.

61. DiNicolantonio, J.J. and J.H. O'Keefe, Myo-inositol for insulin resistance, metabolic syndrome, polycystic ovary syndrome and gestational diabetes. *Open Heart*, 2022. **9**(1): p. e001989.

62. Lien, C.-F., et al., Potential role of protein kinase C in the pathophysiology of diabetes-associated atherosclerosis. *Frontiers in Pharmacology*, 2021. **12**: p. 716332.

63. Evcimen, N.D. and G.L. King, The role of protein kinase C activation and the vascular complications of diabetes. *Pharmacological Research*, 2007. **55**(6): pp. 498–510.

64. Vlassara, H. and G.E. Striker, Advanced glycation endproducts in diabetes and diabetic complications. *Endocrinology and Metabolism Clinics*, 2013. **42**(4): pp. 697–719.

65. Del Turco, S. and G. Basta, An update on advanced glycation endproducts and atherosclerosis. *Biofactors*, 2012. **38**(4): pp. 266–274.

66. Sarfo, F.S., et al., Risk factor control in stroke survivors with diagnosed and undiagnosed diabetes: A Ghanaian registry analysis. *Journal of Stroke and Cerebrovascular Diseases*, 2020. **29**(12): p. 105304.

67. Chooi, Y.C., C. Ding, and F. Magkos, The epidemiology of obesity. *Metabolism*, 2019. **92**: pp. 6–10.

68. Haththotuwa, R.N., C.N. Wijeyaratne, and U. Senarath, Worldwide epidemic of obesity, in *Obesity and Obstetrics*, 2020, Elsevier. pp. 3–8.

69. Kumar, R., M.R. Rizvi, and S. Saraswat, Obesity and Stress: A Contingent Paralysis. *International Journal of Preventive Medicine*, 2022. **13**: p.95.

70. da Fonseca, A.C.P., et al., Genetics of non-syndromic childhood obesity and the use of high-throughput DNA sequencing technologies. *Journal of Diabetes and Its Complications*, 2017. **31**(10): pp. 1549–1561.

71. Gutiérrez-Cuevas, J., A. Santos, and J. Armendariz-Borunda, Pathophysiological molecular mechanisms of obesity: A link between MAFLD and NASH with cardiovascular diseases. *International Journal of Molecular Sciences*, 2021. **22**(21): p. 11629.

72. Heymsfield, S.B. and T.A. Wadden, Mechanisms, pathophysiology, and management of obesity. *New England Journal of Medicine*, 2017. **376**(3): pp. 254–266.

73. Thaker, V.V., Genetic and epigenetic causes of obesity. *Adolescent medicine: State of the Art Reviews*, 2017. **28**(2): p. 379.

74. Lin, X. and H. Li, Obesity: Epidemiology, pathophysiology, and therapeutics. *Frontiers in Endocrinology*, 2021. **12**: p. 706978.

75. Diels, S., W. Vanden Berghe, and W. Van Hul, Insights into the multifactorial causation of obesity by integrated genetic and epigenetic analysis. *Obesity Reviews*, 2020. **21**(7): p. e13019.

76. Stephens, R.W., L. Arhire, and M. Covasa, Gut microbiota: from microorganisms to metabolic organ influencing obesity. *Obesity*, 2018. **26**(5): pp. 801–809.

77. Geng, J., et al., The links between gut microbiota and obesity and obesity related diseases. *Biomedicine & Pharmacotherapy*, 2022. **147**: p. 112678.

78. Wadden, T.A., J.S. Tronieri, and M.L. Butryn, Lifestyle modification approaches for the treatment of obesity in adults. *American Psychologist*, 2020. **75**(2): p. 235.

79. Jacob, J.J. and R. Isaac, Behavioral therapy for management of obesity. *Indian Journal of Endocrinology and Metabolism*, 2012. **16**(1): p. 28.

80. Kaminsky, L.A., et al., The importance of healthy lifestyle behaviors in the prevention of cardiovascular disease. *Progress in Cardiovascular Diseases*, 2022. **70**: pp. 8–15.

81. Yanovski, S.Z. and J.A. Yanovski, Progress in pharmacotherapy for obesity. *JAMA*, 2021. **326**(2): pp. 129–130.

82. Debédat, J., et al., Impact of bariatric surgery on type 2 diabetes: Contribution of inflammation and gut microbiome? in *Seminars in Immunopathology*, 2019, Springer.

83. Arora, T. and F. Bäckhed, The gut microbiota and metabolic disease: Current understanding and future perspectives. *Journal of Internal Medicine*, 2016. **280**(4): pp. 339–349.

84. Anhê, F.F., et al., The gut microbiota as a mediator of metabolic benefits after bariatric surgery. *Canadian Journal of Diabetes*, 2017. **41**(4): pp. 439–447.

85. Kong, L.-C., et al., Gut microbiota after gastric bypass in human obesity: Increased richness and associations of bacterial genera with adipose tissue genes. *The American Journal of Clinical Nutrition*, 2013. **98**(1): pp. 16–24.

86. Šebunova, N., et al., Changes in adipokine levels and metabolic profiles following bariatric surgery. *BMC Endocrine Disorders*, 2022. **22**(1): p. 33.

87. Dyck, D., G.J. Heigenhauser, and C.R. Bruce, The role of adipokines as regulators of skeletal muscle fatty acid metabolism and insulin sensitivity. *Acta Physiologica*, 2006. **186**(1): pp. 5–16.

88. Marino, J.S., Y. Xu, and J.W. Hill, Central insulin and leptin-mediated autonomic control of glucose homeostasis. *Trends in Endocrinology & Metabolism*, 2011. **22**(7): pp. 275–285.

89. Kojta, I., M. Chacińska, and A. Błachnio-Zabielska, Obesity, bioactive lipids, and adipose tissue inflammation in insulin resistance. *Nutrients*, 2020. **12**(5): p. 1305.

90. Wronska, A. and Z. Kmiec, Structural and biochemical characteristics of various white adipose tissue depots. *Acta Physiologica*, 2012. **205**(2): pp. 194–208.

91. Ibrahim, M.M., Subcutaneous and visceral adipose tissue: Structural and functional differences. *Obesity Reviews*, 2010. **11**(1): pp. 11–18.

92. Longo, M., et al., Adipose tissue dysfunction as determinant of obesity-associated metabolic complications. *International Journal of Molecular Sciences*, 2019. **20**(9): p. 2358.

93. Cusi, K., The role of adipose tissue and lipotoxicity in the pathogenesis of type 2 diabetes. *Current Diabetes Reports*, 2010. **10**: pp. 306–315.

94. Rasouli, N., et al., Ectopic fat accumulation and metabolic syndrome. *Diabetes, Obesity and Metabolism*, 2007. **9**(1): pp. 1–10.

95. Sachs, S., et al., Intermuscular adipose tissue directly modulates skeletal muscle insulin sensitivity in humans. *American Journal of Physiology-Endocrinology and Metabolism*, 2019. **316**(5): pp. E866–E879.

96. Feng, B., T. Zhang, and H. Xu, Human adipose dynamics and metabolic health. *Annals of the New York Academy of Sciences*, 2013. **1281**(1): pp. 160–177.

97. Goss, A.M., et al., Effects of weight loss during a very low carbohydrate diet on specific adipose tissue depots and insulin sensitivity in older adults with obesity: A randomized clinical trial. *Nutrition & Metabolism*, 2020. **17**(1): pp. 1–12.

98. Ofori, E.K., et al., Thigh and abdominal adipose tissue depot associations with testosterone levels in postmenopausal females. *Clinical Endocrinology*, 2019. **90**(3): pp. 433–439.

99. Khodabandehloo, H., et al., Molecular and cellular mechanisms linking inflammation to insulin resistance and β-cell dysfunction. *Translational Research*, 2016. **167**(1): pp. 228–256.

100. Soltero-Perez, I., Toward a new definition of atherosclerosis including hypertension: A proposal. *Journal of Human Hypertension*, 2002. **16**(1) Supplement 1: pp. S23–S25.

101. Chung, S.T., et al., The relationship between lipoproteins and insulin sensitivity in youth with obesity and abnormal glucose tolerance. *The Journal of Clinical Endocrinology & Metabolism*, 2022. **107**(6): pp. 1541–1551.

102. Zhong, L., M.J. Simard, and J. Huot, Endothelial microRNAs regulating the NF- κB pathway and cell adhesion molecules during inflammation. *The FASEB Journal*, 2018. **32**(8): pp. 4070–4084.

103. Lusis, A.J., Genetics of atherosclerosis. *Trends in Genetics*, 2012. **28**(6): pp. 267–275.

104. Herrero-Fernandez, B., et al., Immunobiology of atherosclerosis: A complex net of interactions. *International Journal of Molecular Sciences*, 2019. **20**(21): p. 5293.

105. Kalra, S., et al., Metabolic and energy imbalance in dysglycemia-based chronic disease. *Diabetes, Metabolic Syndrome and Obesity: Targets and Therapy*, 2021. **14**: p. 165.

106. Coghlin, C. and G.I. Murray, Current and emerging concepts in tumour metastasis. *The Journal of Pathology*, 2010. **222**(1): pp. 1–15.

107. Lambert, A.W., D.R. Pattabiraman, and R.A. Weinberg, Emerging biological principles of metastasis. *Cell*, 2017. **168**(4): pp. 670–691.

108. Parrinello, G., et al., Blood urea nitrogen to creatinine ratio is associated with congestion and mortality in heart failure patients with renal dysfunction. *Internal and Emergency Medicine*, 2015. **10**(8): pp. 965–972.

109. Cao, W., et al., Changing profiles of cancer burden worldwide and in China: A secondary analysis of the global cancer statistics 2020. *Chinese Medical Journal*, 2021. **134**(07): pp. 783–791.

110. Czene, K., P. Lichtenstein, and K. Hemminki, Environmental and heritable causes of cancer among 9.6 million individuals in the Swedish family-cancer database. *International Journal of Cancer*, 2002. **99**(2): pp. 260–266.

111. Poduri, A., et al., Somatic mutation, genomic variation, and neurological disease. *Science*, 2013. **341**(6141): p. 1237758.

112. Hanahan, D., Hallmarks of cancer: New dimensions. *Cancer Discovery*, 2022. **12**(1): pp. 31–46.

113. Zakhari, S., Overview: How is alcohol metabolized by the body? *Alcohol Research & Health*, 2006. **29**(4): p. 245.

114. Shield, K.D., C. Parry, and J. Rehm, Chronic diseases and conditions related to alcohol use. *Alcohol Research: Current Reviews*, 2014. **35**(2): p. 155.

115. Connor, J., Alcohol consumption as a cause of cancer. *Addiction*, 2017. **112**(2): pp. 222–228.

116. Hosseini, N., J. Shor, and G. Szabo, Alcoholic hepatitis: A review. *Alcohol and Alcoholism*, 2019. **54**(4): pp. 408–416.

117. Singal, A.K., et al., Alcoholic hepatitis: Current challenges and future directions. *Clinical Gastroenterology and Hepatology*, 2014. **12**(4): pp. 555–564.

118. Osna, N.A., T.M. Donohue Jr, and K.K. Kharbanda, Alcoholic liver disease: Pathogenesis and current management. *Alcohol Research: Current Reviews*, 2017. **38**(2): p. 147.

119. Riley, E.P., M.A. Infante, and K.R. Warren, Fetal alcohol spectrum disorders: An overview. *Neuropsychology Review*, 2011. **21**: pp. 73–80.

2 Molecular Basis of Chemical Pathologies

Abigail Aning, Seth Kwabena Amponsah, Kwasi Agyei Bugyei, and Yahwant V. Pathak

2.1 INTRODUCTION

The field of pathology applies science to the study of human diseases [1]. The study of the body's chemical and biochemical processes in relation to disease is known as chemical pathology. The human body is a complex system that relies on chemical reactions to maintain its functionality. These chemical reactions are essential for the body's metabolism, growth, and repair. However, when these reactions go awry, they can lead to chemical pathologies or diseases. Chemical pathologies are the result of disruptions in the normal biochemical processes that occur within the body [2, 3]. Many chemical pathologies are caused by alterations in the molecular pathways that regulate important cellular processes such as metabolism, cell signaling, and gene expression [4]. Molecular pathology involves the study of the molecular mechanisms of diseases. This area of science also aids in the development of new strategies for treating and diagnosing diseases, as well as finding new therapies [4]. Understanding the molecular basis of these diseases is essential for the development of effective treatments. The molecular basis of chemical pathologies has been extensively studied, and several molecular mechanisms have been identified as contributing to the development of various diseases (Figure 2.1). This chapter will provide an overview of the molecular basis of chemical pathologies, including some of the major diseases that are affected by these molecular changes.

2.2 THE MOLECULAR BASIS OF CHEMICAL PATHOLOGIES

2.2.1 Genetic Changes

Genetic changes refer to alterations that occur in the deoxyribonucleic acid (DNA) sequence of an organism. These changes can arise spontaneously, through errors that occur during DNA replication or through exposure to environmental factors such as radiation or chemicals [5]. Genetic changes can also be inherited from parents or acquired during an individual's lifetime. There are several types of genetic changes, including mutations, deletions, insertions, and rearrangements [6]. These changes can have a significant impact on an organism's health, development, and susceptibility to disease (Figure 2.1).

Mutations are the most common type of genetic change. They occur when there is a change in the DNA sequence of a gene, resulting in a different protein being produced. There are different types of mutations, including point mutations, which involve the substitution of one nucleotide for another, and frameshift mutations, which occur when nucleotides are added or deleted, causing a shift in the reading frame of the gene. Mutations can be beneficial, harmful, or neutral, depending on their impact on the protein produced by the gene.

Deletions and insertions are another type of genetic change that can occur. Deletions involve the loss of one or more nucleotides in the DNA sequence, while insertions involve the addition of one or more nucleotides. These changes can cause frameshift mutations, resulting in an altered protein or premature termination in protein synthesis. Rearrangements involve the movement or reordering of DNA sequences within or between chromosomes. This can result in changes in gene expression or protein function, leading to various genetic disorders.

Genetic changes can have a significant impact on an organism's health and development. For example, mutations in the BRCA1 and BRCA2 genes have been linked to an increased risk of breast and ovarian cancer [7]. Similarly, mutations in the CFTR gene can cause cystic fibrosis, a genetic disorder that affects the respiratory, digestive, and reproductive systems [8].

Recent advancements in genetic technologies such as CRISPR/Cas9 have enabled precise gene editing, allowing researchers to study the effects of specific genetic changes in various organisms [9]. These technologies also have the potential to treat genetic disorders by correcting or modifying the genes responsible for the disorder. Genetic changes play a crucial role in an organism's health, development, and susceptibility to disease. Therefore, understanding the various types of genetic changes and their impact on gene expression and protein function is essential for developing new therapies for genetic disorders.

DOI: 10.1201/9781003384823-2

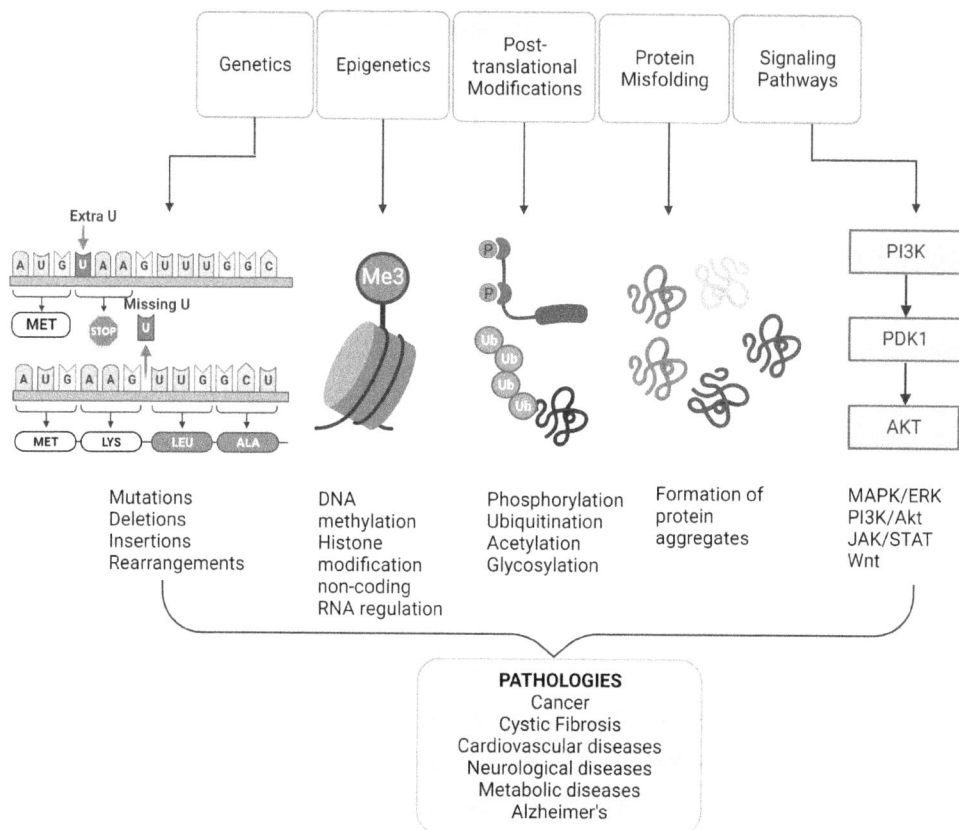

Figure 2.1 Summary of factors leading to chemical pathologies

2.2.2 Epigenetic Changes

Epigenetic changes refer to modifications to the DNA molecule that do not involve alterations to the underlying nucleotide sequence. These modifications can affect the way genes are expressed, leading to changes in an organism's phenotype without altering the DNA sequence itself. Epigenetic changes can be inherited or acquired during an individual's lifetime and are influenced by environmental factors such as diet, stress, and exposure to toxins [10].

There are several types of epigenetic changes, including DNA methylation, histone modification, and non-coding ribonucleic acid (RNA) regulation. DNA methylation is the most well-studied epigenetic modification and involves the addition of a methyl group to the cytosine base of DNA. This modification typically leads to gene silencing, as it interferes with the binding of transcription factors and other proteins necessary for gene expression [10]. Histone modification involves changes to the proteins around which DNA is coiled, which can affect the accessibility of genes to transcriptional machinery. For example, histone acetylation is associated with gene activation, while histone deacetylation is associated with gene repression [11]. Non-coding RNA regulation involves the production of RNA molecules that do not code for proteins but can affect gene expression by targeting messenger RNA molecules or regulating chromatin structure [10]. Non-coding RNAs, such as microRNAs, can also play a role in gene regulation. These small RNAs bind to messenger RNAs and prevent their translation into proteins, leading to gene silencing [12].

Epigenetic changes can have a significant impact on an organism's health and development (Figure 2.1). For example, changes in DNA methylation patterns have been linked to several diseases, including cancer, cardiovascular disease, and neurological disorders [13]. Similarly, alterations in histone modification have been implicated in the development of various types of cancer, including breast cancer and leukemia [14, 15], and have been shown to play a role in aging and age-related diseases [16].

Environmental factors can also influence epigenetic changes. For example, exposure to toxins such as cigarette smoke and air pollution can alter DNA methylation patterns, leading to changes in gene expression and increased risk of disease [10]. Similarly, changes in diet and lifestyle can affect epigenetic modifications, potentially leading to changes in gene expression and increased susceptibility to disease [17].

Recent advancements in epigenetic research have led to the development of new therapies and treatments for various diseases. For example, DNA methyltransferase inhibitors have been approved for the treatment of certain types of cancer, while histone deacetylase inhibitors are being studied as potential treatments for a variety of diseases [18].

In conclusion, epigenetic changes play a critical role in gene regulation and can have a significant impact on an individual's health and development. Understanding the various types of epigenetic modifications and their impact on gene expression is essential for developing new therapies and treatments for epigenetic-related diseases.

2.2.3 Post-translational Modifications

Post-translational modifications (PTMs) are chemical changes that happen to proteins after they have been synthesized. These modifications can alter the function, localization, stability, and interactions of proteins. PTMs play critical roles in many biological processes, and alterations in PTMs can lead to the development of various diseases. Dysregulation of PTMs has been implicated in many human diseases, including cancer, neurological disorders, and metabolic diseases [19].

One of the most common PTMs is phosphorylation, which involves the addition of a phosphate group to specific serine, threonine, or tyrosine residues on a protein [20]. Phosphorylation can activate or deactivate proteins and modulate protein–protein interactions. Aberrant phosphorylation is associated with many diseases, such as cancer, neurodegenerative disorders, and diabetes [21]. For example, abnormal phosphorylation of tau protein is associated with Alzheimer's disease [22].

Another important PTM is ubiquitination, which involves the covalent attachment of ubiquitin molecules to lysine residues on a protein [23]. Ubiquitination can target proteins for degradation by the proteasome or alter their localization or activity. Dysregulation of ubiquitination has been linked to many diseases, including cancer, neurodegenerative disorders, and inflammation [23]. Aberrant ubiquitination of the tumor suppressor protein p53 is associated with cancer [24].

Acetylation is another PTM that involves the addition of an acetyl group to lysine residues on a protein. Acetylation can alter protein activity, stability, and localization. Dysregulation of acetylation has been implicated in many diseases, including cancer, neurodegenerative disorders, and metabolic diseases [25].

Glycosylation is a PTM that involves the addition of carbohydrate molecules to specific amino acid residues on a protein [26]. Glycosylation can modulate protein activity, stability, and interactions. Dysregulation of glycosylation has been associated with many diseases, such as cancer and inflammatory disorders [26].

Other PTMs, such as methylation, SUMOylation, and ADP-ribosylation, also play important roles in regulating protein function and are dysregulated in various diseases [27].

In conclusion, PTMs are crucial for regulating protein function and their dysregulation is associated with a variety of human diseases. Understanding the mechanisms underlying PTMs and their roles in disease pathology could provide new targets for therapeutic intervention.

2.2.4 Protein Misfolding

Protein misfolding is a process by which proteins fail to fold into their correct three-dimensional structure. This can lead to the formation of abnormal protein aggregates and the disruption of biochemical pathways [28]. Protein misfolding is a common feature of many chemical pathologies, including Alzheimer's disease, Parkinson's disease, and Huntington's disease [29].

2.2.5 Signaling Pathways

Signaling pathways play a critical role in the regulation of cellular processes, such as growth, differentiation, and apoptosis [30, 31]. Anomalous signaling can lead to various diseases, including cancer, cardiovascular diseases, and neurodegenerative disorders.

Signal transduction pathways involve a series of events that start with the binding of a ligand to a receptor, leading to the activation of downstream signaling molecules. The most well-known signaling pathways include the MAPK/ERK pathway, the PI3K/Akt pathway, and the JAK/STAT pathway [32].

The MAPK/ERK pathway is involved in the regulation of cell growth, differentiation, and survival [32]. Mutations in this pathway have been implicated in various cancers, such as melanoma and lung cancer [33]. The PI3K/Akt pathway is also critical in cell growth and survival and is frequently dysregulated in cancer, including breast, ovarian, and prostate cancer [34]. The JAK/STAT pathway is involved in immune responses and has been implicated in autoimmune disorders and cancer [35].

Another signaling pathway implicated in disease development is the Wnt pathway, which is critical in embryonic development and tissue homeostasis [36, 37]. Dysregulation of the Wnt pathway has been implicated in cancer and other diseases, including osteoporosis and Alzheimer's disease [37].

In addition to these well-known signaling pathways, recent studies have highlighted the role of non-coding RNAs in regulating signaling pathways and disease development. For instance, microRNAs (miRNAs) have been shown to regulate the MAPK/ERK pathway and have been implicated in various cancers, including breast cancer and hepatocellular carcinoma [38].

2.3 THERAPEUTIC TARGETS AND TREATMENTS

The molecular basis of chemical pathologies has led to the identification of potential therapeutic targets for these diseases. By studying the structure and function of molecules such as proteins, DNA, and RNA, researchers can identify specific targets for drug development. For example, the identification of the HIV and its replication cycle led to the development of antiretroviral drugs that target specific viral proteins, such as reverse transcriptase and protease [39].

Another example of molecular biology in drug discovery is the development of monoclonal antibodies. These are antibodies that are designed to target specific proteins or cells in the body and are used to treat a wide range of conditions, including cancer, autoimmune disorders, and infectious diseases [40]. Monoclonal antibodies are created by isolating a single B-cell that produces a specific antibody and then cloning that cell to produce large quantities of the antibody for therapeutic use [41].

Genetics and genomics have also played a critical role in drug development. By studying the genetic basis of diseases, researchers can identify specific genetic mutations or variations that contribute to the disease, and develop drugs that target those mutations. For example, the development of tyrosine kinase inhibitors for the treatment of chronic myeloid leukemia (CML) was based on the identification of the BCR-ABL fusion protein, which is produced by a specific genetic mutation [42].

Genomics has also revolutionized drug development by allowing for the identification of novel targets for drug development. Genome-wide association studies (GWAS) have identified thousands of genetic variants that are associated with various diseases, providing researchers with new targets for drug development [43]. For example, the identification of the PCSK9 gene as a risk factor for heart disease led to the development of PCSK9 inhibitors, which are used to lower cholesterol levels and reduce the risk of heart disease [44].

2.4 COMMON CHEMICAL PATHOLOGIES

The molecular basis of some diseases has been extensively studied. The molecular basis of some common diseases – Alzheimer's, atherosclerosis, cancer, and diabetes – are discussed and summarized in Table 2.1.

Table 2.1   Summary of some common chemical pathologies

Pathology	Molecular Changes	References
Alzheimer's Disease	Accumulation of low-density lipoproteins (LDL) Mutations in genes involved in lipoprotein metabolism	[56] [63]
Atherosclerosis	Mutations in APP and presenilin genes Tau hyperphosphorylation Dysregulation of calcium homeostasis	[46] [50] [53]
Cancer	Dysregulation of cellular signaling pathways Alteration of cell cycle control Loss of tumor suppressor gene Activation of oncogenes DNA methylation, histone modifications, non-coding RNA expression	[65] [66] [67] [68] [69]
Diabetes	Destruction of pancreatic beta cells Changes in the insulin gene (INS), the solute carrier family 30-member 8 gene (SLC30A8), and the transcription factor 7-like 2 gene (TCF7L2)	[81] [78–80]

2.4.1 Alzheimer's Disease

Alzheimer's disease (AD) is a neurodegenerative disorder characterized by the progressive loss of memory and cognitive function. The molecular basis of Alzheimer's involves the accumulation of beta-amyloid (Aβ) plaques and neurofibrillary tangles (NFTs) in the brain, leading to synaptic dysfunction and neuronal death. In this section, we will discuss the molecular mechanisms underlying Alzheimer's disease.

The accumulation of Aβ plaques is a key feature of Alzheimer's disease. Aβ is a peptide derived from the amyloid precursor protein (APP) through sequential cleavage by β-secretase (BACE1) and γ-secretase [45]. Mutations in the APP and presenilin genes, which encode the components of γ-secretase, can increase the production of Aβ and promote the formation of Aβ plaques [46]. Aβ aggregates can induce oxidative stress and inflammation, leading to synaptic dysfunction and neuronal death [47].

The formation of NFTs is another hallmark of Alzheimer's disease. NFTs are composed of hyperphosphorylated tau protein, which aggregates and forms insoluble fibrils [48]. Tau protein normally stabilizes microtubules, which are crucial for neuronal transport and communication [49]. In Alzheimer's disease, tau protein becomes hyperphosphorylated and detaches from microtubules, leading to their disassembly and dysfunction [50]. The loss of microtubule stability can impair neuronal transport and synaptic function, contributing to cognitive decline.

In addition to Aβ plaques and NFTs, Alzheimer's disease is associated with dysregulation of multiple signaling pathways, including inflammation, oxidative stress, and calcium homeostasis. Chronic inflammation can promote the production of Aβ and tau phosphorylation, leading to neurodegeneration [51]. Oxidative stress can damage neuronal membranes and DNA, leading to cell death [52]. Dysregulation of calcium homeostasis can impair synaptic transmission and neuronal function, contributing to cognitive impairment [53].

Finally, genetic and environmental factors can contribute to the development of Alzheimer's disease. Genetic factors, such as mutations in the APP, presenilin, and tau genes, can increase the risk of developing Alzheimer's disease [54]. Environmental factors, such as exposure to toxins and chronic stress, can also contribute to the development of Alzheimer's disease [55].

In conclusion, the molecular basis of Alzheimer's disease involves the accumulation of Aβ plaques and NFTs, dysregulation of multiple signaling pathways, and the interaction of genetic and environmental factors. Understanding the molecular mechanisms underlying Alzheimer's disease is essential for the development of effective therapies.

2.4.2 Atherosclerosis

Atherosclerosis is a cardiovascular disease characterized by the buildup of plaques in the arteries, which can lead to restricted blood flow and increased risk of heart attack and stroke. The development of atherosclerosis begins with the accumulation of low-density lipoprotein (LDL) particles in the arterial intima. LDL particles can undergo oxidation and become modified, leading to their uptake by macrophages through scavenger receptors [56]. This results in the formation of lipid-laden macrophages, or foam cells, which are a hallmark of early atherosclerotic lesions. Foam cells release pro-inflammatory cytokines and chemokines, which attract more immune cells and contribute to the chronic inflammation observed in atherosclerosis [57].

In addition to immune cells, vascular smooth muscle cells (VSMCs) play a key role in atherosclerosis. VSMCs can proliferate and migrate from the media to the intima, where they contribute to the formation of the fibrous cap of plaques [58]. VSMCs also produce extracellular matrix proteins, such as collagen and elastin, which provide structural support to the plaque [59]. However, VSMCs can undergo phenotypic switching, from a contractile to a synthetic phenotype, in response to inflammatory stimuli [60]. This can lead to the production of matrix-degrading enzymes and further contribute to plaque destabilization.

The immune response in atherosclerosis involves multiple cell types, including macrophages, T cells, and B cells. Macrophages can phagocytose apoptotic cells and cell debris in the plaque, which can activate the immune system through the release of antigens [61]. T cells can recognize these antigens and differentiate into effector cells, which produce pro-inflammatory cytokines and contribute to plaque progression [62]. B cells can also contribute to plaque formation through the production of antibodies against oxidized LDL particles [61].

Finally, genetic and environmental factors can contribute to the development of atherosclerosis. Genetic factors, such as mutations in genes involved in lipoprotein metabolism and inflammation, can increase the risk of developing atherosclerosis [63]. Environmental factors, such as smoking, hypertension, and diabetes, can also contribute to the development of atherosclerosis [64].

In conclusion, the molecular basis of atherosclerosis involves the interplay between lipids, immune cells, and vascular cells, which together contribute to the formation and progression of plaques. Understanding the molecular mechanisms underlying atherosclerosis is essential for the development of effective therapies.

2.4.3 Cancer

Cancer is a group of diseases characterized by the uncontrolled growth and spread of abnormal cells. Cancer can occur in any part of the body and can invade surrounding tissues and metastasize to other parts of the body through the bloodstream or lymphatic system. There are many different types of cancer, each with its own unique molecular characteristics. The molecular basis of cancer is also multifactorial and involves a wide range of genetic and environmental factors. The development of cancer is a multistep process that involves the accumulation of genetic mutations and epigenetic changes that result in the dysregulation of key cellular pathways.

One of the hallmarks of cancer is the deregulation of cellular signaling pathways that control cell proliferation, differentiation, and survival [65]. These pathways include the mitogen-activated protein kinase (MAPK) pathway, the phosphoinositide 3-kinase (PI3K)/Akt pathway, and the tumor suppressor pathways, such as the p53 pathway. Mutations in genes encoding components of these pathways can lead to their activation and drive tumorigenesis.

Another hallmark of cancer is the alteration of the cell cycle control machinery. The cell cycle is regulated by a series of cyclins and cyclin-dependent kinases (CDKs) that coordinate cell growth and division [66]. Mutations in genes encoding these proteins can disrupt the balance between cell growth and cell division and lead to uncontrolled cell proliferation.

The loss of tumor suppressor genes and the activation of oncogenes are also key factors in the development of cancer. Tumor suppressor genes, such as p53, BRCA1, and BRCA2, encode proteins that regulate cell cycle progression, DNA repair, and apoptosis [67]. Mutations in these genes can lead to the loss of their function and promote tumor growth. Oncogenes, on the other hand, encode proteins that promote cell growth and survival, such as the epidermal growth factor receptor (EGFR) and the v-Raf murine sarcoma viral oncogene homolog B (BRAF) [68]. Mutations in these genes can lead to their activation and contribute to tumor growth.

Epigenetic changes, such as DNA methylation, histone modifications, and non-coding RNA expression, are also involved in the molecular basis of cancer [69]. These changes can alter gene expression and promote tumorigenesis by silencing tumor suppressor genes or activating oncogenes.

In addition, cancer cells can modify their microenvironment to promote tumor growth and survival. Tumor-associated stromal cells, such as cancer-associated fibroblasts and immune cells, can secrete growth factors and cytokines that promote tumor growth and angiogenesis [70].

Finally, genetic and environmental factors can contribute to the development of cancer. Genetic factors, such as inherited mutations in tumor suppressor genes or oncogenes, can increase the risk of developing cancer [71]. Environmental factors, such as exposure to carcinogens or chronic inflammation, can also contribute to the development of cancer [72].

In conclusion, the molecular basis of cancer involves multiple genetic and epigenetic changes that disrupt normal cellular processes and promote tumorigenesis. Understanding the molecular mechanisms underlying cancer is essential for the development of effective therapies.

2.4.4 Diabetes

Diabetes is a chronic metabolic disorder characterized by elevated levels of glucose in the blood. The disease is caused by a deficiency of or insensitivity to the hormone insulin, which is produced by the pancreas. Insulin regulates the uptake and utilization of glucose by cells throughout the body. In diabetes, the lack of insulin or its ineffectiveness results in a buildup of glucose in the blood, leading to a variety of complications. There are two main types of diabetes: type 1 diabetes and type 2 diabetes. In type 1 diabetes, the immune system attacks and destroys the insulin-producing cells in the pancreas. In type 2 diabetes, the body becomes resistant to insulin or does not produce enough insulin.

Insulin is a hormone that regulates glucose uptake and metabolism in the body. Insulin secretion from pancreatic beta cells is regulated by a complex interplay of signaling pathways involving glucose, amino acids, and hormones, such as glucagon-like peptide 1 (GLP-1) and glucose-dependent insulinotropic peptide (GIP) [73]. Glucose enters beta cells through glucose transporters, such as GLUT2, and is metabolized to generate ATP, which stimulates insulin secretion via closure of ATP-sensitive potassium channels [74]. In type 1 diabetes, autoimmune destruction of beta cells leads to a lack of insulin secretion, whereas in type 2 diabetes, beta cells fail to secrete adequate amounts of insulin in response to glucose stimulation.

Insulin action is mediated by the insulin receptor, which is a tyrosine kinase receptor that activates multiple downstream signaling pathways, such as the PI3K/Akt pathway and the MAPK pathway [75]. These pathways regulate glucose uptake, glycogen synthesis, and protein synthesis in target tissues, such as muscle, liver, and adipose tissue. Insulin resistance, which is a key feature of type 2 diabetes, is characterized by a decrease in insulin sensitivity in target tissues, leading to impaired glucose uptake and metabolism [76]. Insulin resistance can be caused by multiple factors, such as obesity, inflammation, and genetic factors.

Glucose metabolism is also regulated by multiple enzymes and transporters that control glucose uptake, glycolysis, gluconeogenesis, and glycogen synthesis [77]. In type 2 diabetes, dysregulation of these pathways can lead to impaired glucose tolerance and hyperglycemia. For example, increased gluconeogenesis in the liver can contribute to hyperglycemia in type 2 diabetes.

Genetics also plays a role in the development of diabetes. Several genes have been identified that contribute to the risk of developing diabetes, such as the insulin gene (INS), the solute carrier family 30-member 8 gene (SLC30A8), and the transcription factor 7-like 2 gene (TCF7L2) [78–80].

A key factor in the development of diabetes is the dysfunction of pancreatic beta cells, which secrete insulin. Genetic mutations in genes such as HNF1A and HNF4A can disrupt the function of beta cells, leading to impaired insulin secretion [81]. Additionally, chronic inflammation can lead to insulin resistance, which impairs the ability of cells to respond to insulin. This inflammation can be caused by factors such as obesity and high levels of free fatty acids [82].

In addition to genetic factors, environmental factors, such as diet and physical activity, can contribute to the development of diabetes [83]. High-calorie diets and sedentary lifestyles can lead to obesity and insulin resistance, whereas healthy diets and regular exercise can improve insulin sensitivity and glucose metabolism [83].

Epigenetic changes in genes involved in insulin secretion and glucose metabolism can contribute to the development of diabetes. For example, DNA methylation of the PDX1 gene (an essential transcription factor for beta cell maturation and function as well as pancreas development) has been shown to be associated with impaired insulin secretion in type 2 diabetes [84].

2.5 CONCLUSION

The molecular basis of chemical pathologies remains a complex area of science. In-depth knowledge of genetic mutations, epigenetic modifications, protein misfolding, and signaling pathways are relevant for future progress in chemical pathology. Current advances in our understanding of these molecular mechanisms have led to the identification of potential therapeutic targets for chemical pathologies. Nonetheless, much remains to be discovered about the molecular basis of chemical pathologies, and further research is needed to develop effective treatments for diseases.

REFERENCES

1. Dematteo, R.P., et al., Clinical management of gastrointestinal stromal tumors: before and after STI-571. *Human Pathology*, 2002. **33**(5): pp. 466–477.

2. Takahashi, J.S., et al., The genetics of mammalian circadian order and disorder: Implications for physiology and disease. *Nature Reviews Genetics*, 2008. **9**(10): pp. 764–775.

3. Schug, T.T., et al., Endocrine disrupting chemicals and disease susceptibility. *The Journal of Steroid Biochemistry and Molecular Biology*, 2011. **127**(3–5): pp. 204–215.

4. Coleman, W.B. and G.J. Tsongalis, *Molecular Pathology: The Molecular Basis of Human Disease*, 2009: Academic Press.

5. Moustacchi, E., DNA damage and repair: Consequences on dose-responses. *Mutation Research/Genetic Toxicology and Environmental Mutagenesis*, 2000. **464**(1): pp. 35–40.

6. Stenson, P.D., et al., Human gene mutation database (HGMD®): 2003 update. *Human Mutation*, 2003. **21**(6): pp. 577–581.

7. Sluiter, M.D. and E.J. van Rensburg, Large genomic rearrangements of the BRCA1 and BRCA2 genes: Review of the literature and report of a novel BRCA1 mutation. *Breast Cancer Research and Treatment*, 2011. **125**: pp. 325–349.

8. Cutting, G.R., Cystic fibrosis genetics: from molecular understanding to clinical application. *Nature Reviews Genetics*, 2015. **16**(1): pp. 45–56.

9. Jacinto, F.V., W. Link, and B.I. Ferreira, CRISPR/Cas9-mediated genome editing: From basic research to translational medicine. *Journal of Cellular and Molecular Medicine*, 2020. **24**(7): pp. 3766–3778.

10. Feinberg, A.P., The key role of epigenetics in human disease prevention and mitigation. *New England Journal of Medicine*, 2018. **378**(14): pp. 1323–1334.

11. Ropero, S. and M. Esteller, The role of histone deacetylases (HDACs) in human cancer. *Molecular Oncology*, 2007. **1**(1): pp. 19–25.

12. Green, D., W.D. Fraser, and T. Dalmay, Transfer RNA-derived small RNAs in the cancer transcriptome. *Pflügers Archiv - European Journal of Physiology*, 2016. **468**(6): pp. 1041–1047.

13. Singh, S., B. Murphy, and R. O'Reilly, Involvement of gene–diet/drug interaction in DNA methylation and its contribution to complex diseases: from cancer to schizophrenia. *Clinical Genetics*, 2003. **64**(6): pp. 451–460.

14. Trager, M.H., et al., Control of breast cancer pathogenesis by histone methylation and the hairless histone demethylase. *Endocrinology*, 2021. **162**(8).

15. Zhao, Z. and A. Shilatifard, Epigenetic modifications of histones in cancer. *Genome Biology*, 2019. **20**(1): p. 245.

16. Calvanese, V., et al., The role of epigenetics in aging and age-related diseases. *Ageing Research Reviews*, 2009. **8**(4): pp. 268–276.

17. Abdul, Q.A., et al., Epigenetic modifications of gene expression by lifestyle and environment. *Archives of Pharmacal Research*, 2017. **40**(11): pp. 1219–1237.

18. Gore, S.D., et al., Combined DNA methyltransferase and histone deacetylase inhibition in the treatment of myeloid neoplasms. *Cancer Research*, 2006. **66**(12): pp. 6361–6369.

19. Xu, H., et al., PTMD: A database of human disease-associated post-translational modifications. *Genomics, Proteomics & Bioinformatics*, 2018. **16**(4): pp. 244–251.

20. Tasmia, S.A., et al., Prediction of serine phosphorylation sites mapping on Schizosaccharomyces Pombe by fusing three encoding schemes with the random forest classifier. *Scientific Reports*, 2022. **12**(1): p. 2632.

21. Rudrabhatla, P., Regulation of neuronal cytoskeletal protein phosphorylation in neurodegenerative diseases. *Journal of Alzheimer's Disease*, 2014. **41**: pp. 671–684.

22. Chung, S.H., Aberrant phosphorylation in the pathogenesis of Alzheimer's disease. *BMB Reports*, 2009. **42**(8): pp. 467–474.

23. Mukhopadhyay, D. and H. Riezman, Proteasome-independent functions of ubiquitin in endocytosis and signaling. *Science*, 2007. **315**(5809): pp. 201–205.

24. Brooks, C.L. and W. Gu, Ubiquitination, phosphorylation and acetylation: The molecular basis for p53 regulation. *Current Opinion in Cell Biology*, 2003. **15**(2): pp. 164–171.

25. Choudhary, C., et al., Lysine acetylation targets protein complexes and co-regulates major cellular functions. *Science*, 2009. **325**(5942): pp. 834–840.

26. Reily, C., et al., Glycosylation in health and disease. *Nature Reviews Nephrology*, 2019. **15**(6): pp. 346–366.

27. Wang, H., et al., Protein post-translational modifications in the regulation of cancer hallmarks. *Cancer Gene Therapy*, 2023. **30**(4): pp. 529–547.

28. Gregersen, N., et al., Protein misfolding and human disease. *Annual Review of Genomics and Human Genetics*, 2006. **7**(1): pp. 103–124.

29. Chiti, F. and C.M. Dobson, Protein misfolding, functional amyloid, and human disease. *Annual Review of Biochemistry*, 2006. **75**(1): pp. 333–366.

30. Junttila, M.R., S.-P. Li, and J. Westermarck, Phosphatase-mediated crosstalk between MAPK signaling pathways in the regulation of cell survival. *The FASEB Journal*, 2008. **22**(4): pp. 954–965.

31. Zhou, D., et al., Macrophage polarization and function with emphasis on the evolving roles of coordinated regulation of cellular signaling pathways. *Cellular Signalling*, 2014. **26**(2): pp. 192–197.

32. Peyssonnaux, C. and A. Eychène, The Raf/MEK/ERK pathway: New concepts of activation. *Biology of the Cell*, 2001. **93**(1–2): pp. 53–62.

33. Davies, H., et al., Mutations of the BRAF gene in human cancer. *Nature*, 2002. **417**(6892): pp. 949–954.

34. Engelman, J.A., Targeting PI3K signalling in cancer: Opportunities, challenges and limitations. *Nature Reviews Cancer*, 2009. **9**(8): pp. 550–562.

35. O'Shea, J.J., et al., The JAK-STAT pathway: Impact on human disease and therapeutic intervention. *Annual Review of Medicine*, 2015. **66**(1): pp. 311–328.

36. Clevers, H. and R. Nusse, Wnt/β-Catenin signaling and disease. *Cell*, 2012. **149**(6): pp. 1192–1205.

37. Kahn, M., Can we safely target the WNT pathway? *Nature Reviews Drug Discovery*, 2014. **13**(7): pp. 513–532.

38. Asl, E.R., et al., Interplay between MAPK/ERK signaling pathway and MicroRNAs: A crucial mechanism regulating cancer cell metabolism and tumor progression. *Life Sciences*, 2021. **278**: p. 119499.

39. De Clercq, E., The history of antiretrovirals: Key discoveries over the past 25 years. *Reviews in Medical Virology*, 2009. **19**(5): pp. 287–299.

40. Singh, S., et al., Monoclonal antibodies: A review. *Current Clinical Pharmacology*, 2018. **13**(2): pp. 85–99.

41. Yokoyama, W.M., et al., Production of Monoclonal Antibodies. *Current Protocols in Immunology*, 2013. **102**(1): pp. 2.5.1–2.5.29.

42. Druker, B.J. and N.B. Lydon, Lessons learned from the development of an abl tyrosine kinase inhibitor for chronic myelogenous leukemia. *The Journal Of Clinical Investigation*, 2000. **105**(1): pp. 3–7.

43. Visscher, P.M., et al., Five years of GWAS discovery. *The American Journal of Human Genetics*, 2012. **90**(1): pp. 7–24.

44. Sabatine, M.S., et al., Efficacy and safety of evolocumab in reducing lipids and cardiovascular events. *New England Journal of Medicine*, 2015. **372**(16): pp. 1500–1509.

45. Hardy, J. and D.J. Selkoe, The amyloid hypothesis of Alzheimer's disease: Progress and problems on the road to therapeutics. *Science*, 2002. **297**(5580): pp. 353–356.

46. Heneka, M.T., et al., Neuroinflammation in Alzheimer's disease. *The Lancet Neurology*, 2015. **14**(4): pp. 388–405.

47. Götz, J. and L.M. Ittner, Animal models of Alzheimer's disease and frontotemporal dementia. *Nature Reviews Neuroscience*, 2008. **9**(7): pp. 532–544.

48. A Lasagna-Reeves, C., et al., Tau oligomers as potential targets for immunotherapy for Alzheimer's disease and tauopathies. *Current Alzheimer Research*, 2011. **8**(6): pp. 659–665.

49. Hervy, J. and D.J. Bicout, Dynamical decoration of stabilized-microtubules by Tau-proteins. *Scientific Reports*, 2019. **9**(1): p. 12473.

50. Götz, J., L.M. Ittner, and S. Kins, Do axonal defects in tau and amyloid precursor protein transgenic animals model axonopathy in Alzheimer's disease? *Journal of Neurochemistry*, 2006. **98**(4): pp. 993–1006.

51. Newcombe, E.A., et al., Inflammation: The link between comorbidities, genetics, and Alzheimer's disease. *Journal of Neuroinflammation*, 2018. **15**(1): pp. 1–26.

52. Higuchi, Y., Chromosomal DNA fragmentation in apoptosis and necrosis induced by oxidative stress. *Biochemical Pharmacology*, 2003. **66**(8): pp. 1527–1535.

53. Supnet, C. and I. Bezprozvanny, The dysregulation of intracellular calcium in Alzheimer disease. *Cell Calcium*, 2010. **47**(2): pp. 183–189.

54. Armstrong, R.A., What causes Alzheimer's disease? *Folia Neuropathologica*, 2013. **51**(3): pp. 169–188.

55. Moulton, P.V. and W. Yang, Air pollution, oxidative stress, and Alzheimer's disease. *Journal of Environmental and Public Health*, 2012. **2012**: p. 472751.

56. Libby, P., Inflammation in atherosclerosis. *Arteriosclerosis, Thrombosis, and Vascular Biology*, 2012. **32**(9): pp. 2045–2051.

57. Moore, K.J. and I. Tabas, Macrophages in the pathogenesis of atherosclerosis. *Cell*, 2011. **145**(3): pp. 341–355.

58. Owens, G.K., M.S. Kumar, and B.R. Wamhoff, Molecular regulation of vascular smooth muscle cell differentiation in development and disease. *Physiological Reviews*, 2004. **84**(3): pp. 767–801.

59. Bobryshev, Y.V., Monocyte recruitment and foam cell formation in atherosclerosis. *Micron*, 2006. **37**(3): pp. 208–222.

60. Gomez, D. and G.K. Owens, Smooth muscle cell phenotypic switching in atherosclerosis. *Cardiovascular Research*, 2012. **95**(2): pp. 156–164.

61. Hansson, G.K. and A. Hermansson, The immune system in atherosclerosis. *Nature Immunology*, 2011. **12**(3): pp. 204–212.

62. Saigusa, R., H. Winkels, and K. Ley, T cell subsets and functions in atherosclerosis. *Nature Reviews Cardiology*, 2020. **17**(7): pp. 387–401.

63. Markin, A.M., et al., Cellular mechanisms of human atherogenesis: Focus on chronification of inflammation and mitochondrial mutations. *Frontiers in Pharmacology*, 2020. **11**: p. 642.

64. Hegele, R.A., The pathogenesis of atherosclerosis. *Clinica Chimica Acta*, 1996. **246**(1–2): pp. 21–38.

65. Hanahan, D. and R.A. Weinberg, Hallmarks of cancer: The next generation. *Cell*, 2011. **144**(5): pp. 646–674.

66. Malumbres, M. and M. Barbacid, Cell cycle, CDKs and cancer: A changing paradigm. *Nature Reviews Cancer*, 2009. **9**(3): pp. 153–166.

67. Knudson, A.G., Two genetic hits (more or less) to cancer. *Nature Reviews Cancer*, 2001. **1**(2): pp. 157–162.

68. Sharma, S.V. and J. Settleman, Oncogene addiction: Setting the stage for molecularly targeted cancer therapy. *Genes & Development*, 2007. **21**(24): pp. 3214–3231.

69. Lian, Y., et al., Epigenetic regulation of MAGE family in human cancer progression-DNA methylation, histone modification, and non-coding RNAs. *Clinical Epigenetics*, 2018. **10**: pp. 1–11.

70. Mao, X., et al., Crosstalk between cancer-associated fibroblasts and immune cells in the tumor microenvironment: New findings and future perspectives. *Molecular Cancer*, 2021. **20**(1): pp. 1–30.

71. Knudson, A.G., Cancer genetics. *American Journal of Medical Genetics*, 2002. **111**(1): pp. 96–102.

72. Migliore, L. and F. Coppedè, Genetic and environmental factors in cancer and neurodegenerative diseases. *Mutation Research/Reviews in Mutation Research*, 2002. **512**(2–3): pp. 135–153.

73. Prentki, M. and C.J. Nolan, Islet β cell failure in type 2 diabetes. *The Journal of Clinical Investigation*, 2006. **116**(7): pp. 1802–1812.

74. Ashcroft, F.M. and P. Rorsman, Diabetes mellitus and the β cell: The last ten years. *Cell*, 2012. **148**(6): pp. 1160–1171.

75. White, M.F., IRS proteins and the common path to diabetes. *American Journal of Physiology-Endocrinology and Metabolism*, 2002. **283**(3): pp. E413–E422.

76. Samuel, V.T. and G.I. Shulman, The pathogenesis of insulin resistance: Integrating signaling pathways and substrate flux. *The Journal of Clinical Investigation*, 2016. **126**(1): pp. 12–22.

77. Saltiel, A.R. and C.R. Kahn, Insulin signalling and the regulation of glucose and lipid metabolism. *Nature*, 2001. **414**(6865): pp. 799–806.

78. Liu, M., et al., Proinsulin misfolding and diabetes: Mutant INS gene-induced diabetes of youth. *Trends in Endocrinology & Metabolism*, 2010. **21**(11): pp. 652–659.

79. Rutter, G.A. and F. Chimienti, SLC30A8 mutations in type 2 diabetes. *Diabetologia*, 2015. **58**: pp. 31–36.

80. Huang, Z.-Q., et al., Possible role of TCF7L2 in the pathogenesis of type 2 diabetes mellitus. *Biotechnology & Biotechnological Equipment*, 2018. **32**(4): pp. 830–834.

81. Maestro, M.A., et al., Distinct roles of HNF1 B, HNF1 α, and HNF4 α in regulating pancreas development, B-cell function and growth. *Development of the Pancreas and Neonatal Diabetes*, 2007. **12**: pp. 33–45.

82. Bastard, J.-P., et al., Recent advances in the relationship between obesity, inflammation, and insulin resistance. *European Cytokine Network*, 2006. **17**(1): pp. 4–12.

83. Hu, F.B., Globalization of diabetes: The role of diet, lifestyle, and genes. *Diabetes Care*, 2011. **34**(6): pp. 1249–1257.

84. Rönn, T. and C. Ling, DNA methylation as a diagnostic and therapeutic target in the battle against Type 2 diabetes. *Epigenomics*, 2015. **7**(3): pp. 451–460.

3 Metabolic Changes and Biochemical Monitoring during Pregnancy

Rumi Deori, Chinmoyee Deori, Jitu Das, and Tridip Kutum

3.1 INTRODUCTION: Background and Driving Forces

Pregnancy is a dynamic process that involves metabolic changes required for the growth and development of the foetus and for preparing the mother for delivery and breastfeeding (1). In the life cycle of a woman, pregnancy is the most sensitive stage from the nutritional point of view. It has been observed that nutritional intervention during pregnancy has the greatest potential to influence maternal, foetal, and infant health. It has been found that improved nutrition during gestation and early postnatal life improve overall health and reduce the risk of chronic diseases in adulthood. There is greater metabolic flexibility during pregnancy than in the non-pregnant state to protect foetal growth from maternal nutrient deprivation (2). Pregnancy is a physiological condition that undergoes a series of significant anatomical and biochemical changes to ensure the growth and development of the foetus.

The metabolic changes that occur during pregnancy can be categorized into two types:

(1) Anabolic phase

(2) Catabolic phase

In the early gestational period, it is mostly the anabolic phase that occurs (3). During the anabolic phase, there is insulin resistance, hyperinsulinaemia, and hyperglycaemia, whereas in the catabolic phase there is lipolysis, ketogenesis, and hypoglycaemia in spite of raised glucogenic potential and catabolism of muscle. Metabolic adaptations during pregnancy include increased metabolic adaptation of the mother and the storage of maternal energy to meet the nutritional demands of the foetus. The metabolic changes in pregnancy are shown in the Figure 3.1. Metabolic changes in the mother ensures an adequate supply of nutrients to the developing foetus and these adaptations affect the metabolism of glucose, lipids, and amino acids. The placenta plays a unique role in the transportation of maternal nutrients to the foetus by the diffusion process, as shown in Figure 3.2 (a) and (b).

The hormones secreted from the ovaries are first to change, followed by the hormones secreted by the placenta as the pregnancy progresses. Human chorionic gonadotropin (hCG) is the first hormone to increase after conception, followed by oestrogen, progesterone, prolactin, rennin, and human placental lactogen. Adequate levels of thyroid hormones are of primary importance for normal reproductive functioning and all these changes are accompanied by the growth of the uterus. Pregnancy is associated with increased insulin resistance, predominantly caused by human placental lactogen leading to increased insulin production. This facilitates an increase in maternal plasma glucose and the transfer of glucose to the foetus. Throughout a normal pregnancy, the plasma volume increases. Usually, plasma volume increases (50%) by week 34 of pregnancy and is directly proportional to the foetal birth weight. There is a fall in haemoglobin concentration because of the expansion in plasma volume. During pregnancy, changes in the coagulation system lead to a physiological hypercoagulable state. The concentrations of clotting factors, particularly VIII, IX, X, and fibrinogen, increases during pregnancy; however, fibrinolytic activity is reduced. There is also a decrease in the anticoagulants antithrombin and protein S (4).

Renal blood flow increases during early pregnancy due to renal vasodilatation, which results in an increase in cardiac output (CO), Glomerular Filtration Rate (GFR), and renal plasma flow (RPF), which increases by 50%. There is also an increase in renin and aldosterone levels, which promotes sodium retention, leading to volume overload. Renal functioning faces remarkable demands during pregnancy. GFR reaches a peak increase of 40% to 50% compared to pre-pregnancy levels, which lowers serum uric acid, urea, and creatinine. There is around 1.6-litre retention of water, along with raised sodium (Na^+) and potassium (K^+) levels. The summary of physiological changes is described in Table 3.1 (4). The maternal liver regulates the metabolic effects of fasting during late gestation, including gluconeogenic potential and lipid availability. Liver disorders during pregnancy may influence normal metabolic changes during pregnancy (5). Any abnormality in the metabolic changes during pregnancy may affect the health and wellbeing of the mother, the outcome of pregnancy, and the survival of the foetus.

DOI: 10.1201/9781003384823-3

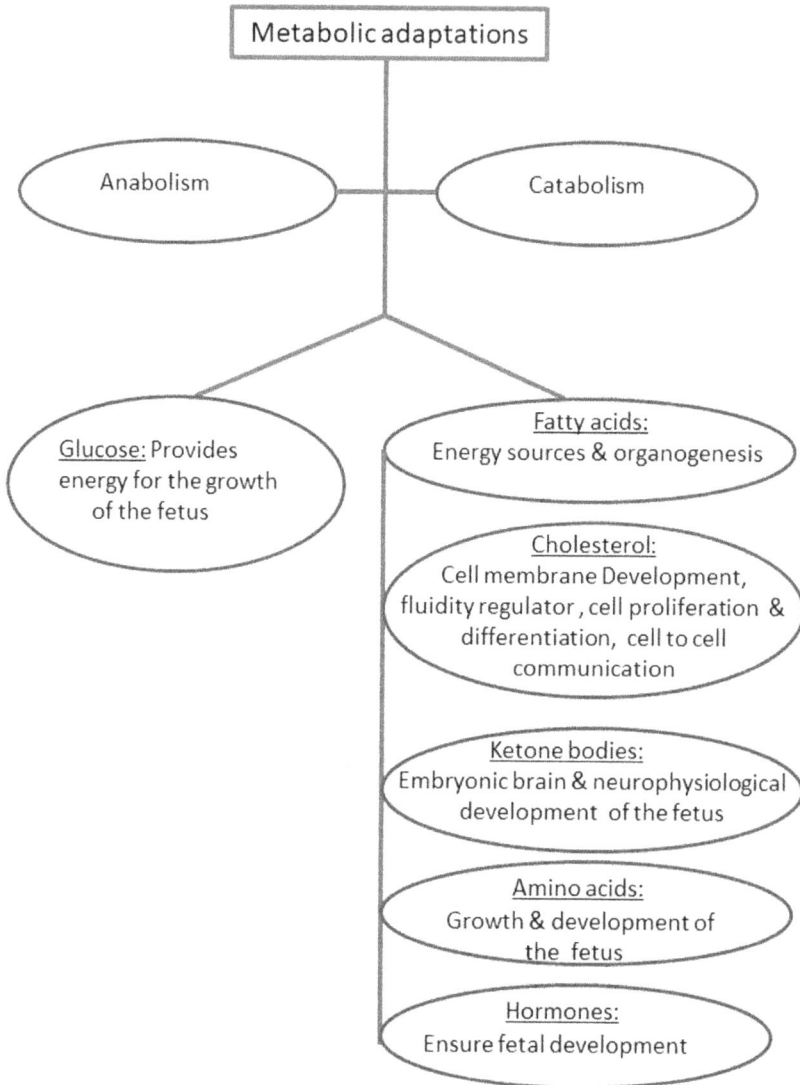

Figure 3.1 Metabolic changes in pregnancy

Complications like pre-term birth, an overweight foetus or growth restriction of the foetus, gestational diabetes, or preeclampsia may arise in pregnancy, leading to immediate or long-term health consequences for both mother and infant (6, 7).

Clinicians should be aware of these physiological changes and accompanied biomarker alterations in pregnancy. Knowing the aforementioned alterations in pregnancy will help clinicians to avoid false result interpretation and misdiagnosis of the physiological state as pathological conditions (8).

Routine investigations should be advised by clinicians to monitor the normal progress of the pregnancy. Additional investigations are to be done in case of high-risk pregnancy or if any abnormality is observed during the monitoring of pregnancy. Specific screening tests should preferably be done for the diseases endemic to the region.

3.2 METABOLIC ADAPTATIONS IN PREGNANCY

Pregnancy is a dynamic process that involves alterations in metabolic adaptations required for the continuous supply of nutrients by the mother to the foetus. The basal metabolic rate (BMR) increases during pregnancy; this is due to the combined effects of increases in tissue synthesis,

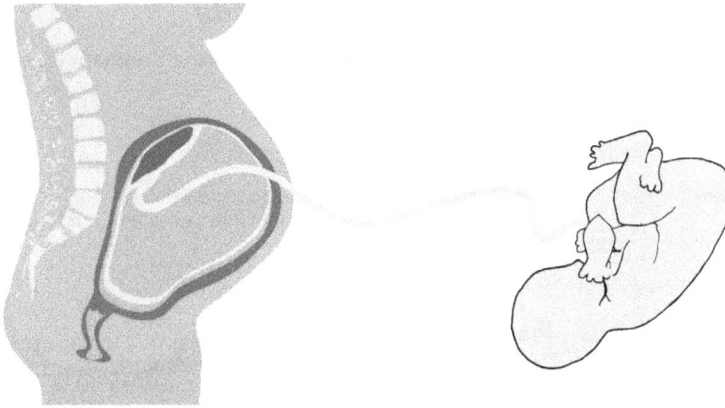

(a)

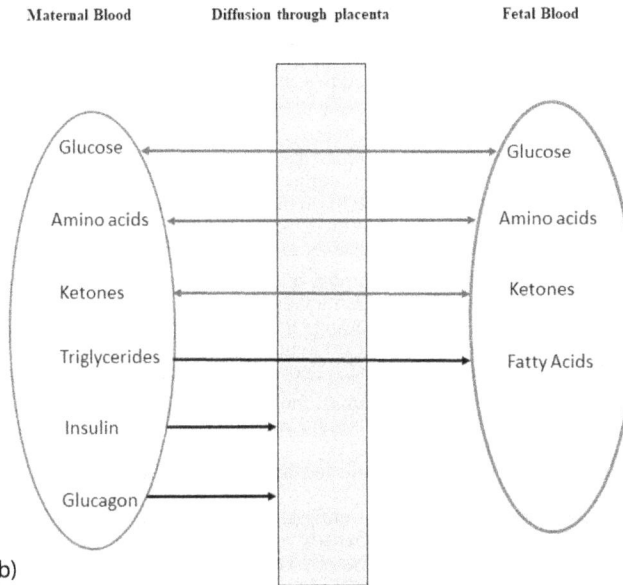

(b)

NB. Maternal insulin and Glucagon do not cross the placenta

Figure 3.2 (a) Fetoplacental unit (b) Maternal nutrients transported to foetus by diffusion

tissue mass, and cardiovascular, respiratory, and renal work (9). Normal metabolic changes are essential as the growing foetus gets all nutrients from (and excretes all wastes to) the mother. The metabolic demand of the growing foetus is mediated by changes in metabolite concentrations or by other secreted factors that directly modify maternal metabolism (10). Foetal metabolic demand is highest during the third trimester, which coincides with the highest basal metabolic rate and energy expenditure in pregnant women. Women with a normal body mass index (BMI) expressed a 28% increase in basal metabolic rate (BMR, kcal/day) and a 13% increase in total energy expenditure (sum of BMR, activity energy expenditure, and thermal effect of food) from pre-pregnancy to 36 weeks of gestation (11). The basal metabolic rate begins to rise gradually from the third month of pregnancy and may have doubled by the time of delivery. There is increase in the utilization of lipids by the mother, which spares glucose and amino acids for foetal uptake (12). As the pregnancy progresses, energy intake and expenditure increase daily, up to 375 kJ (89 kcal) in the first trimester, 1,200 kJ (286 kcal) in the second trimester, and 1,950 kJ (466 kcal) in the third trimester (13). It has been found that variability in total energy expenditure (TEE) in some women has a net negative difference in TEE over the course of pregnancy. Pregnant women use diverse strategies to meet the

Table 3.1   Physiological changes during pregnancy

System/Organ	Changes during Pregnancy
Cardiovascular System	• Tachycardia • Increased cardiac output and heart rate • Increased stroke volume • Enlargement of the heart
Respiratory System	• Displacement of diaphragm superiorly • Increased vascularization of mucosa, edema, and increased glandular secretion • Increased risk of apnoea and dyspnoea • Hyperventilation • Respiratory alkalosis
Gastrointestinal System	• Decrease motility • Decrease tone of gastroesophageal sphincter • Increased absorption of calcium in intestine • Nausea and vomiting • Heartburn and acidity
Nervous System	• Increased activation of prefrontal cortex • Increased proliferation of oligodendrocyte • Increased forebrain olfactory neurogenesis • Brain size and volume is decreased
Hepatic System	• Liver size increases • Increased insulin sensitivity and glycogen content in early pregnancy • Increased insulin resistance and gluconeogenesis in late pregnancy
Renal System	• Renal size increases • Increased glomerular filtration rate • Increased renin-angiotensin-aldosterone system • Increased retention of waste and sodium • Blood flow is increased • Vascular resistance is decreased
Haematological/Haemodynamic	• Increased number of red blood cells • Increased plasma volume • Increased clotting factors • Decreased fibrinolytic activities • Increased width and volume of platelets
Hormonal	• Increased human chorionic gonadotropin • Increased placental lactogen • Increased relaxin • Decreased follicle stimulating hormone (FSH) and luteinizing hormone (LH) • Thyroxine-binding globulin (TBG) rise due to increased oestrogen level • T_4 and T_3 increase over the first half of pregnancy but there is a normal to slightly decreased amount of free hormone due to increased TBG binding. Normal ranges are slightly reduced in the second and third trimesters • Cortisol levels increase, which favours lipogenesis and fat storage • Insulin response increase, so blood sugar should remain normal or low • Peripheral insulin resistance increases after early stages of pregnancy due to increased production of hormones, such as cortisol, prolactin, progesterone, and human placental lactogen
Bone	• Increased bone turnover • Bone mineral density decreases
Skeletal Muscle	• Pelvic floor muscles become stiff • Muscle fibres elongate • Increase in intramuscular extracellular matrix
Adipose Tissue	• Increased adipocyte diameter and volume • Increased leptin • Increased insulin sensitivity and lipid accumulation in early pregnancy • Decreased insulin sensitivity and lipid accumulation/release in late pregnancy

Source: Tina, N., Hannah, E.J.Y., Jourge, L.T., and Amanda, N.S.P. (2018): The role of placental hormones in mediating maternal adaptations to support pregnancy and lactation; *Front physiol.*9:1091. Doi: 10.3389/ fphy.2018.01091. www.frontiersin.org

Modifications of maternal physiology in response to pregnancy.

Anabolism during feeding state   Anabolism during feeding state

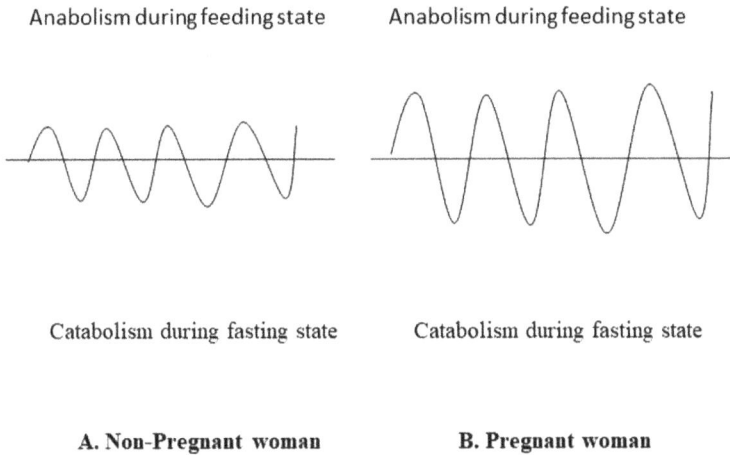

Catabolism during fasting state   Catabolism during fasting state

A. Non-Pregnant woman   **B. Pregnant woman**

Figure 3.3 Metabolic oscillation fuel utilization between fed and fasting states in
A. non-pregnant and B. pregnant women

metabolic demands placed on them. A single recommendation for increased energy intake during pregnancy may not be applicable to all women. In a longitudinal study, it was found that average energy intake increased by 9% from pre-pregnancy to the third trimester; however, in some women, there was no increase in energy intake during pregnancy (14). The changes in the metabolism of macronutrients balance the need for foetal growth (15). The metabolic oscillation fuel utilization between fed and fasting states in non-pregnant and pregnant women is shown in Figure 3.3 (12).

3.2.1 Anabolic Phase

The anabolic phase mostly occurs in early pregnancy. There is an increase in the utilization of lipids by the mother, which spares glucose and amino acids for foetal uptake. Facilitated anabolism during the late gestational period promotes foetal growth. The anabolic phase serves to increase the deposition of lipids in maternal tissues by various factors. Hyperphagia may be one of the factors that increases throughout pregnancy, increasing the exogenous metabolic substrates. During the first and second trimesters, maternal metabolism favours increased fat storage, which is regulated by placental hormones and growth factors. This anabolic phase is significant as the foetal energy demands during the third trimester are not met only by increasing energy intake, but also depend on fat accumulated in the early pregnancy. In the third trimester, an increase in lipolysis leads to a rise in fatty acids and glucose in the blood. This means lipids become the main source of maternal energy during pregnancy and glucose is preserved for the developing foetus (16).

Lipoprotein lipase enzyme activity promotes fat deposition, characterized by hydrolyzing chylomicrons, very low-density lipoproteins (VLDLs) circulating in the plasma leading to the release of non-esterified free fatty acids and glycerol for uptake in adipose tissue.

It has been suggested that early pregnancy anabolism is facilitated by an increase in intracellular glycerol utilization. As the activity of glycerol kinase is negligible in the normal physiological condition, there is minimal conversion of glycerol to glycerol-3-phosphate. Subsequently, during pregnancy, there is decreased lipolytic activity, together with the increased capacity of maternal tissues to convert both glucose and intracellular glycerol for the production of glycerol-3-phosphate, resulting in the accumulation of triglycerides. The overall metabolic adaptation is shown in Figure 3.1 (12).

3.2.2 Catabolic Phase

The catabolic phase occurs mostly in the last trimester of gestation. During this phase, there is accelerated lipolysis. In studies in rats during late pregnancy, increased mRNA expression and increased activity of hormone-sensitive lipase have been observed. Moreover, it has been demonstrated that the levels and activity of LPL are reduced in women and rats in late pregnancy, thereby reducing the deposits of lipids in adipocytes. In the liver, non-esterified fatty acids (NEFA) and glycerol are converted to acyl-CoA and glycerol-3-phosphate, and partial re-esterification takes place for the synthesis of triglycerides. The hepatic triglycerides are transferred to VLDL and released into the maternal circulation. Alternatively, glycerol is used for gluconeogenesis.

Non-esterified fatty acid may be oxidized to acetyl CoA for the production of energy and keto-genesis. During late pregnancy, these metabolic cycles are required as metabolic substrates are greatly augmented for foetal development. In later pregnancy, during fasting periods (for example, during the night) when gluconeogenic substrates are sparse and glucose is vital for the foetus, the need for gluconeogenesis acquires greater importance. Moreover, studies have shown that in early pregnancy, in underfed conditions, plasma ketone bodies are lower in pregnant mice than in non-pregnant mice, which suggests an increased utilization of ketone bodies (3, 12).

Maternal ketogenesis becomes highly accelerated as placental transfer of ketone bodies is highly efficient during fasting periods, allowing the foetus not only to employ these molecules as energy fuels but also to utilize these substrates for brain lipogenesis (3).

3.2.3 Glucose Metabolism

Glucose is the principal molecule for foetal growth. Glucose and oxygen are the two most impor-tant molecules transferred from mother to foetus through the placenta. Glucose metabolism is one of the major factors in a healthy pregnancy. The foetus is unable to produce glucose and there-fore a supply of glucose is required from maternal blood through the placenta. During the first trimester of pregnancy, maternal homeostasis of glucose is regulated by several hormones, such as insulin, oestrogen, cortisol, etc., which leads to increased lipid storage, a reduction in energy expenditure, and a delay in blood glucose clearance (17).

Foetal demand increases by week 26 of gestation. The meeting of this increased demand is facilitated by basal endogenous glucose production via maternal gluconeogenesis. The increase in circulating insulin and the decrease in insulin sensitivity occur simultaneously. Oestrogen helps in the increased glucose production by augmenting cortisol release, which promotes gluconeogen-esis. In spite of an increase in gluconeogenesis, the concentration of plasma glucose may decrease, which suggests that the circulating glucose from the mother is supplied to the foetus via the placenta (12).

3.2.4 Insulin Resistance

Maternal metabolic changes ensure sufficient glucose transport. It has been observed that the mother's tissues become transiently insulin resistant and enhance maternal glucose production by 30% from early to late pregnancy. The blood flow to the uterus increases to 25% of cardiac output to ensure the availability of oxygen and other molecules required for metabolism (18, 19). In a pregnant mother, the metabolism of glucose is altered by an increase in insulin resistance, plasma lipid concentrations, and the expansion of β-cells present in the pancreas due to the hypertro-phy of maternal pancreatic islet cells. Oestrogen and progesterone hormones regulate insulin resistance from the sixth week of gestation. At around ten weeks, a peak in prolactin and human placental lactogen (hPL) hormones is observed, promoting β-cell proliferation, insulin production, and the secretion of insulin to meet higher insulin demands, which increase insulin resistance. Insulin resistance increases in the second trimester and peaks in the last trimester. In adipocytes and skeletal muscles, insulin resistance is further enhanced by an increase in circulating proges-terone, prolactin, cortisol, and hPL hormones. Delayed glucose clearance due to insulin resistance is assisted by high cortisol levels. Glucose uptake is initiated as it attaches to insulin receptors by phosphorylation at β-subunit followed by insulin receptor substrate 1 (IRS-1) phosphorylation at the tyrosine residue. It initiates signal transduction pathways. Decreased phosphorylation of the insulin receptor is observed during pregnancy. As progesterone increases during pregnancy, it decreases IRS-1 expression as insulin-induced translocation of glucose transporter 4 (GLUT4) to the cell membrane decreases. This leads to the reduced cellular uptake of glucose (12, 20).

In the late stage of pregnancy, the cytokine tumour necrosis factor-α (TNF-α) has been identified to be a potential mediator for insulin resistance. Tumour necrosis factor-α (TNF-α) is also associ-ated with insulin resistance in obesity, sepsis, muscle damage, and even ageing. The placenta also produces TNF-α. An increased level of TNF-α is seen during pregnancy in conditions like pre-eclampsia and gestational diabetes, etc. (16).

3.2.5 Role of Glucose Transporter

Glucose is the primary energy source for the growth and development of the foeto-placental unit. Foetal gluconeogenesis is minimal during this period. Glucose demand is facilitated by diffusion via glucose transporter (GLUT) along a concentration gradient. Of the 14 isoforms of the GLUT family, many are present in placental tissue. However, during term pregnancy, GLUT 1 is the only transporter detected as a functional protein in the syncytiotrophoblast (21).

Across the placenta, there is an asymmetrical distribution of GLUT1. In the microvillus membrane, the transporter is three times higher than in the basal part. This suggests that the steps in trans-syncytial glucose flux occur in the basal membrane. The GLUT remains unchanged in the microvillus membrane but expression increases by approximately 50% in the basal membrane during second and third trimesters. Studies have demonstrated that glucose across the basal membrane increases along with the increase in blood flow through the uteroplacental and umbilical unit. This increases the transport of glucose to the foetus during the second half of pregnancy (3). It has been found that in gestational diabetes mellitus (GDM), the placental GLUT1 expression is increased and promotes enhanced glucose transport to the foetus (20). Diabetes alters the expression and activity of the human placental GLUT1 (21).

3.2.6 Lipid Metabolism

In order to meet the demands of foetal growth and development, there is derangement in maternal lipid metabolism. During the "anabolic phase" of pregnancy, that is, in the early trimesters, there is a rise in oestrogen and progesterone levels, and the concentration of insulin favours lipid deposition and inhibits lipolysis. The maternal appetite increases as a result of the increased progesterone, growth hormone (GH), prolactin, etc., leading to extra body fat. With a healthy BMI (18.5–23.9), there is an average weight gain of 25–35 lbs throughout pregnancy. The total surface of the placenta available for exchange during late pregnancy is 10–15 m^2 (approximately) because of the villous nature of the placenta. Maternal non-esterified fatty acid (NEFA) concentrations are elevated during the third trimester of pregnancy, while circulating triglyceride (TG) levels are 250% higher than levels in non-pregnant women. Docosa hexaenoic acid (DHA) is essential for the growth and development of the brain. The requirement of DHA increases from 100 mg/day to 300 mg/day from the second trimester to third trimester. There is an accumulation of DHA in the adipose tissue of the foetus, which is specific to foetal adipose tissue and does not reflect maternal adipose tissue DHA content (22).

Plasma lipid levels decrease during the first few weeks of gestation. Increased sensitivity to insulin promotes fatty acid (FA) production and lipoprotein lipase activity increases. This enhances cellular uptake of circulating triacylglycerols (TAGs). By week 10 of gestation, fatty acids, triacylglycerols, cholesterol, and phospholipid levels increase in the blood, and these continue to increase throughout the last trimester. At week 30 of pregnancy, a catabolic shift of lipid metabolism takes place. As a result, lipids become the energy source for the mother and glucose and amino acids are conserved for the foetus. Insulin resistance during the third trimester promotes lipolysis and decreases lipoprotein lipase activity. Fatty acids are increased and released into circulation to be metabolized into triaceylglycerols before they are absorbed by the placental syncytial layer.

Cholesterol is a major circulating lipid. Circulating cholesterol is either recycled or transported to different tissues, including the placenta. The placenta produces approximately 400–500 mg of steroid hormones daily from cholesterol. Cholesterol plays a significant role in placental membrane formation as well as oxidation. At week 12 of gestation, there is an increase in the level of high density lipoprotein (HDL), which remains elevated throughout the pregnancy. There is about a twofold increase in TAGs and total cholesterol and low-density lipoprotein (LDL) increase by 30% to 50% respectively (16).

Enhanced de novo lipogenesis contributes to anabolism during early pregnancy. It has been demonstrated that in periuterine adipose tissue, there is a progressive increase in the production of fatty acids and glycerol from glucose during pregnancy in rats. Lipoprotein lipase (LPL) promotes fat deposition. It converts chylomicrons and very low-density lipoproteins (VLDLs) circulating in plasma to non-esterified free fatty acids/glycerol for uptake in adipose tissue. In adipose tissue, increased utilization of glycerol facilitates anabolism. Due to the negligible activity of the glycerol kinase enzyme, the conversion of glycerol to glycerol-3-phosphate is minimal for the biosynthesis of triglyceride. The decrease in adipose tissue lipolytic activity, along with the augmented capacity of maternal tissues to employ both glucose and intracellular glycerol for the production of glycerol-3-phosphate, result in a net accumulation of triglycerides (3). The overall metabolic adaptation is shown in Figure 3.1 (3).

3.2.7 Hyperlipidaemia in Pregnancy

In the third trimester, there is enhanced lipolytic activity in the adipose tissue. This precipitates maternal hyperlipidaemia, leading to a marked increase in plasma triglyceride levels. The rise in cholesterol and phospholipids is less marked. As a result, triglyceride content predominantly increases in VLDL. The activity of TAGs peaks during the second trimester of pregnancy and decreases in the third trimester. The changes in cholesteryl ester transfer protein (CETP) activity correlate with the alterations in HDL-triglyceride levels that increase dramatically from the first to the second trimesters of pregnancy. Hepatic lipase converts triglyceride-rich HDL2 sub-fraction into HDL3 particles. This allows increased accumulation of HDL2 in the plasma. During fasting, the circulating lipids are further raised and are available for placental transport (23). There is an early shift from glucose to fat utilization by maternal tissues, and raised levels of circulating lipid metabolites in pregnant women during fasting is called "accelerated starvation" (24). The accelerated fasting response is mostly observed during late gestation. Enhanced maternal utilization of lipids for energy spares glucose and amino acids for foetal uptake. The accelerated fasting response is proportional to the foetal metabolic demand. The intensity of the accelerated fasting response, evidenced by reduced blood glucose, elevated free fatty acids, and ketone bodies, is the same in both lean and obese women (25). It has been found that children born to mothers who fasted in the first trimester had lower birth weights compared to children born to mothers who fasted in the second or third trimesters (26).

The extent to which foetal tissues depend upon lipids for energy metabolism is not clear but the early postnatal switch in nutrition from glucose in utero to lipid-rich milk suggests that late-gestation foetal tissues may have the ability to utilize lipids derived from the mother. The glycogen stored in the foetal liver may be another important source of endogenous glucose at times of nutritional challenge. Glycogen stores are critical for the first hours of postnatal life; glucose is generated from the glycogen stores before the newborn consumes any milk (27).

3.2.8 Role of Fatty Acids

Fatty acids act as a key energy source and play a crucial role in foetal development. Fatty acids are important structural components of cell membranes. They are also the precursors for bioactive signalling compounds. They are of the utmost importance for the development of foetal tissue and organs. The lipoprotein lipase hydrolyzes triglycerides present in chylomicrons that are derived from food and VLDL. HDL-triglycerides are the preferred substrate for endothelial lipase activity. The mRNA required for the expression of endothelial lipases is higher in term placentas than in the first trimester. Fatty acid transport proteins (FATPs) mediate the uptake of long-chain polyunsaturated fatty acids (LCPUFA) into the syncytiotrophoblast. NEFAs are bound by fatty acid-binding proteins (FABPs) and the placenta expresses four different isoforms of FABPs (FABP-1, 3, 4, and 5) within the cytosol of syncytiotrophoblasts that are esterified in cellular sites, beta-oxidation, and subsequently transport to the foetus. Finally, NEFAs that cross the placenta are carried to the foetal liver in α-fetoprotein, are re-esterified, and are released into the foetal circulation in the form of triglycerides (22, 27).

3.2.9 Cholesterol

Cholesterol plays a vital role in embryonic and foetal development. It maintains membrane fluidity and passive permeability of the cell membrane. It also determines cholesterol-rich micro domains called lipid rafts. Lipid rafts are important for plasma membrane-dependent signalling cascades such as that of the sonic hedgehog pathway (a signalling pathway that transmits information to the embryonic cells required for proper cell differentiation). Cholesterol is also required for the production of bile acids and steroid hormones (e.g. glucocorticoids that are actively synthesized in the foetal adrenal gland during late pregnancy). Cholesterol helps in cell proliferation, differentiation, and cell-to-cell communication. Cholesterol and its oxidative derivatives, oxysterols, regulate various metabolic processes. About 1.5–2.0 g of cholesterol accumulates in the body of the developing embryo with every kilogram of tissue gained. As the demand for cholesterol increases, the developing foetus obtains it from de novo biosynthesis and deposits of cholesterol in the yolk sac and the placenta from the mother. Specifically, it has been shown that human placental trophoblasts express LDL receptor (LDLR), VLDL receptor, and scavenger receptor class B type I transmembrane proteins, mediates the removal of cholesteryl esters from maternal plasma lipoproteins, and helps in their transfer to foetal circulation. Apolipoprotein E (ApoE) is also one of the factors required for the maternal–embryonal cholesterol transport system. It is involved in transportation and the receptor-mediated uptake of lipoproteins by various cell types. Several isoforms that have a profound effect on plasma cholesterol level have been identified. A congenital anomaly, Smith–Lemli–Opitz syndrome (SLOS), is characterized by prenatal and postnatal growth restriction: microcephaly, moderate to severe intellectual disability, and multiple major and minor malformations, including characteristic facial features, cleft palate, abnormal gingivae, cardiac defects, hypospadias, and ambiguous genitals (28). Heterozygous mothers with an ApoE2 allele (protein isoforms defective in LDLR binding) have infants with a more severe SLOS phenotype than those without the ApoE2 allele. The placenta expresses Apolipoprotein B (ApoB) and microsomal triglyceride transfer protein and also synthesizes and secretes ApoB-100-containing lipoproteins. These mediate the transport of cholesterol from the basal membrane to the foetus. Adenosine triphosphate-binding cassette transporter A1 (ABCA1) has been identified as a gene that is responsible for the severity of the SLOS phenotype of the infant. This suggests placental cholesterol transport is vital for foetal development and is also a plausible target for prenatal SLOS therapy. Low maternal serum cholesterol levels during pregnancy are associated with reduced birth weights and a raised incidence of microcephaly, while maternal gestational hypercholesterolemia promotes early atherogenesis (3, 23).

3.2.10 Ketone Bodies

Ketone bodies are essential oxidative substrates used as glucose substitutes to fuel the metabolism of both the mother and the foetus. In fasting, accelerated lipolysis and hepatic ketogenesis occur during late pregnancy, which results in increased ketone body formation. The ketone bodies are transported by unfacilitated diffusion down their concentration gradient or by beta-D-hydroxybutyrate placental carrier-dependent transport across the placenta. In a state of nutrient deficiency, ketone bodies guarantee embryonic brain development via unrestricted and rapid transportation from mother to foetal circulation. This adaptation could also have detrimental effects on foetal development, since prolonged maternal hyperketonaemia results in an increased incidence of foetal malformations, impaired neurophysiologic development, and stillbirth (17).

3.2.11. Amino Acids

Amino acids are one of the major nutrients in foetal growth and development. Their plasma concentrations are substantially higher in foetal than maternal circulation, which indicates active transport of these peptides across the syncytiotrophoblast. The human placenta expresses over 15 different amino acid transporters. These are responsible for the uptake of several different amino acids. Amino acids are precursors for the biosynthesis of proteins, nucleotides, neurotransmitters, etc. The amino acids threonine (55%), lysine (45%), isoleucine (63%), and tryptophan (35%) are raised during pregnancy and continue to rise as pregnancy progresses (3).

3.2.12 Water

There is an increase in the total volume of body fluid during pregnancy; nearly 3,500–4,000 ml of fluid is added to the tissues of healthy women during pregnancy. During the end of the pregnancy, a considerable amount of retained fluid accumulates in the lower extremities. The amount of electrolytes (Na^+, K^+, Cl^-) increases during pregnancy (19, 29).

3.3 ENDOCRINE CHANGES AND METABOLIC ADAPTATIONS

Pregnancy is associated with major hormonal and metabolic changes in the mother. It demands a variety of physiological changes that affect all the mother's organ systems and the placenta is the centre of these adaptations as a temporary organ. The placenta mediates maternal–foetal communication and plays a vital role in transfer metabolites. Placental hormones, including growth hormone, prolactin, placental lactogens, and steroid hormones, mediate many of the metabolic changes (30). These are responsible for establishing and maintaining pregnancy, foetal development, and lactation. As early as the first week after ovulation, endocrinal changes appear. Corpus luteum (CL) produces progesterone and oestrogen for approximately 12–14 days during the luteal phase of menstruation. If fertilization occurs, implantation generally takes place between 6 to 12 days after ovulation. To maintain pregnancy, progesterone is needed. After fertilization, human chorionic gonadotropin (hCG) is produced by the trophoblast cells of the implanting blastocyst; hCG is also produced during gestational trophoblastic diseases. Concentrations of hCG begin to rise very rapidly during pregnancy and peak at approximately week 8–12 of pregnancy. There are several qualitative and quantitative assays for detecting hCG in serum or urine. These assays are "sandwich"-type immunoassays (4, 8).

3.3.1 Hormones and Metabolic Adaptations

The insulin sensitivity of the mother is responsible for switching from the anabolic state to catabolic state. In early pregnancy, pancreatic beta cell activity is increased, leading to an increase in insulin, which has an insulinotropic effect on glucose metabolism. Insulin sensitivity remains the same or is even augmented during this period. Thus, hyperinsulinaemia leads to maternal lipogenesis and fat deposition. During the last trimester of gestation, there is progressive insulin resistance that leads to an increase in lipolysis, gluconeogenesis, and ketogenesis (18).

Oestrogen increases throughout the pregnancy. It augments the development of hyperlipidaemia and ensures successful reproduction and foetal growth. Oestrogen enhances the production of light VLDLs. It also reduces the expression and activity of hepatic lipase in the liver. Thus, it inhibits the clearance of circulating triglyceride-rich lipoproteins. Oestrogen administered exogenously increases the levels of HDL-cholesterol and triglycerols and decreases total cholesterol and LDL-cholesterol. Oestrogen increases insulin receptor binding possibly by enhancing insulin sensitivity during pregnancy (22, 23).

Progesterone levels increase throughout gestation. This has a minimal effect on lipoprotein metabolism. Studies on premenopausal women administered a progesterone-only pill have demonstrated minimal reductions in the levels of circulating total cholesterol and triglycerides. It has been suggested that oestrogen-induced adaptations in lipoprotein profiles could not be significantly modified through the administration of progesterone derivatives (12).

Several hormones in the placenta are involved in achieving an insulin-resistant state, altering maternal physiology. There is a thirtyfold increase in human placental lactogen, which activates insulin secretion in islets cells. It interferes with glucose transport; hence, it promotes insulin resistance.

Human placental growth hormone stimulates insulin resistance in late gestation. It is detectable in plasma from the fifth week and increases throughout pregnancy, replacing pituitary growth hormone in maternal circulation. Various studies have shown that transgenic mice overexpressing the human placental growth hormone gene become hyperinsulinaemic, as well as insulin resistant, and are larger than their normal littermates (3).

Leptin and adiponectin are considered to mediate insulin resistance during pregnancy. Tumour necrosis factor alpha (TNF-α) produced by white adipose tissue and the placenta, etc., is inversely related to insulin sensitivity. It is a marker of insulin resistance. Plasma levels of TNF-α are high during advanced gestation in women with gestational diabetes mellitus (GDM) than in normal pregnancies (12).

3.3.2 Insulin

The pancreatic beta cell activity is increased during early pregnancy, leading to hyperinsulinaemia. During the first half of gestation, hyperinsulinaemia is an important factor that enhances lipogenesis and fat deposition. During the last trimester of gestation, there is progressive insulin resistance. The human placental lactogen increases thirtyfold during pregnancy and it stimulates insulin secretion. The human placental growth hormone promotes insulin resistance in late gestation (3).

During normal pregnancy, there is a raised insulin level due to an increase in maternal hormones – HPL, progesterone, prolactin, and cortisol. Hyperinsulinaemia occurs to compensate insulin resistance and also as a result of hyperplasia of beta cells. There are changes in fasting plasma glucose due to increased glucose clearance, increased fasting insulin, and reduced hepatic output of glucose. Therefore, fasting glucose levels may be lower in pregnancy compared to the non-pregnant state (26).

3.3.2.1 Gestational Diabetes Mellitus

Gestational diabetes mellitus (GDM) is defined as a carbohydrate intolerance of variable severity with onset or first recognition during pregnancy. GDM is considered to be the most common metabolic abnormality, affecting 5–9% of pregnant women in the United States (31). There is increased glucose demand for foetal growth and development; the metabolic changes are essential to sustain this high glucose demand while maintaining maternal euglycaemia. GDM has been described as a "disorder of total fuel metabolism" as fasting plasma glucose, NEFA, and TG are higher in women with gestational diabetes than in normal pregnant women (32). The prevalence of GDM ranges from 1% to 15% across the world. The pathophysiology of GDM is due to maladaptive changes in the expression of insulin receptors (33).

During pregnancy, insulin resistance is a physiological phenomenon. It allows glucose to remain for a longer time in the maternal circulation and facilitates the entry of glucose into developing foetus through the placenta by diffusion. Endogenous insulin production increases by more than 60% during pregnancy compared to the non-pregnant state. A pregnant woman who is unable to secrete adequate insulin to overcome the resistance develops GDM (34). The metabolic disorder in pregnant woman mostly affects the organogenesis, growth, and development of the foetus. The stimulation of foetal growth by maternal diabetes mostly occurs during the second and third

Table 3.2   Impact of maternal diabetes

Foetus

1. Effect of foetal hyperinsulinaemia
   - Increased growth of insulin-sensitive tissues
   - Increased deposition of adipose tissue
   - Accelerated skeletal maturation
   - Increased hepatic glycogen content
   - Impaired surfactant production
   - Delay in switch from foetal haemoglobin to adult haemoglobin
   - Increased erythropoietin production
2. Impact on foetal development
   - Excessive growth
   - Macrosomia
   - Stillbirth
3. Potentially teratogenic process
   - Increased production of oxygen-derived free radicals
   - Abnormalities of myo-inositol and arachidonic acid metabolism
   - Abnormalities of basement membrane components
   - Abnormalities of zinc metabolism

Mother

1. Acute complications of diabetes
   - Toxemia of pregnancy
   - Metabolic acidosis
   - Coma
   - Vascular complications
   - Infection
2. Effects on pregnant woman
   - Polyhydromnios
   - Preeclampsia
   - Preterm labour
   - Postpartum bleeding
   - Spontaneous abortion
3. Long-term complications
   - Retinopathy
   - Nephropathy
   - Hypertension
   - Ischaemic heart disease
   - Peripheral vascular disease
   - Autonomic neuropathy

Source: Wenrui Ye, Cong Luo, Jing Huan, Chenglong Li, Zhixiong Liu, and Fangkun Liu: Gestational diabetes mellitus and adverse pregnancy outcomes; *BMJ* 2022; 377. Doi: https://doi.org/10.1136/bmj-2021-067946. BMJ 2022;377:e067946.

trimesters. Maternal insulin deficiency leads to increased catabolism and increased nutrient flux across the placenta, stimulating the secretion of insulin by the foetal pancreas, leading to macrosomia. The impact of maternal diabetes on the mother and the foetus are shown in Table 3.2 (35). Some pregnancy disorders may develop as a result of the mismatch between foetal demands, the maternal response, and the maternal capacity to meet foetal demands (31).

3.3.2.2 *The Effects of Foetal Hyperinsulinaemia*

a) Increased growth of insulin-sensitive tissues

b) Increased deposition of adipose tissue

c) Accelerated skeletal maturation

d) Increased hepatic glycogen content

e) Delay in pulmonary maturation

f) Delay in switch from foetal haemoglobin to adult haemoglobin

g) Polycythaemia (increased erythropoietin production)

There is a risk of stillbirth due to poor metabolic control. Neonatal hypoglycaemia occurs due to increased foetal insulin secretion in response to maternal hyperglycaemia. Excessive growth and foetal macrosomia occur due to overabundances of maternal nutrients, infantile hyperinsulinaemia, and maternal diabetes (31).

3.4 PLACENTAL HORMONES

The placenta acts as a protective barrier against the maternal micro environment and infection. It regulates temperature, establishes the immunologic tolerance of the foetus, and facilitates the exchange of gases, nutrients, and waste products. The hormones produced by the placenta influence the establishment and maintenance of a healthy pregnancy. Alterations in metabolic homeostasis in pregnancy can affect the placenta, leading to reduced functioning and complications during pregnancy, for example, GDM. Placental growth hormone is responsible for the increased placental GLUT1 expression and foetal hyperglycaemia (36, 37).

The placental growth hormone (PGH) regulates maternal gluconeogenesis and lipolysis to modulate maternal adaptations. It replaces pituitary GH in the maternal circulation and increases throughout the pregnancy. It acts as an insulin antagonist. It mediates insulin resistance by directly modulating insulin-like growth factor 1 (IGF-1). It initiates the growth of maternal tissues during pregnancy. It may act independently through IGF-1 to increase the supply of nutrients for

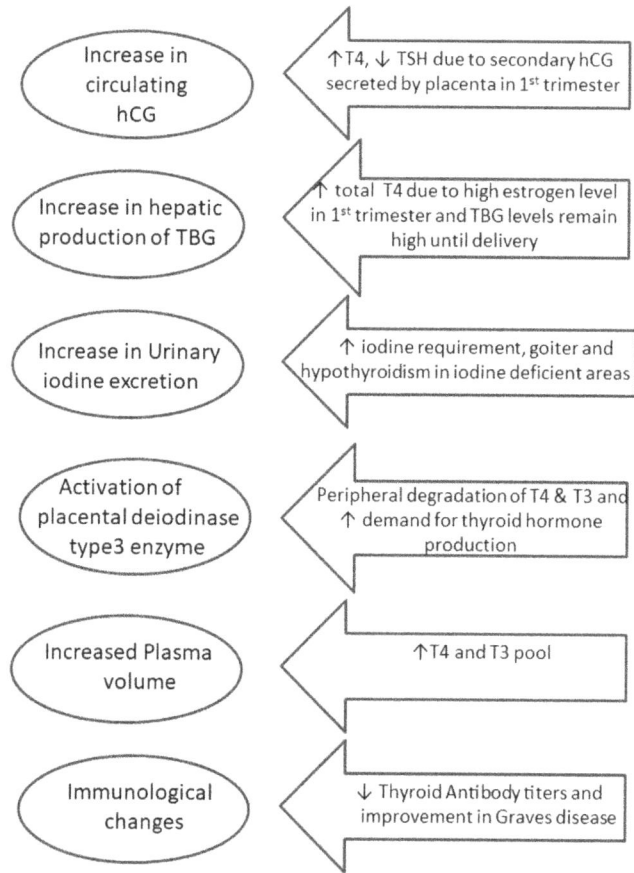

Figure 3.4 Changes in thyroid hormones during pregnancy

the foetus. It stimulates the invasion of trophoblast and placental growth hormone receptor (GHR) on syncytiotrophoblasts. Studies have shown that women with deletions in the PGH gene had children with normal birth weights. This could be explained by other hormones such as GH or hPL acting in overlapping pathways that compensate for PGH insufficiency (16).

3.5 THYROID HORMONE

Hormonal changes, such as changes in the thyroid hormone, are observed during pregnancy. There is an increase in thyroid-binding globulin, which results in increased levels of tri-iodothyronine (T3) and thyroxine (T4). The level of serum TSH is slightly decreased in the first trimester in response to an increased level of human chorionic gonadotropin. At the end of the first trimester, the level of TSH increases again. The levels of T3 and T4 slightly decrease in the second and third trimesters of pregnancy. The changes in thyroid hormones during pregnancy are shown in Figure 3.4 (38).

3.6 IMPORTANCE OF BIOCHEMICAL MONITORING DURING PREGNANCY

The following screening tests are done during pregnancy:

- Alpha-fetoprotein (AFP) test or multiple marker test
- Amniocentesis
- Chorionic villus sampling
- Cell-free foetal DNA testing
- Percutaneous umbilical blood sampling
- Ultrasound scan

Table 3.3 Screening test in antenatal period

Duration of Pregnancy	Test
Early in pregnancy	Blood: • Full blood count • Blood group • Rhesus status • Hepatitis B • Hepatitis C • HIV • Rubella immunity • Syphilis • Thyroid profile • Malaria • G6PD status • Haemoglobin variants Urine: • Analysis for RBCs, WBCs, glucose, albumin, bacteria • Urine culture
6 to 8 weeks of pregnancy	Viability ultrasound scan
8 to 10 weeks of pregnancy	Ultrasound for calculation of EDD

10 to 14 weeks of pregnancy	• OSCAR test (one-stop clinic for assessment of risk for foetal anomalies)
	• USG, fb hCG, PAPP-A (pregnancy-associated plasma protein A), and PLGF (placental growth factor)
	• Foetal scan for anomalies:
	    Anencephaly
	    Spina bifida
	• Haemoglobinopathies:
	    Thalassemia
	    Sickle cell anaemia
	• NIPT
	• Chromosome abnormalities:
	    Trisomy 13
	    Trisomy 21
	    Trisomy 18

11 to 12 weeks of pregnancy	Chorionic villus sampling (for confirmation of chromosomal abnormality detected)
16 to 20 weeks of pregnancy	Amniocentesis (for confirmation of chromosomal abnormality detected)
19 to 22 weeks of pregnancy	Detailed foetal anomaly scan
24 to 28 weeks of pregnancy	OGTT
35 weeks	Group B Streptococcus (Optional)

NB. Repetition of routine test for any abnormality if detected.
Source 1: Hilary Bowman-Smart, Claudia Wiesemann, and Ruth Horn: Non-invasive prenatal testing in Germany: a unique ethical and policy landscape. www.nature.com/ejhg
Source 2: Webpage: A guide to prenatal test and Scans. Dr. Quek Swee Chong, www.parkwayeast.com.sg/healthplus/article/prenatal-test-pregnancy-trimester
Source 3: Vital Glah Abuku, Emmanuel Alote Allotey, and Maxwell Akonde, Clinical and laboratory presentation of first-time antenatal care visits of pregnant women in Ghana, a hospital-based study; https://doi.org/10.1371/journal.pone.0280031; January 4, 2023

Triple test: Down syndrome, trisomy 21, and trisomy 18

The first antenatal screening is performed between weeks 11 and 13 of pregnancy. The test is performed early to determine if a pregnant woman should be considered for first trimester diagnostic tests such as, for example, chorionic villous sampling or amniocentesis in second trimester. The list of screening tests during antenatal period is given in Table 3.3 (39, 40, 41).

3.6.1 Tests Included in the First Antenatal Screening

■ Random blood glucose

■ Complete blood count (CBC)

■ Blood grouping and antibody screen

■ Rubella antibody status

■ Syphilis serology

- Hepatitis B serology

- HIV

Antenatal screening may be requested at any stage of pregnancy if a woman is presenting for the first time.

Random blood glucose: To determine the glycaemic status of the pregnant woman.

Complete blood count: Anaemia is the most common medical disorder seen in underdeveloped countries. It is associated with high maternal morbidity and mortality. There are three main causes of anaemia:

- Decreased erythrocyte production, as in iron, vitamin B12, and folate deficiencies

- Destruction of RBCs, as in haemoglobinopathies

- Loss of RBCs, as in any haemorrhage

While assessing haemoglobin, the gestational age should be considered. Haemoglobin decreases during pregnancy as a result of haemodilution caused by increased plasma volume. In pregnant women, the lower limit of haemoglobin is usually reported as 10 g/dl.

A woman's iron requirement increases two- to threefold during pregnancy. Iron is required for haemoglobin synthesis for both the mother and the foetus and it is also required for the production of iron-containing enzymes. A woman's folate requirement increases ten to 20 times, while her vitamin B12 requirement increases twofold.

During normal pregnancy, the platelet count decreases. The platelet count ranges between $100–150 \times 10^9$ cells/L at term pregnancy (40).

Blood grouping and antibody screen: In pregnant women, ABO blood grouping, rhesus D (RhD) status, and red cell antibodies identification is important to prevent "haemolytic disease of the newborn". If the foetus is rhesus D positive and the mother is negative, the mother may form anti-D antibodies that might affect subsequent rhesus D positive foetuses. In subsequent pregnancies, haemolytic disease of the newborn may occur.

Recently, non-invasive prenatal genetic testing (NIPT) has started to be carried out to determine foetal rhesus D status and prevent rhesus D negative mothers from undergoing unnecessary prophylactic treatment. This allows risk prevention of foetal anaemia and haemolysis when the mother is serologically RhD negative and the foetus is RhD positive (40).

Rubella antibody status: Pregnant women should be screened for rubella antibodies. When the rubella virus infects the developing foetus, especially during the first trimester, congenital rubella syndrome may occur. During this period, 90% of affected neonates will be born with birth defects, e.g. deafness, eye defects, heart defects, mental retardation. After 20 weeks of gestation, the risk of birth defects is reduced (41, 42).

Syphilis serology: Pregnant women should be screened for syphilis. Mothers infected with syphilis may experience long-term morbidity. If a mother is infected with syphilis, about 70–100% of infants will be infected and one-third will be stillborn. A Treponema Elisa Screen assay is carried out for syphilis as it detects both primary and secondary infection (41, 42).

Hepatitis B serology: Up to 85% of infants born to mothers infected with hepatitis B (particularly mothers who are HBeAg positive, i.e., with active infection) will become carriers and will be more likely to develop chronic liver diseases, including cirrhosis of the liver, liver failure, or liver cancer. By administering a hepatitis B vaccine and immunoglobulin to the newborn, transmission of hepatitis B virus infection from mother to infant can be prevented. Therefore, screening for hepatitis B is essential (41, 42).

HIV screening: HIV screening should be carried out on all pregnant women. Treatment of HIV positive mothers reduces the risk of HIV transmission to their infants (the risk is reduced from 32% to less than 1%). Interventions to reduce mother-to-child transmission of HIV infection include antiretroviral therapy, elective caesarean section delivery, and the avoidance of breastfeeding. If a patient is considered at risk for HIV, hepatitis C screening should also be considered (41, 42).

3.6.1.1 Additional Investigation in Early Pregnancy

Varicella antibody status in pregnant women with no (or an uncertain) history of illness (i.e., chicken pox or shingles) or vaccination should be determined through screening. There is a significant risk to both mother and infant if the mother contracts varicella during pregnancy.

Chlamydia and gonorrhoea screening should be considered for women who may be at increased risk based on age (e.g., less than 25 years) and sexual history.

Vitamin D is required for normal bone growth and development in the foetus. Mothers with a vitamin D deficiency or who are at risk of a deficiency (e.g., dark-skinned women, women who wear a veil) should receive vitamin D supplementation (41).

3.6.1.2 Blood Tests Included in the Second Antenatal Screening

At weeks 26–28 of gestation, the second antenatal screening is carried out. This includes:

- 50 gm glucose tolerance test (the "polycose" test)
- Complete blood count (CBC)
- Blood group antibodies

Screening for gestational diabetes: Gestational diabetes affects 5–8% of pregnant women; it is recommended that testing for gestational diabetes be carried out for all women between weeks 26 and 28 of gestation.

A 50 gm glucose tolerance test is used to screen for gestational diabetes. A 50 gm glucose load is given to the non-fasting patient and a blood glucose level is determined after 1 hour. An elevated result should be followed up with a 100 gm oral glucose tolerance test (OGTT) (43).

Repeat CBC and antibody screening: The CBC should be repeated at week 28 of gestation to check haemoglobin and platelet levels. Antibody screening should also be repeated at week 28 of gestation.

Proteinuria in pregnancy can also be a sign of preeclampsia if it is accompanied by high blood pressure. Preeclampsia is a condition that only occurs in pregnancy and causes high blood pressure. It usually occurs after 20 weeks of pregnancy and can happen in women who did not have high blood pressure before pregnancy. It can lead to serious complications for both mother and baby that can sometimes be fatal (41, 42).

3.6.2 Additional Tests during Pregnancy

Sub-clinical urine infection: It is recommended that all women have a midstream urine culture carried out at the time of the first antenatal screen, at the second antenatal screen, and again at week 36 gestation to exclude the possibility of a sub-clinical urine infection (asymptomatic bacteriuria).

Screening for Group B streptococcus: Group B streptococcal (GBS) infection is a significant cause of serious neonatal infection. Approximately 15–25% of women are carriers, and one in 200 of these women will have infants who develop neonatal sepsis.

Women may have a vaginorectal culture collected at week 35–37 of gestation (8, 42).

3.6.2.1 Testing for Down Syndrome and Other Genetic Conditions

Screening for Down syndrome, other chromosomal abnormalities, and neural tube defects is recommended for all pregnant women above the age of 35.

First trimester screening is based on the combination of results of the following.

The pregnancy-associated plasma protein-A (PAPP-A) and βhCG tests must be carried out between weeks 9 and 13 of gestation (ideally between weeks 10 and 12), and the nuchal translucency (NT) scan should be carried out after week 11 and before week 14 of gestation.

Second trimester screening can be offered to all women who present after 14 weeks of gestation but before week 20 of pregnancy and who have not completed first trimester screening (bloods are ideally taken between weeks 14 and 18 of gestation). This serum screen measures βhCG, alpha-fetoprotein (AFP), unconjugated estriol (µE3), and inhibin A (8, 42).

The average human gestation is 280 days (40 weeks), counted from the first day of the last menstrual period (LMP). During this time, a woman undergoes a multitude of normal physiological changes and can be subject to a variety of pregnancy-specific diseases.

3.7 TOOLS FOR MONITORING OF BIOCHEMICAL AND METABOLIC CHANGES DURING PREGNANCY

i) Interpretation of metabolic and biochemical variation during pregnancy.

ii) Interventions for the prevention of metabolic disorders during pregnancy.

iii) Recommendation for the development of health policy for the prevention of metabolic disorders during pregnancy.

3.8 SUMMARY AND CONCLUSION

Metabolic changes are crucial for the development of the foetus. Glucose, fatty acids, cholesterol, ketone bodies, and hormones maintain balance as these metabolic adaptations occur during pregnancy. Any abnormality during these adaptations could hamper the development of the foetus.

The overall health of the mother and the physiological environment determines the ability to undergo normal metabolic changes for foetal growth. Maternal carbohydrate and lipid metabolism and the regulation of this metabolism change with advancing gestation. These trends are characterized by a progressive decrease in maternal glucose sensitivity coinciding with increasing lipolysis, indicating a shift from an anabolic state to a catabolic state in late pregnancy. Numerous placental hormones – including placental growth hormone, placental lactogens, leptin, ghrelin, irisin, and adiponectin – regulate glucose and lipid metabolism, as well as the insulin sensitivity or resistance that occurs throughout anabolic and catabolic states of pregnancy.

Preconception maternal obesity is a risk factor for placental dysfunction, which drives aberrant metabolic control. Altering the normal trends of maternal energy homeostasis can lead to pregnancy-related metabolic disease, such as gestational diabetes mellitus (GDM). This is concerning as two-thirds of pregnancies in the United States involve overweight or obese women, and conditions like GDM can have lasting effects on maternal–foetal health. Gestational diabetes mellitus leads to insufficient insulin levels and aberrant blood glucose concentrations that impair the cognitive, neurological, and endocrine development of the foetus, which negatively impacts the offspring in later life. Besides maternal–foetal co-morbidities, these pregnancy complications pose a large economic burden, costing approximately $1.6 billion per year in the United States.

It is also important to acknowledge that molecular pathways mediated by placental hormones driving the changes in metabolism during normal pregnancy and GDM have not been completely elucidated. This is further complicated by the lack of sensitive methods to detect targets like irisin. Understanding the mechanisms that regulate metabolic trends during pregnancy is critical for better identification, treatment, and prevention of metabolic-related pregnancy complications.

The placenta may additionally secrete as yet undetected factors that might contribute to this process. Future research should focus on determining accurate levels of known factor and global screening approaches that detect novel factors might be beneficial. It is also crucial to determine the full extent to which aberrant hormone expression may be harmful to the placenta, including the regulation of placental function at the molecular level. Finally, research into ways of diminishing the effects of abnormal metabolic trends during metabolic-related pregnancy complications would greatly impact the current treatment methods for alleviating these complications.

REFERENCES

1. Poon LC, Mcintyre HD, Hyett JA, de Fonseca EB, Hod M The first trimester of pregnancy- a window of opportunity for prediction and prevention of pregnancy complications and feature life. *Diabetes Res Clin pract*, 2018. 145: 22–30; doi: 10.1016/ j.diabes.2018.05.002.

2. Barker DJ The foetal and infant origins of adult disease. *BMJ*. 1990 Nov 17;301(6761):1111. doi: 10.1136/bmj.301.6761.1111. PMID: 2252919.

3. Zhandong Z, Fengli L, Shixian L Metabolic adaptations in pregnancy a review. *Ann Nutr Metab*. 2017;70:59–65.

4. Tina N, Hannah EJY, Jourge LT, Amanda NSP The role of placental hormones in mediating maternal adaptations to support pregnancy and lactation. *Front Physiol*. 2018 9:1091. doi: 10.3389/fphy.2018.01091. www.frontiersin.org

5. Liu J, Ghaziani TT, Wolf JL Acute fatty liver disease of pregnancy: Updates in pathogenesis, diagnosis, and management. *Am J Gastroenterol*. 2017;112(6):838–846. doi: 10.1038/ajg.2017.53. PMID: 28291236.

6. Hales CN, Barker DJ The thrifty phenotype hypothesis. *Br Med Bull*. 2001;60:5–20. doi: 10.1093/bmb/60.1.5

7. Fowden AL, Giussani DA, Forhead AJ Intrauterine programming of physiological systems: Causes and consequences. *Physiology (Bethesda)*. 2006;21:29–37. doi: 10.1152/physiol.00050.2005.

8. Adnan A The role of laboratory medicine for health during pregnancy. *Electron J Int Fed Clin Chem Lab Med*. 2018 Dec;29(4):280–283.

9. Forsum E, Löf M Energy metabolism during human pregnancy. *Annu Rev Nutr*. 2007;27:277–292. doi: 10.1146/annurev.nutr.27.061406.093543. PMID: 17465853.

10. Yamashita H, Shao J, Friedman JE Physiologic and molecular alterations in carbohydrate metabolism during pregnancy and gestational diabetes mellitus. *Clin Obstet Gynecol*. 2000 Mar;43(1):87–98. doi: 10.1097/00003081-200003000-00009. PMID: 1069499.

11. Butte NF, Wong WW, Treuth MS, Ellis KJ, O'Brian Smith E Energy requirements during pregnancy based on total energy expenditure and energy deposition. *Am J Clin Nutr*. 2004 Jun;79(6):1078–87. doi: 10.1093/ajcn/79.6.1078. PMID: 15159239.

12. Bowman CE, Zoltan A, Wolfgang MJ Regulation of maternal-foetal metabolic communication: *Cell Mol Life Sci*. 2021 Feb;78(4):1455–1486. doi: 1007/s00018-020-03673.

13. Butte NF, King JC. Energy requirements during pregnancy and lactation. *Public Health Nutr*. 2005;8(7A):1010–1027.

14. Kopp-Hoolihan LE, van Loan MD, Wong WW, King JC Longitudinal assessment of energy balance in well-nourished, pregnant women. *Am J Clin Nutr*. 1999;69(4):697–703. PMID: 10197571.

15. Haig D Genetic conflicts in human pregnancy. *Q Rev Biol*. 1993 Dec;68(4):495–532. doi: 10.1086/418300. PMID: 8115596.

16. Armistead B, Johnson E, VanderKamp R, Kula-Eversole E, Kadam L, Drewlo S, Kohan-Ghadr H-R Placental regulation of energy homeostasis during human pregnancy. *Endocrinology*.2020 July;161(7): 1–13.

17. Battaglia FC, Meschia G Principal substrates of foetal metabolism. *Physiol Rev*. 1978 Apr;58(2):499–527. doi: 10.1152/physrev.1978.58.2.499. PMID: 417347.

18. Kalhan S, Rossi K, Gruca L, Burkett E, O'Brien A Glucose turnover and gluconeogenesis in human pregnancy. *J Clin Invest*. 1997 Oct 1;100(7):1775–81. doi: 10.1172/JCI119703. PMID: 9312177; PMCID: PMC508362.

19. Longo LD Maternal blood volume and cardiac output during pregnancy: A hypothesis of endocrinologic control. *Am J Physiol*. 1983 Nov;245 (5 Pt 1):R720–9. doi: 10.1152/ajpregu.1983.245.5.R720. PMID: 6356942.

20. Illsley NP Glucose transporters in the human placenta. *Placenta*. 2000 Jan; 21(1): 14–22. doi: 10.1053/plac.1999.0448. PMID: 10692246.

21. Gaither K, Quraishi AN, Illsley NP Diabetes alters the expression and activity of the human placental GLUT1 glucose transporter. *J Clin Endocrinol Metab*.1999 Feb;84(2):695–701. doi: 10.1210/jcem.83.2.5438. PMID: 10022440.

22. Haggarty P Fatty acid supply to the human foetus. *Annu Rev Nutr*. 2010 Aug 21;30:237–55. doi: 10.1146/annurev.nutr.0128.9.104742. PMID: 20438366.

23. Herrera E, Amusquivar E, López-Soldado I, Ortega H Maternal lipid metabolism and placental lipid transfer. *Horm Res*. 2006;65 Suppl 3:59–63. doi: 10.1159/000091507. Epub 2006 Apr 10. PMID: 16612115.

24. Boden G Fuel metabolism in pregnancy and in gestational diabetes mellitus. *Obstet Gynecol Clin North Am.*1996;23(1):1–10. PMID: 8684772.

25. Metzger BE, Ravnikar V, Vileisis RA, Freinkel N "Accelerated starvation" and the skipped breakfast in late normal pregnancy. *Lancet (London, England)* 1982;1(8272):588–592.

26. Savitri AI, Yadegari N, Bakker J, van Ewijk RJ, Grobbee DE, Painter RC, Uiterwaal CS, Roseboom TJ Ramadan fasting and newborn's birth weight in pregnant Muslim women in The Netherlands. *Br J Nutr.* 2014;112 (9): 1503–1509. doi:10.1017/s0007114514002219. PMID: 25231606.

27. Girard J, Ferré P, Pégorier JP, Duée PH. Adaptations of glucose and fatty acid metabolism during perinatal period and suckling-weaning transition. *Physiol Rev.* 1992 Apr;72(2):507–62. doi: 10.1152/physrev.1992.72.2.507. PMID: 1557431.

28. Nowaczyk MJM, Wassif CA Smith Lemli Opitz syndrome. 1998 Nov 13 (updated 2020 Jan 30). Ncbi.nlm.nih.gov.

29. Webpage Reference: The basal metabolism before, during, and after pregenancy by irene sandiford and theodora wheeler. Clinical metabolism and obstetrics, division of medicine, mayo clinic and the mayo foundation, rochester.

30. Napso T, Yong HEJ, Lopez-Tello J, Sferruzzi-Perri AN The role of placental hormones in mediating maternal adaptations to support pregnancy and lactation. *Front Physiol.* 2018;9:1091. doi:10.3389/fphys.2018.01091. PMID: 30174608.

31. De Sisto CL, Kim SY, Sharma AJ Prevalence Estimates of Gestational Diabetes Mellitus in the United States, Pregnancy Risk Assessment Monitoring System (PRAMS), 2007–2010. *Prev Chronic Dis.* 2014;11:E103. doi:10.5888/pcd11.130415. PMID: 24945238.

32. Freinkel N Banting lecture 1980. Of pregnancy and progeny. *Diabetes* 1980;29(12):1023–1035. PMID: 7002669.

33. Desoye G, Hauguel-de Mouzon S The human placenta in gestational diabetes mellitus. The insulin and cytokine network. *Diabetes Care* 2007;30(Suppl 2):S120–126. doi: 10.2337/dc07-s203. PMID: 17596459.

34. Seshiah V, Balagi V *Chapter 20- Diabetes and Pregnancy; API text book of Medicine,* Volume 1, page no. 550, 10th edition, 2015.

35. Wenrui Ye, Luo C, Huan J, Li C, Liu Z, Liu F Gestational diabetes mellitus and adverse pregnancy outcomes: *BMJ* 2022;377:e067946. https://doi.org/10.1136/bmj-2021-067946.

36. Simmons D, McElduffa A, Mclntyre HD, Elrish M Gestational diabetes mellitus: NICE for the U.S.? *Diabetes Care* 2010;33:34–337.

37. Kalkhoff RK, Kissebah AH, Kim HJ (1978) Carbohydrate and lipid metabolism during normal pregnancy: Relationship to gestational hormone action. *Semin Perinatol* 2 (4):291–307. PMID: 113883.

38. Marwaha RK, et al. Establishment of reference range for thyroid hormones in normal pregnant Indian women. *BJOG* 2008;115:602–606.

39. Vital GA, Emmanuel AA, Maxwell A Clinical and laboratory presentation of first-time antenatal care visits of pregnant women in Ghana, a hospital-based study: https://doi.org/10.1371/journal.pone.0280031.

40. Webpage Reference: A guide to prenatal test and Scans. Dr. Quek Swee Chong, www.park-wayeast .com.sg/healthplus/article/prenatal-test-preganacy-trimester.

41. Gronowski AM *Handbook of Clinical Laboratory Testing During pregnancy.* Humana Press, Totowa, NJ, 2003.

42. Webpage Reference: Hilary BS, Claudia W, Ruth H *Non-invasive prenatal testing in Germany: a unique ethical and policy landscape.* www.nature.com/ejhg.

43. Webpage Reference: WHO. Definition, Diagnosis and classification of diabetes mellitus and its complication.part-1: *Diagnosis and classification of diabetes mellitus. WHO/ NCD/MCS/99.2ed. Geneva WHO* 1999, pp. 1259. https://apps.who.int>iris>handle.

4 Recent Trends in the Diagnosis of Metabolic Disorders

Jennifer Suurbaar, Zakaria Seidu, and Seth Kwabena Amponsah

4.1 INTRODUCTION

Metabolic disorders are a group of medical conditions that disrupt various aspects of metabolism, including the breakdown, synthesis, and utilization of carbohydrates, proteins, and fats, as well as the regulation of enzymes, hormones, and other substances involved in metabolism [1]. These disorders can occur due to a variety of factors, including genetic mutations, lifestyle factors, and environmental exposures [2]. Metabolic disorders include diabetes, dyslipidemia, obesity, and inborn errors of metabolism (IEMs). Inborn errors of metabolisms are a group of genetic disorders that result from defects in enzymes or other proteins involved in various metabolic pathways in the body and are considered rare diseases [3, 4].

Metabolic disorders impose multi-faceted burdens, including health, economic, emotional, and social burdens, on individuals and families, and on public health systems. For example, diabetes, which is a common metabolic disorder, can lead to complications, such as cardiovascular disease, kidney disease, nerve damage, and eye problems. Other metabolic disorders, such as obesity and dyslipidemia, can also increase the risk of various health issues, including heart disease, stroke, and liver disease [5–9]. Economically, the costs associated with the diagnosis, treatment, and management of metabolic disorders can be high, including expenses related to medications, medical appointments, laboratory tests, and hospitalizations [7, 9, 10]. The need to make lifestyle changes and adhere to medication regimens, the constant monitoring of metabolic markers, and the stigma and discrimination associated with certain metabolic disorders, such as obesity or type 2 diabetes, can result in social and psychological challenges, including negative societal attitudes, bias, and prejudice, which impose an emotional burden on sick individuals and their families [11–13].

Therefore, the early detection and management of these disorders is important in order to prevent or minimize such long-term complications and consequences. Several diagnostic approaches for metabolic disorders have emerged in recent years; these mainly place a greater emphasis on early detection, particularly approaches related to obesity and diabetes.

The diagnosis of metabolic disorders typically involves a combination of medical history, physical examination, and laboratory tests. Some common laboratory tests used to diagnose metabolic disorders include a blood glucose test [14, 15], a lipid profile [16, 17], liver function tests [18, 19], urine tests [20, 21], and genetic testing [20, 22]. In addition to laboratory tests, imaging studies such as x-rays, computerized tomography (CT) scans, and magnetic resonance imaging (MRI) scans, may also be used to help diagnose certain metabolic disorders [23]. In some cases, a biopsy may be necessary to make a definitive diagnosis [24]. It is important to note that the specific tests used to diagnose metabolic disorders will vary depending on the suspected condition and the individual patient's medical history and symptoms. A healthcare provider or specialist can recommend the appropriate tests based on an individual's specific circumstances.

Overall, early detection, more accurate diagnosis, and personalized treatment regimens are what the recent trends in metabolic disorder diagnosis offer. These can contribute to better patient outcomes. Here, we cover current efforts or breakthroughs in the diagnosis of metabolic disorders, such as diabetes, dyslipidemia, obesity, and inherited metabolic disorders, in this context.

4.2 TRENDS IN DIAGNOSING DIABETES

Diabetes, which is characterized by high blood sugar levels, is caused by a lack of insulin or insulin resistance. Type 1 diabetes is caused by a loss of function of the β-cells in the pancreas, typically resulting in a complete lack of insulin [25]. In contrast, type 2 diabetes is caused by a gradual deficiency in insulin secretion against a backdrop of insulin resistance [26]. There are other types of diabetes caused by different factors, such as gestational diabetes mellitus (GDM), which develops during pregnancy, independent of genetic defects in β-cell function and insulin action. There is also drug- or chemical-induced diabetes (such as after organ transplantation or in the treatment of HIV/AIDS). Diseases of the exocrine pancreas can also induce diabetes [27, 28].

Despite the phenotypic heterogeneity of diabetes, as indicated above, the diagnostic criteria for diabetes remain largely the same. The diagnostic modalities of the commonly used diabetes tests are provided in Table 4.1. Mostly, diagnosis of diabetes requires the use of one of these tests, confirmed by repeated testing on different days.

DOI: 10.1201/9781003384823-4

Table 4.1 Modalities of basic tests for diabetes

	Diagnostic test			
HbA1c test	Fasting plasma glucose test	Oral glucose tolerance test*	Random plasma glucose test**	Diagnosis
<5.7%	≤99 mg/dL	≤139 mg/dL	NA	Normal
5.7%–6.4%	100–125 mg/dL	140–199 mg/dL	NA	Prediabetes
≥6.5%	≥126 mg/dL	≥200 mg/dL	≥200 mg/dL	Diabetes

*test is conducted 2 hours after sugar intake
**test is conducted if patient shows symptoms of diabetes
Adapted from: National Institute of Diabetes and Digestive and Kidney Diseases

The fasting plasma glucose (FPG) test measures blood sugar levels after an overnight fast. An FPG level of 126 mg/dL or higher is diagnostic of diabetes [14]. To conduct the oral glucose tolerance test (OGTT), a patient is given a sugary drink after fasting and the patient's blood sugar level is measured after 2 hours. A blood sugar level of 200 mg/dL or higher 2 hours after the sugary drink is diagnostic of diabetes [14]. However, the OGTT has largely been abandoned outside of screening for gestational diabetes, owing to its complexity and low reproducibility in some parts of the United States [29].

The random plasma glucose (RPG) test is a laboratory test that measures blood sugar levels at any time of the day without fasting. An RPG level of 200 mg/dL or higher, plus symptoms of diabetes, is diagnostic of diabetes [15]. Another diagnostic tool is the assessment of glycated hemoglobin (HbA1c). The HbA1c test does not require fasting [30] and is not influenced by changed behavior over a few days or a week, such as engaging in strenuous exercise or adopting a low-calorie diet, in contrast to the fasting plasma glucose test, which can be influenced in this manner [31]. This is the most obvious justification for adopting it as a diagnostic tool, as well as the fact that the test may be carried out on anyone attending a doctor's appointment at any time of the day.

The HbA1c test measures the average blood sugar level over the past two to three months. Blood sugar concentration over the previous weeks to months seems to be best represented by HbA1c concentration. The degree of glucose metabolism control in diabetic patients can be measured through the routine assessment of HbA1c levels, and the relationship between carbohydrate management and the emergence of any complications can be evaluated [32]. Mostly, a HbA1c level of 6.5% or higher is diagnostic of diabetes [33].

One of the drawbacks of adopting this diagnostic tool is that hemoglobin only becomes glycosylated while an erythrocyte circulates in serum; older erythrocytes have more glycosylated hemoglobin, whereas reticulocytes have less. The mixture of older and younger erythrocytes is reflected in total HbA1c. Therefore, observed HbA1c will be lower, regardless of glycemia, if the average life of erythrocytes is abnormally short. However, if the average age of circulating erythrocytes is higher, regardless of glycemia, the older erythrocyte population would have higher HbA1c levels. This might happen, for instance, if erythropoiesis is abruptly interrupted in aplastic anemia. Aside from decreased erythrocyte survival, hemoglobinopathies can also be complicated by aberrant hemoglobins (such as HbF), which can overlap with HbA1c in their electrophoretic peak and negatively impact the outcomes of the assays [31].

Other recent advancements have been made in diagnosing diabetes. These include continuous glucose monitoring (CGM), a method that involves placing a sensor under the skin to continuously measure glucose levels in the interstitial fluid. CGM can help detect diabetes and monitor blood glucose levels in people with diabetes [34, 35]. Point-of-care testing (POCT) refers to diagnostic testing that is performed outside of the laboratory, such as in a doctor's office or clinic. POCT devices are becoming increasingly popular for diagnosing diabetes as they provide quick and reliable results [36, 37].

4.3 TRENDS IN DIAGNOSING DYSLIPIDEMIA

Traditional biomarkers such as low-density lipoprotein (LDL) cholesterol and high-density lipoprotein (HDL) cholesterol are useful in diagnosing lipid disorders. In the standard lipid profile, the LDL cholesterol level is calculated using the Friedewald equation [38, 39] to evaluate the levels of total cholesterol and total triglycerides in serum. Then, all apolipoprotein B (ApoB) lipoproteins are precipitated, and the amount of HDL cholesterol is determined by measuring the amount of cholesterol in the supernatant. The Friedewald equation is then used to determine the LDL cholesterol level [40, 41]. This test may not be sufficient in the context of metabolic disorders. Some of the tests available to clinicians for advanced lipid testing include non–high-density lipoprotein (non-HDL) cholesterol from a standard lipid profile ApoB [42–44], vertical density gradient ultracentrifugation [44, 45], segmented gradient gel electrophoresis [46], and a nuclear magnetic resonance (NMR) lipid profile [47].

Tests such as NMR lipid profiling and the ApoB/ApoA-1 ratio are increasingly being used to assess lipid disorders in metabolic disorders [47]. These tests provide a more detailed picture of lipid metabolism and help identify patients at higher risk of cardiovascular disease. Numerous studies have demonstrated that, particularly in patients with cardiometabolic risk factors like high triglyceride levels, low HDL cholesterol levels, and high numbers of LDL particles, the Friedewald formula-derived LDL cholesterol level is not the most sensitive indicator of lipid- and lipoprotein-associated risk for some disorders. The non-HDL cholesterol level is a better alternative target, but the ApoB level and the number of NMR-measured LDL particles are the most potent single lipid and lipoprotein measurements, and doctors looking to utilize them to enhance lipid-altering medications should be cautious when ordering them [48]. Therefore, health professionals are now using a combination of biomarkers, including triglycerides, apolipoproteins, and inflammatory markers such as C-reactive protein (CRP), to provide a more comprehensive diagnosis.

In addition, the ability of non-invasive imaging techniques, such as ultrasound, CT, MRI, and proton magnetic resonance spectroscopy, to detect concurrent liver inflammation or fibrosis is constrained in comparison to liver biopsy [49]. These techniques can provide a more accurate diagnosis and enable early intervention. Today, ultrasonography is the non-invasive imaging method most frequently utilized in clinical settings to identify fatty infiltration of the liver. Its extensive availability and great tolerability will ensure its continued popularity in the future. Compared to ultrasound, magnetic resonance techniques that use chemical shift imaging and in vivo 1H MRS may detect minute changes in liver fat content [50]. They can be used in conjunction with whole body MRI as part of the same test to compare the distribution of adipose tissue across the body and the amount of hepatic fat in the same person. As a result, it is projected that both will benefit from technology advancements, such as scanning times becoming shorter in the future [51].

Finally, the gut microbiota's potential function in lipid metabolism and dyslipidemia is being increasingly supported by research. The link between lipid abnormalities in metabolic illnesses and the gut microbiota is still being researched, as is the application of this understanding to diagnostics and therapeutic practice [52].

4.4 TRENDS IN DIAGNOSING OBESITY

Obesity is a condition characterized by excess body fat, which can lead to a variety of metabolic and cardiovascular problems [53]. There have been several trends in diagnosing obesity over the years, with the most significant changes occurring in recent times. Body mass index (BMI) has been a widely used tool for measuring obesity since its discovery in the nineteenth century [54], with the term "body mass index" being coined by Keys and his colleagues in 1972 [55]. BMI is a person's weight divided by the square of their height (standard unit of measurement is kg/m^2) [55]. Individuals with BMI values above $30\ kg/m^2$ are considered obese, as illustrated in Figure 4.1.

Although BMI is not a direct measure of body fat percentage, it is so widely used to identify underweight, normal weight, overweight, obese, or morbidly obese individuals because it is easy to measure and calculate. There were concerns about the validity of BMI as a predictor of obesity in the late 1980s and early 1990s [56]. Strong evidence that the World Health Organization (WHO) BMI breakpoints do not accurately reflect the overweight or obese status of all demographic groups comes from the findings of cross-sectional and prospective epidemiological investigations [57]. Thus, BMI has some significant flaws; physical activity and environmental variables including age, gender, and ethnicity have an impact on the link between BMI and body fat percentage. Other obesity measurements may therefore be more accurate and informative, i.e., age and BMI [58], gender and BMI [59], and ethnicity and BMI [60].

Other measures of fatness such as waist circumference, waist-to-hip ratio, mid-upper arm circumference, and skin-fold thicknesses are considered in conjunction with BMI to assess body-specific areas such as the location or distribution of fat in the abdomen [61]. Some other measures used to diagnose obesity include dual-energy x-ray absorptiometry (DXA) [62–64], and underwater weighing [64, 65]. These methods are less commonly used than BMI, waist circumference, and body fat percentage.

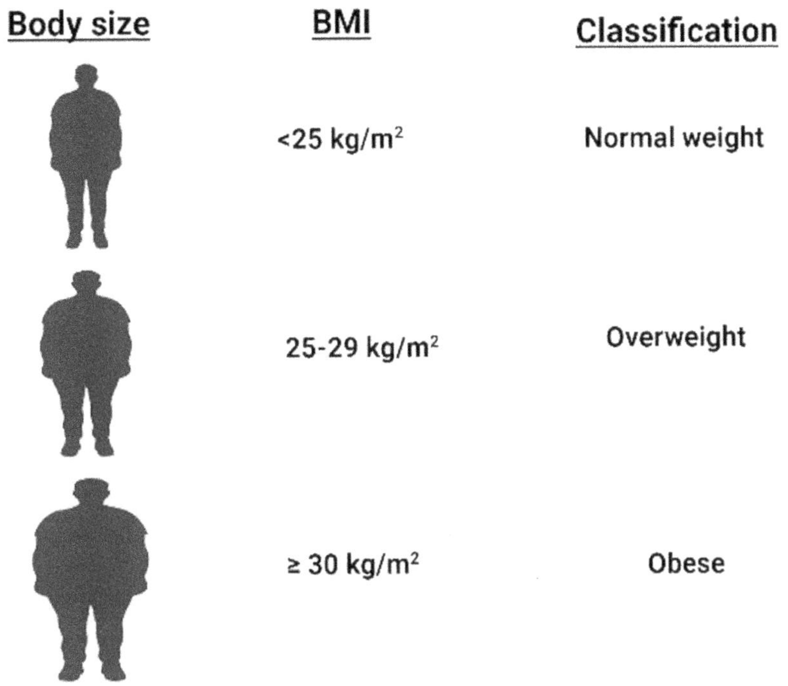

Body size   BMI   Classification

Body size	BMI	Classification
	<25 kg/m²	Normal weight
	25-29 kg/m²	Overweight
	≥ 30 kg/m²	Obese

Figure 4.1   The use of BMI in obesity estimation

4.5 TRENDS IN THE DIAGNOSIS OF INHERITED METABOLIC DISORDERS

Inherited metabolic disorders (IMDs) or inborn errors of metabolism (IEMs) constitute a vast, complex, and important group of rare genetic diseases [66]. They affect various organs and systems in the body, and have symptoms and disease prognoses that vary widely depending on the specific disorder, from slow, progressive disorders that are evident only in adulthood, to acute and potentially lethal effects shortly after birth [67]. Due to the lethality of some of these diseases, some IEMs are included in newborn screening programs in countries like the United States [68, 69], Spain [70], and Ireland [71].

Here, we report on the current diagnosis approaches to IEMs, from biochemical screening tests, metabolomic approaches using mass spectrometry [72], and genomic sequencing approaches such as exome sequencing [73].

4.5.1 Biochemical Tests for the Diagnosis of IEMs

A combination of biochemical tests (urea and electrolytes, liver function tests, blood gases, blood glucose concentrations, plasma ammonia) and certain metabolic investigations (plasma amino acids, acylcarnitine profile, urinary organic acids, and urinary glycosaminoglycans), followed by specific metabolic tests like those for very long-chain fatty acids, lysosomal enzymes, and transferrin isoforms, is reportedly considered a rational approach by many clinicians for the diagnosis of IEMs [74, 75].

Biochemical testing can be performed with a reactive strip or qualitative procedures. Reactive strips are commercially available for quick analysis of several intermediates in urine, including protein, blood, leukocytes, nitrite, glucose, ketones (acetoacetic acid), pH, specific gravity, creatinine, bilirubin, and urobilinogen. Other strips allow the quick determination of reducing substances (glucose, lactose, fructose, galactose, pentoses, sulfite, etc.). Even a simple analysis of urine color and odor could be an indicator of some IEMs [70]. Other basic biochemical tests employed for the diagnosis of IEMs are provided in Table 4.2.

Therefore, despite the availability of advanced techniques, like tandem mass spectrometry and exome sequencing, biochemical assays are still utilized in the diagnosis of IEMs [70, 71], as they play a crucial role in establishing a definitive diagnosis of the diseases. However, in the context of a wider newborn screening program, biochemical testing reportedly has a poor diagnostic yield

Table 4.2 Some basic biochemical tests for the diagnosis of IEMs [70]

Test	Diagnosis
Multistix reagent test	Multiple disorders
Reducing substances	Fructose intolerance (HFI, Fructosemia)
(non-glucose)	Galactosemia (GALT, GALK, or epimerase deficiency) Pentosuria
	Alkaptonuria tyrosinemia 1, 2
Dinitrophenyl-hydrazine (DNPH) test	Maple syrup urine disease (MSUD) Phenylketonuria
	Liver disease, tyrosinemia 1/2, tyrosiluria, histidinemia, methionine malabsorption (Oasthouse syndrome) Ketosis
Ferric chloride test	Phenylketonuria Histidinemia, pheochromocytoma, alkaptonuria MSUD, foriminotransferase deficiency salicylates, methionine malabsorption, DKA phenothiazines, para amino salicylic acid
Nitrosonaphthol test	PKU, direct hyperbilirubinemia, tyrosinemia, INH, L-Dopa
Cyanide nitroprusside test	Tyrosinemia 1/2/transient, tyrosiluria, jistidinemia, methionine malabsorption (Oasthouse syndrome), TPN
	Cystinuria
	Homocystinuria, severe dietary or inherited cobalamin/folate deficiency
Ehrlich's aldehyde test	Porphyria
Sulfite test	Sulfite oxidase, molybdenum cofactor deficiency
Alcian blue, toluidine blue test – MPS screen test on filter paper	Mucopolysaccharide

due to the large volume of blood required to perform such a series of metabolic investigations, as successful phlebotomy is a challenge in the neonatal population [71].

4.5.2 Mass Spectrometry Approaches to the Diagnosis of IEMs

Tandem mass spectrometry is reportedly the main method of clinical screening for neonatal IEMs [76]. As a result, recent applications of mass spectrometry for the diagnosis of IEMs is widely reported [72, 77].

Tandem mass spectroscopy (LC-MS/MS) and gas chromatography–mass spectrometry (GC-MS) are the essential mass spectrometry approaches [72, 77] that can be used to diagnose several IEMs [77, 78] in a range of biological samples, such as plasma, urine, cerebrospinal fluid (CSF), and dried blood spots (DBSs) [79]. LC-MS/MS is highly sensitive; however, it is unable to detect diseases such as mitochondriopathies, purine and pyrimidine disorders, neurotransmitters, congenital disorders of glycosylation, and very long-chain fatty acids. GC-MS makes up for these limitations of LC-MS/MS.

Thus, LC-MS/MS and GC-MS often complement each other, and they are the main diagnostic choices for disorders of amino acids, organic acids, fatty acids, and ketone body metabolism; energy deficiency disorders, such as respiratory chain and congenital lactic acidosis; and the metabolism of vitamins and non-protein cofactors [77].

4.5.3 Exome Sequencing Techniques for the Diagnosis of IEMs

NGS exome sequencing has been successfully used as a cost-effective approach for several years now to detect/diagnose disorders like hyperphenylalaninemia, tetrahydrobiopterin deficiency, phenylketonuria [80, 81], mitochondriopathies [82, 83], and glycogen storage diseases [84]. Two types of exome sequencing approaches have been employed for the detection/diagnosis of IEMs: targeted exome multiplex sequencing [73] and whole exome sequencing (WES) [68].

Their applications have improved the diagnosis and detection of variants of IEMs, and enabled the discovery of new disease genes, providing insight into new IEMs. Examples of such discoveries include the detection of the novel gene CA5A, encoding carbonic anhydrase VA, which contributed to unexplained hyperammonemia, hyperlactatemia, and hypoglycemia in a family [66], and mutations associated with N-acetylneuraminate synthase (NANS) deficiency [66]. As a result, exome sequencing has shown potential utility in newborn screening for IEMs [85]. A classic example of such usage is in the NC NEXUS [69] and BabySeq [68] projects in the United States.

4.6 MILESTONES ACHIEVED IN DIAGNOSTIC STRATEGIES FOR METABOLIC DISORDERS

The trends in metabolic disorder diagnosis are focused on earlier detection, more accurate diagnosis, and personalized treatment plans, all of which can lead to improved outcomes for patients. The clinical diagnosis of metabolic disorders is made using several tests, including biochemical analyses and histologic and genetic studies. Below are some of the new diagnostic tools used in recent times and how they can revolutionize the diagnosis of metabolic disorders.

4.6.1 Next-generation Sequencing (NGS) Technologies

Increased genetic knowledge and better understanding of molecular pathophysiology in recent decades have led to dramatic improvements in therapies using novel methods such as small molecule modulators of defective proteins, gene therapy, and stem cell infusion. One such advanced tool is next-generation sequencing (NGS) technologies [86] in the diagnosis of metabolic disorders; these technologies include whole genome sequencing (WGS), whole exome sequencing, and targeted gene panel sequencing approaches that focus on a specific set of genes known to be associated with metabolic disorders [87].

NGS technologies have revolutionized the field of genetic testing by allowing for the rapid and cost-effective analysis of large amounts of genetic data. This has led to improved diagnostic accuracy and the identification of new genetic variants associated with metabolic disorders. Metabolic disorders are not restricted to diseases that show increased or decreased levels of biochemical parameters in blood and/or urine. Some disorders do not have any biochemical markers and are associated with a wide variety of neurological phenotypes [88]. Genes associated with mitochondrial disease have been identified through WES since the explosion of NGS [89–93].

The first phenylketonuria mutation was found about three decades ago [94] and in 2017, a novel gene underlying this phenotype (DNAJC12) was found through WES [95]. This gene encodes a heat shock co-chaperone family member that interacts with phenylalanine, tyrosine, and tryptophan hydroxylases, catalyzing the BH4-activated conversion of phenylalanine into tyrosine, tyrosine into L-dopa, and tryptophan into 5-hydroxytryptophan. This metabolic deficiency leads to dystonia and intellectual disability, in addition to hyperphenylalaninemia. Again, in 2016, a novel gene was added to the list of genes involved in complex molecule metabolism disorders, which are associated with all the enzymes involved in lysosomal, peroxisomal, and cholesterol metabolism. This gene was ACER3, which hydrolyzes the amide linkage of ceramides, leading to a leukodystrophy phenotype [87].

NGS can be integrated with other diagnostic tools, such as metabolomics or proteomics, to provide a more comprehensive analysis of metabolic function and identify potential targets for treatment or prevention. The use of NGS for the diagnosis of metabolic disorders has the potential to improve the accuracy, efficiency, and cost effectiveness of diagnosis, particularly as the technology becomes more widely available and affordable. However, there are still challenges to be addressed, such as the interpretation of genetic variants and the integration of NGS with other diagnostic tools.

4.6.2 Artificial Intelligence (AI)

Artificial intelligence (AI) has the potential to revolutionize the diagnosis of metabolic disorders by enabling the analysis of large amounts of data, such as electronic health records, genetic information, and biomarker data, to identify patterns and risk factors that may be associated with these disorders [96]. This is discussed in detail in Chapter 6. The prevention and treatment of metabolic disorders are currently the focus of numerous multidisciplinary studies. It is becoming more and more crucial to monitor, treat, and manage metabolic disorders and their consequences using two or more disciplines [97]. One approach is predictive modeling, in which AI is used to identify individuals who are at increased risk of metabolic disorders. These models can take into account a wide range of factors, such as age, sex, family history, lifestyle factors, and biomarkers, to provide personalized risk assessments [98–100]. AI algorithms can be used to analyze medical images, such as MRI scans and CT scans, to identify early signs of metabolic disorders, such as fatty liver disease or atherosclerosis [101]. Similarly, AI algorithms can analyze genetic data to identify genetic variants that may be associated with metabolic disorders, providing a more personalized approach to diagnosis and treatment [102]. Additionally, AI can be combined with other diagnostic tools, such as metabolomics or proteomics, to provide a more comprehensive analysis of metabolic function and identify potential targets for treatment or prevention [103]. In real-time monitoring, AI algorithms can be used to monitor glucose levels, blood pressure, and other biomarkers in real time, providing continuous feedback and enabling early detection and intervention for metabolic disorders [104].

REFERENCES

1. Heindel, J.J., et al., Metabolism disrupting chemicals and metabolic disorders. *Reproductive Toxicology*, 2017. **68**: pp. 3–34.

2. Gilbert-Barness, E. and P.M. Farrell, Approach to diagnosis of metabolic diseases. *Translational Science of Rare Diseases*, 2016. **1**: pp. 3–22.

3. Mukherjee, S. and S.K. Ray, Inborn errors of metabolism screening in neonates: Current perspective with diagnosis and therapy. *Current Pediatric Reviews*, 2022. **18**(4): pp. 274–285.

4. Hoffmann, G.F., Selective screening for inborn errors of metabolism—past, present and future. *European Journal of Pediatrics*, 1994. **153**(Supplement 1): pp. S2–S8.

5. James, P.T., et al., The obesity epidemic, metabolic syndrome and future prevention strategies. *European Journal of Cardiovascular Prevention & Rehabilitation*, 2004. **11**(1): pp. 3–8.

6. Sandilands, K., A. Williams, and A.J. Rylands, Carer burden in rare inherited diseases: A literature review and conceptual model. *Orphanet Journal of Rare Diseases*, 2022. **17**(1): pp. 1–20.

7. Centorrino, F., et al., Health and economic burden of metabolic comorbidity among individuals with bipolar disorder. *Journal of Clinical Psychopharmacology*, 2009. **29**(6): pp. 595–600.

8. Crisóstomo, L., et al., The burden of metabolic diseases on male reproductive health. *International Journal of Diabetology & Vascular Disease Research*, 2017. **5**(1e): pp. 1–2.

9. Piero, M., G. Nzaro, and J. Njagi, Diabetes mellitus-a devastating metabolic disorder. *Asian Journal of Biomedical and Pharmaceutical Sciences*, 2015. **5**(40): p. 1.

10. Bikbov, B., et al., Global, regional, and national burden of chronic kidney disease, 1990–2017: A systematic analysis for the global burden of disease study 2017. *The Lancet*, 2020. **395**(10225): pp. 709–734.

11. Kesavadev, J., et al., Challenges in type 1 diabetes management in South East Asia: Descriptive situational assessment. *Indian Journal of Endocrinology and Metabolism*, 2014. **18**(5): p. 600.

12. Kumar, K.P., et al., Type 1 diabetes: Awareness, management and challenges: Current scenario in India. *Indian Journal of Endocrinology and Metabolism*, 2015. **19**(Suppl 1): p. S6.

13. Holt, R.I. and S. Kalra, A new DAWN: Improving the psychosocial management of diabetes. *Indian Journal of Endocrinology and Metabolism*, 2014. **17**(Suppl 1): p. S95.

14. Group, D.S. and E.D.E. Group, Glucose tolerance and cardiovascular mortality: Comparison of fasting and 2-hour diagnostic criteria. *Archives of Internal Medicine*, 2001. **161**(3): pp. 397–405.

15. Sumathy, M., et al., Diagnosis of diabetes mellitus based on risk factors. *International Journal of Computers and Applications*, 2010. **10**(4): pp. 1–4.

16. Boehm, B.O. and S. Claudi-boehm, The metabolic syndrome. *Scandinavian Journal of Clinical and Laboratory Investigation*, 2005. **65**(Suppl 240): pp. 3–14.

17. de Asua, D.R., et al., Evaluation of the impact of abdominal obesity on glucose and lipid metabolism disorders in adults with down syndrome. *Research in Developmental Disabilities*, 2014. **35**(11): pp. 2942–2949.

18. Hamaguchi, M., et al., The metabolic syndrome as a predictor of nonalcoholic fatty liver disease. *Annals of Internal Medicine*, 2005. **143**(10): pp. 722–728.

19. Lidofsky, S.D., Nonalcoholic fatty liver disease: Diagnosis and relation to metabolic syndrome and approach to treatment. *Current Diabetes Reports*, 2008. **8**(1): pp. 25–30.

20. Guerrero, R.B., D. Salazar, and P. Tanpaiboon, Laboratory diagnostic approaches in metabolic disorders. *Annals of Translational Medicine*, 2018. **6**(24): p. 470.

21. Liu, H., et al., Untargeted metabolomic analysis of urine samples for diagnosis of inherited metabolic disorders. *Functional & Integrative Genomics*, 2021. **21**: pp. 645–654.

22. Chen, B., et al., Good laboratory practices for biochemical genetic testing and newborn screening for inherited metabolic disorders. *Morbidity and Mortality Weekly Report: Recommendations and Reports*, 2012. **61**(2): pp. 1–44.

23. Lovibond, S., et al., The promise of metabolic imaging in diffuse midline glioma. *Neoplasia*, 2024. **39**: p. 100896.

24. Kalmar, J.R. and K.K. McNamara, Differential diagnosis of oral disease, in *Peterson's Principles of Oral and Maxillofacial Surgery*. 2022, Springer. pp. 873–889.

25. Syed, F.Z., Type 1 diabetes mellitus. *Annals of Internal Medicine*, 2022. **175**(3): pp. ITC33–ITC48.

26. Mahler, R.J. and M.L. Adler, Type 2 diabetes mellitus: Update on diagnosis, pathophysiology, and treatment. *The Journal of Clinical Endocrinology & Metabolism*, 1999. **84**(4): pp. 1165–1171.

27. Steck, A.K., et al., CGM metrics predict imminent progression to type 1 diabetes: Autoimmunity screening for kids (ASK) study. *Diabetes Care*, 2022. **45**(2): pp. 365–371.

28. Gollapalli, M., et al., A novel stacking ensemble for detecting three types of diabetes mellitus using a Saudi Arabian dataset: Pre-diabetes, T1DM, and T2DM. *Computers in Biology and Medicine*, 2022. **147**: p. 105757.

29. Inzucchi, S.E., Diagnosis of diabetes. *New England Journal of Medicine*, 2012. **367**(6): pp. 542–550.

30. Rahbar, S., O. Blumenfeld, and H.M. Ranney, Studies of an unusual hemoglobin in patients with diabetes mellitus. *Biochemical and Biophysical Research Communications*, 1969. **36**(5): pp. 838–844.

31. Saudek, C.D. and J.C. Brick, The clinical use of hemoglobin A1c. *Journal of Diabetes Science and Technology*, 2009. **3**(4): pp. 629–634.

32. Koenig, R.J., et al., Correlation of glucose regulation and hemoglobin AIc in diabetes mellitus. *New England Journal of Medicine*, 1976. **295**(8): pp. 417–420.

33. Standards of medical care in diabetes--2010. *Diabetes Care*, 2010. **33** (Suppl 1): pp. S11–S61.

34. Kleiman, D., et al., Simple continuous glucose monitoring in freely moving mice. *JoVE (Journal of Visualized Experiments)*, 2023. **192**: p. e64744.

35. Monisha, G., et al., A smart novel approach of blood glucose monitoring system using Arduino board. *International Journal of Intelligent Systems and Applications in Engineering*, 2024. **11**(2): pp. 495–502.

36. Florkowski, C., et al., Point-of-care testing (POCT) and evidence-based laboratory medicine (EBLM)–does it leverage any advantage in clinical decision making? *Critical Reviews in Clinical Laboratory Sciences*, 2017. **54**(7–8): pp. 471–494.

37. Luppa, P.B., et al., Point-of-care testing (POCT): Current techniques and future perspectives. *TrAc Trends in Analytical Chemistry*, 2011. **30**(6): pp. 887–898.

38. Friedewald, W.T., R.I. Levy, and D.S. Fredrickson, Estimation of the concentration of low-density lipoprotein cholesterol in plasma, without use of the preparative ultracentrifuge. *Clinical Chemistry*, 1972. **18**(6): pp. 499–502.

39. Tremblay, A.J., et al., Validation of the Friedewald formula for the determination of low-density lipoprotein cholesterol compared with β-quantification in a large population. *Clinical Biochemistry*, 2004. **37**(9): pp. 785–790.

40. Puavilai, W. and D. Laoragpongse, Is calculated LDL-C by using the new modified Friedewald equation better than the standard Friedewald equation? *Journal-Medical Association of Thailand*, 2004. **87**(6): pp. 589–594.

41. Bairaktari, E., et al., Estimation of LDL cholesterol based on the Friedewald formula and on apo B levels. *Clinical Biochemistry*, 2000. **33**(7): pp. 549–555.

42. Sniderman, A.D., et al., A meta-analysis of low-density lipoprotein cholesterol, non-high-density lipoprotein cholesterol, and apolipoprotein B as markers of cardiovascular risk. *Circulation: Cardiovascular Quality and Outcomes*, 2011. **4**(3): pp. 337–345.

43. Holewijn, S., et al., Apolipoprotein B, non-HDL cholesterol and LDL cholesterol for identifying individuals at increased cardiovascular risk. *Journal of Internal Medicine*, 2010. **268**(6): pp. 567–577.

44. Islam, S.T., et al., Methods of low-density lipoprotein-cholesterol measurement: Analytical and clinical applications. *Ejifcc*, 2022. **33**(4): p. 282.

45. Erkens, M., et al., Ultrasonication-induced extraction of inner shells from double-wall carbon nanotubes characterized via in situ spectroscopy after density gradient ultracentrifugation. *Carbon*, 2021. **185**: pp. 113–125.

46. Kosmas, C.E., et al., The Triglyceride/High-Density Lipoprotein Cholesterol (TG/HDL-C) Ratio as a risk marker for metabolic syndrome and cardiovascular disease. *Diagnostics*, 2024. **13**(5): p. 929.

47. Gholizadeh, N., et al. Nuclear magnetic resonance spectroscopy of human body fluids and in vivo magnetic resonance spectroscopy: Potential role in the diagnosis and management of prostate cancer. in *Urologic Oncology: Seminars and Original Investigations*, 2020. Elsevier.

48. Lau, J.F. and D.A. Smith, Advanced lipoprotein testing: Recommendations based on current evidence. *Endocrinology and Metabolism Clinics of North America*, 2009. **38**(1): pp. 1–31.

49. Mehta, S.R., et al., Non-invasive means of measuring hepatic fat content. *World Journal of Gastroenterology*, 2008. **14**(22): p. 3476.

50. Cannet, C., et al., Ex vivo proton spectroscopy (1H–NMR) analysis of inborn errors of metabolism: Automatic and computer-assisted analyses. *NMR in Biomedicine*, 2024. **36**(4): p. e4854.

51. Mehta, S.R., et al., Non-invasive means of measuring hepatic fat content. *World Journal of Gastroenterology*, 2008. **14**(22): pp. 3476–84.

52. Wang, Z., et al., Gut microbiome and lipid metabolism: from associations to mechanisms. *Current Opinion in Lipidology*, 2016. **27**(3): pp. 216–224.

53. Kim, S.Y., The definition of obesity. *Korean Journal of Family Medicine*, 2016. **37**(6): pp. 309–309.

54. Nuttall, F.Q., Body mass index: obesity, BMI, and health: a critical review. *Nutriton Today*, 2015. **50**(3): pp. 117–128.

55. Keys, A., et al., Indices of relative weight and obesity. *Journal of Chronic Diseases*, 1972. **25**(6): pp. 329–44.

56. Kuskowska-Wolk, A., et al., The predictive validity of body mass index based on self-reported weight and height. *International Journal of Obesity*, 1989. **13**(4): pp. 441–454.

57. Simmonds, M., et al., The use of measures of obesity in childhood for predicting obesity and the development of obesity-related diseases in adulthood: A systematic review and meta-analysis. *Health Technology Assessment (Winchester, England)*, 2015. **19**(43): pp. 1–336.

58. Hall, D.M. and T.J. Cole, What use is the BMI? *Archives of Disease in Childhood*, 2006. **91**(4): pp. 283–286.

59. Gallagher, D. and M. Visser, D. Sepulveda , R.N. Pierson, T. Harris, S.B. Heymsfield, How useful is body mass index for comparison of body fatness across age, sex, and ethnic groups, 1996. **143**(3): pp. 228–239.

60. Fernández, J.R. and D.B. Allison, Understanding racial differences in obesity and metabolic syndrome traits. *Nutrition Reviews*, 2004. **61**(9): pp. 316–319.

61. Nowak-Szczepanska, N., A. Gomula, and S. Koziel, Mid-upper arm circumference and body mass index as different screening tools of nutritional and weight status in Polish schoolchildren across socio-political changes. *Scientific Reports*, 2019. **9**(1): p. 12399.

62. Messina, C., et al., Body composition with dual energy x-ray absorptiometry: from basics to new tools. *Quantitative Imaging in Medicine and Surgery*, 2020. **10**(8): p. 1687.

63. Curtin, F., et al., Body mass index compared to dual-energy x-ray absorptiometry: Evidence for a spectrum bias. *Journal of Clinical Epidemiology*, 1997. **50**(7): pp. 837–844.

64. Czeck, M.A., et al., Total and regional dual x-ray absorptiometry derived four-compartment model. *Clinical Nutrition Espen*, 2023. **5**: pp. 185–190.

65. Mohajan, D. and H.K. Mohajan, A study on body fat percentage for physical fitness and prevention of obesity: A two compartment model. *Journal of Innovations in Medical Research*, 2024. **2**(4): pp. 1–10.

66. van Karnebeek, C.D., et al., The role of the clinician in the multi-omics era: Are you ready? *Journal of Inherited Metabolic Disease*, 2018. **41**: pp. 571–582.

67. Saudubray, J.-M. and À. Garcia-Cazorla, Inborn errors of metabolism overview: Pathophysiology, manifestations, evaluation, and management. *Pediatric Clinics*, 2018. **65**(2): pp. 179–208.

68. Holm, I.A., et al., The BabySeq project: Implementing genomic sequencing in newborns. *BMC Pediatrics*, 2018. **18**(1): pp. 1–10.

69. Milko, L.V., et al., Evaluating parents' decisions about next-generation sequencing for their child in the NC NEXUS (North Carolina Newborn Exome Sequencing for Universal Screening) study: A randomized controlled trial protocol. *Trials*, 2018. **19**(1): pp. 1–14.

70. Bijarnia-Mahay, S., and S. Kapoor Testing modalities for inborn errors of metabolism – What a clinician needs to know? *Indian Pediatrics*, 2019: **56**(9): pp. 757–766.

71. Dunne, E., et al., Biochemical testing for inborn errors of metabolism: Experience from a large tertiary neonatal centre. *European Journal of Pediatrics*, 2022. **181**(10): pp. 3725–3732.

72. Meiouet, F., et al., Moroccan experience of targeted screening for inborn errors of metabolism by tandem mass spectrometry. *Pediatric Reports*, 2024. **15**(1): pp. 227–236.

73. Adhikari, A.N., et al., The role of exome sequencing in newborn screening for inborn errors of metabolism. *Nature Medicine*, 2020. **26**(9): pp. 1392–1397.

74. Civallero, G., R.D. Kremer, and R. Giugliani, High-risk screening and diagnosis of inborn errors of metabolism: A practical guide for laboratories. *Journal of Inborn Errors of Metabolism and Screening*, 2018. **6**: pp. 1–6.

75. Laikind, P.K., J. Seegmiller, and H.E. Gruber, Detection of 5′-phosphoribosyl-4-(N-su ccinylcarboxamide)-5-aminoimidazole in urine by use of the Bratton-Marshall reaction: Identification of patients deficient in adenylosuccinate lyase activity. *Analytical Biochemistry*, 1986. **156**(1): pp. 81–90.

76. He, X., et al., A retrospective analysis of MS/MS screening for IEM in high-risk areas. *Bmc Medical Genomics*, 2024. **16**(1): p. 57.

77. Patial, A., et al., Detection of IEMs by mass spectrometry techniques in high-risk children: A pilot study. *Indian Journal of Pediatrics*, 2022. **89**(9): pp. 885–894.

78. Al-Riyami, S., et al., Establishment and validation of reference values for amino acids and acylcarnitines in dried blood spots for omani newborns using tandem mass spectrometry. *Oman Medical Journal*, 2022. **37**(5): p. e426.

79. Casado, M., et al., A targeted metabolomic procedure for amino acid analysis in different biological specimens by ultra-high-performance liquid chromatography–tandem mass spectrometry. *Metabolomics*, 2018. **14**: pp. 1–12.

80. Gu, Y., et al., Mutation spectrum of six genes in Chinese phenylketonuria patients obtained through next-generation sequencing. *PLOS One*, 2014. **9**(4): p. e94100.

81. Trujillano, D., et al., Accurate molecular diagnosis of phenylketonuria and tetrahydrobi-opterin-deficient hyperphenylalaninemias using high-throughput targeted sequencing. *European Journal of Human Genetics*, 2014. **22**(4): pp. 528–534.

82. Carroll, C., V. Brilhante, and A. Suomalainen, Next-generation sequencing for mitochondrial disorders. *British Journal of Pharmacology*, 2014. **171**(8): pp. 1837–1854.

83. Mahmud, S., et al., Use of next-generation sequencing for identifying mitochondrial disorders. *Current Issues in Molecular Biology*, 2022. **44**(3): pp. 1127–1148.

84. Wang, J., et al., Clinical application of massively parallel sequencing in the molecular diagnosis of glycogen storage diseases of genetically heterogeneous origin. *Genetics in Medicine*, 2014. **15**(2): pp. 106–114.

85. Huang, X., et al., Application of a next-generation sequencing (NGS) panel in newborn screening efficiently identifies inborn disorders of neonates. *Orphanet Journal of Rare Diseases*, 2022. **17**(1): p. 66.

86. Fernandez-Marmiesse, A., S. Gouveia, and M.L. Couce, NGS technologies as a turning point in rare disease research, diagnosis and treatment. *Current Medicinal Chemistry*, 2018. **25**(3): pp. 404–432.

87. Edvardson, S., et al., Deficiency of the alkaline ceramidase ACER3 manifests in early childhood by progressive leukodystrophy. *Journal of Medical Genetics*, 2016. **53**(6): pp. 389–396.

88. Falabella, M., et al., Gene therapy for primary mitochondrial diseases: Experimental advances and clinical challenges. *Nature Reviews Neurology*, 2022. **18**(11): pp. 689–698.

89. Kanako, K.-I., et al., BCS1L mutations produce Fanconi syndrome with developmental disability. *Journal of Human Genetics*, 2022. **67**(3): pp. 143–148.

90. Dong, X., et al., Precision medicine via the integration of phenotype-genotype information in neonatal genome project. *Fundamental Research*, 2022. 2(6): pp. 873–884.

91. Haack, T.B., et al., Exome sequencing identifies ACAD9 mutations as a cause of complex I deficiency. *Nature Genetics*, 2010. **42**(12): pp. 1131–1134.

92. Haack, T.B., et al., Molecular diagnosis in mitochondrial complex I deficiency using exome sequencing. *Journal of Medical Genetics*, 2012. **49**(4): pp. 277–284.

93. Calvo, S.E., et al., Molecular diagnosis of infantile mitochondrial disease with targeted next-generation sequencing. *Science Translational Medicine*, 2012. **4**(118): pp. 118ra10–118ra10.

94. DiLella, A.G., et al., An ammo-acid substitution involved in phenylketonuria is in linkage disequilibrium with DNA haplotype 2. *Nature*, 1987. **327**(6120): pp. 333–336.

95. Schiff, M., et al., Bi-allelic mutations in DNAJC12 cause hyperphenylalaninemia, neurotransmitter deficiencies, dystonia and intellectual disability. *European Journal of Paediatric Neurology*, 2017. **21**: p. e175.

96. Saberi-Karimian, M., et al., Potential value and impact of data mining and machine learning in clinical diagnostics. *Critical Reviews in Clinical Laboratory Sciences*, 2021. **58**(4): pp. 275–296.

97. Chen, H., S. Xiong, and X. Ren, Evaluating the risk of metabolic syndrome based on an artificial intelligence model. in *Abstract and Applied Analysis*, 2014. Hindawi.

98. Fregoso-Aparicio, L., et al., Machine learning and deep learning predictive models for type 2 diabetes: A systematic review. *Diabetology & Metabolic Syndrome*, 2021. **13**(1): pp. 1–22.

99. Kaur, H. and V. Kumari, Predictive modelling and analytics for diabetes using a machine learning approach. *Applied Computing and Informatics*, 2022. **18**(1/2): pp. 90–100.

100. Wong, G.L.H., et al., Artificial intelligence in prediction of non-alcoholic fatty liver disease and fibrosis. *Journal of Gastroenterology and Hepatology*, 2021. **36**(3): pp. 543–550.

101. Pickhardt, P.J., et al., Automated CT biomarkers for opportunistic prediction of future cardiovascular events and mortality in an asymptomatic screening population: A retrospective cohort study. *The Lancet Digital Health*, 2020. **2**(4): pp. e192–e200.

102. Quazi, S., Artificial intelligence and machine learning in precision and genomic medicine. *Medical Oncology*, 2022. **39**(8): p. 120.

103. Cammarota, G., et al., Gut microbiome, big data and machine learning to promote precision medicine for cancer. *Nature Reviews Gastroenterology & Hepatology*, 2020. **17**(10): pp. 635–648.

104. AlZu'bi, S., et al., Diabetes monitoring system in smart health cities based on big data intelligence. *Future Internet*, 2024. **15**(2): p. 85.

5 The Role of Mitochondrial Dysfunction in Metabolic Syndrome

Emmanuel A. Tagoe and Sheila A. Santa

5.1 INTRODUCTION

Metabolism (from the Greek word *metabolē*, implying "to change") is the total of all the chemical reactions that take place within a cell and that are necessary for the proper functioning of a living organism (1). Metabolism comprises both the synthesis (anabolism) and degradation (catabolism) of complex macromolecules. Catabolic reactions involve the breakdown of large biomolecules, such as glucose, through the process of cellular respiration, resulting in the release of energy (2). The body makes use of the energy that is released as a byproduct of catabolic reactions to carry out the anabolic activities that are necessary for the synthesis of macromolecules, such as proteins, carbohydrates, lipids, and nucleic acids (2).

Chemical reactions of metabolism are usually organized into distinct metabolic pathways to ensure efficiency and reduce wastage (1). Catabolic pathways, for instance, are ordered to ensure that energy is slowly released in discrete quanta stored in the form of adenosine triphosphate (ATP) and guanosine triphosphate (GTP) (1). The synthesis of ATP is usually through substrate-level phosphorylation or oxidative phosphorylation (3). By oxidizing electron carriers like nicotinamide adenine dinucleotide (NADH) and flavin adenine dinucleotide (FADH2), these pathways allow electrons to be released into the electron transport chain (ETC), which is located on the outer membrane of mitochondria (4). ATP is the main form of cellular energy necessary for all biological processes and, together with nicotinamide adenine dinucleotide phosphate (NADPH), it drives the synthesis of biomolecules required for the growth and maintenance of oxidative balance (5). The biomolecules needed for growth include protein, carbohydrates, nucleic acid, and lipids, and the basic units of these molecules, except for nucleic acids, are metabolized to produce energy or converted to other biomolecules (6). De novo synthesis of the units of these biomolecules, except nucleic acids, is usually due to an inadequate exogenous supply or the lack of an exogenous supply.

Proteins are polymers of amino acids. Peptide bonds hold the amino acid units together to form linear primary structures (7). The complexity of the protein structure is a result of several forces, including ionic interaction, hydrogen bonding, Van der Waals forces, and disulfide bridges, that exist between the side chains of the individual amino acids (8). Proteins, including enzymes, catalyze several chemical reactions in the body, while the structural types of proteins, such as actin, are involved in cytoskeletal or scaffolding systems that maintain cell shape and structure (9, 10). Some other important functions of protein include immune responses, cell adhesion, the cell cycle, cell signalling, and the active transport of substances across cell membranes (11). Catabolism of protein begins with the hydrolysis of the peptide bonds to yield free amino acids, followed by deamination to produce a carbon skeleton. Utilization of the carbon skeleton for cellular energy through the citric acid cycle (tricarboxylic acid cycle) occurs during metabolic stress or periods of glucose depletion (7). Carbon skeletons obtained from amino acids are usually channelled through a process known as gluconeogenesis to produce glucose.

Generally, carbohydrates are the commonest biological molecules involved in the storage of energy. Carbohydrates are polymers with monosaccharide units, such as galactose, fructose, and glucose (12). The monosaccharides are joined together by a glycosidic bond to form different kinds of polysaccharides and serve as the major source of chemical energy in cells (7), as well as serving as structural components in plants (cellulose) and animals (chitin) (12). The catabolism of carbohydrates yields acetyl-CoA which is a precursor for fatty acid synthesis and is dependent on glucose availability and ATP levels (13).

Additionally, lipids are a great source of cellular energy; they are a diverse group of biochemical molecules composed of long chains of fatty acids (14). The fatty acid chains consist of a long, non-polar hydrocarbon chain and a carboxylic group (14). Lipid units are heterogenous, unlike other biomolecules, and are a major component of biological membranes (14). In addition to the structural lipids, some lipids can be found in circulation. These lipids include triacylglycerol, low-density lipoprotein, high-density lipoprotein, very low-density lipoprotein, and cholesterol. Triacylglycerols are mostly used for chemical energy at times when glucose levels are low (7, 15). During starvation, the stored triacylglycerols are mobilized from the adipocytes and finally metabolized in the mitochondrion to generate energy in the form of ATP (7).

DOI: 10.1201/9781003384823-5

Nucleic acids – ribonucleic acid (RNA) and deoxyribonucleic acids (DNA) – however, are not directly involved in cellular energy production. They are polymers of nucleotides that are essential for the storage of genetic information and the synthesis of proteins (7). The mitochondrion is the central energy production hub of a cell; it is for this reason that it is termed the "powerhouse" (16). Over 90% of the ATP that is necessary for cellular activity is generated within the mitochondria through the citric acid cycle, fatty acid beta-oxidation, and oxidative phosphorylation. The mitochondrion has a double membrane that consists of an outer and inner membrane, creating an inter-membrane space (17). The inner membrane surrounds the matrix, which is the site of cellular respiration and ATP production and contains protein complexes and cytochromes required for electron transfer during oxidative phosphorylation (18). The inner membrane has many folds that bend inwards, forming a structure called cristae, and is selectively permeable only to oxygen (19). Enzymes necessary for fatty acid elongation and adrenaline oxidation are housed in the mitochondrial outer membrane, along with porins, a kind of protein that allows ions to enter and exit the mitochondria (17). Mitochondria are the only other cellular organelles outside of the nucleus that are thought to have their own genome (20).

As well as their involvement in the synthesis of ATP, mitochondria play an important part in facilitating cellular adaptation during times of cellular stress, such as nutritional deprivation, oxidative stress, DNA damage, etc. (21). In addition to its role in the creation of lipids, proteins, nucleic acids, glucose, and heme, the mitochondrion is responsible for the generation of metabolic byproducts, such as reactive oxygen species (ROS) and ammonia, both of which are essential for the continued existence and expansion of the cell (22). The mitochondria play a role in controlling calcium homeostasis, programmed cell death, and the creation of iron-sulfur clusters (23). Mitochondria need calcium for two different functions: buffering fluctuations in cytosolic calcium and regulating their intrinsic metabolism (24). Mitochondria that are healthy are dependent on a delicate equilibrium in the processes of mitochondrial dynamics, known as fission and fusion. These processes involve the production of an extended organelle by the fusion of two or more mitochondria, as well as the division of a single mitochondrion into two daughter mitochondria (25). The dysregulation of these biochemical pathways, which is most commonly caused by dysfunction in the mitochondria, has been linked to several disorders, one of which is metabolic syndrome (26–28).

The term "metabolic syndrome" (MetS) refers to a cluster of comorbid disorders that increases a person's risk of developing cardiovascular disease. These conditions include obesity, high blood pressure, and poor glucose and lipid metabolism (29). Different groups of people have different ways of defining metabolic syndrome. For instance, a recent definition by Dobrowolski et al. considers metabolic syndrome to be present when obese individuals also have any two of the following three conditions: high blood pressure, impaired glucose metabolism, and/or an elevated non-high-density lipoprotein (non-HDL) cholesterol level (atherogenic dyslipidaemia) (30). However, the most commonly cited definition of MetS is the presence of three or more concurrent risk factors, as outlined by the National Cholesterol Education Programme Adult Treatment Panel III (31). MetS is also associated with an increased risk of cardiovascular disease that can be caused by several diseases and conditions, including poor kidney function, hepatic steatosis, obstructive sleep apnoea, heart failure with maintained ejection fraction, polycystic ovary syndrome, chronic inflammation, sympathetic activation, and hyperuricaemia (30). Causes of MetS include poor dietary habits, insufficient physical activity, excessive alcohol usage, and inadequate amounts of sleep (30). Despite this, mitochondrial dysfunction has been deemed the primary causative factor in the pathophysiology of almost all the consequences of MetS, including obesity, type 2 diabetes, dyslipidaemia, and cardiovascular illnesses. This is because mitochondrial dysfunction causes an imbalance between the production of energy and its utilization (32). The partial reduction of oxygen in the mitochondria during OXPHOS generates ROS, such as superoxide anion ($\cdot O_2^-$), hydrogen peroxide (H_2O_2), and hydroxyl radicals ($\cdot OH$), designated as "primary" ROS (33). The excessive generation of superoxide anions leads to the interaction of the anions with other compounds to generate "secondary" ROS (34). These ROS are beneficial in cell signalling pathways and regulate biological and physiological processes. The cell's antioxidant systems keep ROS levels at safe concentrations (35) and include enzyme-based systems, such as superoxide dismutase (SOD), peroxiredoxins, catalase, glutathione peroxidase, and non-enzyme-based systems, including several vitamins, polyphenols, and coenzyme Q_{10} (CoQ_{10}) (33). Sometimes, due to disrupted mitochondrial processes, such as impaired fission/fusion, imbalances arise between ROS production and the ROS scavenging capacity of the antioxidant systems, resulting in the excessive generation of ROS and a state of oxidative stress (OS) (36). Cigarette smoke, ultraviolet (UV) radiation, heavy metal ions, ozone, allergies, medicines, poisons, pollutants, pesticides, and insecticides are all examples of exogenous sources that have been linked to ROS production and oxidative stress (OS) (37, 38).

Reduced ATP synthesis, disturbed calcium homeostasis, and other alterations in energy metabolism, all of which are implicated in type 2 diabetes, obesity, and cardiovascular disease (CVD), have been linked to oxidative stress (39). ROS, during periods of oxidative stress, are also able to interact with mitochondrial DNA (mtDNA) molecules, causing damage to the nitrogenous bases, purine and pyrimidine, and the deoxyribose backbone (27).

So far, therapies for the management of mitochondrial dysfunction have shown promise in reversing MetS. Antioxidant therapies have been reported to manage the overproduction of ROS and reduce ROS-related toxicity in the mitochondria; hence, these therapies are mostly used for the treatment of mitochondrial diseases (40). For instance, the powerful ubiquinone antioxidant CoQ10 has been shown to have considerable protective effects on the mitochondria of pancreatic beta cells when they are subjected to oxidative stress (41). It has also been claimed that taking CoQ10 supplements can relieve clinical symptoms of metabolic disorders and restore electron flow in the body, both of which are related to a lack of CoQ10 (42). Another antioxidant that is typically utilized in the treatment of mitochondrial dysfunction is vitamin B1 (also known as thiamine). It has been demonstrated that vitamin B1 raises the activity level of the enzyme pyruvate dehydrogenase and causes the oxidative breakdown of pyruvate. Vitamin B1 may be used alone or in conjunction with other medications. It has been observed that giving adult patients with Leigh syndrome who also have subacute severe brainstem encephalopathy a combination supplement that contains CoQ10, carnitine, thiamine, and vitamins C and E results in a considerable improvement in the patient's clinical symptoms (43). In addition, restoring glutathione levels through cysteine supplementation in patients with glutathione deficiency was shown to eliminate excessive ROS production and improve mitochondrial function (44). Another powerful antioxidant, lipoic acid is a cofactor of pyruvate dehydrogenase and alpha-ketoglutarate dehydrogenase. Its primary purpose is to lower oxidative stress indicators (45, 46). In individuals with mitochondrial disorders, lipoic acid is typically used in combination with other antioxidants (47). It has been demonstrated in some studies that taking lipoic acid, creatine monohydrate, and CoQ10 together is an effective method for lowering oxidative stress indicators (42, 46, 48). It has been demonstrated that the production of nitric oxide (NO) can be revived with the help of NO precursors, like citrulline and arginine. Therefore, citrulline and arginine have a curative effect on symptoms associated with a lack of NO in mitochondrial disorders (49). Nevertheless, a large cohort of subjects with mitochondrial diseases that are not related to antioxidant deficiencies do not respond well to antioxidant therapy (50). For the treatment of these disorders, further treatments, such as gene therapy, mitochondria replacement therapy, cell replacement therapy, mitochondrial augmentation therapy, hypoxia therapy, and mtDNA base editing are being researched (51).

5.2 BIOCHEMICAL AND GENETIC PLAYERS IN MITOCHONDRIAL DYSFUNCTION

The mtDNA is circular (approximately 16.5 kb) with no introns and requires about 100 nuclear-encoded proteins for transcription and translation (52). The limited repair mechanisms of mtDNA predispose it to damage with a higher mutation rate (about 100–1,000 times greater) than the nuclear genome (53, 54). Additionally, the proximity of mtDNA to the source of oxidants, and the absence of histone-like protective proteins predispose it to further mutations (55). Mitochondrial DNA is almost exclusively maternally transmitted; hence, acquired mutations are likely to be transferred to the offspring (56), causing mitochondrial dysfunction and diseases (57). Several mtDNA mutations have been implicated in mitochondria diseases such as mitochondrial encephalopathy, lactic acidosis, and stroke-like episodes (MELAS) syndrome; myoclonic epilepsy with ragged red fibres (MERRF) syndrome; neuropathy ataxia retinitis pigmentosa (NARP) syndrome; and Leber's hereditary optic neuropathy (LHON) syndrome. For example, mutations in the transfer RNA (tRNA) genes, such as MTTL1, POLG, and BCS1L, have been implicated in MELAS syndrome, a mitochondrial disease of the nervous system and muscles (58). Furthermore, mutations of the mtDNA lysine tRNA gene, such as m.8344A>G, m.8356T>C, m.8363G>A, m.3243A>G, m.3255G>A, and m.3291T>C, have been implicated in MERRF syndrome, a multisystem mitochondrial syndrome characterized by progressive myoclonus and seizure (59). A thymine to guanine and thymine to cytosine point mutation at nucleotide 8993 position of the MT-ATP6 gene (m.8993T>G) and (m.8993T>C), and a guanine to adenine substitution at nucleotide 14459 position of the MT-ND6 gene (m.14459G>A), have both been linked to NARP syndrome, a progressive neurodegenerative disease characterized by neurological and cognitive impairments and seizures (60). Moreover, mtDNA missense point mutations at nucleotide positions m.3460G>A, m.11778G>A, and m.14484T>C have been implicated in LHON syndrome, one of the most prevalent forms of hereditary optic neuropathy that results in a loss of central vision on both sides (61). Likewise, heterozygous missense mutations in the LIAS, LIPT1, and LIPT2 genes have been implicated in aberrant lipoic acid metabolism as a consequence of mitochondrial dysfunction and diseases (62). Other mutations such as those in peroxin genes have also been associated with both non-functional peroxisomes and mitochondrial dysfunction, resulting in peroxisomal biogenesis disorders (PBDs), characterized by profound developmental and neurological phenotypes (63).

Segregation of mtDNA before transcription is usually affected by mitochondrial dynamics such as fusion, fission, movement, and mitophagy; thus, variance exists in the severity of possible mutations in potential offspring who can become heteroplasmic (presence of both normal and mutant mtDNA) or homoplasmic (presence of a pure population of either normal or mutant mtDNA) (64). The clinical severity of mitochondrial illnesses is determined by several factors, including the types of mutations present, as well as the degree of heteroplasmy that is present. Therefore, the illness phenotype will manifest itself once the biochemical threshold for the percentage of mutant mtDNA has been exceeded (65). The cell and tissue types also contribute to the threshold value, which is usually between 60% and 90% (66). Errors in the OXPHOS pathway of the mitochondria may result in increased ROS production and consequently changes in gene expression (67). A switch from respiration to glycolysis to compensate for the ATP shortfall has been reported to be caused by genetic or functional deficiencies in the ETC of cells. This results in higher-than-normal lactate levels, which predispose tissues to acidification (68). Mutations in some nuclear genes, such as *COQ2*, *PDSS1/2*, and *ADCK3/CABC1*, which encode for enzymes involved in the biosynthesis of mitochondrial CoQ$_{10}$, have been implicated in CoQ$_{10}$ deficiencies leading to several mitochondrial diseases (69). Recent data also highlights the role of spontaneous mtDNA mutations in the onset of insulin resistance through disruption of the mitochondrial ETC, which increases the NADH/NAD$^+$ ratio and reduces muscle oxidative capacity, thus impairing β-oxidation and increasing fatty acid levels, which consequently result in insulin resistance and type 2 diabetes (70, 71). Environmental factors, such as ultraviolet (UV) exposure, smoking, alcohol consumption, pesticide exposure, use of antiretroviral drugs, exposure to industrial toxins, and exposure to other chemicals, may contribute to mitochondrial dysfunction (67). Mitochondrial DNA (mtDNA) can be epigenetically modified by environmental influences via methylation, long and short noncoding RNAs, and post-translational alterations of nucleoid proteins, making them more susceptible to a wide range of illnesses (72). The types of mtDNA damage mostly implicated in mitochondrial dysfunction include alkylation damage (may result from the interaction of DNA with endogenous molecules), hydrolytic damage (through the action of N-glycosylases), the formation of adducts (endogenous factors, such as reactive intermediate products of diethylstilbestrol metabolization), mismatches (mostly during replication), and DNA strand breaks (due to ineffective base excision repair or through oxidative stress) (53, 73–75).

5.3 ENVIRONMENTAL FACTORS IN MITOCHONDRIAL DYSFUNCTION

Research suggests that mitochondrial damage and dysfunction can be caused by environmental toxicants, such as polycyclic aromatic hydrocarbons (PAHs), air pollutants, heavy metals, endocrine-disrupting substances, pesticides, UV radiation, nanomaterials, and infection (37, 38, 76). Markers of mitochondrial dysfunction, such as changes in mtDNA copy number (mtDNAcn), higher mtDNA mutation load (heteroplasmy), increased cardiolipin and calcium levels, circulating cell-free mitochondria and cell-free mtDNA fragments, and increased 8-hydroxy-2-deoxyguanosine (8-OHdG) levels, have been observed in persons exposed to these environmental toxicants (37, 37, 76). A summary of how environmental factors cause mitochondrial dysfunction is shown in Table 5.1.

Tobacco use, vehicle exhaust fumes, the production of coke and coal tar, and emissions from industrial power generators and incinerators are the primary sources of PAHs. PAHs are a leading cause of persistent environmental pollution. PAHs primarily originate from the incomplete combustion of fossil fuels, wood, and petroleum products (77). PAHs are organic and are made up of multiple aromatic rings containing only carbons and hydrogens (78). PAHs such as benzo[a]pyrene, anthracene, benz[a]anthrancene, fluoranthene, fluorene, pyrene, naphthalene, and chrysene may come into contact with humans through dietary sources, soil, drinking water, air, etc. (79). PAH exposure has been linked to many different disorders that affect humans, including cancer, obstructive lung diseases, cardiovascular disease, reproductive toxicity, carcinogenicity, genotoxicity, immunotoxicity, teratogenicity, systemic inflammation, endocrine-disrupting effects, and mitochondrial dysfunction (79–81). The lipophilic nature of PAHs results in them being easily

63

Table 5.1 A summary of how environmental factors cause mitochondrial dysfunction

Factor	Mechanism	Refs
Polycyclic aromatic hydrocarbons	Generation of ROS causing changes in mtDNAcn	(83)
Toxic heavy metals	Production of excess ROS, decreasing the transmembrane potential and ATP levels of the mitochondria	(96)
Endocrine-disrupting chemicals	Alterations in mitochondrial biogenesis, bioenergetics, the rate of decline in the mitochondrial membrane potential, mitophagy, and apoptosis	(109)
Pesticides	Increase the mRNA expression of induced nitric oxide synthase (iNOS), and further increase NO levels in the plasma	(124)
Ultraviolet radiations	mtDNA deletion	(128)
Nanomaterials	ROS generation, and inhibition of mitochondrial membrane potential	(140)
Pathogens	Damage mitochondria, causing high levels of mitochondrial cell-free DNA	(147)

attracted to the mitochondria, where they bind to the mtDNA, causing damage (82). In the mitochondria, the cytochrome P450, aldo-keto reductase, and/or manganese superoxide dismutase systems, in an attempt to bioactivate PAHs, make them more toxic, leading to further organelle damage and the production of ROS (76). In their study, Bhargava et al. found that PAH exposure caused oxidative damage in blood cells, as well as having an impact on the mitochondrial redox machinery. This led to an increased accumulation of reactive oxygen species (ROS) (83). The accumulation of ROS and the resultant oxidative stress within the mitochondria triggers mtDNAcn changes in populations affected by PAH exposure (84).

Similarly, toxic heavy metals such as mercury, cadmium, arsenic, chromium, nickel, copper, and lead are very common in the environment (85). The accumulation of these metals in the body compromises health. Lead poisoning, for example, can cause disturbances in the central nervous system, as well as seizures and coma. Lead also suppresses heme production (86). Copper poisoning has been associated with liver and gastrointestinal diseases (87). Nickel has been implicated in fibrosis, chronic bronchitis and emphysema (88), and cobalt in severe cardiomyopathy (89). Humans are particularly vulnerable to the toxic effects of heavy metals because these substances alter the structure and function of essential cellular components, such as mitochondria, nuclei, lysosomes, cell membranes, and enzymes (90). Heavy metal toxicity resulting from the utilization of metals in industrial operations has been linked to mitochondrial dysfunction (91). For example, prolonged mercury exposure has been reported to cause an accumulation of mercury in the mitochondria, resulting in ultrastructural mitochondrial changes and depolarization of the mitochondria membrane, with a concomitant reduction in the ATP production and Ca^{2+} buffering capacity of the mitochondria (92, 93). Mercury is also thought to increase ROS production, further disrupting mitochondrial structure and function (94).

In humans, higher 8-OHd levels have been observed in populations with high cadmium exposure (95). Cadmium has also been shown to stimulate the production of excess ROS and a decrease in the transmembrane potential and ATP levels of the mitochondria (96), possibly through the suppression of ADP, which is known to stimulate ion permeability of the inner mitochondrial membrane (97). The loss of mitochondrial membrane potential results in the release of cytochrome c and the activation of caspases, leading to apoptosis of the mitochondria (98). Additionally, it has been observed that treatment with cadmium inhibits the enzymes involved in the mitochondrial respiratory chain in human osteoblasts (99), thus causing organelle swelling and respiratory difficulties in rats (100). Heavy metals have also been reported to interact with proteins and DNA, resulting in alterations in protein synthesis, enzyme activity, nucleic acid functions, DNA repair, DNA stability, protein phosphatase 2 A (PP2A) activity, cellular iron homeostasis, nuclear factor kappa B (NF-kB), p53 (TP53), and Jun N-terminal kinase (JNK) pathways, eventually causing mutations and cell death (101).

Endocrine-disrupting chemicals (EDCs) are yet another group of exogenous chemicals that have been implicated in mitochondrial dysfunction. It is well established that they inhibit the functioning of hormones, which raises the probability of unfavourable effects on one's health (102). EDCs, such as phthalates, parabens, and bisphenols, are mostly used in pharmaceuticals, cosmetics, personal care products, and as plasticizers (103–105). EDCs have been reported to affect different cellular processes, including those responsible for energy production and utilization, thus contributing to the disruption of energy homeostasis and the subsequent loss of mitochondrial function (106). Phthalates and bisphenols exposure has also been associated with changes in mtDNA methylation (107). Di(2-ethylhexyl) phthalate (DEHP), monoethyl hexyl phthalate (MEHP), and bisphenol A (BPA) have all been linked with elevated oxidative stress and changes in redox homeostasis, resulting in the production of extracellular superoxide and changes in mtDNAcn (76, 107, 108). Similarly, BPA exposure has been linked to changes in mitochondrial biogenesis, bioenergetics, the reduction of the mitochondrial membrane potential (MMP), mitophagy, and apoptosis (109). The expression of regulatory genes associated with mitochondrial energy metabolism, fusion and fission, and mitochondrial fatty acid metabolism is thought to be altered as a result of BPA exposure as well, according to a recent study (110).

Furthermore, pesticides have been reported to have effects on the membrane potential of the mitochondria, cause mtDNA and oxidative damage, and deregulate mitochondrial ATP production (111). Pesticides are highly lipophilic chemicals that are known to have a strong affinity for the mitochondria (112). It has been established that the pesticide rotenone can prevent oxidative phosphorylation and interfere with ATP synthesis. It does this by preventing the transport of electrons from iron-sulfur clusters to ubiquinone in the mitochondrial respiratory chain, which results in the creation of reactive oxygen species (ROS) (113, 114). Rotenone was also shown to destabilize the activity of microtubules, which disrupted microtubule assembly (115), and consequently apoptosis and cellular senescence (116). Paraquat, at high concentrations, was reported to cause mitophagy and apoptosis by increasing free radicals and oxidative stress levels, which resulted in cytochrome c release and caspase-9 recruitment (117). Dichlorodiphenyltrichloroethane (DDT) was also shown to upregulate p53, NFκB, and caspase 3 in PC12 cells, and depress the transmembrane potential of the mitochondria, resulting in the release of Ca2+ into the cytosol and causing apoptosis (118–120). Diquat (1,1-ethylene-2,2-bipyridinium ion) (DQ) has been shown to generate oxidative stress, resulting from ROS and reactive nitrogen species in hepatocytes (121, 122). It was also found that exposure to permethrin (PER) enhanced the mRNA expression of induced nitric oxide synthase (iNOS), which in turn increased the levels of NO in the plasma of rats that had been given a modest dose (123, 124). The presence of NO and NO metabolites in the blood may trigger the generation of RNS, leading to multiple organ damage (122). Exposure to the insecticide cypermethrin (CYP) was similarly shown to cause a significant increase in the plasma concentration of 8-nitroguanine (8-NO2Gua) in rats when compared with the control group (125).

Ultraviolet radiations (UVRs) form a large component of the electromagnetic waves emitted by the sun and are subdivided into UVA radiation (320–400 nm), UVB radiation (280–320 nm), and UVC radiation (100–280 nm (126)). UVR wavelengths less than 200 nm are effectively eliminated by the earth's atmospheric ozone layer. A fraction of wavelengths of approximately 300–320 nm, however, can penetrate the ozone to reach the earth's surface (127). Exposure to these UVRs can cause substantial damage to the skin via direct DNA damage or oxidative stress and has been implicated in several health outcomes, including cancer and photoageing (128). A hallmark of photoageing, mostly not observed in chronological ageing, is large-scale mtDNA deletion (128). An earlier study reported a tenfold increase in mtDNA deletion in photoaged skin cells compared to skin cells protected from the sun (129); these UV-induced deletions were observed to linger on for several years, increasing thirty- to fortyfold even in the absence of further exposure (129, 130). Similarly, Powers et al. observed significantly higher mtDNA deletions in subjects in high sun exposure habitats compared to low sun exposure habitats (131). According to a recent study, the DNA of primary mouse embryonic fibroblasts, human foreskin fibroblasts, and human epidermal keratinocytes can be irreversibly altered by UV nail polish dryer radiation (132). DNA damage in mitochondria has thus been proposed as a biomarker of ultraviolet radiation (UVR) exposure in human skin (133, 134).

Nanomaterials are also deeply implicated in mitochondrial dysfunction. They consist of particles ranging from 1 to 100 nm in size; they usually occur naturally or are synthesized, and can be found in cosmetics, tires, and electronics (76). The toxic effects of nanomaterials (silver nanoparticles, hydroxyapatite nanoparticles, cadmium telluride quantum dots, and carbon nanotubules) are thought to be caused by physical stress rather than chemical stress. This causes the mitochondria to enlarge, the mitochondrial membrane potential to be disrupted, the intracellular calcium levels to change, the cellular respiration to be impaired, and the levels of adenosine triphosphate to drop (135–137). Several other studies support the deleterious effect of nanomaterials on the mitochondria (138–140). Skalska et al. demonstrated that exposure to low-dose silver nanoparticles led to the induction of autophagy in adult rat brains as a result of partial mitochondrial dysfunction (139). Additionally, titanium dioxide nanoparticles were observed to facilitate ROS generation and inhibit mitochondrial membrane potential, causing mitochondrial dysfunction (140).

Interestingly, pathogens, especially bacteria, have also been implicated in mitochondrial dysfunction. Bacteria have been reported to manipulate or subvert the mitochondria to ensure their intracellular survival, thus leading to mitochondria-induced cell death (141). For instance, the mitochondrial dysfunction that results from the formation of reactive oxygen species (ROS), the depolarization of mitochondrial membrane potential, and the depletion of the ATP pool can be caused by the N-acetylglucosamine-binding protein of *Vibrio cholerae* (142). Likewise, the primary quorum-sensing molecule, N-(3-Oxododecanoyl)-L-homoserine lactone, of *Pseudomonas aeruginosa* has been shown to disrupt mitochondrial morphology, attenuate mitochondrial bioenergetics, and induce mitochondrial DNA oxidative injury by impairing the expression of peroxisome proliferator-activated receptor-γ coactivator-1α (PGC-1α), and its downstream effectors in primary lung epithelial cells (143). *Escherichia coli*'s mitochondrial-associated protein (MAP) has also been reported to target the mitochondrion and disrupt the mitochondrial membrane potential, causing the discharge of mitochondrial Ca^{2+} into the host cell cytoplasm, leading to apoptosis (144). Macrophages exposed to the outer membrane vesicles of *Neisseria gonorrhoeae*, *Escherichia coli*, and *Pseudomonas aeruginosa* were shown to present with mitochondrial apoptosis and nucleotide-binding oligomerization domain (NOD), leucine-rich repeats (LRR), and pyrin domain-containing protein 3 inflammasome activation (145). Additionally, the vacuolating cytotoxin-A (VacA) protein of *Helicobacter pylori* was demonstrated to cause mitochondrial depolarization, retard the import of PTEN-induced kinase 1 into the damaged mitochondria, and evoke mitophagy (146). High levels of mitochondrial cell-free DNA were also observed in pulmonary tuberculosis, which decreased after treatment (147). Thus, controlling the negative effects of these environmental factors on mitochondrial function will reduce the incidence of diseases, including MetS, associated with mitochondrial dysfunction and improve overall health.

5.4 METABOLIC SYNDROME: A Collapsed Link between the Powerhouse and the Consumers

MetS involves a cascade of molecular events, including insulin resistance, chronic inflammation, and neurohormonal activation, which results from increased caloric intake and reduced physical activity, encouraging the storage of lipids and obesity (29). Abnormalities in pancreatic β-cell function and insulin uptake by adipocytes, myocytes, and hepatocytes have been linked to diabetes and related complications (148). Type 2 diabetes, which typically manifests in middle age or later, results from a complicated interaction between obesity, insufficient physical activity, food, and genetic predisposition, resulting in decreased tissue sensitivity to insulin and inadequate insulin secretion (148). Excess lipids, especially diacylglycerol (DAG) and ceramides, can cause insulin resistance by suppressing insulin signalling in the skeletal muscle and liver (149, 149, 150).

Under optimal conditions, insulin increases the entry of glucose into muscle and liver cells, thus suppressing lipolysis and hepatic gluconeogenesis (151). Insulin resistance, however, creates a state of hyperinsulinaemia, increased lipase activity, and lipolysis in adipose tissue, with a resultant increase in free fatty acid (FFA) levels in the plasma (152). The excess FFAs are transported to the liver, where an increased synthesis of very low-density lipoprotein (VLDL) and triglycerides occurs, further inhibiting the antipolytic effect of insulin (153). FFAs are also able to suppress the activation of protein kinase in the muscle, while increasing protein kinase activation in the liver, thus reducing glucose uptake and promoting gluconeogenesis and lipogenesis, which ultimately results in hyperglycaemia (154). Recurrent hyperglycaemia is known to overstimulate pancreatic beta cells, which causes pancreatic beta cell failure and type 2 diabetes mellitus (T2DM) (155). Chronic hyperglycaemia causes excessive ROS formation, oxidative stress, and ultimately apoptosis of beta cells, all of which have been implicated in reduced beta cell mass, insulin resistance, and T2DM (156). The decrease in insulin's vasodilatory impact and the vasoconstriction generated by FFAs have both been linked to insulin resistance, which has been linked to hypertension (157). An increased risk of CVD has also been linked to insulin resistance, which has been shown to enhance the following: sympathetic activity; salt reabsorption in the kidneys; serum viscosity; the induction of a prothrombotic state; and the release of pro-inflammatory cytokines from adipose tissue (158–160).

The available literature suggests that intra-abdominal fat (visceral fat) is more associated with insulin resistance than subcutaneous fat, possibly because of the higher lipolytic activity, lower adiponectin levels, leptin resistance, and increased inflammatory cytokines of intra-abdominal fat (161–163). Because of its central location, visceral fat is thought to be more metabolically active and to constantly release free fatty acids (FFAs) into the portal circulation, putting one at risk of certain conditions associated with metabolic syndrome. These include, but are not limited to, type 2 diabetes, dyslipidaemia (hypertriglyceridaemia, a high level of small dense low-density lipoprotein (LDL) particles, and a low level of high-density lipoprotein (HDL) cholesterol), insulin resistance, and non-alcoholic fatty liver disease (NAFLD) (164). Increases in NADH and $FADH_2$ production as a result of the accumulation of fat in adipocytes has been observed to cause a subsequent increase in electron supply to the ETC of the mitochondria, which can lead to the generation of ROS (165). When ROS production overwhelms the antioxidant defence systems, oxidative stress occurs, which further predisposes a person to MetS (166). Inflammatory signalling mechanisms, including canonical NF-kB activation and downstream inflammatory gene induction, proteasome activity, antioxidant gene transcription, inflammasome activation, and cytokine secretion, are disrupted when there is an excessive amount of ROS production (167). If the issue is not rectified, the persistent buildup of lipids in adipocytes will, over time, lead to adipocyte stress, as well as hypoxia, in the surrounding tissue. This will eventually result in the necrosis of adipocytes and the infiltration of macrophages, which will result in systemic inflammation (168).

Aside from their role in fat storage, adipose tissues are also endocrine glands that modulate metabolism (169). Adipose tissues are known to secrete adipokines, which function at the autocrine/paracrine and endocrine levels, and also express numerous receptors that facilitate their interaction with signals from traditional hormone systems and the central nervous system (CNS) (169). Thus, adipose tissues are closely involved in energy metabolism, neuroendocrine function, and immune function (169). A deregulated adipokine secretory pattern has been observed in hypertrophied and stressed adipocytes; this is marked by the increased secretion of proinflammatory and prothrombic adipokines, such as leptin, interferon-γ, and resistin, and a decrease in anti-inflammatory adipokine, such as adiponectin, which can increase insulin sensitivity (170, 171). Eventually, the imbalances between pro-inflammatory and anti-inflammatory adipokines make the local and systemic inflammatory state worse, which in turn causes insulin resistance, hepatic steatosis, endothelial dysfunction, hypertension, and atherosclerosis, which are the classic components of metabolic syndrome (MetS) (172, 173). Adipose tissue has also been implicated in obesity-associated renin–angiotensin–aldosterone system (RAAS) overactivity and has been shown to contribute to increased circulating levels of Ang II and aldosterone and potential impairment of the metabolism of Ang II to Ang (1–7) (174). In addition to causing sodium retention and sympatho-excitation, it is believed that the raised levels of Ang II and aldosterone impair (insulin-associated) microvascular function and modify arterial stiffness, leading to hypertension (174).

The role of mitochondrial dysfunction in the pathophysiology of type 2 diabetes, obesity, cardiovascular disease, and stroke has been well documented (71, 175, 176). There are over 20 mtDNA mutations implicated in diabetes; the commonest is the A to G replacement at position 3243 (A3243G), which encodes the tRNA Leu (UUR) gene (177). Maturity-onset diabetes of the young (MODY) types 1, 3, and 4 have also been closely associated with mitochondrial dysfunction (178). Mitochondrial diseases such as MELAS syndrome and maternally inherited diabetes (MIDD), both characterized by the same A3243G mutation in the mtDNA, have been implicated in mitochondrial diabetes (179, 180). A study by Park et al. showed that an mtDNA 16189 T>C variation, found in the control region of mtDNA transcription and replication, is strongly associated with an increased risk of type 2 diabetes among Asians (181). It is believed that the mutations in mtDNA are responsible for insulin resistance due to their effect on the efficiency of oxidative phosphorylation. This, in turn, leads to decreased membrane potential and ATP synthesis, as well as the increased formation of reactive oxygen species (ROS) (182). Generally, type 2 diabetic patients are found to have reduced mitochondrial respiration, reduced ATP production, and reduced mitochondrial density (183).

Adipose tissue is one of the tissues that is most negatively altered during mitochondria dysfunction because it strongly relies on mitochondrial function for optimal activity (184). Mounting evidence supports the role of obesity in defective mitochondrial biogenesis, which presents as mitochondrial dysfunction, oxidative metabolism, low mitochondrial gene expression, and reduced ATP generation (185–187). A study by Cioffi et al. reported increased mitochondrial reactive oxygen species (ROS) production, mitochondrial DNA (mtDNA) damage, reduced mitochondrial biogenesis, reduced mtDNA copy numbers, reduced mtDNA repair, altered mitochondrial fusion, and impaired mitophagy in obesity (188). An earlier study conducted by Valerio and colleagues indicates that TNF-α inhibits mitochondrial synthesis and function in the tissues of obese rats by downregulating endothelial nitric oxide synthase (eNOS) expression. This finding hints at a unique pathophysiological pathway that contributes to the maintenance of obesity (189). A reduction in mtDNA, respiratory protein, and mtDNA transcription factor A (Tfam) gene expressions was also observed in obese mice (32).

Mitochondrial dysfunction has been associated with numerous cardiac diseases, including atherosclerosis, heart failure, and hypertension, usually through insufficient cellular energy production and uncontrolled production of ROS, which eventually create a state of oxidative stress (175). It is believed that stress or the presence of vasoactive substances might impact the uncoupling of eNOS, the primary producer of nitric oxide (NO). This results in the generation of superoxide anion in place of NO, which leads to an increase in the number of reactive oxygen species produced in vascular endothelial cells (175). Additionally, oxidative stress originating from NADPH oxidases, xanthine oxidase, and mitochondrial ETC has been implicated in the pathogenesis of atherosclerosis through its signalling role in endothelial cells, smooth muscular cells, and fibroblasts (190). It was observed in an earlier study that a malfunction in mitochondrial ATP synthase and mitochondrial Ca^{2+} overload in cardiomyocytes were strongly associated with the onset of hypertension (191). Mutations in mitochondrial DNA (mtDNA) have been linked to a variety of diseases, including heart disease. Patients with a history of cardiovascular disease-related adverse clinical events had significantly lower mtDNA copy numbers (192). Similarly, mutations $16145\,G > A$ and m.16311 T > C (both fixed and in heteroplasmy) in the mtDNA control region were found to be significantly different when stroke and myocardial infarction patients were compared to healthy subjects (193). A study conducted by Zhang et al. also reported a possible link between a 15910C > T tRNA[Thr] mutation and coronary heart disease (194). Thus, mitochondrial dysfunction can be seen to play a vital role in the pathophysiology of insulin resistance, T2DM, obesity, and cardiovascular disease, which are classic risk factors for MetS and may therefore be considered a therapeutic target in metabolic syndrome.

5.5 CURRENT RECOMMENDATIONS FOR IMPROVING METABOLIC SYNDROME

The most important strategy in the management of MetS involves aggressive lifestyle changes such as non-smoking, increased physical activity, and a healthy diet. According to a paper by Pérez-Martnez et al. on lifestyle guidelines for the prevention and management of metabolic syndrome, an individual-centred weight loss programme based on a strict diet plan and exercise, taking into consideration the fitness level and comorbidities of the individual, must be adopted for the prevention or management of MetS (195). Moderate consumption of olive oil (20–40 g/d), along with a wide variety of legumes, cereals (whole grains), fruits, vegetables, fish, nuts, and dairy products, as well as a small amount of red wine and/or beer, has been shown to help manage metabolic syndrome (MetS) (195). Alternatively, dietary patterns including the Dietary Approaches to Stop Hypertension (DASH), new Nordic, and vegetarian diets have all shown considerable promise in the management of MetS (195). Likewise, the American Diabetes Association (ADA) recommends ≥5% weight loss for overweight and obese persons with type 2 diabetes, with additional weight loss usually proving beneficial (196).

5.6 MANAGEMENT OPTIONS FOR TYPE 2 DIABETES

In addition to lifestyle changes, some individuals may require pharmacological interventions for the management of type 2 diabetes. Such interventions include sulfonylureas, meglitinides, metformin (a biguanide), thiazolidinediones (TZDs), alpha-glucosidase inhibitors, dipeptidyl peptidase IV (DPP-4) inhibitors, bile acid sequestrants, dopamine agonists, sodium-glucose transport protein 2 (SGLT2) inhibitors, and oral glucagon-like peptide. Injectable versions of amylin and other glucagon-like peptide 1 (GLP-1) receptor agonists are available, however. Treatment of type 2 diabetes might involve a single medicine from one of these categories (monotherapy) or two or more treatments from separate classifications, each of which works in a slightly different way (197–199). High-efficacy glucose-lowering pharmacological agents, such as the GLP-1 RAs dulaglutide (high dose), semaglutide, GIP, GLP-1 RA tirzepatide, and insulin, have proven to be very effective in the management of type 2 diabetes (200). Metformin, on the other hand, is a medicine that is widely used because it is effective, safe, and economical. It can reduce the risk of cardiovascular events as well as the risk of death, and it is available in two different formulations: an immediate-release version that is taken twice daily and an extended-release form that is taken once daily (201, 202). Metformin, when used as first-line therapy, has benefits for glycated haemoglobin, weight, and cardiovascular disease-related mortality. This is in contrast to the effects of sulfonylureas, which are negative (203, 204). Insulin, on the other hand, is particularly successful in situations when other agents are ineffective and is used as part of a combination regimen when hyperglycaemia is severe. It is particularly favoured when catabolic traits, such as weight loss, hypertriglyceridaemia, or ketosis, are present. Insulin therapy may be started in patients who present with blood glucose levels of less than 300 mg/dL (16.7 mmol/L), an A1C of more than 10% (86 mmol/mol), polyuria or polydipsia, and indications of catabolism (weight loss). Polyuria and polydipsia are also symptoms of diabetes (200).

5.7 MANAGEMENT OPTIONS FOR HYPERTENSION AND CARDIOVASCULAR DISEASES

According to the report published in 2019 by the American College of Cardiology and the American Heart Association on the prevention, detection, evaluation, and management of high blood pressure in adults, prehypertensive patients who do not have comorbidities such as heart failure, prior myocardial infarction or stroke, high coronary risk status, diabetes mellitus, or chronic renal disease may respond well to lifestyle measures such as maintaining a normal body weight and a diet that is rich in vegetable content. Alterations to one's way of life, in addition to medical treatment, are strongly advised for individuals who have hypertension (205).

Classes of antihypertensive agents currently in use for the management of hypertension include drugs targeting the renin–angiotensin–aldosterone system (angiotensin-converting enzyme inhibitors (ACEi), angiotensin receptor blockers (ARBs), renin inhibitors, calcium channel blockers (CCBs), and diuretics); drug classes targeting adrenergic receptors (α-blockers, combined α/β-blockers, α2-adrenergic receptor agonists); and vasodilators (206). Among these drug therapies, diuretics, CCBs, ACEi, and ARBs are highly recommended for the management of high blood pressure (207), and ACEi have become the first choice for managing hypertension in diabetic patients struggling with glycaemic control (206).

5.8 MANAGEMENT OPTIONS FOR DYSLIPIDAEMIA

The European Society of Cardiology (ESC) and the European Atherosclerosis Society (EAS) recommend an LDL-C < 55 mg/dL for those at very high risk in primary and secondary prevention (Class I recommendation), and a goal of <40 mg/dL for those with a second atherosclerotic CVD event within 2 years of the incident event (Class IIb) (207, 208, 208). A wide range of therapies is available for lowering cholesterol to the recommended levels. These include statins, ezetimibe, proprotein convertase subtilisin/kexin type 9 (PCSK9) inhibitors, fibrates, niacin, lomitapide, and mipomersen (209). Statins, which are HMG-CoA reductase inhibitors, are the gold standard therapy for lowering LDL cholesterol and triglyceride levels, followed by ezetimibe, fibrates, and nicotinic acid, which are mostly used as second-choice drugs in combination with statins if the lipid target cannot be reached in high cardiovascular risk patients or statin-intolerant patients (209, 210). Anti-PCSK9 drugs are an alternative option for high cardiovascular risk patients with familial hypercholesterolemia (FH) and statin intolerance (211). Lomitapide and mipomersen, however, are indicated for use in patients with homozygous familial hypercholesterolemia; thus, they have a very narrow scope of use (212, 213).

5.9 MANAGEMENT OPTIONS FOR MITOCHONDRIAL DYSFUNCTION

Standard therapies for mitochondrial dysfunction rely on metabolic interventions like dietary changes, healthy lifestyle choices, medication, and exposure to hypoxia. These interventions typically aim to promote mitochondrial biogenesis, the nitric oxide synthase pathway, ATP synthesis, antioxidant defence, and the mitochondrial quality control pathway by promoting dynamics (fission/fusion events), as well as the degradation of damaged mitochondria (autophagy) (50). So far, these metabolic therapies have been ineffective in a large cohort of patients because of their non-selectiveness, low mitochondrial targeting, and the poor overlap of their action with disease-causing mechanisms (214, 215). Among all the approved drugs for mitochondrial dysfunction, none has succeeded in curing or slowing the progression of mitochondrial diseases (216). Thus, there is an urgent need for more effective therapies for treating mitochondrial disorders. Gene therapy approaches have therefore been proposed as suitable therapeutic alternatives for treating mitochondria diseases (214, 216, 217). Various approaches to gene therapy include replacing a mutant gene with a healthy gene, "knocking out" or inactivating a mutated gene that is dysfunctional, and introducing new genes into cells to protect the cells from illnesses (218).

So far, gene delivery approaches in gene therapy use viral and non-viral delivery systems. The non-viral delivery approach uses natural or synthetic compounds (non-viral vectors), which are complexed with DNA, proteins, polymers, or lipids to form particles that can efficiently transfer genes into cells (219). These genes may be transferred into the cell using either physical or chemical methods. The physical methods (hydrodynamic or ballistic injection of DNA) mostly use a physical force to overcome cells' membrane barrier to enable intracellular gene transfer (220). The most straightforward and risk-free approach is to use physical means; nevertheless, these methods are linked to inefficient gene transport and a certain amount of cell damage at the discharge site (221). Alternatively, chemical methods use micelles of cationic surfactants, nanoparticles, and liposomes to effect the intracellular transfer of genes (222). Non-viral vectors are preferred to viral vectors because of their ease of production, reduced pathogenicity, low toxicity, and low cost (219). Currently, there is no approved non-viral vector for managing mitochondrial dysfunction, and viral gene delivery is still the mainstay (217).

Gene therapy approaches using viral vectors involve modifying some viruses, such as retrovirus, adenovirus, adeno-associated virus (AAV), herpes simplex virus, and lentiviruses, in the laboratory for use in gene therapy applications (218). A viral vector usually consists of the protein capsid and/or envelope that encapsulates the genetic cargo, the genetic payload of interest, and the "regulatory expression cassette", including enhancer/promoter/auxiliary elements that control the expression of the genes (217). Viral vectors are generally considered safe and effective delivery vehicles for clinical gene therapy; however, some viral vectors are considered potentially hazardous (223). Thus, engineering strategies geared towards the avoidance of viral replication, the promotion of viral inactivation, and the attenuation of the natural toxicity of viruses have been employed to ensure the safety of viral vectors without compromising their efficiency (224). Among all the viral vectors in preclinical and clinical trials, adeno-associated virus (AAV) has shown great promise (225). So far, the US Food and Drug Administration (FDA) has approved two AAV vector-based gene therapy products, namely, Luxturna and Zolgensma, for the management of some mitochondrial diseases (225). Since the year 2000, there has been a rise in the number of AAV vector-based gene therapy clinical trials initiated every year (226), so the probability of FDA approval for more gene therapy products for the management of mitochondria diseases is very high.

5.10 FUTURE PERSPECTIVE

Metabolic syndrome continues to be a significant risk factor for public health all over the world. It is projected that by the year 2050, obesity will be the leading cause of death (a 102.8% increase from 2019), followed by hypertension (a 61.4% increase), hyperlipidaemia (a 60.8% increase), type 2 diabetes (a 158.6% increase), and non-alcoholic fatty liver disease (a 158.4% increase), with men continuing to be disproportionately affected by all metabolic diseases (227). Notwithstanding the huge burden of metabolic syndrome, there is currently no effective therapy for the treatment of the condition, partly because of the numerous contributing factors implicated in the onset and progression of the disease. Central to these contributing factors is the issue of mitochondrial dysfunction, as outlined in this chapter.

Thus, to manage metabolic syndrome, effective therapies for the treatment of mitochondria dysfunction will be necessary. To this end, several advances have been made over the years and gene therapy approaches seem to hold great promise for the treatment of mitochondrial dysfunctions. Despite the challenges encountered by researchers in this area, we anticipate that the few successes will stimulate more studies that will be directed at understanding precisely how gene therapy can alter defective mitochondria and nuclear genes to mitigate the onset and progression of metabolic syndrome. We also envisage the identification of effective treatment options that could help in the management of persons with metabolic syndrome or persons who are at risk of metabolic syndrome. We believe that such interventions will close the gaps in the race to reduce the burden of metabolic syndrome.

REFERENCES

1. Judge A, Dodd MS. Metabolism. *Essays Biochem.* 2020 Aug 24;64(4):607–47.

2. Bartee L, Shriner W, Creech C. *Metabolism.* 2017 [cited 2023 Feb 2]; Available from: https://openoregon.pressbooks.pub/mhccmajorsbio/chapter/7-3-metabolism/

3. Panawala L. *Difference Between Substrate Level Phosphorylation and Oxidative Phosphorylation.* 2017 Oct 20.

4. Ahmad M, Wolberg A, Kahwaji CI. Biochemistry, electron transport chain. In: *StatPearls* [Internet]. Treasure Island (FL): StatPearls Publishing; 2022 [cited 2023 Feb 2]. Available from: http://www.ncbi.nlm.nih.gov/books/NBK526105/

5. Lee H, Jose PA. Coordinated contribution of NADPH oxidase- and mitochondria-derived reactive oxygen species in metabolic syndrome and its implication in renal dysfunction. *Front Pharmacol.* 2021 May 4;12:670076.

6. Zohoori FV. Chapter 1: Nutrition and diet. *Monogr Oral Sci.* 2020;28:1–13.

7. Nelson DL, Cox MM. *Lehninger Principles of Biochemistry.* W.H. Freeman; 2017, p. 1328.

8. Rehman I, Kerndt CC, Botelho S. Biochemistry, tertiary protein structure. In: *StatPearls* [Internet]. Treasure Island (FL): StatPearls Publishing; 2022 [cited 2023 Feb 2]. Available from: http://www.ncbi.nlm.nih.gov/books/NBK470269/

9. Alberts B, Johnson A, Lewis J, Raff M, Roberts K, Walter P. *Protein Function. Mol Biol Cell* 4th Ed [Internet]. 2002 [cited 2023 Feb 2]; Available from: https://www.ncbi.nlm.nih.gov/books/NBK26911/

10. Muñoz-Lasso DC, Romá-Mateo C, Pallardó FV, Gonzalez-Cabo P. Much more than a scaffold: Cytoskeletal proteins in neurological disorders. *Cells.* 2020 Feb;9(2):358.

11. Morris R, Black KA, Stollar EJ. Uncovering protein function: From classification to complexes. *Essays Biochem.* 2022 Aug 10;66(3):255–85.

12. Holesh JE, Aslam S, Martin A. Physiology, carbohydrates. In: *StatPearls* [Internet]. Treasure Island (FL): StatPearls Publishing; 2022 [cited 2023 Feb 2]. Available from: http://www.ncbi.nlm.nih.gov/books/NBK459280/

13. Hao Y, Yi Q, XiaoWu X, WeiBo C, GuangChen Z, XueMin C. Acetyl-CoA: An interplay between metabolism and epigenetics in cancer. *Front Mol Med [Internet].* 2022 [cited 2023 Feb 2];2. Available from: https://www.frontiersin.org/articles/10.3389/fmmed.2022.1044585

14. Ahmed S, Shah P, Ahmed O. Biochemistry, lipids. In: *StatPearls* [Internet]. Treasure Island (FL): StatPearls Publishing; 2022 [cited 2023 Feb 2]. Available from: http://www.ncbi.nlm.nih.gov/books/NBK525952/

15. Boucheniata C, Tessier N, Martel C. Editorial: Highlights in lipids in cardiovascular disease: 2021. *Front Cardiovasc Med [Internet].* 2022 [cited 2023 Feb 2];9. Available from: https://www.frontiersin.org/articles/10.3389/fcvm.2022.915262

16. Javadov S, Kozlov AV, Camara AKS. Mitochondria in health and diseases. *Cells.* 2020 May 9;9(5):1177.

17. Kühlbrandt W. Structure and function of mitochondrial membrane protein complexes. *BMC Biol.* 2015 Oct 29;13(1):89.

18. Chen MM, Li Y, Deng SL, Zhao Y, Lian ZX, Yu K. Mitochondrial function and reactive oxygen/nitrogen species in skeletal muscle. *Front Cell Dev Biol [Internet].* 2022 [cited 2023 Feb 2];10. Available from: https://www.frontiersin.org/articles/10.3389/fcell.2022.826981

19. Glancy B, Kim Y, Katti P, Willingham TB. The functional impact of mitochondrial structure across subcellular scales. *Front Physiol [Internet].* 2020 [cited 2023 Jan 16];11. Available from: https://www.frontiersin.org/articles/10.3389/fphys.2020.541040

20. Paraskevaidi M, Martin-Hirsch PL, Kyrgiou M, Martin FL. Underlying role of mitochondrial mutagenesis in the pathogenesis of a disease and current approaches for translational research. *Mutagenesis.* 2017 May 1;32(3):335–42.

21. Sainero-Alcolado L, Liaño-Pons J, Ruiz-Pérez MV, Arsenian-Henriksson M. Targeting mitochondrial metabolism for precision medicine in cancer. *Cell Death Differ.* 2022 Jul;29(7):1304–17.

22. Spinelli JB, Haigis MC. The multifaceted contributions of mitochondria to cellular metabolism. *Nat Cell Biol.* 2018 Jul;20(7):745–54.

23. Mohsen AW, Hatch GM, Leipnitz G, Wanders R, editors. Mitochondrial disorders: Biochemical and molecular basis of disease [Internet]. *Frontiers Media SA*; 2022 [cited 2023 Feb 16]. (Frontiers Research Topics). Available from: https://www.frontiersin.org/research-topics /13266/mitochondrial-disorders-biochemical-and-molecular-basis-of-disease

24. Dard L, Blanchard W, Hubert C, Lacombe D, Rossignol R. Mitochondrial functions and rare diseases. *Mol Aspects Med.* 2020 Feb;71:100842.

25. Tilokani L, Nagashima S, Paupe V, Prudent J. Mitochondrial dynamics: Overview of molecular mechanisms. *Essays Biochem.* 2018 Jul 20;62(3):341–60.

26. Avram VF, Merce AP, Hâncu IM, Bătrân AD, Kennedy G, Rosca MG, et al. Impairment of mitochondrial respiration in metabolic diseases: An overview. *Int J Mol Sci.* 2022 Aug 9;23(16):8852.

27. Li A, Zheng N, Ding X. Mitochondrial abnormalities: A hub in metabolic syndrome-related cardiac dysfunction caused by oxidative stress. *Heart Fail Rev.* 2022 Jul 1;27(4):1387–94.

28. Yang J, Guo Q, Feng X, Liu Y, Zhou Y. Mitochondrial Dysfunction in cardiovascular diseases: Potential targets for treatment. *Front Cell Dev Biol [Internet].* 2022 [cited 2023 Jan 16];10. Available from: https://www.frontiersin.org/articles/10.3389/fcell.2022.841523

29. Fahed G, Aoun L, Bou Zerdan M, Allam S, Bou Zerdan M, Bouferraa Y, et al. Metabolic syndrome: Updates on pathophysiology and management in 2021. *Int J Mol Sci.* 2022 Jan 12;23(2):786.

30. Dobrowolski P, Prejbisz A, Kuryłowicz A, Baska A, Burchardt P, Chlebus K, et al. Metabolic syndrome – A new definition and management guidelines. A joint position paper by the Polish Society of Hypertension, Polish Society for the Treatment of Obesity, Polish Lipid Association, Polish Association for Study of Liver, Polish Society of Family Medicine, Polish Society of Lifestyle Medicine, Division of Prevention and Epidemiology Polish Cardiac Society, "Club 30" Polish Cardiac Society, and Division of Metabolic and Bariatric Surgery Society of Polish Surgeons. *Arch Med Sci.* 2022 Sep 1;18(5):1133–56.

31. Expert Panel on Detection E and Treatment of High Blood Cholesterol in Adults. Executive summary of the third report of the National Cholesterol Education Program (NCEP) expert panel on detection, evaluation, and treatment of high blood cholesterol in adults (Adult treatment panel III). *JAMA.* 2001 May 16;285(19):2486–97.

32. Bhatti JS, Bhatti GK, Reddy PH. Mitochondrial dysfunction and oxidative stress in metabolic disorders - A Step towards mitochondria based therapeutic strategies. *Biochim Biophys Acta.* 2017 May;1863(5):1066–77.

33. Aranda-Rivera AK, Cruz-Gregorio A, Arancibia-Hernández YL, Hernández-Cruz EY, Pedraza-Chaverri J. RONS and oxidative stress: An overview of basic concepts. *Oxygen.* 2022 Oct 10;2(4):437–78.

34. Collin F. Chemical basis of reactive oxygen species reactivity and involvement in neurode-generative diseases. *Int J Mol Sci.* 2019 May 15;20(10):2407.

35. Checa J, Aran JM. Reactive oxygen species: Drivers of physiological and pathological processes. *J Inflamm Res.* 2020 Dec 2;13:1057–73.

36. Li D, Yang S, Xing Y, Pan L, Zhao R, Zhao Y, et al. Novel insights and current evidence for mechanisms of atherosclerosis: Mitochondrial dynamics as a potential therapeutic target. *Front Cell Dev Biol.* 2021 Jul 7;9:673839.

37. Iakovou E, Kourti M. A comprehensive overview of the complex role of oxidative stress in aging, The contributing environmental stressors and emerging antioxidant therapeutic interventions. *Front Aging Neurosci.* 2022 Jun 13;14:827900.

38. Sharifi-Rad M, Anil Kumar NV, Zucca P, Varoni EM, Dini L, Panzarini E, et al. Lifestyle, oxidative stress, and antioxidants: back and forth in the pathophysiology of chronic diseases. *Front Physiol [Internet].* 2020 [cited 2023 Feb 3];11. Available from: https://www.frontiersin.org/articles/10.3389/fphys.2020.00694

39. Raut SK, Khullar M. Oxidative stress in metabolic diseases: Current scenario and therapeutic relevance. *Mol Cell Biochem.* 2023 Jan;478(1):185–96.

40. Zhong G, Venkatesan JK, Madry H, Cucchiarini M. Advances in human mitochondria-based therapies. *Int J Mol Sci.* 2022 Dec 29;24(1):608.

41. Luo K, Yu JH, Quan Y, Shin YJ, Lee KE, Kim HL, et al. Therapeutic potential of coenzyme Q10 in mitochondrial dysfunction during tacrolimus-induced beta cell injury. *Sci Rep.* 2019 May 29;9:7995.

42. Hernández-Camacho JD, Bernier M, López-Lluch G, Navas P. Coenzyme Q10 supplementation in aging and disease. *Front Physiol.* 2018 Feb 5;9:44.

43. Mermigkis C, Bouloukaki I, Mastorodemos V, Plaitakis A, Alogdianakis V, Siafakas N, et al. Medical treatment with thiamine, coenzyme Q. *Vitamins E and C, and carnitine improved obstructive sleep apnea in an adult case of Leigh disease. Sleep Breath Schlaf Atm.* 2013 Feb 7;17.

44. Strutynska N, Goshovska Y, Mys L, Strutynskyi R, Luchkova A, Fedichkina R, et al. Glutathione restores the mitochondrial redox status and improves the function of the cardiovascular system in old rats. *Front Physiol [Internet].* 2023 [cited 2023 Jan 20];13. Available from: https://www.frontiersin.org/articles/10.3389/fphys.2022.1093388

45. Maciejczyk M, Żebrowska E, Nesterowicz M, Żendzian-Piotrowska M, Zalewska A. α-Lipoic acid strengthens the antioxidant barrier and reduces oxidative, nitrosative, and glycative damage, as well as inhibits inflammation and apoptosis in the hypothalamus but not in the cerebral cortex of insulin-resistant rats. *Oxid Med Cell Longev.* 2022;2022:7450514.

46. Rodriguez MC, MacDonald JR, Mahoney DJ, Parise G, Beal MF, Tarnopolsky MA. Beneficial effects of creatine, CoQ10, and lipoic acid in mitochondrial disorders. *Muscle Nerve.* 2007;35(2):235–42.

47. Rezaei Zonooz S, Hasani M, Morvaridzadeh M, Beatriz Pizarro A, Heydari H, Yosaee S, et al. Effect of alpha-lipoic acid on oxidative stress parameters: A systematic review and meta-analysis. *J Funct Foods.* 2021 Dec 1;87:104774.

48. Lin WY, Rehfuss A, Schuler C, Levin RM. Effect of co-enzyme Q10 and alpha-lipoic acid on response of rabbit urinary bladder to repetitive stimulation and In vitro ischemia. *Urology.* 2008 Jul 1;72(1):214–9.

49. El-Hattab AW, Almannai M, Scaglia F. Arginine and citrulline for the treatment of MELAS syndrome. *J Inborn Errors Metab Screen*. 2017 Jan;5:10.1177/2326409817697399.

50. Bottani E, Lamperti C, Prigione A, Tiranti V, Persico N, Brunetti D. Therapeutic approaches to treat mitochondrial diseases: "one-size-fits-all" and "precision medicine" strategies. *Pharmaceutics*. 2020 Nov 11;12(11):1083.

51. Tinker RJ, Lim AZ, Stefanetti RJ, McFarland R. Current and emerging clinical treatment in mitochondrial disease. *Mol Diagn Ther*. 2021 Mar 1;25(2):181–206.

52. Rubalcava-Gracia D, García-Villegas R, Larsson NG. No role for nuclear transcription regulators in mammalian mitochondria? *Mol Cell [Internet]*. 2022 Sep 30 [cited 2023 Feb 17]; Available from: https://www.sciencedirect.com/science/article/pii/S1097276522008991

53. García-Lepe UO, Bermúdez-Cruz RM, García-Lepe UO, Bermúdez-Cruz RM. Mitochondrial genome maintenance: Damage and repair pathways [Internet]. *DNA Repair- An Update*. IntechOpen; 2019 [cited 2023 Feb 17]. Available from: https://www.intechopen.com/chapters/65844

54. Wallace DC, Chalkia D. Mitochondrial DNA genetics and the heteroplasmy Conundrum in evolution and disease. *Cold Spring Harb Perspect Biol*. 2013 Nov;5(11):a021220.

55. Singh G, Pachouri UC, Khaidem DC, Kundu A, Chopra C, Singh P. Mitochondrial DNA damage and diseases. *F1000Research*. 2015 Jul 1;4:176.

56. Chiaratti MR, Macabelli CH, Augusto Neto JD, Grejo MP, Pandey AK, Perecin F, et al. Maternal transmission of mitochondrial diseases. *Genet Mol Biol*. 2020;43(1 suppl. 1):e20190095.

57. Ryzhkova AI, Sazonova MA, Sinyov VV, Galitsyna EV, Chicheva MM, Melnichenko AA, et al. Mitochondrial diseases caused by mtDNA mutations: A mini-review. *Ther Clin Risk Manag*. 2018 Oct 9;14:1933–42.

58. Pia S, Lui F. Melas syndrome. In: *StatPearls* [Internet]. Treasure Island (FL): StatPearls Publishing; 2022 [cited 2023 Feb 21]. Available from: http://www.ncbi.nlm.nih.gov/books/NBK532959/

59. Hameed S, Tadi P. Myoclonic epilepsy and ragged red fibers. In: *StatPearls* [Internet]. Treasure Island (FL): StatPearls Publishing; 2022 [cited 2023 Feb 21]. Available from: http://www.ncbi.nlm.nih.gov/books/NBK555923/

60. Juaristi L, Irigoyen C, Quiroga J. Neuropathy, ataxia, and retinitis pigmentosa syndrome: A multidisciplinary diagnosis. *Retin Cases Brief Rep*. 2021 Jul;15(4):486–9.

61. Peverelli L, Catania A, Marchet S, Ciasca P, Cammarata G, Melzi L, et al. Leber's hereditary optic neuropathy: A report on novel mtDNA pathogenic variants. *Front Neurol [Internet]*. 2021 [cited 2023 Feb 21];12. Available from: https://www.frontiersin.org/articles/10.3389/fneur.2021.657317

62. Cronan JE. Progress in the enzymology of the mitochondrial diseases of lipoic acid requiring enzymes. *Front Genet [Internet]*. 2020 [cited 2023 Feb 21];11. Available from: https://www.frontiersin.org/articles/10.3389/fgene.2020.00510

63. Nuebel E, Morgan JT, Fogarty S, Winter JM, Lettlova S, Berg JA, et al. The biochemical basis of mitochondrial dysfunction in Zellweger Spectrum Disorder. *EMBO Rep*. 2021 Oct 5;22(10):e51991.

64. Aryaman J, Bowles C, Jones NS, Johnston IG. Mitochondrial network state scales mtDNA genetic dynamics. *Genetics*. 2019 Aug;212(4):1429–43.

65. Gorman GS, Chinnery PF, DiMauro S, Hirano M, Koga Y, McFarland R, et al. Mitochondrial diseases. *Nat Rev Dis Primer*. 2016 Oct 20;2(1):1–22.

66. Holt IJ, Harding AE, Petty RK, Morgan-Hughes JA. A new mitochondrial disease associated with mitochondrial DNA heteroplasmy. *Am J Hum Genet*. 1990 Mar;46(3):428–33.

67. Nissanka N, Moraes CT. Mitochondrial DNA damage and reactive oxygen species in neuro-degenerative disease. *FEBS Lett*. 2018 Mar;592(5):728–42.

68. McInnes J. Mitochondrial-associated metabolic disorders: Foundations, pathologies and recent progress. *Nutr Metab*. 2013 Oct 12;10(1):63.

69. Santos-Ocaña C, Cascajo MV, Alcázar-Fabra M, Staiano C, López-Lluch G, Brea-Calvo G, et al. Cellular models for primary CoQ deficiency pathogenesis study. *Int J Mol Sci [Internet]*. 2021 Oct [cited 2023 Feb 22];22(19). Available from: https://www.ncbi.nlm.nih.gov/pmc/articles/PMC8508219/

70. Cortés-Rojo C, Vargas-Vargas MA, Olmos-Orizaba BE, Rodríguez-Orozco AR, Calderón-Cortés E. Interplay between NADH oxidation by complex I, glutathione redox state and sirtuin-3, and its role in the development of insulin resistance. *Biochim Biophys Acta BBA - Mol Basis Dis*. 2020 Aug 1;1866(8):165801.

71. Takano C, Ogawa E, Hayakawa S. Insulin resistance in mitochondrial diabetes. *Biomolecules*. 2023 Jan;13(1):126.

72. Sharma N, Pasala MS, Prakash A. Mitochondrial DNA: Epigenetics and environment. *Environ Mol Mutagen*. 2019 Oct;60(8):668–82.

73. De Bont R, van Larebeke N. Endogenous DNA damage in humans: A review of quantitative data. *Mutagenesis*. 2004 May;19(3):169–85.

74. Lindahl T. DNA Repair Enzymes. *Annu Rev Biochem*. 1982;51(1):61–87.

75. Sykora P, Wilson DM, Bohr VA. Repair of persistent strand breaks in the mitochondrial genome. *Mech Ageing Dev*. 2012 Apr;133(4):169–75.

76. Reddam A, McLarnan S, Kupsco A. Environmental chemical exposures and mitochondrial dysfunction: A review of recent literature. *Curr Environ Health Rep*. 2022 Dec 1;9(4):631–49.

77. Olasehinde TA, Olaniran AO. Neurotoxicity of polycyclic aromatic hydrocarbons: A systematic mapping and review of neuropathological mechanisms. *Toxics*. 2022 Jul 25;10(8):417.

78. Suman S, Sinha A, Tarafdar A. Polycyclic aromatic hydrocarbons (PAHs) concentration levels, pattern, source identification and soil toxicity assessment in urban traffic soil of Dhanbad, India. *Sci Total Environ*. 2016 Mar 1;545–546:353–60.

79. Chen YY, Chen WL. The relationship between polycyclic aromatic hydrocarbons exposure and serum klotho among adult population. *BMC Geriatr*. 2022 Mar 14;22(1):198.

80. Abedini E. A systematic review on the effects of polycyclic aromatic hydrocarbons on cardio-metabolic impairment. *Int J Prev Med*. 2017 Apr 11;8.

81. Mallah MA, Changxing L, Mallah MA, Noreen S, Liu Y, Saeed M, et al. Polycyclic aromatic hydrocarbon and its effects on human health: An overeview. *Chemosphere*. 2022 Jun;296:133948.

82. Backer JM, Weinstein IB. Mitochondrial DNA is a major cellular target for a dihydrodiol-epoxide derivative of benzo[a]pyrene. *Science*. 1980 Jul 11;209(4453):297–9.

83. Bhargava A, Kumari R, Khare S, Shandilya R, Gupta P, Tiwari R, et al. Mapping the mitochondrial regulation of epigenetic modifications in association with carcinogenic and non-carcinogenic polycyclic aromatic hydrocarbon exposure. *Int J Toxicol*. 2020 Jun 26;39.

84. Hori A, Yoshida M, Shibata T, Ling F. Reactive oxygen species regulate DNA copy number in isolated yeast mitochondria by triggering recombination-mediated replication. *Nucleic Acids Res*. 2009 Feb;37(3):749–61.

85. Hazrat MA, Rasul MG, Khan MMK, Ashwath N, Rufford TE. Emission characteristics of waste tallow and waste cooking oil based ternary biodiesel fuels. *Energy Procedia*. 2019 Feb;160:842–7.

86. Kumar SB, Padhi RK, Mohanty AK, Satpathy KK. Distribution and ecological- and health-risk assessment of heavy metals in the seawater of the southeast coast of India. *Mar Pollut Bull*. 2020 Dec 1;161:111712.

87. Delahaut V, Rašković B, Salvado MS, Bervoets L, Blust R, Boeck GD. Toxicity and bioaccumulation of Cadmium, Copper and Zinc in a direct comparison at equitoxic concentrations in common carp (Cyprinus carpio) juveniles. *PLOS ONE*. 2020 Apr 9;15(4):e0220485.

88. Lee HW, Jose CC, Cuddapah S. Epithelial-mesenchymal transition: Insights into nickel-induced lung diseases. *Semin Cancer Biol*. 2021 Nov 1;76:99–109.

89. Jenkinson MRJ, Meek RMD, Tate R, MacMillan S, Grant MH, Currie S. Cobalt-induced cardiomyopathy – Do circulating cobalt levels matter? *Bone Jt Res*. 2021 May 31;10(6):340–7.

90. Briffa J, Sinagra E, Blundell R. Heavy metal pollution in the environment and their toxicological effects on humans. *Heliyon*. 2020 Sep 8;6(9):e04691.

91. Mitra S, Chakraborty AJ, Tareq AM, Emran TB, Nainu F, Khusro A, et al. Impact of heavy metals on the environment and human health: Novel therapeutic insights to counter the toxicity. *J King Saud Univ - Sci*. 2022 Apr 1;34(3):101865.

92. Atchison WD, Hare MF. Mechanisms of methylmercury-induced neurotoxicity. *FASEB J*. 1994;8(9):622–9.

93. Grabowska M, Gumińska M. The effect of lead on lactate formation, ATP level and membrane ATPase activities in human erythrocytes in vitro. *Int J Occup Med Environ Health*. 1996;9(3):265–74.

94. Jia G, Aroor AR, Martinez-Lemus LA, Sowers JR. Mitochondrial functional impairment in response to environmental toxins in the cardiorenal metabolic syndrome. *Arch Toxicol*. 2015 Feb;89(2):147.

95. Ventura C, Gomes BC, Oberemm A, Louro H, Huuskonen P, Mustieles V, et al. Biomarkers of effect as determined in human biomonitoring studies on hexavalent chromium and cadmium in the period 2008–2020. *Environ Res*. 2021 Jun 1;197:110998.

96. Branca JJV, Fiorillo C, Carrino D, Paternostro F, Taddei N, Gulisano M, et al. Cadmium-Induced Oxidative Stress: Focus on the Central Nervous System. *Antioxidants*. 2020 Jun 5;9(6):492.

97. Genchi G, Sinicropi MS, Lauria G, Carocci A, Catalano A. The effects of cadmium toxicity. *Int J Environ Res Public Health*. 2020 Jun;17(11):3782.

98. Chen Q, Gong B, Almasan A. Distinct stages of cytochrome c release from mitochondria: Evidence for a feedback amplification loop linking caspase activation to mitochondrial dysfunction in genotoxic stress induced apoptosis. *Cell Death Differ*. 2000 Feb;7(2):227–33.

99. Monteiro C, Ferreira de Oliveira JMP, Pinho F, Bastos V, Oliveira H, Peixoto F, et al. Biochemical and transcriptional analyses of cadmium-induced mitochondrial dysfunction and oxidative stress in human osteoblasts. *J Toxicol Environ Health A*. 2018 Aug 3;81(15):705–17.

100. Al-Nasser IA, Al-Nasser I. Cadmium hepatotoxicity and alterations of the mitochondrial function. *J Toxicol Clin Toxicol*. 2000 Jan 1;38(4):407–13.

101. Rahimzadeh MR, Rahimzadeh MR, Kazemi S, Amiri RJ, Pirzadeh M, Moghadamnia AA. Aluminum poisoning with emphasis on its mechanism and treatment of intoxication. *Emerg Med Int*. 2022 Jan 11;2022:e1480553.

102. La Merrill MA, Vandenberg LN, Smith MT, Goodson W, Browne P, Patisaul HB, et al. Consensus on the key characteristics of endocrine-disrupting chemicals as a basis for hazard identification. *Nat Rev Endocrinol*. 2020 Jan;16(1):45–57.

103. Gao CJ, Kannan K. Phthalates, bisphenols, parabens, and triclocarban in feminine hygiene products from the United States and their implications for human exposure. *Environ Int*. 2020 Mar;136:105465.

104. Lucas A, Herrmann S, Lucas M. The role of endocrine-disrupting phthalates and bisphenols in cardiometabolic disease: The evidence is mounting. *Curr Opin Endocrinol Diabetes Obes*. 2022 Apr;29(2):87–94.

105. Marroqui L, Tudurí E, Alonso-Magdalena P, Quesada I, Nadal Á, Dos Santos RS. Mitochondria as target of endocrine-disrupting chemicals: Implications for type 2 diabetes. *J Endocrinol*. 2018 Nov 1;239(2):R27–45.

106. Papalou O, Kandaraki EA, Papadakis G, Diamanti-Kandarakis E. Endocrine disrupting chemicals: An occult mediator of metabolic disease. *Front Endocrinol*. 2019 Mar 1;10:112.

107. Zhou Z, Goodrich JM, Strakovsky RS. Mitochondrial epigenetics and environmental health: Making a case for endocrine disrupting chemicals. *Toxicol Sci*. 2020 Nov 1;178(1):16–25.

108. Zhang Q, Zhao Y, Talukder M, Han Y, Zhang C, Li XN, et al. Di(2-ethylhexyl) phthalate induced hepatotoxicity in quail (Coturnix japonica) via modulating the mitochondrial unfolded protein response and NRF2 mediated antioxidant defense. *Sci Total Environ*. 2019 Feb 15;651(Pt 1):885–94.

109. Nayak D, Adiga D, Khan NG, Rai PS, Dsouza HS, Chakrabarty S, et al. Impact of bisphenol a on structure and function of mitochondria: A critical review. *Rev Environ Contam Toxicol*. 2022 Nov 9;260(1):10.

110. Azevedo LF, Porto Dechandt CR, Cristina de Souza Rocha C, Hornos Carneiro MF, Alberici LC, Barbosa F. Long-term exposure to bisphenol A or S promotes glucose intolerance and changes hepatic mitochondrial metabolism in male Wistar rats. *Food Chem Toxicol*. 2019 Oct 1;132:110694.

111. Chen T, Tan J, Wan Z, Zou Y, Kessete Afewerky H, Zhang Z, et al. Effects of commonly used pesticides in china on the mitochondria and ubiquitin-Proteasome system in Parkinson's disease. *Int J Mol Sci*. 2017 Nov 23;18(12):2507.

112. Zolkipli-Cunningham Z, Falk MJ. Clinical effects of chemical exposures on mitochondrial function. *Toxicology*. 2017 Nov 11;391:90.

113. Heinz S, Freyberger A, Lawrenz B, Schladt L, Schmuck G, Ellinger-Ziegelbauer H. Mechanistic investigations of the mitochondrial complex I inhibitor rotenone in the context of pharmacological and safety evaluation. *Sci Rep.* 2017 Apr 4;7:45465.

114. Palmer G, Horgan DJ, Tisdale H, Singer TP, Beinert H. Studies on the respiratory chain-linked reduced nicotinamide adenine dinucleotide dehydrogenase. XIV. Location of the sites of inhibition of rotenone, barbiturates, and piericidin by means of electron paramagnetic resonance spectroscopy. *J Biol Chem.* 1968 Feb 25;243(4):844–7.

115. Passmore JB, Pinho S, Gomez-Lazaro M, Schrader M. The respiratory chain inhibitor rotenone affects peroxisomal dynamics via its microtubule-destabilising activity. *Histochem Cell Biol.* 2017;148(3):331–41.

116. Won JH, Park S, Hong S, Son S, Yu JW. Rotenone-induced impairment of mitochondrial electron transport chain confers a selective priming signal for NLRP3 inflammasome activation. *J Biol Chem.* 2015 Nov 6;290(45):27425–37.

117. Jang YJ, Won JH, Back MJ, Fu Z, Jang JM, Ha HC, et al. Paraquat induces apoptosis through a mitochondria-dependent pathway in RAW264.7 cells. *Biomol Ther.* 2015 Sep;23(5):407–13.

118. Giorgi C, Baldassari F, Bononi A, Bonora M, De Marchi E, Marchi S, et al. Mitochondrial Ca2+ and apoptosis. *Cell Calcium.* 2012 Jul;52(1):36–43.

119. Huang SH, Jacinto JCK, O'Sullivan B, Su J, Kim J, Ringash J, et al. Clinical presentation and outcome of human papillomavirus-positive nasopharyngeal carcinoma in a North American cohort. *Cancer.* 2022 Aug 1;128(15):2908–21.

120. Jin X, Song L, Liu X, Chen M, Li Z, Cheng L, et al. Protective efficacy of vitamins C and E on p,p′-DDT-induced cytotoxicity via the ROS-mediated mitochondrial pathway and NF-κB/FasL pathway. *PLoS ONE.* 2014 Dec 2;9(12):e113257.

121. Fu Y, Sies H, Lei XG. Opposite roles of selenium-dependent glutathione peroxidase-1 in superoxide generator diquat- and peroxynitrite-induced apoptosis and signaling. *J Biol Chem.* 2001 Nov 16;276(46):43004–9.

122. Sule RO, Condon L, Gomes AV. A common feature of pesticides: Oxidative stress—the role of oxidative stress in pesticide-induced toxicity. *Oxid Med Cell Longev.* 2022 Jan 19;2022:e5563759.

123. Fedeli D, Carloni M, Nasuti C, Gambini A, Scocco V, Gabbianelli R. Early life permethrin exposure leads to hypervitaminosis D, nitric oxide and catecholamines impairment. *Pestic Biochem Physiol.* 2013 Sep 1;107:93–7.

124. Jin Y, Liu J, Wang L, Chen R, Zhou C, Yang Y, et al. Permethrin exposure during puberty has the potential to enantioselectively induce reproductive toxicity in mice. *Environ Int.* 2012 Jul 1;42:144–51.

125. Afolabi OK, Aderibigbe FA, Folarin DT, Arinola A, Wusu AD. Oxidative stress and inflammation following sub-lethal oral exposure of cypermethrin in rats: Mitigating potential of epicatechin. *Heliyon.* 2019 Aug 1;5(8):e02274.

126. Fitsiou E, Pulido T, Campisi J, Alimirah F, Demaria M. Cellular senescence and the senescence-associated secretory phenotype as drivers of skin photoaging. *J Invest Dermatol.* 2021 Apr;141(4S):1119–26.

127. Pfeifer GP. Mechanisms of UV-induced mutations and skin cancer. *Genome Instab Dis.* 2020 May 1;1(3):99–113.

128. Brand RM, Wipf P, Durham A, Epperly MW, Greenberger JS, Falo LD. Targeting mitochondrial oxidative stress to mitigate UV-induced skin Damage. *Front Pharmacol.* 2018 Aug 20;9:920.

129. Berneburg M, Gattermann N, Stege H, Grewe M, Vogelsang K, Ruzicka T, et al. Chronically ultraviolet-exposed human skin shows a higher mutation frequency of mitochondrial DNA as compared to unexposed skin and the hematopoietic system. *Photochem Photobiol.* 1997 Aug;66(2):271–5.

130. Fisher GJ, Wang Z, Datta SC, Varani J, Kang S, Voorhees JJ. Pathophysiology of premature skin aging induced by ultraviolet light. *N Engl J Med.* 1997 Nov 13;337(20):1419–29.

131. Powers JM, Murphy G, Ralph N, O'Gorman SM, Murphy JEJ. Mitochondrial DNA deletion percentage in sun exposed and non sun exposed skin. *J Photochem Photobiol B.* 2016 Dec 1;165:277–82.

132. Zhivagui M, Hoda A, Valenzuela N, Yeh YY, Dai J, He Y, et al. DNA damage and somatic mutations in mammalian cells after irradiation with a nail polish dryer. *Nat Commun.* 2023 Jan 17;14(1):276.

133. Birch-Machin MA, Russell EV, Latimer JA. Mitochondrial DNA damage as a biomarker for ultraviolet radiation exposure and oxidative stress. *Br J Dermatol.* 2013 Jul;169 Suppl 2:9–14.

134. Park J, Baruch-Torres N, Iwai S, Herrmann GK, Brieba LG, Yin YW. Human mitochondrial DNA polymerase metal dependent UV lesion bypassing ability. *Front Mol Biosci [Internet].* 2022 [cited 2023 Feb 14];9. Available from: https://www.frontiersin.org/articles/10.3389/fmolb.2022.808036

135. Cameron SJ, Sheng J, Hosseinian F, Willmore WG. Nanoparticle effects on stress response pathways and nanoparticle–protein interactions. *Int J Mol Sci.* 2022 Jan;23(14):7962.

136. Ma DD, Yang WX. Engineered nanoparticles induce cell apoptosis: Potential for cancer therapy. *Oncotarget.* 2016 Apr 2;7(26):40882–903.

137. Nguyen K, Rippstein P, Tayabali A, Willmore W. Mitochondrial toxicity of cadmium telluride quantum dot nanoparticles in mammalian hepatocytes. *Toxicol Sci.* 2015 Jul 1;146:31–42.

138. Gallud A, Klöditz K, Ytterberg J, Östberg N, Katayama S, Skoog T, et al. Cationic gold nanoparticles elicit mitochondrial dysfunction: A multi-omics study. *Sci Rep.* 2019 Mar 13;9(1):4366.

139. Skalska J, Dąbrowska-Bouta B, Frontczak-Baniewicz M, Sulkowski G, Strużyńska L. A low dose of nanoparticulate silver induces mitochondrial dysfunction and autophagy in adult rat brain. *Neurotox Res.* 2020 Oct 1;38(3):650–64.

140. Wilson CL, Natarajan V, Hayward SL, Khalimonchuk O, Kidambi S. Mitochondrial dysfunction and loss of glutamate uptake in primary astrocytes exposed to titanium dioxide nanoparticles. *Nanoscale.* 2015 Nov 5;7(44):18477–88.

141. Tiku V, Tan MW, Dikic I. Mitochondrial functions in infection and immunity. *Trends Cell Biol.* 2020 Apr;30(4):263–75.

142. Mandal S, Chatterjee NS. Vibrio cholerae GbpA elicits necrotic cell death in intestinal cells. *J Med Microbiol.* 2016 Aug;65(8):837–47.

143. Maurice NM, Bedi B, Yuan Z, Goldberg JB, Koval M, Hart CM, et al. Pseudomonas aeruginosa Induced Host Epithelial Cell Mitochondrial Dysfunction. *Sci Rep.* 2019 Aug 15;9(1):11929.

144. Ramachandran RP, Spiegel C, Keren Y, Danieli T, Melamed-Book N, Pal RR, et al. Mitochondrial targeting of the enteropathogenic escherichia coli map triggers calcium mobilization, ADAM10-MAP kinase signaling, and host cell apoptosis. *mBio*. 2020 Sep 15;11(5):e01397-20.

145. Deo P, Chow SH, Han ML, Speir M, Huang C, Schittenhelm RB, et al. Mitochondrial dysfunction caused by outer membrane vesicles from Gram-negative bacteria activates intrinsic apoptosis and inflammation. *Nat Microbiol*. 2020 Nov;5(11):1418–27.

146. Wang L, Yi J, Yin XY, Hou JX, Chen J, Xie B, et al. Vacuolating cytotoxin a triggers mitophagy in helicobacter pylori-infected human gastric epithelium cells. *Front Oncol [Internet]*. 2022 [cited 2023 Feb 15];12. Available from: https://www.frontiersin.org/articles/10.3389/fonc.2022.881829

147. Pan SW, Syed RR, Catanzaro DG, Ho ML, Shu CC, Tsai TY, et al. Circulating mitochondrial cell-free DNA dynamics in patients with mycobacterial pulmonary infections: Potential for a novel biomarker of disease. *Front Immunol [Internet]*. 2022 [cited 2023 Feb 15];13. Available from: https://www.frontiersin.org/articles/10.3389/fimmu.2022.1040947

148. Galicia-Garcia U, Benito-Vicente A, Jebari S, Larrea-Sebal A, Siddiqi H, Uribe KB, et al. Pathophysiology of type 2 diabetes mellitus. *Int J Mol Sci*. 2020 Aug 30;21(17):6275.

149. Park SS, Seo YK. Excess accumulation of lipid impairs insulin sensitivity in skeletal muscle. *Int J Mol Sci*. 2020 Jan;21(6):1949.

150. Sokolowska E, Blachnio-Zabielska A. The role of ceramides in insulin resistance. *Front Endocrinol*. 2019 Aug 21;10:577.

151. Santoro A, McGraw TE, Kahn BB. Insulin action in adipocytes, adipose remodeling, and systemic effects. *Cell Metab*. 2021 Apr 6;33(4):748–57.

152. Freeman AM, Pennings N. Insulin Resistance. In: *StatPearls* [Internet]. Treasure Island (FL): StatPearls Publishing; 2022 [cited 2023 Feb 27]. Available from: http://www.ncbi.nlm.nih.gov/books/NBK507839/

153. Arvind A, Osganian SA, Cohen DE, Corey KE. Lipid and lipoprotein metabolism in liver disease. In: Feingold KR, Anawalt B, Blackman MR, Boyce A, Chrousos G, Corpas E, et al., editors. Endotext [Internet]. South Dartmouth (MA): MDText.com, Inc.; 2000 [cited 2023 Feb 27]. Available from: http://www.ncbi.nlm.nih.gov/books/NBK326742/

154. Lee SH, Park SY, Choi CS. Insulin resistance: From mechanisms to therapeutic strategies. *Diabetes Metab J*. 2021 Dec 30;46(1):15–37.

155. Oberhauser L, Maechler P. Lipid-Induced adaptations of the pancreatic beta-cell to glucotoxic conditions sustain insulin secretion. *Int J Mol Sci*. 2022 Jan;23(1):324.

156. Eguchi N, Vaziri ND, Dafoe DC, Ichii H. The role of oxidative stress in pancreatic β cell dysfunction in diabetes. *Int J Mol Sci*. 2021 Feb 3;22(4):1509.

157. Sinha S, Haque M. Insulin resistance is cheerfully hitched with hypertension. *Life*. 2022 Apr 10;12(4):564.

158. Juhan-Vague I, Alessi MC, Mavri A, Morange PE. Plasminogen activator inhibitor-1, inflammation, obesity, insulin resistance and vascular risk. *J Thromb Haemost JTH*. 2003 Jul;1(7):1575–9.

159. Rochlani Y, Pothineni NV, Kovelamudi S, Mehta JL. Metabolic syndrome: Pathophysiology, management, and modulation by natural compounds. *Ther Adv Cardiovasc Dis.* 2017 Aug;11(8):215–25.

160. Tripathy D, Mohanty P, Dhindsa S, Syed T, Ghanim H, Aljada A, et al. Elevation of free fatty acids induces inflammation and impairs vascular reactivity in healthy subjects. *Diabetes.* 2003 Dec;52(12):2882–7.

161. Bergman RN, Kim SP, Catalano KJ, Hsu IR, Chiu JD, Kabir M, et al. Why visceral fat is bad: mechanisms of the metabolic syndrome. *Obesity.* 2006;14(S2):16S–19S.

162. Hocking S, Samocha-Bonet D, Milner KL, Greenfield JR, Chisholm DJ. Adiposity and insulin resistance in humans: The role of the different tissue and Cellular lipid depots. *Endocr Rev.* 2013 Aug 1;34(4):463–500.

163. Wang H, Cao H, Cao J, Zhang L. The Visceral Adiposity Index (VAI) and Lipid Accumulation Product (LAP) are predictors of insulin resistance and hyperandrogenaemia in obesity/overweight women with polycystic ovary syndrome. *BioMed Res Int.* 2023 Feb 13;2023:e1508675.

164. Yki-Järvinen H. Non-alcoholic fatty liver disease as a cause and a consequence of metabolic syndrome. *Lancet Diabetes Endocrinol.* 2014 Nov;2(11):901–10.

165. Masschelin PM, Cox AR, Chernis N, Hartig SM. The impact of oxidative stress on adipose tissue energy balance. *Front Physiol.* 2020 Jan 22;10:1638.

166. Masschelin PM, Cox AR, Chernis N, Hartig SM. The impact of oxidative stress on adipose tissue energy balance. *Front Physiol [Internet].* 2020 [cited 2023 Feb 28];10. Available from: https://www.frontiersin.org/articles/10.3389/fphys.2019.01638

167. Checa J, Aran JM. <p>Reactive Oxygen Species: Drivers of Physiological and Pathological Processes</p>. *J Inflamm Res.* 2020 Dec 2;13:1057–73.

168. Cinti S, Mitchell G, Barbatelli G, Murano I, Ceresi E, Faloia E, et al. Adipocyte death defines macrophage localization and function in adipose tissue of obese mice and humans. *J Lipid Res.* 2005 Nov 1;46(11):2347–55.

169. Kershaw EE, Flier JS. Adipose tissue as an endocrine organ. *J Clin Endocrinol Metab.* 2004 Jun 1;89(6):2548–56.

170. MB. Adipose tissue dysfunction contributes to obesity related metabolic diseases. *Best Pract Res Clin Endocrinol Metab [Internet].* 2013 Apr [cited 2023 Feb 28];27(2). Available from: https://pubmed.ncbi.nlm.nih.gov/23731879/

171. Mathis D. Immunological goings-on in visceral adipose tissue. *Cell Metab.* 2013 Jun 4;17(6):851–9.

172. Guh DP, Zhang W, Bansback N, Amarsi Z, Birmingham CL, Anis AH. The incidence of co-morbidities related to obesity and overweight: A systematic review and meta-analysis. *BMC Public Health.* 2009 Mar 25;9:88.

173. Schelbert KB. Comorbidities of obesity. *Prim Care Clin Off Pract.* 2009 Jun 1;36(2):271–85.

174. Schütten MTJ, Houben AJHM, de Leeuw PW, Stehouwer CDA. The link between adipose tissue renin-angiotensin-aldosterone system signaling and obesity-associated hypertension. *Physiology.* 2017 May;32(3):197–209.

175. Poznyak AV, Ivanova EA, Sobenin IA, Yet SF, Orekhov AN. The role of mitochondria in cardiovascular diseases. *Biology.* 2020 Jun;9(6):137.

176. Wen B, Xu K, Huang R, Jiang T, Wang J, Chen J, et al. Preserving mitochondrial function by inhibiting GRP75 ameliorates neuron injury under ischemic stroke. *Mol Med Rep.* 2022 May 1;25(5):1–11.

177. Maechler P, Wollheim CB. Mitochondrial function in normal and diabetic β-cells. *Nature.* 2001 Dec;414(6865):807–12.

178. Kwak SH, Park KS, Lee K, Lee HK. Mitochondrial metabolism and diabetes. *J Diabetes Investig.* 2010 Oct 19;1(5):161–9.

179. Chae HW, Na JH, Kim HS, Lee YM. Mitochondrial diabetes and mitochondrial DNA mutation load in MELAS syndrome. *Eur J Endocrinol.* 2020 Nov 1;183(5):505–12.

180. Maassen JA, Jahangir Tafrechi RS, Janssen GMC, Raap AK, Lemkes HH, 't Hart LM. New insights in the molecular pathogenesis of the maternally inherited diabetes and deafness syndrome. *Endocrinol Metab Clin North Am.* 2006 Jun;35(2):385–96, x–xi.

181. Park KS, Chan JC, Chuang LM, Suzuki S, Araki E, Nanjo K, et al. A mitochondrial DNA variant at position 16189 is associated with type 2 diabetes mellitus in Asians. *Diabetologia.* 2008 Apr;51(4):602–8.

182. Vidoni S, Zanna C, Rugolo M, Sarzi E, Lenaers G. Why mitochondria must fuse to maintain their genome integrity. *Antioxid Redox Signal.* 2013 Aug 1;19(4):379–88.

183. Grubelnik V, Zmazek J, Marković R, Gosak M, Marhl M. Mitochondrial dysfunction in pancreatic alpha and beta cells associated with type 2 diabetes mellitus. *Life.* 2020 Dec;10(12):348.

184. Murri M, el Azzouzi H. MicroRNAs as regulators of mitochondrial dysfunction and obesity. *Am J Physiol-Heart Circ Physiol.* 2018 Aug;315(2):H291–302.

185. Boudina S, Sena S, O'Neill BT, Tathireddy P, Young ME, Abel ED. Reduced mitochondrial oxidative capacity and increased mitochondrial uncoupling impair myocardial energetics in obesity. *Circulation.* 2005 Oct 25;112(17):2686–95.

186. de Mello AH, Costa AB, Engel JDG, Rezin GT. Mitochondrial dysfunction in obesity. *Life Sci.* 2018 Jan 1;192:26–32.

187. Yin X, Lanza IR, Swain JM, Sarr MG, Nair KS, Jensen MD. Adipocyte mitochondrial function is reduced in human obesity independent of fat cell size. *J Clin Endocrinol Metab.* 2014 Feb;99(2):E209–16.

188. Cioffi F, Giacco A, Petito G, de Matteis R, Senese R, Lombardi A, et al. Altered mitochondrial quality control in rats with Metabolic Dysfunction-Associated Fatty Liver Disease (MAFLD) Induced by high-fat feeding. *Genes.* 2022 Feb;13(2):315.

189. Valerio A, Cardile A, Cozzi V, Bracale R, Tedesco L, Pisconti A, et al. TNF-α downregulates eNOS expression and mitochondrial biogenesis in fat and muscle of obese rodents. *J Clin Invest.* 2006 Oct 2;116(10):2791–8.

190. Batty M, Bennett MR, Yu E. The role of oxidative stress in atherosclerosis. *Cells.* 2022 Jan;11(23):3843.

191. Postnov IV. The role of mitochondrial calcium overload and energy deficiency in pathogenesis of arterial hypertension. *Arkh Patol.* 2001 May 1;63(3):3–10.

192. Ruipeng W, Ying N, Peter B, Sneha G, Janet W, Li Samuel T, et al. Mitochondrial DNA content is linked to cardiovascular disease patient phenotypes. *J Am Heart Assoc.* 2021 Feb 16;10(4):e018776.

193. Umbria M, Ramos A, Aluja MP, Santos C. The role of control region mitochondrial DNA mutations in cardiovascular disease: Stroke and myocardial infarction. *Sci Rep.* 2020 Feb 17;10(1):2766.

194. Zhang Z, Liu M, He J, Zhang X, Chen Y, Li H. Maternally inherited coronary heart disease is associated with a novel mitochondrial tRNA mutation. *BMC Cardiovasc Disord.* 2019 Dec 16;19(1):293.

195. Pérez-Martínez P, Mikhailidis DP, Athyros VG, Bullo M, Couture P, Covas MI, et al. Lifestyle recommendations for the prevention and management of metabolic syndrome: An international panel recommendation. *Nutr Rev.* 2017 May;75(5):307–26.

196. ElSayed NA, Aleppo G, Aroda VR, Bannuru RR, Brown FM, Bruemmer D, et al. 8. Obesity and weight management for the prevention and treatment of type 2 diabetes: Standards of care in diabetes—2023. *Diabetes Care.* 2022 Dec 12;46 (Supplement_1):S128–39.

197. American Diabetes Association. 9Pharmacologic Approaches to glycemic treatment: Standards of medical care in diabetes-2020. *Diabetes Care.* 2020 Jan;43(Suppl 1):S98–110.

198. Buse JB, Wexler DJ, Tsapas A, Rossing P, Mingrone G, Mathieu C, et al. 2019 Update to: Management of hyperglycemia in type 2 diabetes, 2018. A consensus Report by the American Diabetes Association (ADA) and the European Association for the Study of Diabetes (EASD). *Diabetes Care.* 2020 Feb;43(2):487–93.

199. Davies MJ, D'Alessio DA, Fradkin J, Kernan WN, Mathieu C, Mingrone G, et al. Management of Hyperglycemia in Type 2 Diabetes, 2018. A consensus report by the American Diabetes Association (ADA) and the European Association for the Study of Diabetes (EASD). *Diabetes Care.* 2018 Dec;41(12):2669–701.

200. ElSayed NA, Aleppo G, Aroda VR, Bannuru RR, Brown FM, Bruemmer D, et al. 9. Pharmacologic approaches to glycemic treatment: Standards of care in diabetes—2023. *Diabetes Care.* 2023 Jan;46(Suppl 1):S140–57.

201. Han Y, Xie H, Liu Y, Gao P, Yang X, Shen Z. Effect of metformin on all-cause and cardiovascular mortality in patients with coronary artery diseases: A systematic review and an updated meta-analysis. *Cardiovasc Diabetol.* 2019 Jul 30;18(1):96.

202. Holman RR, Paul SK, Bethel MA, Matthews DR, Neil HAW. 10-year follow-up of intensive glucose control in type 2 diabetes. *N Engl J Med.* 2008 Oct 9;359(15):1577–89.

203. Christofides EA. Practical insights into improving adherence to metformin therapy in patients with type 2 diabetes. *Clin Diabetes Publ Am Diabetes Assoc.* 2019 Jul;37(3):234–41.

204. Maruthur NM, Tseng E, Hutfless S, Wilson LM, Suarez-Cuervo C, Berger Z, et al. Diabetes medications as monotherapy or metformin-based combination therapy for type 2 diabetes: A systematic review and meta-analysis. *Ann Intern Med.* 2016 Jun 7;164(11):740–51.

205. Whelton PK, Carey RM, Aronow WS, Casey DE, Collins KJ, Dennison Himmelfarb C, et al. 2017 ACC/AHA/AAPA/ABC/ACPM/AGS/APhA/ASH/ASPC/NMA/PCNA Guideline for the prevention, detection, evaluation, and management of high blood pressure in adults: A report of the American college of cardiology/American heart association task force on clinical practice guidelines. *J Am Coll Cardiol.* 2018 May 15;71(19):e127–248.

206. Ojha U, Ruddaraju S, Sabapathy N, Ravindran V, Worapongsatitaya P, Haq J, et al. Current and emerging classes of pharmacological agents for the Management of hypertension. *Am J Cardiovasc Drugs.* 2022 May 1;22(3):271–85.

207. Mach F, Baigent C, Catapano AL, Koskinas KC, Casula M, Badimon L, et al. 2019 ESC/EAS guidelines for the management of dyslipidaemias: Lipid modification to reduce cardiovascular risk. *Eur Heart J*. 2020 Jan 1;41(1):111–88.

208. Knuuti J, Wijns W, Saraste A, Capodanno D, Barbato E, Funck-Brentano C, et al. 2019 ESC guidelines for the diagnosis and management of chronic coronary syndromes. *Eur Heart J*. 2020 Jan 14;41(3):407–77.

209. Zodda D, Giammona R, Schifilliti S. Treatment strategy for dyslipidemia in cardiovascular disease prevention: Focus on old and new drugs. *Pharm J Pharm Educ Pract*. 2018 Jan 21;6(1):10.

210. Feingold KR. Cholesterol lowering drugs. In: Feingold KR, Anawalt B, Blackman MR, Boyce A, Chrousos G, Corpas E, et al., editors. Endotext [Internet]. South Dartmouth (MA): *MDText .com*, Inc.; 2000 [cited 2023 Mar 8]. Available from: http://www.ncbi.nlm.nih.gov/books/NBK395573/

211. Alnouri F, Santos RD. New trends and therapies for familial hypercholesterolemia. *J Clin Med*. 2022 Jan;11(22):6638.

212. Chambergo-Michilot D, Alur A, Kulkarni S, Agarwala A. <p>Mipomersen in Familial Hypercholesterolemia: An Update on Health-Related Quality of Life and Patient-Reported Outcomes</p>. *Vasc Health Risk Manag*. 2022 Feb 21;18:73–80.

213. D'Erasmo L, Gallo A, Cefalù AB, Di Costanzo A, Saheb S, Giammanco A, et al. Long-term efficacy of lipoprotein apheresis and lomitapide in the treatment of homozygous familial hypercholesterolemia (HoFH): A cross-national retrospective survey. *Orphanet J Rare Dis*. 2021 Sep 8;16(1):381.

214. Tinker RJ, Lim AZ, Stefanetti RJ, McFarland R. Current and emerging clinical treatment in mitochondrial disease. *Mol Diagn Ther*. 2021 Mar 1;25(2):181–206.

215. Viscomi C, Bottani E, Zeviani M. Emerging concepts in the therapy of mitochondrial disease. *Biochim Biophys* Acta BBA - Bioenerg. 2015 Jun 1;1847(6):544–57.

216. Faria R, Boisguérin P, Sousa Â, Costa D. Delivery systems for mitochondrial gene therapy: A review. *Pharmaceutics*. 2023 Feb;15(2):572.

217. Di Donfrancesco A, Massaro G, Di Meo I, Tiranti V, Bottani E, Brunetti D. Gene therapy for mitochondrial diseases: Current status and future perspective. *Pharmaceutics*. 2022 Jun 17;14(6):1287.

218. Sung Y, Kim S. Recent advances in the development of gene delivery systems. *Biomater Res*. 2019 Mar 12;23(1):8.

219. Zu H, Gao D. Non-viral vectors in gene therapy: Recent development, challenges, and prospects. *AAPS J*. 2021 Jun 2;23(4):78.

220. Yasuzaki Y, Yamada Y, Ishikawa T, Harashima H. Validation of mitochondrial gene delivery in liver and skeletal muscle via hydrodynamic injection using an artificial mitochondrial reporter DNA vector. *Mol Pharm*. 2015 Dec 7;12(12):4311–20.

221. Du X, Wang J, Zhou Q, Zhang L, Wang S, Zhang Z, et al. Advanced physical techniques for gene delivery based on membrane perforation. *Drug Deliv*. 2018 Jul 3;25(1):1516–25.

222. Gao Y, Liu X, Chen N, Yang X, Tang F. Recent advance of liposome nanoparticles for nucleic acid therapy. *Pharmaceutics*. 2023 Jan;15(1):178.

223. Fears R, ter Meulen V. Assessing security implications of genome editing: emerging points from an international workshop. *Front Bioeng Biotechnol [Internet]*. 2018 [cited 2023 Mar 13];6. Available from: https://www.frontiersin.org/articles/10.3389/fbioe.2018.00034

224. Lundstrom K. Viral Vectors in Gene Therapy. Dis Basel Switz. 2018 May 21;6(2):42.

225. Hanaford AR, Cho YJ, Nakai H. AAV-vector based gene therapy for mitochondrial disease: Progress and future perspectives. *Orphanet J Rare Dis*. 2022 Jun 6;17(1):217.

226. Kuzmin DA, Shutova MV, Johnston NR, Smith OP, Fedorin VV, Kukushkin YS, et al. The clinical landscape for AAV gene therapies. *Nat Rev Drug Discov*. 2021 Mar;20(3):173–4.

227. Chong B, Kong G, Shankar K, Chew HSJ, Lin C, Goh R, et al. The global syndemic of metabolic diseases in the young adult population: A consortium of trends and projections from the Global Burden of Disease 2000–2019. *Metab - Clin Exp [Internet]*. 2023 Apr 1 [cited 2023 Mar 13];141. Available from: https://www.metabolismjournal.com/article/S0026-0495(23)00005-7/fulltext

6 Artificial Intelligence in Metabolic Disorders

Surovi Saikia, AK Unais, Vishnu Prabhu Athilingam, Aparna Anandan, Partha P Kalita, V. Vijaya Padma, and Yashwant Pathak

6.1 INTRODUCTION

John McCarthy, in his 2004 article, explained artificial intelligence (AI) as the science and engineering of making intelligent machines, especially intelligent computer programs. It is related to the similar task of using computers to understand human intelligence, but AI does not have to confine itself to methods that are biologically observable [1]. The various use of artificial intelligence in healthcare has gained significant attention in recent times. The challenges related to putting AI into practice have not been thoroughly resolved, but the use of AI in medical practices is slowly evolving [2]. The advancements in digitized data acquisition, machine learning, and modern computing infrastructure have led to the expansion of AI applications into domains that were earlier considered exclusive to human experts. AI has improved clinical diagnosis and decision-making in various medical fields. Many medical specialities, including ophthalmology, radiology, pathology, and dermatology, have successfully applied AI in detecting different diseases that depend on image-based diagnosis [3, 4]. It is also used in genome interpretation [5], biomarker discovery [3, 6], clinical outcome prediction and patient monitoring [7, 8], autonomous robotic surgery [9], and inferring health status through wearable devices, etc. [10, 11]. The impact of AI on medical practice, such as in disease detection and treatment, will rely on the ability of AI applications to adapt to the demanding healthcare sector, though a large amount of AI research in healthcare focuses on a few areas, like cancer [12], neurology [13], cardiology, etc. [14].

Metabolic disorder is a global public health threat. The correlation between metabolic disorder and its physical symptoms is quite challenging, and research in this area is limited. It is crucial to identify individuals who are at high risk of progressing to metabolic disorder without relying exclusively on biochemical markers using cost-effective technology [15]. The use of AI in this context would be helpful as it may be cost-effective, as well as less time-consuming. Gaucher disease, Wilson disease, type 1 diabetes, phenylketonuria, obesity, and glucose galactose malabsorption (GGM) are some of the metabolic disorders studied in context of AI technology worldwide [16, 17]. A machine learning (ML) analysis of the Spanish registry of those with Gaucher disease (GD) has identified the level of IgA as a potent risk factor [18]. A study has shown the application of the Gated Recurrent Unit Cooperation-Attention-Network (GCAN) model to evaluate the therapeutic use of two drugs cyclopropavir and AZD0837 in type I Gaucher disease, which proved to be effective [19]. A study used a support vector machine (SVM) classifier with a radial basis function kernel to evaluate the impact of abnormal rs-fMRI parameters in distinguishing between Wilson disease (WD) patients and healthy controls. Regional homogeneity (ReHo) and amplitude of low-frequency fluctuations (ALFF) values between groups showed that WD patients exhibited increased ReHo in the inferior frontal gyrus, postcentral gyrus, and insula, and decreased ReHo in the superior frontal gyrus. Additionally, ALFF was elevated in the pallidum and thalamus but decreased in the orbital part of the inferior frontal gyrus, cingulum, and medial frontal gyrus in WD patients [20]. There are many models that support the use of AI in managing diabetes. Samadi and Cinar developed a fuzzy logic estimated controller for detecting meals by utilizing glucose trends and insulin dosages to identify the shape of glycemic profiles and estimate meal content [21]. Another meal-detection algorithm was developed by Mahmoudi et al. utilizing a Kalman filter, and evaluated in the UVA-Padova *in-silico* simulator [22]. Toffanin et al., in their run-2-run algorithm, could modify insulin dosage settings [23]. A study by Zhu et al. used a supervised machine learning approach to design diagnostic screening methods for phenylketonuria in pediatrics using high-dimensional metabolic data [24]. Artificial intelligence has the potential to simplify interactive programming for analyzing body composition imaging, offering behavior coaching, suggesting personalized nutritional interventions, and recommending physical activity regimens. AI can also help in predicting the risk of obesity-related complications through predictive modeling and assist clinicians in providing precision medicine to their patients [25].

6.2 ETIOPATHOGENESIS FROM METABOLIC SYNDROME

Metabolic syndrome is a complex condition that is influenced by a variety of factors, including lifestyle choices, genetics, and environmental factors. It includes a cluster of conditions that

DOI: 10.1201/9781003384823-6

increase the risk of developing cancer, cardiovascular disease, stroke, PCOS, diabetes, etc. In the context of metabolic syndrome, these variables typically encompass blood pressure, measures of central obesity, insulin levels or sensitivity, glycemic measures, and lipid levels. The etiopathologies, or underlying causes, of metabolic syndrome include the following.

6.2.1 Insulin Resistance

Insulin resistance occurs when the body's cells become less responsive to the effects of insulin, a hormone that regulates blood sugar levels. This can lead to high blood glucose levels, which can contribute to the development of metabolic syndrome [26]. While insulin resistance and hyperinsulinemia are possible shared underlying causes for one or more of the components of metabolic syndrome, the degree and nature of this relationship can vary greatly between different populations. Western diet and lifestyle, through their impact on the insulin–IGF-I system, could potentially play a significant role in the development of metabolic syndrome. Lipid accumulation product (LAP) with insulin resistance serves as a novel biomarker that can indicate the presence of lipid build-up in central regions of the body and is therefore linked to heightened risks of cardiovascular disease and diabetes [27].

6.2.2 Obesity

Excess body fat, particularly around the waist, is a significant risk factor for metabolic syndrome. Obesity can cause insulin resistance and increase the risk of developing other conditions associated with metabolic syndrome, such as high blood pressure and high cholesterol. While plasma leptin levels do exhibit a positive correlation with obesity measures, the degree of obesity cannot be solely used to predict the levels of leptin, as there is a wide variation [28]. Other factors such as insulin, reproductive hormones, renal function, and diurnal rhythms may also influence leptin levels. As such, it has been suggested that hyperleptinemia, in addition to hyperinsulinemia/insulin resistance, could be another significant factor driving the development of metabolic syndrome [29].

6.2.3 Physical Inactivity

A lack of physical activity can lead to weight gain, insulin resistance, and other metabolic abnormalities that contribute to metabolic syndrome. Incorporating lifestyle modifications such as engaging in at least 1 hour of daily physical activity, avoiding smoking, reducing sodium and alcohol intake, and maintaining a healthy body weight can potentially yield supplementary benefits that alter the occurrence and frequency of metabolic syndrome, as well as its associated consequences. While multiple studies have established a link between physical activity and metabolic syndrome, the specific types and frequencies of physical activity that offer the most significant preventative benefits remain largely unexplored [30].

6.2.4 Genetics

Certain genetic factors can increase the risk of developing metabolic syndrome, including a family history of diabetes or obesity. The candidate gene approach, genome-wide linkage analysis, and genome-wide association studies (GWAS) are the commonly used genetic approaches for the discovery of metabolic syndrome [31].

6.2.5 Aging

As we age, our metabolism slows down, and we may become less active, which can contribute to the development of metabolic syndrome. Reactive oxygen species (ROS), which are produced as by-products of biological oxidations, cause incidental and cumulative oxidative damage to macromolecules, leading to cellular malfunction with aging and ultimately cell death, according to the free radical hypothesis of aging. In fact, oxidative stress contributes significantly to the pathophysiology of vascular changes by inducing or aggravating the metabolic syndrome's associated biochemical processes. Additionally, laboratory and clinical findings suggest that oxidative stress plays a significant role in the development of diabetes and its consequences, obesity-associated metabolic syndrome, and "satellite" diseases such non-alcoholic steatohepatitis (NASH) [32].

6.2.6 Hormonal Imbalances

Hormonal imbalances, such as those seen in polycystic ovary syndrome (PCOS), can contribute to the development of metabolic syndrome. The global prevalence of metabolic syndrome caused by androgen deprivation in males is on the rise. Epidemiological research demonstrates a link between metabolic syndrome and low testosterone levels, according to the National Institutes of Health, showing the symptoms of decreased muscle and bone mass, loss of libido, erectile dysfunction, etc. [33].

6.2.7 Sleep Disorders

Sleep apnea and other sleep disorders can disrupt hormone levels and contribute to insulin resistance, obesity, and other metabolic abnormalities.

6.2.8 Chronic Inflammation

Chronic inflammation, which can be caused by a variety of factors, including infections, stress, and a poor diet, can contribute to the development of metabolic syndrome [34].

6.3 RISK FACTORS FOR METABOLIC DISORDERS

Abdominal obesity and insulin resistance are the chief risk factors for the appearance of metabolic syndrome; other contributing factors include aging, being physically inactive, and hormonal imbalances [35]. Another risk enhancer is a diet rich in cholesterol and saturated fat, although it is not listed as an underlying risk factor for developing CVD in individuals with the syndrome [36], even though insulin resistance is considered the critical cause that predisposes individuals to type 2 diabetes mellitus (hyperglycemia). This is evident from the studies showing how multiple metabolic pathways are linked to compensatory hyperinsulinemia and insulin resistance [37]. People who are not obese but are insulin resistant with abnormal levels of metabolic risk factors are typically individuals with type 2 diabetic parents or with a first- or second-degree relative or with one parent of South Asian ethnicity [38]. Clinical obesity is not the primary criterion for insulin-resistant individuals but such individuals commonly exhibit abnormal fat distribution, characterized the upper body fat deposited either as subcutaneous or visceral fat. As claimed by many studies, the surplus visceral fat is related to insulin resistance as compared to other adipose tissue [39], while others claim that truncal fat is directly related to insulin resistance [40]. A high-level release of nonesterified fatty acids from adipose tissue is an important feature of the obesity related to the upper body that leads to lipid accumulation in places other than adipose tissue [41]. The abnormalities that arise in adipose tissue metabolism lead to insulin resistance in individuals, thereby raising the nonesterified levels of fatty acids, which further disturb the insulin resistance scenario. Obese individuals also exhibit fluctuations in the adipokinase production, which affects insulin resistance or the risk of atherosclerotic cardiovascular disease (ASCVD) [42]. Table 6.1 shows the criteria previously used for metabolic syndrome diagnosis [43].

Factors that directly affect atherosclerotic disease are known as the metabolic risk factors. These consist of high levels of apoB and serum triglyceride, abnormalities in lipoprotein aggregation, low levels of HDL-C, and elevated small LDL [36]. It has been shown by studies that the greatest atherogenicity is carried by the smallest LDL particles and the common association of small LDL with the atherogenic potential of lipoprotein functioning leads to an increased level of circulating apoB lipoprotein [44]. Other atherogenic factors that are included in metabolic factors are a high level of plasma glucose, a proinflammatory and prothrombotic state, and hypertension [45]. Table 6.2 shows the recent norms for clinical diagnosis of metabolic syndrome [43].

6.4 METABOLIC SYNDROME CLINICAL DIAGNOSIS

A group of interrelated biochemical and anthropometric characteristics, such as central obesity, glucose intolerance or diabetes, hypertension, and dyslipidemia, define metabolic syndrome. Increased levels of inflammatory markers, hyperuricemia, microalbuminuria, elevated alanine transaminase (ALT), and hemostatic abnormalities are other test findings associated with metabolic syndrome. The World Health Organization (WHO), the International Diabetes Federation (IDF), the National Cholesterol Education Programme Adult Treatment Panel III (NCEP ATPIII), the European Group for the Study of Insulin Resistance (EGIR), and the American Association of Clinical Endocrinologists (AACE) have all made attempts to define metabolic syndrome [46].

Since insulin resistance is a key component of metabolic syndromes like type 2 diabetes and cardiovascular disease, a quick, reliable, objective test that can be repeated would be perfect for diagnosing the condition. Methods used to measure insulin sensitivity are the oral glucose tolerance test, serum insulin concentration, the insulin tolerance test, the homoeostatic model assessment, and the hyperinsulinemic euglycemic clamp. Non-alcoholic fatty liver disease (NAFLD), another metabolic syndrome, is diagnosed by the good predictive biomarker gamma-glutamyl-transpeptidase (c-GT). It has been claimed that measuring ALT and AST activities as well as the

Table 6.1 Previously used criteria for metabolic syndrome diagnosis [43]

Measure	WHO	EGIR	ATP III	AACE	IDF
Glucose	T2DM, IGT, IGF	IFG or IGT (without diabetes)	>110 mg/dL (with diabetes)	IFG or IGT (without diabetes)	>100 mg/dL (without diabetes)
Lipid	**Men:** TG ≥150 mg/dL or HDL-C <35 mg/dL; **Women:** <39 mg/dL	**Men:** TG ≥150 mg/dL HDL-C <39 mg/dL; **Women:** <39 mg/dL	**Men:** TG ≥150 mg/dL HDL-C <40 mg/dL; **Women:** <50 mg/dL	**Men:** TG ≥150 mg/dL HDL-C <40 mg/dL; **Women:** <50 mg/dL	**Men:** TG ≥150 mg/dL or on TG Rx HDL-C <40 mg/dL; **Women:** <50 mg/dL HDL-C Rx
Blood pressure	≥140/90 mm Hg	≥140/90 mm Hg or on Rx hypertension	≥130/85 mm Hg	≥130/85 mm Hg	≥130 mm Hg systolic ≥85 mm Hg diastolic or Rx hypertension
Insulin resistance	Low insulin sensitivity, IFG, T2DM, IGT, and any two of other factors	Insulin in plasma >75%, and any two of the factors	Three factors following five features	IFG and IFT and any one factor on clinical judgment	NIL
Weight	**Men:** Waist–hip >0.90 **Women:** Waist–hip >0.90 BMI >30 kg/m²	**Men:** Waist circumference ≥94 cm **Women:** Waist circumference ≥80 cm	**Men:** Waist circumference ≥102 cm **Women:** Waist circumference≥ 88 cm	BMI >25 kg/m²	Increased waist circumference + any two factors
Other factors	Microalbuminuria			Insulin resistance	

Abbreviations: WHO – World Health Organization; EGIR – European Group for Study of Insulin Resistance; ATP III –Adult Treatment Panel III; AACE – American Association of Clinical Endocrinologists; IDF – The International Diabetes Foundation

Table 6.2   Recent norms for clinical diagnosis of metabolic syndrome [43]

Criteria (three out of five needed for diagnosis of metabolic syndrome)	Cutoff
Fasting glucose (raised)	≥100 mg/dL; or may be elevated due to drug use
HDL-C (reduced)	Men: <40 mg/dL; Women: <50 mg/dL; decreased due to drug use
Blood pressure (reduced)	≥130 mm/Hg systolic; ≥85 mm/Hg diastolic; antihypertensive treatment
Waist circumference (increased)	Men: ≥40 inches; Women: ≥35 inches
Triglycerides (increased)	≥ 150 mg/dL; or on drug treatment

AST:ALT ratio can help in assessing fibrosis (AST:ALT increases). Additionally, in NAFLD, plasma/serum apolipoprotein-A1 decreases, while haptoglobin, a2 macroglobulin, hyaluronic acid, amino-terminal propeptide of type III collagen, and tissue inhibitor of tissue matrix metalloproteinase 1 increase [47]. PCOS is a prevalent metabolic syndrome commonly found in the endocrinopathy in women of reproductive age. Usually, ovulatory dysfunction, clinical and/or biochemical hyperandrogenism, and polycystic ovaries on ultrasound are all characteristics of PCOS [48].

6.5 MANAGEMENT OF METABOLIC SYNDROME

The management of metabolic syndrome involves two main therapeutic goals: a) the treatment of underlying causes, such a sedentary lifestyle, central obesity; b) curing CVD risk factors that exist even after modification of lifestyle.

6.5.1 Modification of Lifestyle

6.5.1.1 Physical Activity

The risk of metabolic syndrome is reduced by between 11% and 42% with moderate to high physical activity. A study has shown that people who practiced physical activity for one week as compared to others who had not practiced physical activity, had a low risk of developing metabolic syndrome [49]. Both sexes demonstrated a similar improvement in the components of metabolic syndrome, with the exception of triglyceride levels [49]. In another similar study, men showed a decrease of 30% in triglyceride levels and women showed a 2% decrease; while postmenopausal women (overweight) who walked for 5 minutes or stood, thereby interrupting long hours of sitting, reduced postprandial levels of glucose without showing any changes in triglyceride levels. A 47% reduction in proneness to metabolic syndrome was shown in a randomized control study involving a 30-minute daily exercise routine; a follow-up 4.3 years later demonstrated the sustainability of the results [50]. Another trial called the Finnish Diabetes Prevention Study found a reduction of 52% in diabetes with follow-up of 3.2 years; the study included counseling at an individual level and factors such as physical activity, a reduction in weight, increased intake of fiber, and reduced intake of saturated fat [51].

6.5.2 Management of Diet

Diet management mainly relates to the amount of fat, carbohydrate, and sodium consumed.

Fatty acid diet: Eicosapentaenoic acid (EPA) and docosahexaenoic acid (DHA) are the omega-3 polyunsaturated fatty acids; a diet rich in these fatty acids lowers cardiovascular mortality. Studies have shown that following an omega-3 fatty acid rich diet that includes fish oil, fatty fish, flaxseed oil, and walnuts results in a fall in plasma proinflammatory cytokines such as TNF-α, IL-6, and C-reactive protein. Cardiovascular mortality is also prevented by a recommended daily intake of 250 mg of EPA and DHA [52].

Moderate–high protein diet: is the usual recommended normal diet constitution is 55% carbohydrate, 15% protein, and 30% fat. For obese individuals, in order to lower carbohydrate content, a protein diet of >20% is recommended; this is considered a moderate–high protein rich diet. High levels of fullness and thermogenesis are achieved through this type of diet, and it is preferable to increase the protein content when a hypocaloric diet is recommended in order to reach the energy requirements [53].

Carbohydrate quality: Glycemic index determines the quality of carbohydrates. A diet with a high glycemic index promptly increases the blood glucose level, resulting in a rapid insulin response and thereby leading to hypoglycemia, which is observed as an increased feeling of hunger and greater caloric intake.

Low-calorie diet: This is the most recommended diet as it an energy-restricted diet, which produces less energy than the body requires, resulting in a disproportionate energy balance. Obesity and metabolic syndrome are strongly associated with inflammation, and weight loss may lower inflammatory markers, such as IL-6 in plasma. The overall inflammatory state of the body, including insulin sensitivity and transduction, is improved by calorie restriction.

Other diet recommendations include the Mediterranean diet, an antioxidant-rich diet, and more frequent meals. Increasing meal frequency is associated with low glucose level fluctuations and stable insulin secretion, with much better appetite control. A diet rich in antioxidants aids in scavenging free radicals and the WHO recommends that people eat at least 400 g of vegetables and fruits per day. Herbs and spices are other sources of antioxidants, and the Mediterranean diet, which is rich in olive oil, fruits, and vegetables, and involves only small amounts of red meat and sweets, is associated with a lower incidence of coronary heart disease [54].

6.6 RESEARCH OVERVIEW USING RELATED METABOLIC SYNDROME DATA

New study methods, such as empirical, investigative, comparative, and experimental studies, have been developed recently. Due to the availability of large data sets relating to medical information and examinations, early-stage disease prediction is possible in metabolic syndrome. The classification of metabolic data involves a novel approach using classification methods such as JRip classifiers, random forests, and C 4.5 classifiers, including information such as blood tests. Feature selection is carried out using chi-square to leave out the unnecessary details of the data. This leads to the final inference that waist circumference, triglycerides, and HDL cholesterol are the critical factors for metabolic syndrome [55]. Another study used the WEKA tool to create a framework using genetic and clinical data from the Korean community. The group used machine learning classifiers such as random forests, naive Bayes, neural networks, support vector machines, and decision trees using the data from 10,349 individuals. Alcohol intake, levels of triglycerides, and levels of high-density lipoprotein cholesterol are detailed in this study. Of all the classifiers, naive Bayes was the most efficient as it covered the largest area under the curve value of 0.69 [56]. Table 6.3 shows the different methods employed for the collection of indicators of metabolic syndrome.

6.7 FRAMEWORK FOR METABOLIC CLASSIFICATION FOR AI APPLICATION

Metabolic syndrome is a multifactorial condition that increases the risk of developing a variety of diseases. Although the precise cause of metabolic syndrome is unknown, it is caused by a combination of genetic, environmental, and lifestyle factors. Several strategies for managing metabolic syndrome and lowering the risk of complications are currently practiced. Early detection and management of metabolic syndrome can halt or delay the onset of associated diseases. A prediction model is needed that helps restrict the onset of metabolic syndrome and provide a better life for people [66]. Metabolic syndrome frequency is projected to range from 20% to 25% across the globe [67]. Disease risk prediction models are used to predict metabolic syndrome early on the basis of many variables, such as sex, age, and family history, so it can be treated as early as possible [68]. For the classification of data, we need a proper framework. Several frameworks are currently used; one such framework used to predict metabolic syndrome in the Mexican population combines random forests, C 4.5 classifiers, and JRip classifiers [69]. Choe et al. created a framework using the WEKA tool to predict metabolic syndrome using the data from non-obese healthy people in Korea. Saffarian et al. created a continuous metabolic syndrome (cMetS) score predictor framework, which improved predictions [70, 71]. Yang et al. used the Shapley Additive Explanations (SHAP) framework to predict metabolic syndrome after a long 3-year study [72]. Tavares et al. used a combination of three metrics – the lowest Brier score, the highest receiver operator characteristic-area under the curve (ROC-AUC), and the highest precision-recall-rea under the curve (PR-AUC) – to predict metabolic syndrome and also for early prevention based on the conditional average treatment effect (CATE) [73]. Karimi-Alavijeh et al. used SVM and decision tree methods in the prediction of the 7-year incidence of metabolic syndrome [74]. Kim et al. used nine machine learning models: decision tree, Gaussian Naive Bayes, K-nearest neighbors, eXtreme gradient boosting (XGBoost), random forest, logistic regression, support vector machine, multi-layer perceptron, and 1D convolutional neural network in the prediction of metabolic syndrome and pre-metabolic syndrome in Korean populations [75]. Apart from the nine machine learning classifiers, categorical boosting (CatBoost) can also be used to predict MS at an early stage using

Table 6.3 Various methods applied for collection of indicators metabolic syndrome

Classifiers Used	Dataset Volume	Indicators	Metaheuristics Use	Inferences	Ref.
LG, GBT, RFs	Japanese Metabolic Syndrome dataset	None	No	None	[57]
RFs, JRip, C 4.5	2,942 patients	Waist circumference Triglycerides HDL cholesterol	No	RFs is best performer	[58]
DTs, SVM	Cohort Isfahan dataset	None	No	SVM with 75% accuracy	[59]
ANN, SVM, DTs, RFs, NB	1,039 Korean patients	None	No	NB with AUC 69%	[56]
ANN, SVM, XGBoost, LG, KNNs, RFs, 1D NN, DTs	1,991 Korean medical test reports	BMI Waist–hip ratio	No	XGBoost with AUC 85%	[60]
SVM, ANN, CART	3,577 student data	HDL cholesterol Waist circumference	No	CART outperforms others	[61]
DTs, KNNs, LGB, XGBoost, linear analysis, LG	17,182 patients	HDL cholesterol Waist circumference Triglycerides	No	LGB with AUC 86%	[62]
LG, RFs, XGBoost	39,134 patients	Systolic blood pressure Fasting triglycerides Central adiposity	No	XGBoost 99.7% accuracy	[63]
Stacking, XGBoost, RFs	67,730 patients	Body mass index Fasting triglycerides Abdominal Obesity	No	XGBoost with AUC 93%	[64]
RFs	5,646 patients	Triglycerides	No	RFs with 98.11% accuracy	[65]

Abbreviations: ANN – Artificial Neural Network; CART –Classification and Regression Tree; DTs – Decision Trees; KNNs – K-Neural Networks; NN – Neural Network; RFs – Random Forests; SVM – Support Vector Machine; XGBoost – eXtreme Gradient Boosting

AI. Apart from the machine learning models, we also use the five metaheuristics algorithms in prediction and detection: particle swarm optimization, genetic algorithms, the Bat algorithm, the firefly algorithm, and ant colony optimization. So, through the use of AI algorithms, we can create different frameworks that can predict, detect, or help in prevention of metabolic syndrome.

6.8 AI ALGORITHMS USED FOR INBORN METABOLISM ERRORS IN NEWBORNS

Inborn metabolism errors (IEMs) are a serious issue that can lead to non-standard growth and death in later stages. A number of clinical symptoms brought on by the build-up of intermediate, bypass, or terminal metabolites are the result of enzyme defects, membrane dysfunction, or receptor defects [76, 110], so early detection, screening, and treatment are necessary in bringing up a healthy individual [77]. Zhou et al. have demonstrated the use of tandem mass spectrometry in screening IEMs in a more efficient and economical way [78]. Yang et al. have developed an auxiliary diagnosis system to predict IEMs in newborns; the model is based on the construction and selection of model indicators, model selection and training, and model evaluation [79]. Enhancing Data-driven Disease Detection in Newborns (ED3N) is a pilot program designed to enhance newborn disease detection through dried blood spot (DBS) screening using both biochemical and molecular analytical techniques. It is expected that disease prediction tests will be greatly improved and expanded by the use of both genomic data and biochemical results to provide phenotypic information [80]. Shirwaikar et al. used the heightened eight-layer multilayer perceptron (MLP) prototypical tool to develop a framework to reduce complex neural networks to simpler ones, which is helpful in apnea prediction in newborns [81]. Uryu et al. developed a deep neural-network model based on AI algorithms to detect cases of Fabry disease in newborns using their urine samples [82]. Kaur et al. combined AI techniques in predicting congenital diseases in newborns based on PRISMA guidelines; resulting insights relate to fetal health, chromosome anomalies, congenital heart disease (CHD), cytomegalovirus (CMV), Zika virus, sepsis, and preeclampsia (PE) hypertension [83]. For the prediction of fetal health, several algorithms are used, including Kalman filtering, Gaussian model selection, convolutional neural network (CNN), type-2 fuzzy logic system classifier [84], deep neural networks (DNN), ensemble learning [85], averaged perceptron, decision tree (DT), decision jungle, SVM, neural network, locally deep SVM [86], and image-based ML [87]. For chromosomal anomalies, the frequently used algorithms are CNN [88], artificial neural network (ANN), feed-forward ANN [89], deep CNN [90], YOLOv2 convolutional neural network (CNN) [91], and L1-norm-based support vector regression (L1-SVR) [92]. For congenital heart disease, the most commonly used algorithms are GG16-based neural network for transfer learning [93], backward propagation neural network (BPNN) [94], deep neural network [95], k-nearest neighbors (KNN), SVM, logistic regression [96], ensemble neural network [97], and explainable boosting machine (EBM) [98]. Intrauterine growth restriction (IUGR) detection in newborns can be carried out by artificial neural networks (ANNs), K-means clustering [99], bagging with naive Bayesian (NB), KNN, C4.5, and SMO [100], Matthews correlation coefficient (MCC) [101], radial basis function (RBF)-SVM [102], stochastic gradient descent, KNN, radio frequency (RF), and logistic regression [103]. Cytomegalovirus (CMV) can be detected using hierarchical ranking CNN (HR-CNN), K-means clustering, high SVM (HSVM) [104], Kalman filtering, and Gaussian model selection [105], and Zika virus can be detected using backward propagation neural network (BPNN), glioblastoma multiforme (GBM), RF [106], multilayer perceptron neural network (MLPNN) using the cloud [107], cubic support vector classifier [108], and multilayer perceptron with a probabilistic optimization strategy. Sepsis in newborns was detected using logistic regression, NB, SVM with radial basis function kernel, KNN, RF, adaptive boosting (AdaBoost), gradient boosting, Gaussian Naive Bayes (GNV), decision tree, bagging classifier, and ultilayer perceptron, and hypertensive complication can be detected using ANN, adaptive neuro fuzzy inference system (ANFIS), fuzzy logic, particle swarm optimization, deep learning, neural network (NN), cost-sensitive DNN (CSDNN), and Bayesian optimization. With the help of these AI algorithms, we can easily predict metabolism errors in newborns [108].

6.9 ABDOMINAL ADIPOSE TISSUE ANALYSIS USING AI METHODS

6.9.1 The Importance of Adipose Tissue

It was once thought that adipose tissue served as a long-term energy storage organ from which the body could quickly release free fatty acids when necessary [109, 110]. According to recent research, adipose tissue should in fact be viewed as an endocrine organ whose dynamic and complicated activity is aimed at controlling whole-body homeostasis. Numerous adipokines secreted by the adipocytes are involved in the regulation of appetite, glucose, and lipid metabolism, cardiovascular homeostasis, inflammatory, immune, and reproductive functions, as well as other essential biological and physiological processes [111, 112]. Visceral adipose tissue (VAT) and subcutaneous adipose tissue (SAT) are both primary compartments of abdominal adipose tissue. With their diverse molecular, biological, and anatomical makeup, these two compartments have various characteristics. SAT is involved in more long-term storage of energy, whereas VAT exhibits greater metabolic and hormonal activity through the discharge of adipokines [113, 114]. Increased VAT influences health because it is linked to a wide range of illnesses, including cardiovascular diseases. For instance, a link between hypercoagulability and peripheral artery disease, increased intima–media thickness, and increased plasminogen activator inhibitor 1 (PAI-1) production was discovered [115, 116]. Additionally, coronary artery disease is predicted by hyperinsulinemia in a clinical picture of visceral obesity [117]. Type 2 diabetes and cardiovascular illnesses are more likely to occur in obese people with elevated VAT [118]. The development of obesity-related tumors is thought to be mediated by adipokines, growth factors, and proinflammatory cytokines released by VAT [119, 120]. In fact, distinct signatures of the quantity and distribution of abdominal adipose tissue have been linked to several diseases (including oncological ones) in terms of risk, intra-tumoral genetic alterations, prognosis, and side effects and complications following therapy [121–126].

6.9.1.1 Artificial Neural Network and Linear Regression-Based Equation for Estimating Visceral Adipose Tissue Volume

Numerous techniques have been developed to assess visceral fat. The most clinically expedient are those that can be performed quickly, provide instant results, and can be carried out by the bedside without extensive technical training. Anthropometric measures and bioelectrical impedance analysis (BIA) are designed to provide expedient, albeit crude, measures of body composition; however, VAT is only an indirect measure when using these approaches. Only computed tomography (CT) and magnetic resonance imaging (MRI) can provide direct measures of cross-sectional areas or volumetric measures of VAT.

Researchers created and tested novel equations to calculate the amount of abdominal visceral adipose tissue in 5,772 UK Biobank participants using only basic anthropometric measurements. To estimate the abdomen's VAT volume, they evaluated the effectiveness of linear regression with artificial neural network-based equations. In this study, the derivation sample and the validation sample both produced favorable results for the basic and expanded regression models and ANN-based equations. Although there were statistical differences between the estimated visceral adipose tissues (eVATs) produced by ANN-based equations and those based on linear regression, the mean differences were small. When adjusted R^2 and error measurements were considered, ANN-based equations showed somewhat better performances than linear regression equations, with higher adjusted R^2, lower root-mean-square error (RMSE), and lower mean absolute error (MAE). When compared to linear regression equations, ANN models showed only modest improvements in estimation accuracy. A recent systematic analysis that examined comparable phenomena found no performance advantage for clinical prediction models for machine learning over logistic regression [127]. The ANN-based equations may therefore potentially provide the optimum estimation of VAT based on adjusted R^2 and error measurements, whilst regression equations may produce competent estimations based on ROC analysis. Given this, we suggest that either equation can be used in clinical practice.

The fact that ANN-based equations in this investigation did not significantly outperform linear regression in terms of accuracy does not diminish the potential benefits of using ANN for other medical applications. A recent work that used an ANN-based equation to calculate maximum oxygen uptake showed that it was more accurate than a traditional linear regression equation [128]. The percentage of non-linearity in the relationship between the dependent and independent variables, as well as the properties of the training data, play a significant role in determining the level of improvements produced by ANN models in comparison with linear regression. ANN may be a potential alternative for clinical parameters for which linear regression cannot provide adequate estimation accuracy. The performance of the fundamental linear regression and ANN-based equations was marginally worse than that of the expanded ones.

However, the extended equations' performance was not noticeably enhanced by the addition of waist circumference (WC) and hip circumference (HC). There were significant variations in WC, waist–hip ratio (WHR), and VAT between males and females, even though in this study's ANN-based equations, the enlarged equation, which accounted for 75% of the validation sample, showed greater accuracy. Therefore, whenever WC and HC can be attained without a disproportionate workload, the enlarged equation is advised. Several equations have been established for the calculation of VAT; however, only one equation accurately predicted abdominal VAT volume using a volumetric MRI of the abdomen (adjusted $R^2 = 0.47$ [9]). Nonetheless, in this equation, WC and WHR had a strong correlation with VAT ($r = 0.83$, $r = 0.73$). As a result, the greater coefficient of "sex" in the fundamental equation accounted for nearly all the variance in VAT associated with WC and WHR. Meanwhile, the WC and HC intra- and inter-observer variation may be detrimental to the performance of the enlarged equations. Due to tissue composition (such as the quantity of subcutaneous fat, intestines, etc.) [129], measurement site [130], and the wall's tension, previous researchers have revealed that circumference measurements are less reliable than weight and height indices [131], which is due to the tissue composition (e.g., amount of subcutaneous fat, intestines, abdominal wall tension [132] and measurement site) [133].

Most previous equations were constructed using the cross-sectional VAT areas of different measurement sites, such as the lumbar vertebrae L3–L5. Although single-slice images may not accurately depict an individual's VAT [134, 135], and VAT volume is more closely linked with the risk factors of metabolic syndrome than VAT area within the L4–L5 level [136, 137], cross-sectional VAT area continues to be used as a proxy for volumetric VAT in numerous studies [138, 139]. No such previous studies have evaluated the performance of the estimation equation by ROC analysis. It has been discovered that there is no concordance between anatomical sites and the determination coefficient (R^2) of cross-sectional VAT area in the assessment of entire abdominal VAT volume. In a study of 59 healthy female volunteers, the R^2 for the VAT area at the level of L2–L3 was 0.31 and for L4–L5 it was 0.58 [140]. R^2 for VAT regions assessed at multiple vertebral levels from L1 to S1 varied from 0.76 to 0.98 in research involving 200 patients from the Framingham Heart Study [141]. Another study found that in 142 healthy Caucasians, VAT regions evaluated at several lumbar vertebral levels from L1 to L5 had R^2 values ranging from 0.78 to 0.97 [142]. A sample of 197 people ranging from overweight to severely obese were studied and it was found that R^2 for numerous lumbar intervertebral levels from L1 to S1 ranged from 0.58 to 0.95 for single-slice VAT volumes and 0.63 to 0.92 for five-slice VAT volumes [142]. It is important to note that all four equations in this investigation showed adjusted R^2 values greater than 0.71, with 0.78 being the best. This suggests that our equations may be able to estimate VAT volumes similar to those from cross-sectional VAT regions obtained from a single CT/MRI slice. Our equation may therefore be a more affordable option for investigations when CT/MRI scans are simply used to measure the cross-sectional VAT area. Our estimating equations were constructed using data from persons aged 45 to 76 and solely from white participants, taking into account the age distribution and ethnic mixture of the UK Biobank participants. This limits the applicability of our equations to other age groups and ethnicities. It is also probable that the estimating capacity of our equations would differ with external samples because of the inter- and intra-variability of the anthropometric factors, as well as the inter-study disagreement of MRI/CT-derived VAT volumes, which is a topic for further study. Another drawback is the fact that in the validation sample, 16.7% of very slim females (body mass index [BMI] < 20 kg/m^2) had eVATs computed by linear regression models that were less than zero. This is inevitable given the characteristics of linear regression, whereas ANN-based equations do not show this flaw. Finally, the study did not use several parameters (such as dual-energy X-ray absorptiometry, android percentage fat, bioelectrical impedance analysis, skin fold, and sagittal diameter) due to their contentious relevance for estimating VAT [143], uncertainties relating to their applicability [144], and the need for specialized equipment for measurement.

6.10 PRECISION MEDICINE FOR CHRONIC DISEASES WITH AI USE

Precision medicine is "an emerging approach for disease treatment and prevention that takes into account individual variability in genes, environment, and lifestyle for each person", according to the National Institutes of Health [145]. This method enables medical professionals and researchers to make more precise predictions about which preventative and treatment options for a specific disease will be most effective for which demographics. It calls for powerful computers (supercomputers), algorithms that can learn on their own at a previously unheard-of rate (deep learning), and, generally, an approach that makes use of doctors' cognitive talents on a new level (AI). Supercomputers' computing capacity has turned into a battlefield where nations can show off their might [146]. In the fields of dermatology [147], cancer [148], and cardiology [149], it has been demonstrated that deep learning algorithms can diagnose patients at least as effectively as doctors. However, we must stress how crucial it is to combine these algorithms with medical expertise. For the International Symposium on Biomedical Imaging's grand challenge, competitors developed computational techniques for detecting metastatic breast cancer in entire slide pictures of sentinel lymph node biopsies. The success rate of the winning algorithm was 92.5%. The success rate was 96.6% when a pathologist independently examined the same photos. Combining the diagnosis of a human pathologist with the predictions of a deep learning system raised the pathologist's success rate to 99.5%, reducing human mistake rates by about 85% [150].

Although the terms AI and ML have frequently been used interchangeably, it is crucial to know the distinctions between them. A group of technologies known as artificial intelligence (AI) allow a machine to mimic human behaviors. ML and natural language processing (NLP) are two areas of AI that are particularly pertinent to the healthcare industry [151, 152]. While NLP enables robots to read, understand, and infer meaning from human languages, ML enables software or algorithms to automatically learn from prior data without explicit programming. As most AI applications in the healthcare industry are built on ML, we will mostly concentrate on ML in this evaluation. It is well known that traditional statistical methods, like linear and logistic regression, which are frequently used to predict clinical outcomes, have many drawbacks. These methods struggle with non-linear relationships or high-dimensional data and are unable to consider the unknowable interactions between the input variables. They are also excessively labor-intensive in the age of big data [153].

6.10.1 Artificial Intelligence in Chronic Heart Failure

Chronic heart failure (CHF) is a disorder in which the patient's heart weakens over time, leading to higher rates of death, morbidity, and a lower quality of life. Heart failure (HF) incidents are happening more frequently [154]. The most frequent type of left-sided failure occurs when the left ventricle fails to properly pump blood out to the body. There are two different types of failure: systolic HF and diastolic failure. Congestive heart failure symptoms include fatigue, swelling, weight gain, and fast breathing. Blood tests, MRIs, and ECGs are a few examples of HF diagnostic tools; however, HF prediction accuracy is still being studied. Numerous AI-based methods have been released over the years for the accurate prediction and diagnosis of HF. These will be discussed in this section. Up to 2014, many authors used their own datasets. The approaches employed in these articles with SVM as their classification algorithm have an accuracy range of 77% to 100%. The highest accuracy rates (98.97% and 100%, respectively) for the CNN approaches, with z-score normalization, regularization, and kernel function computation as pre-processing steps [155], and with normalization as pre-processing steps, were obtained in 2019 and 2021, respectively [156]. Measures of HRV were crucial in the identification of CHF. The first approach to the detection of HF was based on heart rate variability (HRV), in which the frequency domain determines the frequency components, and the time domain calculates the beat-to-beat intervals. Additionally, a model for CHF detection based on HRV measurements has been developed [157–159].

Işer and Kuntalp (2007) employed KNN for classification and GA as a feature selector. Their model's accuracy was 96.39% when tested on the MIT/BIH/PhysioBank dataset. Elfadil and Ibrahim (2011) presented a similar strategy using two neural networks: an unsupervised self-organizing neural network and a supervised multi-perceptron [160]. They used 53 normal individuals and 17 with CHF to train their supervised model, while they used 1,000 random normal individuals and 1,000 random individuals with CHF to train their unsupervised model. Unsupervised accuracy (92.90%) was higher than supervised accuracy (83.65%). Two strategies based on HRV measurements were put forward in 2014 by Narin et al. Using the PhysioBank dataset, the authors [161] tested five classifications based on LDA, KNN, SVM, RBF, and MLP. Based on their testing, SVM had the best scores, at 91.56% accuracy, 82.75% sensitivity, and 96.29% specificity, while Liu et al. (2014) achieved 100% sensitivity, precision, and accuracy. This research has shown that HRV can be identified and distinguished from other HF detection methods, but HRV is losing value. In the article [162], an innovative approach employing deep CNN was used to predict congestive HF. The authors suggested an architecture for the automatic diagnosis of HFs that combined deep neural networks with ECG signals. Four sets, A, B, C, and D, were used to test the model. The congestive HF database, the Fantasia Database, and the MIT-BIH Normal Sinus Rhythm Database (NSRDB) were three sets of data that were made available to the public. Several techniques, including z-score normalization, regularization, and kernel functions, were used during the pre-processing stage.

It was suggested that an 11-layer deep CNN model be used to determine the possibility that a person has congestive HF signals. The model's accuracy for set B was 98.97%, which was higher than any other work suggested. The analysis suggested another CNN-based strategy for predicting congestive HF. The MIT-BIH NSRDB, which is a part of PhysioNet, provided the dataset used by the model. The redundant data from the beats was removed from the ECG recordings of all the data after they had been normalized. The model's innovative feature utilized raw ECG signals as opposed to HRV characteristics. Since clinical patients oversee the congestive HF measures, their input is essential. The model's accuracy was 100% [162].

6.11 FUTURE RESEARCH

AI has already started changing the healthcare system. It has been extensively tested in different pathology and radiology laboratories. As the health-based data repositories are increasing day by day, AI will play a crucial role in disease prediction, diagnosis, and the provision of precision medicine to the patients. The development of different chatbots and wearables will also help in the management of different diseases. With the help of the available disease distribution data, it may be possible to predict any epidemic outbreak. However, there could be many challenges in implementing AI or other machine learning approaches in healthcare due to various ethical issues.

CONCLUSIONS

In this chapter, we have discussed the different factors and causes of metabolic syndrome and the various AI models employed to deduce the critical causes and symptoms.

CONFLICT OF INTEREST

Declared none.

ACKNOWLEDGMENTS

We thank the Vice Chancellor, Bharathiar University, Coimbatore-641046, Tamil Nadu for providing the necessary facilities. We also thank UGC-New Delhi for the Dr D.S. Kothari Fellowship

((No. F-2/ 2006 (BSR) / BL / 20-21 / 0396)), TANSCHE (RGP/ 2019-20/BU /HECP-0005; No.C3/ CRTD/995/ 2021), DST-INSPIRE (DST/INSPIRE/2019/IF190185), and RUSA (BU/RUSA2.0/ BCTRC/2020/BCTRC-CT03).

REFERENCES

1. Tai MC. The impact of artificial intelligence on human society and bioethics. *Tzu Chi Medical Journal* 2020;32(4):339–343.

2. Shaw J, Rudzicz F, Jamieson T, Goldfarb A. Artificial intelligence and the implementation challenge. *Journal of Medical Internet Research* 2019;21(7):e13659.

3. Yu K-H, Beam AL, Kohane IS. Artificial intelligence in healthcare. *Nature Biomedical Engineering* 2018;2(10):719–731.

4. Litjens G, Kooi T, Bejnordi BE, Setio AAA, Ciompi F, Ghafoorian M, et al. A survey on deep learning in medical image analysis. *Medical Image Analysis* 2017;42:60–88.

5. Quang D, Xie X. DanQ: A hybrid convolutional and recurrent deep neural network for quantifying the function of DNA sequences. *Nucleic Acids Research* 2016;44(11):e107–e107.

6. Wallden B, Storhoff J, Nielsen T, Dowidar N, Schaper C, Ferree S, et al. Development and verification of the PAM50-based Prosigna breast cancer gene signature assay. *BMC Medical Genomics* 2015;8(1):1–14.

7. Altman RB. Artificial intelligence (AI) systems for interpreting complex medical datasets. *Clinical Pharmacology & Therapeutics* 2017;101(5):585–586.

8. Churpek MM, Yuen TC, Winslow C, Robicsek AA, Meltzer DO, Gibbons RD, et al. Multicenter development and validation of a risk stratification tool for ward patients. *American Journal of Respiratory and Critical Care Medicine* 2014;190(6):649–655.

9. Elek R, Nagy TD, Nagy DÁ, Kronreif G, Rudas IJ, Haidegger T. Recent trends in automating robotic surgery. In 2016 IEEE 20th Jubilee International Conference on Intelligent Engineering Systems (INES), pp. 27–32. IEEE, 2016.

10. Li X, Jessilyn D, Salins D, Zhou G, Zhou W, Miryam S, et al. Digital health: tracking physiomes and activity using wearable biosensors reveals useful health-related information. *PLoS Biology* 2017;15(1):e2001402.

11. Majumder S, Mondal T, Deen MJ. Wearable sensors for remote health monitoring. *Sensors* 2017;17(1):130.

12. Esteva A, Kuprel B, Novoa RA, Ko J, Swetter SM, Blau HM, et al. Dermatologist-level classification of skin cancer with deep neural networks. *Nature* 2017;542:115–118.

13. Farina D, Vujaklija I, Sartori M, Kapelner T, Negro F, Jiang N, et al. Man/machine interface based on the discharge timings of spinal motor neurons after targeted muscle reinnervation. *Nature Biomedical Engineering* 2017;1(2):0025.

14. Dilsizian SE, Siegel EL. Artificial intelligence in medicine and cardiac imaging: Harnessing big data and advanced computing to provide personalized medical diagnosis and treatment. *Current Cardiology Reports* 2014;16:1–8.

15. Chen H, Xiong S, Ren X. Evaluating the risk of metabolic syndrome based on an artificial intelligence model. In *Abstract and Applied Analysis* (Vol. 2014). Hindawi, 2014.

16. National Center for Biotechnology Information (US). Genes and disease [Internet]. Bethesda (MD): National Center for Biotechnology Information (US); 1998–. Nutritional and Metabolic Diseases. Available from: https://www.ncbi.nlm.nih.gov/books/NBK22259/

17. Sghaireen MG, Al-Smadi Y, Al-Qerem A, Srivastava KC, Ganji KK, Khursheed Alam M, et al. Machine learning approach for metabolic syndrome diagnosis using explainable data-augmentation-based classification. *Diagnostics* 2022;12(12):3117.

18. Andrade-Campos MM, López de Frutos L, Cebolla JJ, Serrano-Gonzalo I, Medrano-Engay B, Roca-Espiau M, et al. Identification of risk features for complication in Gaucher's disease patients: A machine learning analysis of the Spanish registry of Gaucher disease. *Orphanet Journal of Rare Diseases* 2020;15(1):1–11.

19. Cao H, Zhang L, Jin B, Cheng S, Wei X, Che C. Enriching limited information on rare diseases from heterogeneous networks for drug repositioning. *BMC Medical Informatics and Decision Making* 2021;21(Supplement 9):1–9.

20. Wu Y, Kan H, Hu S, Lu H, Jin L. Predictive value of different rs-fMRI parameters in Wilson disease based on SVM. In 2022 IEEE 6th Advanced Information Technology, Electronic and Automation Control Conference (IAEAC), pp. 1534–15. IEEE, 2022.

21. Samadi S, Rashid M, Turksoy K, Feng J, Hajizadeh I, Hobbs N, et al. Automatic detection and estimation of unannounced meals for multivariable artificial pancreas system. *Diabetes Technology & Therapeutics* 2018;20:235–246.

22. Mahmoudi Z, Cameron F, Kjølstad Poulsen N, Madsen H, Bequette BW, Jørgensen JB. Sensor-based detection and estimation of meal carbohydrates for people with diabetes. *Biomedical Signal Processing and Control* 2019;48:12–25.

23. Toffanin C, Messori M, Cobelli C, Magni L. Automatic adaptation of basal therapy for type 1 diabetic patients: A run-to-run approach. *Biomedical Signal Processing and Control* 2017;31:539–549.

24. Zhu Z, Gu J, Genchev GZ, Cai X, Wang Y, Guo J, Tian G, Lu H. Improving the diagnosis of phenylketonuria by using a machine learning–based screening model of neonatal MRM data. *Frontiers in Molecular Biosciences* 2020;7:115.

25. Bays HE, Fitch A, Cuda S, Rickey E, Hablutzel J, Coy R, Censani M. Artificial intelligence and obesity management: An Obesity Medicine Association (OMA) Clinical Practice Statement (CPS) 2023. *Obesity Pillars* 2023:100065.

26. Kim T, Kang J. Relationship between obstructive sleep apnea, insulin resistance, and metabolic syndrome: A nationwide population-based survey. *Endocrine Journal*, 2023;70(1):107–119.

27. Janssen JA. The impact of westernization on the insulin/IGF-I signaling pathway and the metabolic syndrome: It is time for change. *International Journal of Molecular Sciences* 2023;24(5):4551.

28. Zimmet P, Boyko EJ, Collier GR, de Courten M. Etiology of the metabolic syndrome: Potential role of insulin resistance, leptin resistance, and other players. *Annals of the New York Academy of Sciences* 1999;892(1):25–44.

29. De Courten M, Zimmet P, Hodge A. Hyperleptinaemia: The missing link in the Metabolic Syndrome? *Diabetic Medicine* 1997;14:200–208.

30. Hastert TA, Gong J, Campos H, Baylin A. Physical activity patterns and metabolic syndrome in Costa Rica. *Preventive Medicine* 2015;70:39–45.

31. Abou Ziki MD, Mani A. Metabolic syndrome: Genetic insights into disease pathogenesis. *Current Opinion in Lipidology* 2016;27(2):162–171.

32. Bonomini F, Rodella LF, Rezzani, R. Metabolic syndrome, aging and involvement of oxidative stress. *Aging and Disease* 2015;6(2):109.

33. Ziaei S, Mohseni, H. Correlation between hormonal statuses and metabolic syndrome in postmenopausal women. *Journal of Family & Reproductive Health* 2013;7(2), 63.

34. Furukawa S, Fujita T, Shimabukuro M, Iwaki M, Yamada Y,Nakajima Y et al. Increased oxidative stress in obesity and its impact on metabolic syndrome. *Journal of Clinical Investigation* 2004;114:1752–1761.

35. Apridonidze T, Essah PA, Iuorno MJ, Nestler JE. Prevalence and characteristics of the metabolic syndrome in women with polycystic ovary syndrome. *The Journal of Clinical Endocrinology and Metabolism* 2004;90:1929–1935.

36. National Cholesterol Education Program (NCEP). Expert panel on detection, evaluation, and treatment of high blood cholesterol in adults (Adult Treatment Panel III). Third Report of the National Cholesterol Education Program (NCEP) expert panel on detection, evaluation, and treatment of high blood cholesterol in adults (Adult Treatment Panel III) final report. *Circulation* 2002;106:3143–3421.

37. Eckel RH, Grundy SM, Zimmet PZ. The metabolic syndrome. *Lancet* 2005;365:1415–1428.

38. Abate N, Chandalia M, Snell PG, Grundy SM. Adipose tissue metabolites and insulin resistance in nondiabetic Asian Indian men. *The Journal of Clinical Endocrinology and Metabolism* 2004;89:2750–2755.

39. Carr DB, Utzschneider KM, Hull RL, Kodama K, Retzlaff BM, Brunzell JD, Shofer JB, Fish BE, Knopp RH, Kahn SE. Intra-abdominal fat is a major determinant of the national cholesterol education program adult treatment panel III criteria for the metabolic syndrome. *Diabetes.* 2004; 53:2087–2094.

40. Nielsen S, Guo Z, Johnson CM, Hensrud DD, Jensen MD. Splanchnic lipolysis in human obesity. *Journal of Clinical Investigation* 2004;113:1582–1588.

41. Abate N, Chandalia M, Snell PG, Grundy SM. Adipose tissue metabolites and insulin resistance in nondiabetic Asian Indian men. *The Journal of Clinical Endocrinology and Metabolism* 2004;89:2750–2755.

42. You T, Yang R, Lyles MF, Gong D, Nicklas BJ. Abdominal adipose tissue cytokine gene expression: Relationship to obesity and metabolic risk factors. *American Journal of Physiology-Endocrinology and Metabolism* 2005;288:E741–E747.

43. Grundy SM, Cleeman JI, Daniels SR, Donato KA, Eckel RH, Franklin BA, et al. Diagnosis and management of the metabolic syndrome: An American Heart Association/National Heart, Lung, and Blood Institute Scientific Statement. *Circulation* 2005 Oct 25;112(17):2735–2752. Doi: 10.1161/CIRCULATIONAHA.105.169404. Epub 2005 Sep 12. Erratum in: Circulation. 2005 Oct 25;112(17):e297. Erratum in: Circulation. 2005 Oct 25;112(17):e298. PMID:16157765.

44. Brunzell JD. Increased apo B in small dense LDL particles predicts premature coronary artery disease. *Arteriosclerosis, Thrombosis, and Vascular Biology* 2005;25:474–475.

45. Chobanian AV, Bakris GL, Black HR, Cushman WC, Green LA, Izzo JL Jr, et al. National heart, lung, and blood institute joint national committee on prevention, detection, evaluation, and treatment of high blood pressure; national high blood pressure education program

coordinating committee. The seventh report of the joint national committee on prevention, detection, evaluation, and treatment of high blood pressure: The JNC 7 report. *JAMA* 2003;289:2560–2572.

46. Alberti KG, Zimmet P, Shaw J. Metabolic syndrome—A new world-wide definition. A consensus statement from the international diabetes federation. *Diabetic Medicine* 2006;23:469–480.

47. Olufadi R, Byrne CD. Clinical and laboratory diagnosis of the metabolic syndrome. *Journal of Clinical Pathology* 2008;61(6):697–706.

48. Amanti-Kandarakis E. Insulin resistance in PCOS. *Endocrine* 2006;30:13–17.

49. Lee J, Kim Y, Jeon JY. Association between physical activity and the prevalence of metabolic syndrome: From the Korean National Health and Nutrition Examination Survey, 1999–2012. *SpringerPlus* 2016;5(1):1870. DOI: 10.1186/s40064-016-3514-5.

50. Henson J, Davies MJ, Bodicoat DH, Edwardson CL, Gill JMR, Stensel DJ, et al. Breaking up prolonged sitting with standing or walking attenuates the postprandial metabolic response in postmenopausal women: A randomized acute study. *Diabetes Care* 2016;39(1):130–138. DOI: 10.2337/dc15-1240.

51. Pérez-Martínez P, Mikhailidis DP, Athyros VG, Bullo M, Couture P, Covas MI, et al. Lifestyle recommendations for the prevention and management of metabolic syndrome: An international panel recommendation. *Nutrition Reviews* 2017;75(5):307–326.

52. Iglesia R, Loria-Kohen V, Zulet M, Martinez J, Reglero G, Ramirez de Molina A. Dietary strategies implicated in the prevention and treatment of metabolic syndrome. *International Journal of Molecular Sciences* 2016;17(11):1877.

53. Akbaraly TN, Tabak AG, Shipley MJ, Mura T, Singh-Manoux A, Ferrie JE, et al. Little change in diet after onset of type 2 diabetes, metabolic syndrome, and obesity in middle-aged adults: 11-year follow-up study. *Diabetes Care* 2016;39(3):e29–e30.

54. Lee J, Kim Y, Jeon JY. Association between physical activity and the prevalence of metabolic syndrome: from the Korean National Health and Nutrition Examination Survey, 1999–2012. *SpringerPlus* 2016;5(1):1870.

55. Gutiérrez-Esparza GO, Vázquez OI, Vallejo M, Hernández-Torruco J. Prediction of metabolic syndrome in a Mexican population applying machine learning algorithms. *Symmetry* 2020;12:581.

56. Choe EK, Rhee H, Lee S, Shin E, Oh S-W, Lee J-E, et al. Metabolic syndrome prediction using machine learning models with genetic and clinical information from a nonobese healthy population. *Genomics & Informatics* 2018;16:e31.

57. Shimoda A, Ichikawa D, Oyama H. Prediction models to identify individuals at risk of metabolic syndrome who are unlikely to participate in a health intervention program. *International Journal of Medical Informatics* 2018;111:90–99.

58. Gutiérrez-Esparza GO, Vázquez OI, Vallejo M, Hernández-Torruco J. Prediction of metabolic syndrome in a Mexican population applying machine learning algorithms. *Symmetry* 2020;12:581.

59. KarimiAlavijeh F, Jalili S, Sadeghi M. Predicting metabolic syndrome using decision tree and support vector machine methods. *ARYA Atherosclerosis* 2016;12:146–152.

60. Kim J, Mun S, Lee S, Jeong K, Baek Y. Prediction of metabolic and pre-metabolic syndromes using machine learning models with anthropometric, lifestyle, and biochemical factors from a middle-aged population in Korea. *BMC Public Health* 2022;22:664.

61. Saffarian M, Babaiyan V, Namakin K, Taheri F, Kazemi T. Developing a novel continuous metabolic syndrome score: A data mining based model. *Journal of Artificial Intelligence and Data Mining* 2021;9:193–202.

62. Tavares LD, Manoel A, Donato THR, Cesena F, Minanni CA, Kashiwagi NM, et al. Prediction of metabolic syndrome: A machine learning approach to help primary prevention. *Diabetes Research and Clinical Practice* 2022;191:110047.

63. Zhang Y, Zhang X, Razbek J, Li D, Xia W, Bao L, et al. Opening the black box: Interpretable machine learning for predictor finding of metabolic syndrome. *BMC Endocrine Disorders* 2022;22;214.

64. Yang H, Yu B, Ouyang P, Li X, Lai X, Zhang G, et al. Machine learning-aided risk prediction for metabolic syndrome based on 3 years study. *Scientific Reports* 2022;12:2248.

65. Worachartcheewan A, Shoombuatong W, Pidetcha P, Nopnithipat W, Prachayasittikul V, Nantasenamat C. Predicting metabolic syndrome using the random forest method. *The Scientific World Journal* 2015;2015:581501.

66. Sghaireen MG, Al-Smadi Y, Al-Qerem A, Srivastava KC, Ganji KK, Alam MK, et al. Machine learning approach for metabolic syndrome diagnosis using explainable data-augmentation-based classification. *Diagnostics* 2022;12(12):3117.

67. Tanner RM, Brown TM, Muntner P. Epidemiology of obesity, the metabolic syndrome, and chronic kidney disease. *Current Hypertension Reports* 2012;14:152–159.

68. Ibrahim MS, Pang D, Randhawa G, Pappas Y. Risk models and scores for metabolic syndrome: Systematic review protocol. *BMJ Open* 2019;9(9):e027326.

69. Gutiérrez-Esparza GO, Infante Vázquez O, Vallejo M, Hernández-Torruco J. Prediction of metabolic syndrome in a Mexican population applying machine learning algorithms. *Symmetry* 2020;12(4):581.

70. Choe EK, Rhee H, Lee S, Shin E, Oh SW, Lee JE, Choi SH. Metabolic syndrome prediction using machine learning models with genetic and clinical information from a nonobese healthy population. *Genomics & Informatics* 2018;16(4): e31.

71. Saffarian M, Babaiyan V, Namakin K, Taheri F, Kazemi T. Developing a novel continuous metabolic syndrome score: A data mining based model. *Journal of AI and Data Mining* 2021;9(2):193–202.

72. Yang H, Yu B, OUYang P, Li X, Lai X, Zhang G, et al. Machine learning-aided risk prediction for metabolic syndrome based on 3 years study. *Scientific Reports*, 2022;12(1):2248.

73. Tavares, LD, Manoel, A, Donato, THR, Cesena F, Minanni CA, Kashiwagi NM, et al. Prediction of metabolic syndrome: A machine learning approach to help primary prevention. *Diabetes Research and Clinical Practice* 2022;191:110047.

74. Karimi-Alavijeh F, Jalili S, Sadeghi M. Predicting metabolic syndrome using decision tree and support vector machine methods. *ARYA Atherosclerosis* 2016;12(3):146.

75. Kim J, Mun S, Lee S, Jeong K, Baek Y. Prediction of metabolic and pre-metabolic syndromes using machine learning models with anthropometric, lifestyle, and biochemical factors from a middle-aged population in Korea. *BMC Public Health* 2022;22(1):664.

76. Aliu E, Kanungo S, Arnold GL. Amino acid disorders. *Annals of Translational Medicine* 2018;6(24):471.

77. Blau N, Duran M, Gibson KM, Vici CD (Eds.). *Physician's Guide to the Diagnosis, Treatment, and Follow-Up of Inherited Metabolic Diseases* (Vol. 213). 2014. Berlin/Heidelberg: Springer.

78. Zhou M, Deng L, Huang Y, Xiao Y, Wen J, Liu, N, et al. Application of the artificial intelligence algorithm model for screening of inborn errors of metabolism. *Frontiers in Pediatrics* 2022;10:855–943.

79. Yang RL, Yang YL, Wang T, Xu WZ, Yu G, Yang JB, et al. Establishment of an auxiliary diagnosis system of newborn screening for inherited metabolic diseases based on artificial intelligence technology and a clinical trial. *Zhonghua er ke za zhi= Chinese Journal of Pediatrics* 2021;59(4):286–293.

80. la Marca G, Carling RS, Moat SJ, Yahyaoui R, Ranieri E, Bonham JR, et al. Current state and innovations in newborn screening: Continuing to do good and avoid harm. *International Journal of Neonatal Screening* 2023;9(1):15.

81. Shirwaikar RD, Acharya D, Makkithaya K, Surulivelrajan M, Srivastava S. Optimizing neural networks for medical data sets: A case study on neonatal apnea prediction. *Artificial Intelligence in Medicine* 2019;98:59–76.

82. Uryu H, Migita O, Ozawa M, Kamijo C, Aoto S, Okamura K, et al. Automated urinary sediment detection for Fabry disease using deep-learning algorithms. *Molecular Genetics and Metabolism Reports* 2022;33:100921.

83. Kaur K, Singh C, Kumar Y. Diagnosis and detection of congenital diseases in new-borns or foetuses using artificial intelligence techniques: A systematic review. *Archives of Computational Methods in Engineering* 2023;30:3031–3058.

84. Haghpanahi M, Borkholder DA. Fetal QRS extraction from abdominal recordings via model-based signal processing and intelligent signal merging. *Physiological Measurement* 2014;35(8):1591.

85. Abbasi H, Bennet L, Gunn AJ, Unsworth CP. Robust wavelet stabilized 'Footprints of Uncertainty'for fuzzy system classifiers to automatically detect sharp waves in the EEG after hypoxia ischemia. *International Journal of Neural Systems* 2017;27(03):1650051.

86. Miao JH, Miao KH. Cardiotocographic diagnosis of fetal health based on multiclass morphologic pattern predictions using deep learning classification. *International Journal of Advanced Computer Science and Applications* 2018;9(5):1–11.

87. Akbulut A, Ertugrul E, Topcu V. Fetal health status prediction based on maternal clinical history using machine learning techniques. *Computer Methods and Programs in Biomedicine* 2018;163:87–100.

88. Pisapia JM, Akbari H, Rozycki M, Goldstein H, Bakas S, Rathore S, et al. Use of fetal magnetic resonance image analysis and machine learning to predict the need for postnatal cerebrospinal fluid diversion in fetal ventriculomegaly. *JAMA Pediatrics* 2018;172(2):128–135.

89. Feng B, Samuels DC, Hoskins W, Guo Y, Zhang Y, Tang J, et al. Down syndrome prediction/screening model based on deep learning and illumina genotyping array. In 2017 IEEE International Conference on Bioinformatics and Biomedicine (BIBM), pp. 347–352. IEEE, November 2017.

90. Neocleous AC, Syngelaki A, Nicolaides KH, Schizas CN. Two-stage approach for risk estimation of fetal trisomy 21 and other aneuploidies using computational intelligence systems. *Ultrasound in Obstetrics & Gynecology* 2018;51(4):503–508.

91. Sharma M, Vig L. Automatic chromosome classification using deep attention based sequence learning of chromosome bands. In 2018 International joint conference on neural networks (IJCNN), pp. 1–8. IEEE July 2018.

92. Al-Kharraz MS, Elrefae LA, Fadel MA. Automated system for chromosome karyotyping to recognize the most common numerical abnormalities using deep learning. *IEEE Access* 2020;8:157727–157747.

93. Jaganathan M, Gopal R, Kiruthika VR. Modelling an effectual feature selection approach for predicting down syndrome using machine learning approaches. *International Journal of Aquatic Science* 2021;12:1238–1249.

94. Nimitha N, Abbiraamavallee S, Elakiya E, Harini J, Kotishree Y. Supervised chromosomal anomaly detection using VGG-16 CNN model. In *AIP Conference Proceedings* (Vol. 2405, No. 1, p. 030010). AIP Publishing LLC, April 2022.

95. Li H, Luo M, Zheng J, Luo J, Zeng R, Feng N, et al. An artificial neural network prediction model of congenital heart disease based on risk factors: A hospital-based case-control study. *Medicine* 2017;96(6):e6090.

96. Du Y, Huang S, Huang C, Maalla A, Liang H. Recognition of child congenital heart disease using electrocardiogram based on residual of residual network. In 2020 IEEE International Conference on Progress in Informatics and Computing (PIC), pp. 145–148. IEEE, December 2020.

97. Yoon, SA, Hong, WH, Cho, HJ. Congenital heart disease diagnosed with echocardiogram in newborns with asymptomatic cardiac murmurs: A systematic review. *BMC Pediatrics* 2020;20:1–10.

98. Arnaout R, Curran L, Zhao Y, Levine JC, Chinn E, Moon-Grady AJ. An ensemble of neural networks provides expert-level prenatal detection of complex congenital heart disease. *Nature Medicine* 2021;27(5):882–891.

99. Qu Y, Deng X, Lin S, Han F, Chang HH, Ou Y, et al. Using innovative machine learning methods to screen and identify predictors of congenital heart diseases. *Frontiers in Cardiovascular Medicine* 2022;8:2087.

100. Buscema M, Grossi E, Montanini L, Street ME. Data mining of determinants of intrauterine growth retardation revisited using novel algorithms generating semantic maps and prototypical discriminating variable profiles. *PLoS One* 2015;10(7):e0126020.

101. Sufriyana H, Wu YW, Su ECY. Prediction of preeclampsia and intrauterine growth restriction: Development of machine learning models on a prospective cohort. *JMIR Medical Informatics* 2020;8(5), e15411.

102. Pini N, Lucchini M, Esposito G, Tagliaferri S, Campanile M, Magenes G, et al. A machine learning approach to monitor the emergence of late intrauterine growth restriction. *Frontiers in Artificial Intelligence* 2021;4:622616.

103. Crockart IC, Brink LT, Du Plessis C, Odendaal HJ. Classification of intrauterine growth restriction at 34–38 weeks gestation with machine learning models. *Informatics in Medicine Unlocked* 2021;23:100533.

104. Rogers R, Saharia K, Chandorkar A, Weiss ZF, Vieira K, Koo S, et al. Clinical experience with a novel assay measuring cytomegalovirus (CMV)-specific CD4+ and CD8+ T-cell immunity by flow cytometry and intracellular cytokine staining to predict clinically significant CMV events. *BMC Infectious Diseases* 2020;20(1):1–11.

105. Eisenberg L, XplOit consortium, Brossette C, Rauch J, Grandjean A, Ottinger H, et al. Time-dependent prediction of mortality and cytomegalovirus reactivation after allogeneic hematopoietic cell transplantation using machine learning. *American Journal of Hematology* 2022;97(10):1309–1323.

106. Jiang D, Hao M, Ding F, Fu J, Li M. Mapping the transmission risk of Zika virus using machine learning models. *Acta Tropica* 2018;185:391–399.

107. Mahalakshmi B, Suseendran G. Prediction of zika virus by multilayer perceptron neural network (MLPNN) using cloud. *International Journal of Recent Technology and Engineering (IJRTE)* 2019;8:1–6.

108. Tahir M, Badriyah T, Syarif I. Classification algorithms of maternal risk detection for preeclampsia with hypertension during pregnancy using particle swarm optimization. *EMITTER International Journal of Engineering Technology* 2018;6(2):236–253.

109. Galic S, Oakhill JS, Steinberg GR. Adipose tissue as an endocrine organ. *Molecular and Cellular Endocrinology* 2010;316:129–139.

110. Scherer PE. Adipose tissue: from lipid storage compartment to endocrine organ. *Diabetes* 2006;55:1537–45.

111. Frühbeck G, Gómez-Ambrosi J. Control of body weight: A physiologic and transgenic perspective. *Diabetologia* 2003;46:143–172.

112. Rodríguez A, Ezquerro S, Méndez-Gimenez L, Becerril S, Frühbeck G. Revisiting the adipocyte: A model for integration of cytokine signaling in the regulation of energy metabolism. *American Journal of Physiology-Endocrinology and Metabolism* 2015;309:E691–714.

113. Ibrahim MM. Subcutaneous and visceral adipose tissue: Structural and functional differences. *Obesity Reviews* 2010;11:11–18.

114. Fox CS, Massaro JM, Hoffmann U, Pou KM, MaurovichHorvat P, Liu CY, et al. Abdominal visceral and subcutaneous adipose tissue compartments: Association with metabolic risk factors in the Framingham Heart Study. *Circulation* 2007;116:39–48.

115. Harris MM, Stevens J, Thomas N, Schreiner P, Folsom AR. Association of fat distribution and obesity with hypertension in a bi-ethnic population: The ARIC study. Atherosclerosis Risk in Communities Study. *Obesity Research* 2000;8:516–524.

116. Planas A, Clará A, Pou JM, Vidal-Barraquer F, Gasol A, de Moner A, et al. Relationship of obesity distribution to peripheral arterial occlusive disease in elderly men. *International Journal of Obesity and Related Metabolic Disorders* 2001;25:1068–1070.

117. Fontbonne A, Charles MA, Thibult N, Richard JL, Claude JR, Warnet JM, et al. Hyperinsulinemia as a predictor of coronary heart disease mortality in a healthy population: The Paris Prospective Study, 15-year follow-up. *Diabetologia* 1991;34:356–361.

118. McFarlane SI, Banerji M, Sowers JR. Insulin resistance and cardiovascular disease. *The Journal of Clinical Endocrinology and Metabolism* 2001;86:713–738.

119. Després JP, Lemieux I. Abdominal obesity and metabolic syndrome. *Nature* 2006;444:881–887.

120. Zhang HP, Zou J, Xu ZQ, Ruan J, Yang SD, Yin Y, Mu HJ. Association of leptin, visfa-tin, apelin, resistin and adiponectin with clear cell renal cell carcinoma. *Oncology Letters* 2017;13:463–468.

121. Seguro LPC, Paupitz JA, Caparbo VF, Bonfa E, Pereira RMR. Increased visceral adipose tissue and altered adiposity fistribution in premenopausal lupus patients: Correlation with cardio-vascular risk factors. *Lupus* 2018;27:1001–1006.

122. Greco F, Cirimele V, Mallio CA, Beomonte Zobel B, Grasso RF. Increased visceral adipose tissue in male patients with clear cell renal cell carcinoma. *Clinical Cancer Investigation Journal* 2018;7:132–136. 31. Greco F, Mallio CA, Grippo R, Messina L, Vallese S, Rabitti C, Quarta LG, Grasso RF, Beomonte Zobel B. Increased visceral adipose tissue in male patients with non-clear cell renal cell carcinoma. *La radiologia medica* 2020;125:538–543.

123. Greco F, Quarta LG, Grasso RF, Beomonte Zobel B, Mallio CA. Increased visceral adipose tissue in clear cell renal cell carcinoma with and without peritumoral collateral vessels. *The British Journal of Radiology* 2020;93:20200334.

124. Greco F, Mallio CA, Cirimele V, Grasso RF, Beomonte Zobel B. Subcutaneous adipose tissue as a biomarker of pancreatic cancer: A pilot study in male patients. *Clinical Cancer Investigation Journal* 2019;8:10–19.

125. Mallio CA, Greco F, Pacella G, Schena E, Beomonte Zobel B. Gender-based differences of abdominal adipose tissue distribution in non-small cell lung cancer patients. *Shanghai Chest* 2018;2:20.

126. Greco F, Mallio CA. Relationship between visceral adipose tissue and genetic mutations (VHL and KDM5C) in clear cell renal cell carcinoma. *La Radiologia Medica* 2021;126:645–651.

127. Ruiz JR, Ramirez-Lechuga J, Ortega FB, Castro-Pinero J, Benitez JM, Arauzo-Azofra A, et al. Artificial neural network-based equation for estimating VO2max from the 20 m shuttle 402 run test in adolescents. *Artificial Intelligence in Medicine* 2008;44:233–245.

128. Christodoulou E, Ma J, Collins GS, Steyerberg EW, Verbakel JY, van Calster B. A systematic review shows no performance benefit of machine learning over logisticregression for clinical prediction models. *Journal of Clinical Epidemiology* 2019;110:12–22.

129. Ruiz JR, Ramirez-Lechuga J, Ortega FB, Castro-Pinero J, Benitez JM, Arauzo-Azofra A, et al. Artificial neural network-based equation for estimating VO2max from the 20 m shuttle run test in adolescents. *Artificial Intelligence in Medicine* 2008;44:233–245.

130. Arnold TB. kerasR: R interface to the keras deep learning library. *The Journal of Open Source Software* 2017;415:2.

131. Nadas J, Putz Z, Kolev G, Nagy S, Jermendy G. Intraobserver and interobserver 420 variabil-ity of measuring waist circumference. *Medical Science Monitor* 2008;14:CR15–CR8.

132. Oka R, Miura K, Sakurai M, Nakamura K, Yagi K, Miyamoto S, et al. Comparison of waist circumference with body mass index for predicting abdominal adipose tissue. *Diabetes Research and Clinical Practice* 2009;83:100–105. 424

133. Bosy-Westphal A, Booke C-A, Blöcker T, Kossel E, Goele K, Later W, et al. Measurement 425 site for waist circumference affects its accuracy as an index of visceral and abdominal 426 subcutaneous fat in a caucasian population. *The Journal of Nutrition* 2010;140:954–961.

134. World Health Organization. *Waist Circumference and Waist-Hip Ratio: Report of a WHO Expert Consultation*, Geneva, 8–11 December 2008. 2011.

135. Thomas EL, Bell JD. Influence of undersampling on magnetic resonance imaging measurements of intra-abdominal adipose tissue. *International Journal of Obesity* 2003;27:211.

136. Demerath EW, Reed D, Rogers N, Sun SS, Lee M, Choh AC, et al. Visceral adiposity, and its anatomical distribution as predictors of the metabolic syndrome and cardiometabolic risk factor levels. *The American Journal of Clinical Nutrition* 2008;88:1263–1271.

137. So, R, Matsuo T, Sasai H, Eto M, Tsujimoto T, Saotome K, et al. Best single-slice measurement site for estimating visceral adipose tissue volume after weight loss in obese, Japanese men. *Nutrition & Metabolism* 2012;9:56.

138. Thomas EL, Bell JD. Influence of undersampling on magnetic resonance imaging measurements of intra-abdominal adipose tissue. *International Journal of Obesity* 2003;27:211.

139. Irlbeck T, Massaro JM, Bamberg F, O'Donnell CJ, Hoffmann U, Fox CS. Association between single-slice measurements of visceral and abdominal subcutaneous adipose tissue with volumetric measurements: The Framingham Heart Study. *International Journal of Obesity* 2010;34:781.

140. Geisler C, Schweitzer L, Pourhassan M, Braun W, Müller MJ, Bosy-Westphal A, et al. What is the best reference site for a single MRI slice to assess whole-body skeletal muscle and adipose tissue volumes in healthy adults. *The American Journal of Clinical Nutrition* 2015;102:58–65.

141. Schaudinn A, Linder N, Garnov N, Kerlikowsky F, Bluher M, Dietrich A, et al. Predictive accuracy of single- and multi-slice MRI for the estimation of total visceral adipose tissue in overweight to severely obese patients. *NMR in Biomedicine* 2015;28:583–590.

142. Hill AM, LaForgia J, Coates AM, Buckley JD, Howe PRC. Estimating abdominal adipose tissue with DXA and Anthropometry. *Obesity* 2012;15:504.

143. Ball SD, Swan PD. Accurary estimating intra-abdominal fat in obese women. *Journal of Exercise Physiology Online* 2003;6:1–7.

144. Kyle UG, Bosaeus I, De Lorenzo AD, Deurenberg P, Elia M, Manuel Gómez J, et al. 457 Bioelectrical impedance analysis—part II: utilization in clinical practice. *Clinical Nutrition* 2004;23:1430–1453.

145. Molarius A, Seidell JC. Selection of anthropometric indicators for classification of abdominal fatness—A critical review. *International Journal of Obesity*. 1998;22:719.

146. Collins F. Precision Medicine Initiative | National Institutes of Health(NIH) [Internet]. National Institutes of Health.2015. Accessed online on the 25th of July 2017 from:https://www.nih.gov/precision-medicine-initiative-cohort-program.

147. Top 500 Supercomputers [Internet]. Accessed online on the 25th of July, 2017 from: https://www.top500.org/.

148. Luo G, Sun G, Wang K, et al. A novel left ventricular volumes prediction method based on deep learning network in cardiac MRI. *Computer Cardiology [Internet]* 2010;2017:2–5. Available from: http://www.cinc.org/archives/2016/pdf/028-224.pdf.

149. Esteva A, Kuprel B, Novoa RA, et al. Dermatologist-level classification of skin cancer with deep neural networks. *Nature [Internet]* 2017;542(7639):115–118. Available from: http://www.nature.com/doifinder/10.1038/nature21056.

150. Wang D, Khosla A, Gargeya R, et al. Deep learning for identifying metastatic breast cancer. eprint arXiv:1606.05718, Publication Date:06/2016.

151. Nadkarni PM, Ohno-Machado L, Chapman WW. Natural language processing: An introduction. *Journal of the American Medical Informatics Association* 2011;18:544–551.

152. Ray S. (Ed.). A quick review of machine learning algorithms. *2019 International Conference on Machine Learning, Big Data, Cloud and Parallel Computing (COMIT Con)*, 2019.

153. Krittanawong C, Zhang H, Wang Z, et al. Artificial intelligence in precision cardiovascular medicine. *Journal of the American College of Cardiology* 2017;69:2657–2664.

154. Francis EU, Mashor MY, Hassan R, Abdullah AA. Screening of bone marrow slide images for leukemia using multilayer perceptron (mlp). In 2011 IEEE Symposium on Industrial Electronics and Applications, 2011 pp. 643–648.

155. Acharya UR, Fujita H, Oh SL, Hagiwara Y, Tan JH, Adam M, et al. Deep convolutional neural network for the automated diagnosis of congestive heart failure using ecg signals. *Applied Intelligence* 2019;1:16–27.

156. Porumb M, Iadanza E, Massaro S, Pecchia L. A convolutional neural network approach to detect congestive heart failure. *Biomedical Signal Processing and Control* 2020;55:101597.

157. Asyali MH. Discrimination power of long-term heart rate variability measures. In *Proceedings of the 25th Annual International Conference of the IEEE Engineering in Medicine and Biology Society (IEEE Cat. No.03CH37439)* (Vol. 1, pp. 200–203), 2003.

158. İşer Y, Kuntalp M. Combining classical HRV indices with wavelet entropy measures improves to performance in diagnosing congestive heart failure. *Computers in Biology and Medicine* 2007;37(10):1502–1510. QT Variability & Heart Rate Variability.

159. Elfadil N, Ibrahim I. Self-organizing neural network approach for identification of patients with heart failure. In *2011 International Conference on Multimedia Computing and Systems*, pp. 1–6. IEEE, 2011.

160. Liu G, Wang L, Wang Q, Zhou G, Wang Y, Jiang Q. A new approach to detect congestive heart failure using short-term heart rate variability measures. *PLOS One* 2014;9(4):1–8.

161. Goldberger AL, Amaral LA, Glass L, Hausdorff JM, Ivanov PC, Mark RG, et al. Physiobank physiotoolkit, and physionet: Components of a new research resource for complex physiologic signals. *Circulation* 2000;101(23):215–220.

162. Narin A, Isler Y, Ozer M. Investigating the performance improvement of hrv indices in chf using feature selection methods based on backward elimination and statistical significance. *Computers in Biology and Medicine* 2014;45:72–79.

7 The Burden of Diabetes Mellitus

Biochemical and Nutritional Aspects

Chinmoyee Deori, Raktim Borgohain, Gaurab Kumar Gogoi, and Migom Doley

7.1 INTRODUCTION

Diabetes mellitus is a metabolic disorder characterized by high blood glucose due to endogenous insulin deficiency with or without resistance to insulin. Insulin is a hormone secreted by the endocrine part of pancreas (β cells) that regulates the blood glucose levels. The increasing burden of the disease can be attributed to current dietary trends and sedentary lifestyles. Poor adherence to nutritional recommendations, an increased intake of carbohydrates, a lack of high fiber intake, a lack of awareness among certain populations, and fast foods with a high sugar content have made diabetes more prominent. Stress, a lack of physical activity, inadequate sleep, smoking, and alcohol intake are also contributory factors. Though different studies have shown relationships between sugar consumption, obesity, heart diseases, and diabetes mellitus, several studies show that 40% of patient suffering from diabetes are non-obese (1). The etiology of diabetes is multi-factorial and includes genetic, environmental, and lifestyle factors.

As the economic burden caused by diabetes mellitus increases, there has been a rising trend of preventing diabetes mellitus by decreasing daily sugar intake, keeping the blood sugar index under control (2). Other evidence suggests that diabetes mellitus, as a chronic disorder, needs continuous treatment in order for patients to maintain a healthy blood sugar level. An important parameter in measuring glycemic index is fasting blood glucose (FBG), which is measured after an overnight fast. Recently, it has been observed that fasting blood sugar as a parameter helps to diagnose heart diseases in asymptomatic individuals. The median age of onset of diabetes has shifted due to numerous factors related to lifestyle (1).

Overall, women are more sensitive to insulin as compared to males and are thus at a reduced risk of vascular disease. This can be explained by high levels of estrogen production in females, which has a protective effect against inflammation, oxidation, fibrosis, constriction of vessels, and abnormal lipid profile. Hence, following menopause, women are at higher risk of developing diabetes due to decreased estrogen levels.

In diabetes, the risk of developing heart disease is associated with plasma lipid profile. A deranged lipid profile is related to insulin resistance, an important component of type 2 diabetes mellitus. Some studies suggest that insulin resistance is associated with factors such as high very low-density lipoprotein (VLDL) levels, high levels of serum triglycerides, and lower levels of high density lipoprotein (HDL). Hence, lipid profile is an important component of follow-up in type 2 diabetes mellitus. Another important component in managing diabetes mellitus is the assessment of renal function as diabetics are predisposed to develop chronic kidney disease (CKD), as seen in 25–40% of type 2 diabetes mellitus cases (3). Patients are at higher risk of premature mortality if they have concurrent chronic kidney disease with hypertension and obesity (4).

An important factor in the diagnosis and management of diabetes mellitus patients is the measurement of different biochemical parameters through various laboratory tests, like glycemic index, hepatic and renal function tests (creatinine, sodium, potassium, urea, uric acid), etc. Awareness of diabetes and its management are still big challenges faced globally. The main reason for this is poor insight among populations in developing countries. This is also aggravated by non-compliance of patients with medical therapy in developing countries. The American Diabetes Association (ADA) has defined self-management of diet as a key factor, along with awareness, treatment, nutritional aspects, and complications, in the control of diabetes. Contrary to popular belief that diabetes is a disease of the rich, reports suggest that lower-income countries contribute to a higher diabetes burden globally.

7.2 EPIDEMIOLOGY OF DIABETES MELLITUS

According to the International Diabetes Federation (IDF), the number of adults worldwide between the ages of 20 and 79 years with diabetes was 463 million and is expected to rise to 700 million by 2045 (Figure 7.1) (5, 6). Type 2 diabetes is more prevalent in geriatric populations, but in younger generations, the number of diabetics is also rising day by day. Type 2 diabetes mellitus cases constitute 8% of total cases among those below 44 years of age in developed countries and

DOI: 10.1201/9781003384823-7

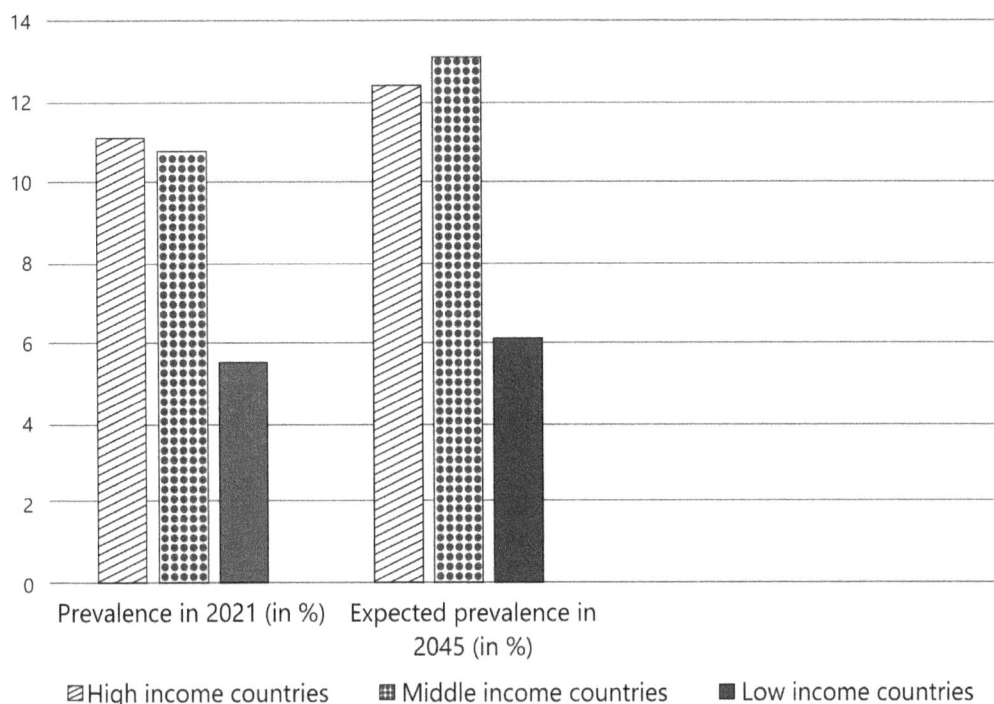

Figure 7.1 Number of adults (20–79 years) with diabetes per World Bank income classification in 2021 and 2045

25% in developing countries (7). Approximately 10,145 deaths occurred as a result of diabetes in the year 2017 (8).

Of the total number of deaths, 21% were due to ischemic heart disease and 13% were due to stroke (9). Diabetes leads to several complications, like nephropathy, retinopathy, neuropathy, heart diseases, and stroke if not diagnosed early. China is the country with the highest number of diabetics worldwide, with around 140.9 million people suffering from the disease. By the year 2045, it is predicted that China will have around 174.4 million people with diabetes. The IDF Diabetes Atlas (tenth edition) states that in 2021 approximately 537 million adults (20–79 years) were living with diabetes (Table 7.1). Diabetes may lead to the alteration of our normal physiological system and can increase various complications and disability rates, resulting in a heavy economic burden for society (10).

Table 7.1   Top ten countries for number of adults (20–79 years) with diabetes in 2021

Rank	Name of country	Number of people with diabetes (in millions)
1	China	140.9
2	India	74.2
3	Pakistan	33.0
4	United States	32.2
5	Indonesia	19.5
6	Brazil	15.7
7	Mexico	14.1
8	Bangladesh	13.1
9	Japan	11.0
10	Egypt	10.9

7.3 BIOCHEMICAL CHANGES IN DIABETES MELLITUS

7.3.1 Insulin

The maintenance of the glucose level in the blood within narrow limits, on account of variation in the supply and demand of the body, is a very finely and efficiently regulated system mediated by neuro-hormonal feedback mechanisms. This is important, because it is essential to have a continuous supply of glucose to the brain, which only uses glucose, although in an insulin-independent fashion, as its source of energy and consumes 20% of all energy required by the human body. Insulin, an anabolic hormone, promotes the uptake, use, and storage of carbohydrate and fat, as well as promoting protein synthesis (Figure 7.2).

Insulin is synthesized in the beta cells within the islets of Langerhans in the pancreas. The insulin molecule consists of two polypeptide chains, linked by two disulphide bridges; the A chain contains 21 amino acids and the B chain 30 amino acids (11). The insulin gene, which is located on the short arm of chromosome 11, encodes for preproinsulin (110 amino acids). The synthesis of insulin is genetically regulated at transcriptional and translation levels. The rate of the synthesis of insulin may be increased or decreased by many factors, including the availability of nutrients. Preproinsulin is synthesized in the endoplasmic reticulum of the beta cells in the islets of Langerhans in the pancreas (12). It is then cleaved by peptidase activity to proinsulin (86 amino acids), which is packaged into vesicles in the Golgi apparatus. Inside the vesicles, proinsulin is converted by enzymes into insulin and connecting peptide (C-peptide). Insulin exists within the vesicles as hexamers until it is secreted from the β-cell by exocytosis. Once in the blood, insulin dissociates into its active monomeric form and diffuses throughout the body down its concentration gradient. The biosynthesis of insulin is controlled by multiple factors, but the most important is blood glucose, which stimulates insulin gene transcription and mRNA translation and consequently insulin production.

Insulin secretion is increased by increases in blood glucose, free fatty acids, or amino acids. Gastrointestinal hormones that promote insulin secretion are gastrin, cholecystokinin, secretin, and gastric inhibitory peptide. Glucagon, growth hormone, thyroxine, and cortisol, which are known as hyperglycemic hormones, increase insulin secretion by increasing blood glucose. Parasympathetic and beta-adrenergic stimulation increases, whereas alpha adrenergic stimulation decreases, insulin secretion. Other factors that inhibit insulin release are fasting (hypoglycemia) and the hormones somatostatin and leptin.

Diabetes mellitus (DM) is a metabolic condition characterized by a decrease in insulin secretion or insulin action. In type 1 DM, there may be a complete absence of endogenous insulin due to the destruction of beta cells in the pancreas by CD4+ and CD8+ T cells and macrophages that infiltrate the pancreatic islets. Though insulin primarily has hypoglycemic action, alterations in lipid and

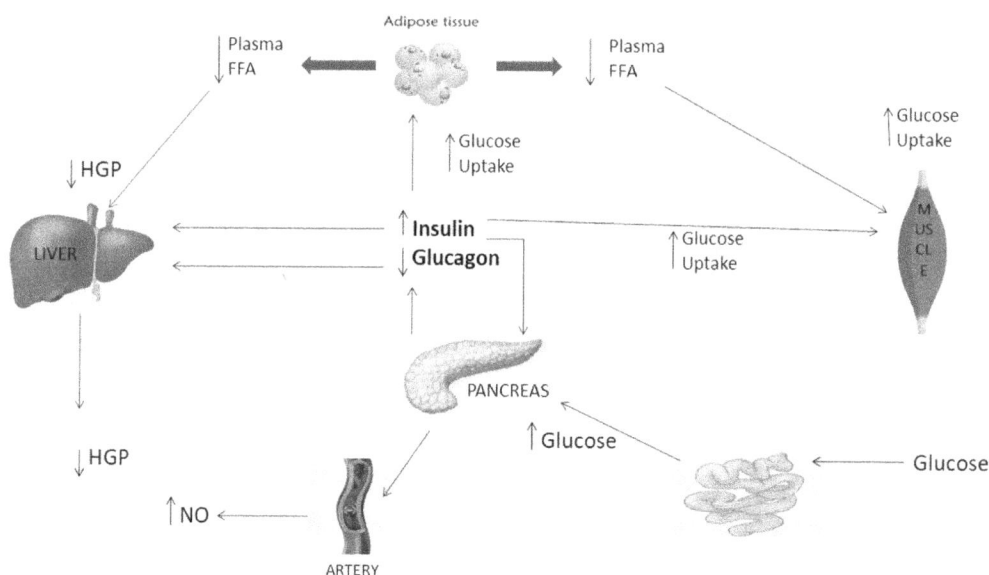

Figure 7.2   Role of insulin in glucose, lipid, and protein metabolism

protein metabolism also occur due to diverse actions of insulin. The actions of insulin on lipid metabolism are particularly important as many of the long-term complications of DM are associated with lipid metabolism. Abnormalities in the lipid profile of patients with type 2 diabetes are fairly common, even in those with reasonable glycemic control.

7.3.2 Lipids

In diabetics, visceral fat in particular, and adipose tissues in general, show decreased inhibition of lipolysis and increased lipoprotein lipase activity, together with increased hepatic cholesterol synthesis. Hyperlipidemia in diabetes mellitus involves increased levels of triglycerides and very low-density lipoprotein (VLDL), along with decreased levels of high density lipoprotein (HDL). Low density lipoprotein (LDL) levels may increase or remain within range as a result of a decrease in the formation of LDL, along with a decreased number and decreased sensitivity of LDL receptors (13). However, the profile of LDL subfractions in patients with type 2 diabetes is deranged in such a way that the proportion of small dense LDL particles (known as the "type B" pattern) is greater. These small dense LDL particles are more atherogenic as they are more susceptible to oxidation by free radicals and thereby atherogenic as they are readily taken up by macrophages compared to unoxidized fraction. Insulin has diverse effects on liver apoprotein production, lipoprotein lipase, cholesterol ester transfer protein (CETP), as well as on peripheral tissues like adipose and muscle tissue. A decrease in the activity of lipoprotein lipase (HSL>ATGL, MGL), together with the increased production of apolipoprotein B by the liver, causes an increase in the release of fatty acids (non-esterified fatty acids (NEFAs)/free fatty acids (FFAs)) from peripheral tissues and subsequently their transport to the liver. The FFAs reaching the liver are converted to TG and secreted in VLDL. In diabetics, a higher level of triglycerides leads to the production of larger VLDL particles, causing hypertriglyceridemia. The excess deposition of triglycerides in adipose tissue accounts for the obesity prevalent in type 2 diabetes patients. The cholesteryl ester transfer protein (CTEP)-mediated exchange of cholesteryl ester in HDL with triglyceride in VLDL causes a decrease in HDL levels (13). Raised FFA levels in the blood along with an increase in acetyl CoA carboxylase activity in insulin deficiency causes a surge in acetyl CoA levels in the blood, which is diverted to form ketone bodies, leading to diabetic ketoacidosis. This tendency is seen more in type 1 diabetes mellitus. Other vital enzymes involved in lipid metabolism stimulated by insulin are glycerol kinase and HMG CoA reductase.

Elevated levels of free fatty acids ("lipotoxicity") and chronic hyperglycemia (glucotoxicity), along with systemic and local elevations in pro-inflammatory cytokines that occur in chronic uncontrolled diabetes mellitus, in turn impair beta cell function, resulting in further degradation of the disease. High free fatty acids levels are known to inhibit glucose utilization, as demonstrated by Randle (glucose-fatty acid cycle).

There is also increased local lipolysis in adipose tissue in diabetics. This occurs as a result of increased amounts of 11 beta hydroxysteroid dehydrogenase in adipose tissue, leading to increased levels of cortisol. Additionally, adipose tissue promotes insulin resistance by secreting TNF alpha and interleukins. Resistin is another hormone that is secreted by abdominal adipose tissue and responsible for insulin resistance.

Physical exercise, which increases the insulin sensitivity of peripheral tissues and pharmacotherapy with lipid-lowering agents, along with strict glycemic control, thus have the potential to reduce long-term macrovascular complications of diabetes mellitus, such as cardiovascular and cerebrovascular events.

7.3.3 Carbohydrate

Insulin plays a central role in carbohydrate metabolism and the ADA/IDF criteria for the diagnosis of diabetes are based on blood sugar level. Carbohydrate metabolism is deranged in insulin deficient (beta cell dysfunction) and insulin resistant (Glut4 receptor dysfunction) persons, depending on the severity. Insulin inhibits phosphoenolpyruvate-carboxykinase and fructose 1,6-biphosphatase involved in gluconeogenesis and glucose 6-phosphatase and glycogen phosphorylase involved in glycogenolysis. Thus, in diabetes, gluconeogenesis and glycogenolysis occur unrestricted. Glycogenesis in the liver also decreases as glycogen synthase remains inhibited in the absence of insulin. These factors – viz, the reduced uptake of glucose by peripheral tissues, an increase in the breakdown of stored glycogen, and reduced glucose storage in liver cells – lead to the elevation of blood sugar in diabetes mellitus.

Chronic hyperglycemia causes microvascular complications, such as retinopathy, neuropathy, and nephropathy. The skeletal muscle glucose utilization is impaired to a greater degree than adipose tissue in type 2 diabetes. High free fatty acid concentration in the myocytes also leads to severe impairment in non-oxidative glucose disposal, like that in the hexose monophosphate (HMP) shunt. Thus, instead of high blood glucose, there is cellular starvation. Sustained hyperglycemia can produce glucotoxicity through the enhancement of the hexosamine pathway, leading to increased glucosamine levels. In turn, increased glucosamine levels can produce insulin resistance in adipose tissue and skeletal muscle. Sustained hyperinsulinemia also down-regulates the insulin receptor and further aggravates insulin resistance. This forms a vicious cycle until appropriate medical intervention is taken to increase insulin sensitivity and the level of insulin in the blood. Exercise increases glucose transporter activity, improves capillary density, increases mitochondrial mass, and increases type 2 A muscle fibers, which are involved in the glycolytic process.

Hyperglycemia also causes irreversible and nonenzymatic glycation of the small dense sub-fraction of LDL by promoting the binding of glucose or its metabolites to lysine residues of apolipoprotein apoB-100. Glycated LDL is a major factor contributing to diabetic atherosclerosis.

7.3.4 Protein

A lack or deficiency of insulin produces a catabolic state in diabetics. There is an increase in the breakdown of proteins to amino acids in order to produce substrates for gluconeogenesis. In diabetes, glucogenic amino acids such as alanine, glutamic acid, and aspartic acid are transaminated to corresponding carbon skeletons. They then enter the tricarboxylic acid cycle (TCA) cycle, form oxaloacetate or pyruvate, and are diverted to glycolytic pathways. Alanine released from the muscle is the major substrate for gluconeogenesis, which is responsible for the wasting of muscles. This occurs as a result of the unopposed actions of enzymes – transaminases and ornithine transcarbamoylase – along with a reduction in RNA polymerase-mediated protein synthesis in the absence of insulin or when there is an insulin deficiency.

7.3.5 Complications

Chronic complications arising due to diabetes type 1 and type 2 can broadly be divided into vascular and nonvascular complications. Vascular complications are further divided into microvascular and macrovascular. Microvascular complications are retinopathy, nephropathy, and neuropathy, while macrovascular complications are coronary heart disease, cerebrovascular disease, and peripheral arterial disease (14). Nonvascular complications include infections, skin changes, hearing loss, glaucoma, periodontal disease, and an increased risk of dementia and impaired cognitive function. Microvascular complications are specific to diabetes, while macrovascular complications have additional features that are common in the general population, such as dyslipidemia and hypertension.

Biochemical changes that occur due to hyperglycemia, leading to microvascular complications, are diverse in etiology and involve multiple pathways. Hyperglycemia acts as the key driving force in the development of microvascular complications. Four major cellular signaling pathways related to the metabolic and/or redox state of the cell that are activated by hyperglycemia in endothelial cells and other cell types vulnerable to hyperglycemic attack have been documented. Though each pathway is injurious alone, collectively they cause an imbalance in the mitochondrial redox state of the cell, leading to the excessive formation of reactive oxygen species (ROS). The pathways are: i) increased advanced glycation end product (AGE) formation and receptor for AGE (RAGE) activation, ii) increased polyol pathway flux, iii) increased hexosamine pathway flux, and iv) activation of protein kinase C (PKC) (via diacylglycerol).

i) Increased advanced glycation end product (AGE) formation and activation of RAGE

AGEs (e.g., pentosidine, glucosepane, and carboxymethyllysine) are heterogenous irreversibly modified biomolecules that may be intracellular or extracellular, formed as a result of persistent hyperglycemia. They are formed as a consequence of nonenzymatic reactions between reducing sugars or oxaldehydes and proteins or lipids. The reactive bicarbanyls that are the precursors of AGE are derivatives of aberrant glucose metabolism. They are glyoxal, methyl glyoxal, and offshoots of Amadori products (fructose lysine adducts). Inside the cells, protein and DNA adducts disrupt cell function and transport. Extracellularly, AGEs formed from plasma protein and matrix proteins are deposited in the extracellular matrix which alters cell adhesion and activates receptors for AGE (RAGE). RAGE is a member of the immunoglobulin family and binds many ligands besides AGE. The signals transmitted by the AGE-RAGE combination include transforming growth factor (TGF)-beta, NF K-beta, and NADPH dependent oxidases (NOX). They induce vascular adhesion molecule 1, E-selectin, VEGF, and proinflammatory cytokines and oxidative stress, leading to vascular inflammation, fibrosis, calcification, and prothrombotic effects that ultimately lead to vascular damage. AGEs are also antigenic and trigger an autoimmune response (15).

ii) Activation of polyol pathway

In persistent hyperglycemia, a disproportionate amount of glucose is diverted to the polyol pathway. The pathway has two major steps. Firstly, glucose is converted to sorbitol by aldose reductase enzyme and NADPH+ is converted to NADP, and secondly, sorbitol is oxidized to fructose by sorbitol dehydrogenase and NAD+ is converted to NADH. The polyol pathway induces vascular damage by i) increasing fructose and its metabolites, e.g., triose phosphate, methylglyoxal, fructose 3-phosphate, and 3-deoxyglucosone, which are potent glycating agents, leading ultimately to more AGEs, ii) depleting NADPH, leading to decreased glutathione (an potent antioxidant) formation and subsequently increased oxidative stress, iii) activating protein kinase C by DAG, which is increased as a result of the increase in NADH and iv) effecting an efflux of taurine and myoinositol from the cell (16).

iii) Activation of the hexosamine pathway

In hyperglycemia, fructose 6 phosphate is diverted from the glycolytic pathway to the hexosamine pathway and converted to glucosamine 6 phosphate by glutamine fructose 6 phosphate amidotransferase enzyme, which leads to the formation of uridine diphosphate-N-acetyl glucosamine (UDP-GlcNAc). It binds to transcription factors and modifies gene expression, leading to the overexpression of plasminogen activator inhibitor 1 and TGF-beta 1. Together, they cause vascular smooth muscle mitosis and endothelial fibrosis. Increased levels of glutamine fructose 6 phosphate amidotransferase, along with glucosamine, also increase hydrogen peroxide, leading to oxidative damage.

iv) PKC pathway

Hyperglycemia increases intracellular DAG and activates the PKC pathway, which in turn induces VEGF, NF K-B, PAI-1, and TGF-beta. As a result, there is basement membrane thickening, endothelial proliferation, the activation of NOX, vasoconstriction due to decreased NO production, and increased capillary permeability, leading to vascular damage. PKC is mainly implicated in retinopathy, nephropathy, and coronary heart disease.

The poly (ADP-ribose) polymerase (PARP) pathway is another pathway that leads to the generation of free radicals and an increase in oxidants by cleaving NAD+ to nicotinamide and ADP ribose residues. Increased activation of PARP causes NAD+ depletion, changes in gene transcription and expression, increase in ROS levels, and the diversion of glycolytic intermediates to AGE formation and PKC pathways (16).

The augmented activation of the AGEs-RAGE axis, the enhanced polyol pathway, the increased flux into the hexosamine pathway, and increased PKC activation, together with increased glucose autooxidation and activation of other pathways, finally leads to increased oxidative stress in diabetics. The free radicals are normally deactivated in the mitochondria by agents like superoxide dismutase, catalase, glutathione, taurine, etc. In diabetics, the natural capacity to neutralize the ROS is overwhelmed, resulting in damage to nucleic acids, proteins, and lipids. Mitochondrial DNA is more susceptible to damage as it is not protected by histones. Damage to mitochondrial DNA results in the depletion of ATP, cell death, and tissue necrosis. Apart from degenerating lipids, proteins, and nucleic acids, ROS also causes aberrations in many genes, leading to their erroneous expression, which includes genes coding for antioxidant enzymes like catalase, stress response proteins like metalloproteins and heme oxygenase, cellular growth factors like VEGF, epidermal growth factor, platelet-derived growth factor, basic fibroblast growth factor, connective tissue growth factor, along with those coding for proinflammatory cytokines (17).

The macrovascular complications of diabetes mellitus result from the constant exposure of vasculature to high blood sugar, along with other factors like hypertension, dyslipidemia, inflammation, and impaired fibrinolysis, which promotes atherosclerosis. Coronary heart disease, which is a major cause of morbidity and mortality among diabetics, is caused by the synergism of hyperglycemia and other cardiovascular risk factors such as dyslipidemia (elevated triglycerides, low HDL cholesterol, and high small dense LDL), hypertension, obesity, reduced physical activity, and cigarette smoking. Other risk factors include abnormal platelet function, increased markers of inflammation, and endothelial dysfunction (Figure 7.3).

113

MICROVASCULAR COMPLICATION

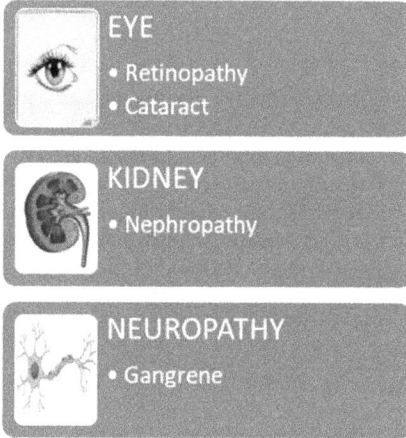

EYE
• Retinopathy
• Cataract

KIDNEY
• Nephropathy

NEUROPATHY
• Gangrene

MACROVASCULAR COMPLICATION

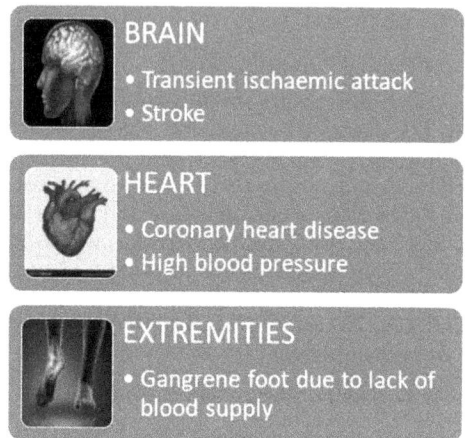

BRAIN
• Transient ischaemic attack
• Stroke

HEART
• Coronary heart disease
• High blood pressure

EXTREMITIES
• Gangrene foot due to lack of blood supply

Figure 7.3 Microvascular and macrovascular complications of diabetes

The key mechanism involved in macrovascular complications is atherosclerosis, which leads to narrowing of the arteries. The components of atherosclerosis are inflammation, lipid deposition, remodeling, thrombosis, and fibrosis. The endothelium of blood vessels contains vasodilators (nitric oxide (NO) and prostacyclin) and vasoconstrictors (endothelin 1 and angiotensin II). The balance between vasoconstrictors and vasodilators is finely maintained in normal persons. However, in diabetics, due to decreased NO synthesis, this balance is lost. As a result of hyperlipidemia and the prevailing proinflammatory state in diabetics, monocytes, T lymphocytes, and lipids infiltrate the endothelium and form a fatty streak that progresses into atheromatous plaque. Oxidative stress promotes further vascular damage. Subsequently, leucocytes that accumulate in the sub-endothelium and smooth muscle cells proliferate, leading to the formation of atheromatous plaques. The rupture of atheromatous plaque is a major cause of cardiovascular and cerebrovascular events, mortality, and morbidity among diabetics.

The interplay of the narrowing of arteries, high blood sugar, and neuropathy leads to peripheral arterial diseases. Increased susceptibility to infection is also due to neutrophil dysfunction occurring at blood sugar levels >200mg/dl.

7.4 NUTRITIONAL BURDEN

Nutritional deficiencies are seen in all types of diabetes (type 1, type 2, and gestational diabetes). Type 2 diabetes is a bigger challenge for the healthcare system worldwide. According to the 2019 Diabetes Atlas of the International Diabetes Federation, 463 million adults are suffering from diabetes currently, which accounts for 1 in 11 individuals worldwide, but 1 in 5 are over 65 years old (18). The increasing number of diabetics, with the associated high costs of treatment and complications, also contributes indirectly to disability costs. This huge nutritional burden due to diabetes may amount to a huge economic burden globally.

Nutritional deficiencies are more common in diabetes mellitus. A sedentary lifestyle may result in overeating, leading people to become overweight and obese. These multiple factors add to genetic defects in the pathophysiology of the disease. Dietary modifications are advised to reduce the incidence of type 2 diabetes, as well to improve metabolic control. In diabetics, weight loss is seen due to a negative nitrogen balance, and sarcopenia adds to muscle wasting with increasing age. National and international guidelines for nutritional and lifestyle modifications, together with protocols for losing weight, aim to produce long-term diabetes remission (Figure 7.4).

7.4.1 Micronutrient Deficiency

In patients who have poor control of diabetes mellitus, there may be a deficiency of micronutrients, which necessitates counseling patients on adequate intake of vitamins and minerals from diet. The micronutrients that are deficient in these patients include zinc, chromium, magnesium, manganese, vitamin B6, copper, etc.

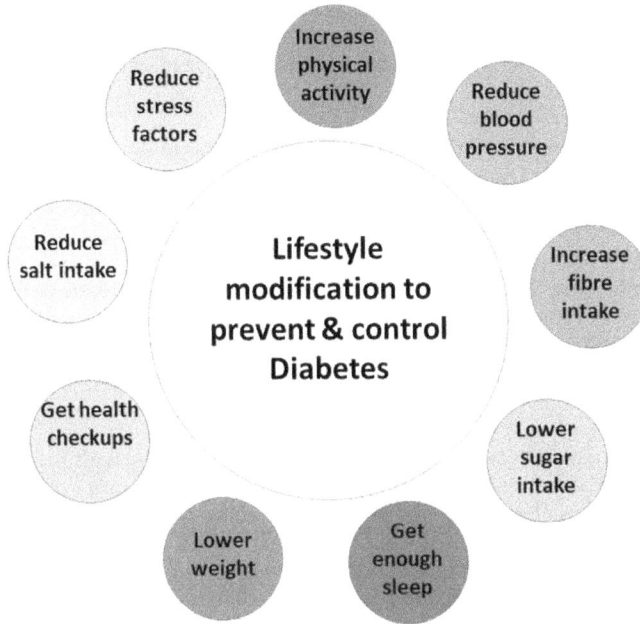

Figure 7.4 Lifestyle modifications to prevent and control diabetes mellitus

7.4.2 Zinc

Zinc, an element in the structure of insulin, is involved in various metabolic processes as it is needed for the activity of many enzymes related to carbohydrate metabolism, heme biosynthesis, carbonic anhydrase transport, and other reactions. Insufficient levels of zinc in diabetic patients promote atherosclerotic vascular changes and decreases bone mineralization (19).

7.4.3 Manganese

Manganese is a cofactor for several enzymatic pathways. Reduced levels of manganese in the blood is seen in diabetes and pancreatectomy patients. In diabetic patients, levels of manganese in hair and blood are reduced due to increased urinary excretion. A deficiency of manganese causes decreased glucose tolerance and granulation of pancreatic cells in guinea pig and also affects lactation and fetal development (rats), as well as causing a fatty liver. Manganese supplementation can improve glucose tolerance in animals (20).

7.4.4 Chromium

Chromium is one of the most important elements for oxidative reactions. Most food contains trivalent chromium, which is essential for normal glucose metabolism. A deficiency of chromium can cause decreased glucose tolerance, along with impaired lipid metabolism. Studies have shown that chromium supplementation has improved HbA1C levels in diabetics (21).

7.4.5 Magnesium

Magnesium acts as an important cofactor in many enzymatic reactions involving energy metabolism. Magnesium plays an important role in glucose homeostasis and insulin action. In type 1 and type 2 diabetes, there is a decreased level of serum magnesium due to increased urinary loss of magnesium. Magnesium deficiency in patients suffering from diabetes can cause muscle weakness, seizures, anorexia, and vomiting. Magnesium deficiency is also related to the presence of hypertension, insulin resistance, glucose intolerance, dyslipidemia, with increased complications seen in pregnancy – this aspect needs further research. An impaired magnesium status can lead to diabetic retinopathy and polyneuropathy.

7.4.6 Selenium

Selenium is a known antioxidant, having anti-inflammatory properties that are helpful in patients with insulin resistance and diabetes. Selenium can also inhibit hyperglycemia and hyperinsulinemia caused by the expression of adhesion molecules, as well as reducing inflammation, C-reactive protein, and L-selectin (22). A selenium deficiency can lead to reproductive disorders, diminished food intake, muscular dystrophy, subcutaneous edema, and mineralization of the kidneys.

7.4.7 Vitamin D

Vitamin D has been in the papers in the recent years in relation to its possible role in chronic disease like diabetes. Vitamin D deficiency can affect glucose metabolism, reduce beta cell function, and increase glucose intolerance. A meta-analysis by Song et al. found that there is a relevant association between serum vitamin D levels and type 2 diabetes.

Vitamin D deficiency has been linked to the onset of diabetes. This review summarizes the role of vitamin D in maintaining the normal release of insulin by the pancreatic beta cells. Diabetes is initiated by the onset of insulin resistance. It has also been noted that people newly diagnosed with type 2 diabetes tend to have lower vitamin D levels than people without diabetes. Vitamin D deficiency can cause rickets, costochondral enlargement, osteomalacia, and osteoporosis (21).

7.4.8 Vitamin C

The antioxidant status of a diabetic can be significantly improved through the targeted administration of vitamin C, which reduces protein glycosylation through competitive displacement of glucose from amino groups of proteins that further prevents endothelial damage by the glycosylated reaction products. Vitamin C inhibits the enzyme aldose reductase, thereby slowing the process of intracellular accumulation of sorbitol and thus slowing the damage to eyes, nerves, and kidneys. Oxidized vitamin C is significantly lower in diabetics than non-diabetics. Cellular uptake of vitamin C is impeded by high blood sugar levels. The risk of hyperglycemia can be decreased to a third by increasing vitamin C levels by 20 micromoles per liter (23).

7.4.9 Vitamin E

Vitamin E is an important antioxidant that protects hormones, enzymes, and polyunsaturated fatty acids present in biological membranes against reactive oxygen species. It lowers thrombocyte aggregation and hence the risk of thrombosis is reduced and protein glycosylation is reduced (24). Vitamin E also slows down the inflammatory processes and the proliferation of vascular connective tissues, thereby preventing diabetic complications.

7.4.10 Vitamin B Complex

Vitamin B complex consist of B1, B2, B6, B12, niacin, biotin, pantothenic acid, folic acid, and vitamin C. In carbohydrate metabolism, vitamin B acts as an essential cofactor of enzymes and it plays a crucial role in the mechanism of nerve impulses. Vitamin B2 mediates in the transfer of energy from protein, fat, and carbohydrates to ATP. Vitamin B6 (pyridoxine) has an important role in the transmission of nerve impulses, hemoglobin formation, and amino acid metabolism, and maintains the stability and integrity of the nervous system. Niacin plays a role in the formation of energy and skin integrity, as well as having a function in nervous tissue and the gastrointestinal tract. Biotin helps in the production of fatty acids and the conversion of nutrients into energy. In an elderly population with high homocysteine levels, the rate of brain atrophy was significantly delayed by regular intake of vitamin B12, vitamin B6, and folic acid.

7.4.11 Vitamin B1

Vitamin B1 deficiency can cause anorexia, loss of weight, ataxia, polyneuritis, ventriflexion in cats, paresis, and cardiac hypertrophy in dogs. Studies have shown that diabetics have reduced vitamin B1 supplies and also deranged vitamin B1 metabolism.

7.4.12 Vitamin B6

Reduced vitamin B6 availability might also contribute to the pancreatic islet autoimmunity in T1DM. This idea is based on the consideration that pyridoxal 5′ phosphate (PLP), the active form of vitamin B6, is a cofactor for glutamic acid decarboxylase (GAD-65), which represents an important autoantigen implicated in the pathogenesis of T1DM. Lack of vitamin B6 intake can also impact insulin resistance. Furthermore, vitamin B6 has an effect on the metabolism of lipids. It was proposed that reduced levels of vitamin B6 might increase levels of homocysteine, as PLP is a cofactor for cystamethioninesynthase (CBS) and cystamethionine lyase (CGL), which are involved in the metabolism of this compound. Elevated homocysteine levels are associated with obesity, and they can also impair endothelial function and lead to lipid accumulation in the liver. People with diabetes have a high risk of developing many serious health issues: persistent high glucose levels in the blood can damage the heart, blood vessels, eyes, kidneys, and nerves. In diabetes, the accumulation of AGEs is caused by hyperglycemia through a spontaneous chemical change of amine-containing molecules (25).

7.4.13 Vitamin B12

Neuropathies are more common in diabetics with vitamin B12 deficiency compared to non-diabetics.

7.4.14 Omega 3 Fatty Acids

These are long-chain, polyunsaturated fatty acids that can lower lipid levels, protect the endothelium, and prevent thrombotic events. Omega 3 fatty acids help in increasing the levels of adiponectin in the blood, which helps in controlling metabolic processes like the regulation of blood sugar levels and the containment of inflammation (26). Diabetic patients can benefit from the intake of omega-3 fatty acids, which help to prevent the occurrence of micro- and macroangiopathies. Supplementary intake of omega-3 fatty acids enhances the composition of the nerve cell myelin sheath and essential fatty acids in the cell membrane and thereby prevents diabetic neuropathy.

7.4.15 Coenzyme Q10

In diabetic patients, the levels of coenzyme Q10 are frequently lower than in normal individuals. Reduced coenzyme Q10 levels are an indicator of increased oxidative stress. These reduced levels are observed in diabetic patients suffering from cardiomyopathy and retinopathy. Some clinical studies have indicated that coenzyme Q10 lowers blood pressure levels in type 2 diabetes mellitus.

7.4.16 Niacin

Niacin deficiency in diabetics may lead to diarrhea, mucosal ulcers, anorexia, tongue necrosis (dogs and cats), and cheilosis (21).

7.4.17 Folate

A deficiency of folic acid in diabetics impairs amino acid metabolism and is associated with high homocysteine levels in the blood. An increased homocysteine level is associated with a high risk of stroke, dementia, heart attack, and macular degeneration. Diabetics with a folate deficiency are more likely to suffer from stroke compared to non-diabetics (27).

7.5 NUTRACEUTICALS

Nutraceuticals ("nutrition" + "pharmaceutical") are foods or fortified food products that could have beneficial effects for the consumer. The term "nutraceuticals" was coined in 1989 by Stephen DeFelice, founder and chairman of the Foundation for Innovation in Medicine.
Sources of nutraceuticals:

- Plants: garlic, tomato, tea, soya.

- Animals: shark liver oil, cod liver oil.

- Minerals: calcium, iron, magnesium, phosphorus, iodine.

- Microorganisms: bifido-bacterium, lacto-bacilli.

Coenzyme Q10 is a nutraceutical that is obtained from flax seeds, garlic, bitter gourd, spirulina, garlic, turmeric, tomato, and fenugreek (Table 7.2 and Table 7.3) (28).

Table 7.2 Beneficial herbs in diabetes mellitus management

Sl no.	Herb	Scientific name	Benefit
1.	Bitter gourd	*Momordica charantia*	Anti-diabetic property
2.	Fenugreek seeds	*Trigonella foenum graecum*	Hypoglycemic agent
3.	Java plum	*Syzygium cumini*	Anti-diabetic property
4.	Cinnamon	*Cinnamonium zeylanicum*	Anti-diabetic property
5.	Nigella seeds	*Nigella sativa*	Hypoglycemic agent
6.	Garlic	*Allium sativum*	Anti-diabetic property
7.	Gurmar	*Gymnema sylvestre*	Hypoglycemic agent

Table 7.3   Vitamins and their health benefits

Sl no.	Vitamins	Benefits	Source
1.	Vitamin B1	Reduces blood sugar and neurological symptoms.	Fruits and potatoes, rice, sweet potatoes, green peas, sunflower seeds, nuts.
2.	Vitamin B6	Maintains blood sugar level.	Meat, fish, beef liver, beans, avocado, potatoes.
3.	Vitamin B12	Useful in diabetic neuropathy, prevents megaloblastic anemia.	Milk, banana, apple, orange, fish, egg.
4.	Vitamin C	Anti-oxidant, reduces heart diseases, dementia, increases iron absorption, lowers blood pressure.	Citrus fruits, tomato, broccoli, strawberry, kiwi.
5.	Vitamin D	Improves tolerance of glucose, reduces insulin resistance.	Fish liver oil, egg, beef, chicken breast.
6.	Vitamin E	Antioxidant, maintains skin and eye health.	Pumpkin, milk, mango, almonds, red bell pepper.
7.	Omega 3 fatty acids	Regulates carbohydrate metabolism, stimulates skin and hair growth, lowers cholesterol level.	Walnuts, eggs, salmon, tuna, flax seeds.
8.	Niacin	Decreases blood sugar levels, increases good cholesterol levels.	Dalia, poha, mushroom, roasted groundnut, sunflower seeds.
9.	Biotin	Improves blood sugar control in patients with diabetes, cardioprotective, improves immunity.	Egg yolk, milk, yoghurt, nuts, soyabean.

ACKNOWLEDGMENTS

Dr Nandita Deka

Dr Neelomjyoti Gohain

REFERENCES

1. Le AM, Do AT, Khaiat A. A randomized, double-blind, monocentric, and placebo-controlled blood glycemic response evaluation of Sweetch, a natural sugar replacement blend, on healthy volunteers. *Int J Diabetes Clin Res.* 2023;10(1):165.

2. Thabuis C, Rodriguez B, Gala T, Salvi A, Parashuraman M, Wils D, Guérin-Deremaux L. Evaluation of glycemic and insulinemic responses of maltitol in Indian healthy volunteers. *Int J Diabetes Dev Ctries.* 2015;35:482–487.

3. Remuzzi G, Schieppati A, Ruggenenti P. Clinical practice. Nephropathy in patients with type 2 diabetes. *N Engl J Med.* 2002; 346: 1145–1151.

4. Keith DS, Nicolas GA, Gullion CM, et al. Longitudinal follow-up and outcomes among a population with chronic kidney disease in a large managed care organization. *Arch Intern Med.* 2004;164:659–663.

5. Prakash S, Yadav OP, Sah VK, Singh JK, Jha B. Correlation of biochemical parameters among diabetes patients attending medicine OPD of Janaki Medical College Teaching Hospital. *Janaki Medical College Journal of Medical Science.* 2022 Aug 28;10(2):11–22.

6. IDF: International Diabetes Federation. *Diabetes Atlas 2019*, 9th edn, Brussels, Belgium, 2019. http://www.idf.org/diabetesatlas

7. WHO. *Management of Substance Abuse Unit. Global Status Report On Alcohol And Health.* World Health Organization, 2014; 1:1.

8. Khanal P, Nielsen MO. Is foetal programming by mismatched pre- and postnatal nutrition contributing to the prevalence of obesity in Nepal? *Prev Nutr Food Sci.* 2019;24(3):235–244.

9. World Health Organization. Data and statistics: The challenge of diabetes. https://www.euro .who.int/en/health-topics/noncommunicablediseases/diabetes/data-and-statistics.

10. International Diabetes Federation. *IDF Diabetes Atlas*, 10th edn. Brussels, Belgium: International Diabetes Federation, 2021.

11. Grozavescu M, Butnariu M. Biochemical aspects of diabetes mellitus. *J Diabetes Res.* 2021 Apr;3:1–7.

12. Vasudevan DM, Sreekumari S. *Regulation of Blood Glucose, Insulin and Diabetes Mellitus. Textbook of Biochemistry (For Medical Students)*, 9th edition. Delhi: Jaypee Brothers Medical Publishers(P) Ltd., 2019, pp. 167–168.

13. Goldberg IJ. Diabetic dyslipidemia: Causes and consequences. *J Clin Endocrinol Metab.* 2001 March 1;86(3):965–971. https://doi.org/10.1210/jcem.86.3.7304

14. Jameson JL, Fauci A, Kasper D, Hauser S, Longo D, Loscalzo J. *Harrison's Principles of Internal Medicine*, 20th ed. New York: Mc Graw Hill Education, 2018. Chapter 398, Diabetes mellitus: Complications; p. 2875.

15. Bunza JM, Alhassan AJ. Complications of diabetes mellitus: An insight in to biochemical basis. *Eur J Pharm Med Res.* 2019 Feb;6:114–120.

16. Edwards JL, Vincent AM, Cheng HT, Feldman EL. Diabetic neuropathy: Mechanisms to management. *Pharmacol Ther.* 2008 Oct;120(1):1–34. doi: 10.1016/j.pharmthera.2008.05.005. Epub 2008 Jun 13. PMID: 18616962; PMCID: PMC4007052

17. Asmat U, Abad K, Ismail K. Diabetes mellitus and oxidative stress-A concise review. *Saudi Pharm J.* 2016 Sep;24(5):547–553. doi: 10.1016/j.jsps.2015.03.013. Epub 2015 Mar 21. PMID: 27752226; PMCID: PMC5059829

18. Prakash S, Yadav OP, Sah VK, Singh JK, & Jha B. Correlation of biochemical parameters among diabetes patients attending medicine OPD of Janaki Medical College Teaching Hospital. *Janaki Med Coll J Med Sci.* 2022;10(2):11–22. https://doi.org/10.3126/jmcjms.v10i2 .47852

19. Guo Y, Huang Z, Sang D, Gao Q, Li Q. The role of nutrition in the prevention and intervention of type 2 diabetes. *Front Bioeng Biotechnol.* 2020 Sep 15;8:575442. doi: 10.3389/ fbioe.2020.575442. PMID: 33042976; PMCID: PMC7523408.

20. Kazi TG, Afridi HI, Copper KN. Chromium, manganese, iron, nickel, and zinc levels in biological samples of diabetes mellitus patients. *Biol Trace Elem Res.* 2008;122(1):1–18.

21. Nur Rosyid F. Micronutrient deficiency in type 1 and 2 diabetes mellitus: Diagnosis and therapy. *Int J Res Med Sci.* 2022 Mar 28;10(4):973–979.

22. Battin EE, Brumaghim JL. Antioxidant activity of sulfur and selenium: A review of reactive oxygen species scavenging, glutathione peroxidase, and metal-binding antioxidant mechanisms. *Cell Biochem Biophys.* 2009;55(1):1–23.

23. Meredith ME et al. Ascorbate reverses high glucose- and RAGE-induced leak of the endothelial permeability barrier. *Biochem Biophys Res Commun.* 2014;445:30–35.

24. Ceriello A et al. Vitamin E reduction of protein glycosylation in diabetes: New prospect for prevention of diabetic complications? *Diabetes Care.* 1991;14(1):68–72.

25. Mascolo E, Vernì F. Vitamin B6 and diabetes: Relationship and molecular mechanisms. *Int J Mol Sci.* 2020 May 23;21(10):3669. doi: 10.3390/ijms21103669. PMID: 32456137; PMCID: PMC7279184.

26. Wu JH et al. Effect of fish oil on circulating adiponectin: A systematic review and meta-analysis of randomized controlled trials. *J Clin Endocrinol Metab.* 2013;98(6):2451–2459.

27. Wu JH et al. Effect of fish oil on circulating adiponectin: A systematic review and meta-analysis of randomized controlled trials. *J Clin Endocrinol Metab.* 2013;98(6):2451–2459.

28. Padmaja U. *Medical Pharmacology*, 7th ed. New Delhi: CBS Publishers and Distributors Pvt Ltd, 2021: Chapter 62 Dietary supplements, nutraceuticals, vitamins, herbal medicines and enzymes in therapy; pp. 723–724.

8 Clinical Management of Diabetes Mellitus

Patricia Underwood, Jordan Keels, and Andrew A. Dwyer

Key Terms	Definitions
Self-care	managing chronic illness through a set of health-promoting practices [1]
Self-management	engagement in daily activities in collaboration with families, communities, and healthcare professionals to manage chronic disease [2]
Diabetes technology	refers to the software, devices, and hardware that individuals use to assist with diabetes self-management [3]

8.1 INTRODUCTION: Diabetes Epidemiology and Population Health

Diabetes mellitus (DM) is a chronic disease affecting more than 500 million adults worldwide and is a leading cause of mortality, contributing to annual US healthcare costs exceeding $500 billion [4, 5]. Globally, the incidence of DM is increasing. Currently, 1 in 10 adults between the ages of 20 and 79 years is living with DM [4]. Rates of DM are projected to rise, with an estimated 783 million individuals affected by 2045. The prevalence of DM is disproportionately high in both low- and middle-income countries, where 3 in 4 adults are living with DM [4]. Further, individuals from racial and ethnic minority groups experience higher rates of DM and worse clinical outcomes – including higher rates of mortality compared to non-Hispanic White counterparts [6].

Poorly controlled DM is characterized by high glucose variability and elevated hemoglobin A1c (HbA1c). Importantly, poorly glycemic control is associated with an increased risk of developing micro- and macrovascular complications [7–11]. Microvascular complications from DM (i.e., small blood vessel disease) can be devastating and include diabetic retinopathy, nephropathy, and neuropathy [12]. The incidence of DM-related microvascular complications is declining in the United States and worldwide. However, microvascular complications remain the leading cause of blindness, chronic kidney disease (CKD), and limb amputation. Estimated lifetime rates are variable for retinopathy (30–90%) [13], peripheral neuropathy and lower extremity DM foot disease (6–51%) [14], nephropathy (25–40%) [15, 16], and erectile dysfunction (20–30%) [17]. Macrovascular complications (i.e., large blood vessel disease) include cerebrovascular events (stroke), myocardial infarction (MI), peripheral vascular disease (PVD), and congestive heart failure (CHF). Recent evidence suggests that achieving guideline-based treatment goals (e.g., glycemic control) has helped mitigate macrovascular complications and decrease macrovascular-related deaths among individuals with DM [18]. Despite improvements, macrovascular complications are still the leading cause of death in individuals with DM. Overall, DM-related complications are declining, as evidenced by falling rates of hospitalizations for hyperglycemia, vascular complications, and cardiac death [19–21]. However, gains have not benefited all populations equally. Traditionally marginalized and underserved groups, including Black and Indigenous people of color (BIPOC), experience higher rates of DM and a greater disease burden from complications, including mortality [19, 21]. Poorer outcomes for BIPOC communities are thought to relate to differences in access to care and social determinants of health [6].

Social determinants of health (SDoH) refer to the constellation of factors that influence overall health, including education access and quality, healthcare access and quality, neighborhood and built environment, social and community context (i.e., cultural drivers), and economic stability [6, 22]. Race, ethnicity, and SDoH all contribute significantly to clinical outcomes in patients with DM [6, 23]. When developing a DM treatment plan, clinicians should assess aspects of SDoH, including educational attainment, income/employment status, access to healthy foods, social support, and levels of distress/depression, as all these factors are associated with DM self-care and glycemic control. Data indicate that BIPOC individuals are more likely to have higher HbA1c measurements, hypertension (HTN), and dyslipidemia compared to their non-Hispanic White counterparts [24, 25].

Given the scope and complexity of DM management, significant effort has focused on developing evidence-based approaches to care. Some posit that a multi-level, systemic approach to DM care is needed, including interventions targeting healthcare policy, healthcare systems, and individual patients with DM [26]. The American Diabetes Association (ADA) advocates the Chronic

DOI: 10.1201/9781003384823-8

Care Model (CCM) as a framework guiding the delivery of high-quality DM care [27]. Key aspects of the CCM include collaborative, multi-disciplinary clinical teams with well-defined roles and interventions to support patient self-management, including health behaviors that promote and maintain health. Given the robust body of literature supporting the effectiveness of the CCM for DM management, we employ this framework to guide our discussion of DM interventions. Moreover, DM self-management behavior is essential for achieving tight glycemic control and reducing the risk of micro- and macrovascular complications. Accordingly, significant attention is given to therapeutic education (i.e., DM self-management education, DSME). Importantly, DSME delivered in person or virtually is an effective strategy for improving glycemic control, health-related quality of life (HR-Qol), and patient well-being [28–30].

8.2 GLUCOSE HOMEOSTASIS AND DIABETES PATHOPHYSIOLOGY

Diabetes results from disrupted glucose homeostasis (i.e., impaired insulin secretion and insulin resistance) leading to chronic hyperglycemia. The pathophysiologic underpinnings of DM include reduced mass of insulin-secreting β cells, impaired insulin signaling and glucose metabolism (insulin resistance), defects in incretin hormone response, and disrupted renal tubular glucose reabsorption capacity contributing to increased plasma glucose levels (hyperglycemia) [31].

8.2.1 Pancreas

The pancreas is both an endocrine and exocrine gland, with the vast majority of the pancreatic tissue dedicated to its exocrine function [32]. Acinar cells make up about 85% of the pancreas and produce digestive enzymes trypsin, lipase, and amylase, which are critical for protein, fat, and carbohydrate digestion [32]. Pancreatic secretions enter the duodenum via the main pancreatic duct [32]. The islets of Langerhans are the endocrine secretory cells of the pancreas and are located between the clusters of acinar cells [32]. Insulin is a peptide hormone necessary for energy metabolism, including glucose, fat, and protein metabolism [33]. Insulin-secreting beta cells (β cells) make up approximately 40–60% of the endocrine cells in the pancreas. The remaining pancreatic endocrines are alpha (α α), delta, epsilon, and F cells [32]. These cell types secrete factors critical for glucose homeostasis, including glucagon, somatostatin, ghrelin, and pancreatic polypeptide (PP) respectively [32].

8.2.2 Impaired Pancreatic β Cell Function and Insulin Secretion

Studies demonstrate that individuals with DM have reduced β cell mass and corresponding decreased insulin secretion. Histologic studies of organ donors and autopsies performed on individuals with type 2 DM (T2DM) reveal 40% fewer β cells compared to healthy individuals [34]. Chronic hyperglycemia and the pro-inflammatory state of DM lead to β cell apoptosis, decreased insulin secretion, and chronic hyperglycemia [31, 35]. The mechanism(s) underlying decreased beta cell mass has yet to be determined, but is thought to be a slow, progressive β cell loss following an initial phase of β cell hypertrophy with concurrent hyperinsulinemia and hyperglycemia [35]. Loss of β cell function and diminished insulin secretion decreases insulin availability causing altered glucose metabolism with hyperglycemia, insulin resistance, and DM [36].

8.2.3 Impaired Pancreatic α Cell Function and Glucagon Secretion

Glucagon is a hormone secreted from the pancreatic α cells that plays a key role in glucose homeostasis by triggering glucose production from hepatic glycogen stores. In healthy individuals, glucagon is secreted in response to hypoglycemia and spurs gluconeogenesis. In individuals with T2DM, α cells are dysregulated and secrete glucagon despite chronic hyperglycemia contributing to fasting hyperglycemia observed in T2DM [34]. Recent studies suggest that glucagon dysregulation is a key contributor not only to hyperglycemia but also to non-alcoholic fatty liver disease (NAFLD) [37].

8.2.4 Impaired Insulin Signaling and Insulin Resistance

Insulin secretion and insulin signaling are key components of cellular glucose uptake and glucose homeostasis. Insulin is secreted in a biphasic pattern. The first phase inhibits hepatic glucose production and lipolysis, while the second phase increases glucose utilization in the muscle, fat, and white adipose tissue [33]. Insulin signaling promotes glucose utilization and storage in adipose and muscle tissue – a key process for whole body glucose homeostasis [36]. Individuals with DM have inadequate insulin secretion, increased hepatic glucose production, and altered insulin signaling, leading to altered glucose metabolism. Specifically, altered intracellular insulin signaling and/or altered insulin-stimulated glucose uptake (in the muscle or adipose tissue) lead to insulin resistance, poor glucose utilization, and hyperglycemia [38]. The insulin signaling pathway has been studied extensively, demonstrating a strong interplay between different signaling proteins and sub-pathways, including phosphoinositide 3-kinase (PI-3 kinase), protein kinase B (AKT), and glycogen synthase kinase 3 (GSK3). Pathway alterations underlie insulin resistance in DM [39]. Further, glucose transporter type 4 (GLUT4) is an intracellular transport molecule required for insulin-stimulated glucose uptake. Decreased GLUT4 expression on the plasma membrane results in decreased glucose uptake in the muscle and insulin resistance [40, 41].

Alterations in fatty acid metabolism, lipid accumulation, and insulin desensitization also contribute to insulin resistance in the muscle [42]. Increased free fatty acids and disruptions in AMP kinase (AMPK) and glut-4 translocation lead to alterations in intracellular glucose metabolism and the inhibition of insulin-stimulated glucose uptake, resulting in hyperglycemia and worsening insulin resistance in the muscle [42, 43].

8.2.5 Altered Hepatic Glucose Production and Lipid Homeostasis

In healthy individuals, insulin regulates hepatic glucose production (gluconeogenesis) and lipid homeostasis (lipogenesis, lipolysis) [42]. Individuals with DM have decreased hepatic insulin sensitivity so insulin secretion no longer suppresses hepatic gluconeogenesis and lipolysis, leading to hyperglycemia, free fatty acid (FFA) liberation, and hypertriglyceridemia [44]. Further, increased circulating FFAs inhibit hepatic insulin signaling, contributing to insulin resistance, hyperinsulinemia, and hyperglycemia [45].

8.2.6 Altered Incretin Hormone Function

The incretin hormones are gastrointestinal hormones released in response to food intake and play key roles in glucose-dependent insulin secretion [46]. After food is ingested and glycemia increases, the incretin hormones induce insulin synthesis and secretion, suppress glucagon, decelerate gastric emptying, and increase satiety [46]. The incretins include glucagon-like peptide-1 (GLP-1) and gastric inhibitory polypeptide (GIP). Dipeptidyl peptidase 4 (DDP-4) is an enzyme that inactivates GLP-1 and GIP. Both GLP-1 and GIP activity is reduced in individuals with DM. The result is decreased insulin secretion, as well as diminished suppression of hepatic gluconeogenesis and lipolysis, resulting in hyperglycemia. Further, decreased incretin activity results in reduced satiety, increased food intake, and resulting weight gain – contributing to worsening insulin resistance [34]. Pharmacologic agents that mimic incretin hormone function, GLP-1 receptor agonists (GLP-1 RA) and *DPP-4 inhibitors, effectively induce insulin secretion, suppress glucagon, and increase satiety, leading to both improved glycemic control and the promotion of weight loss (thereby improving insulin sensitivity)* [47]. Such pharmacologic agents are highly effective at targeting the two key aspects of DM (i.e., impaired insulin secretion and insulin resistance). A subsequent chapter specifically covers pharmacotherapy for DM.

8.2.7 Altered Renal Tubular Glucose Reabsorption

The kidney contributes to glucose homeostasis via renal gluconeogenesis, glucose uptake from circulation, and tubular reabsorption regulated by sodium/glucose cotransporter-2 (SGLT-2) in the proximal convoluted tubule [48]. In healthy individuals, glucose is filtered in the glomerulus until the maximal resorptive capacity is exceeded (>11 mmol/l) [49]. Beyond this threshold, glucose is excreted in the urine (glucosuria). In individuals with DM, the renal threshold for glucosuria is disturbed and glucosuria is initiated at higher glucose levels, contributing to chronic hyperglycemia and microvascular renal damage (nephropathy) [50–52]. Pharmacologic agents targeting renal aspects of glucose homeostasis – specifically, SGLT2 inhibitors – improve glycemic control, improve blood pressure, promote weight loss, and have been shown to have beneficial effects on micro- and macrovascular complications of DM, including nephropathy and cardiovascular disease [53]. Further, studies show that SGLT-2 inhibitor use is associated with reduced hospitalizations in individuals with T2DM and comorbid CHF [54]. SGLT2 inhibitor mechanisms of action and benefit are discussed in detail in a subsequent chapter of this textbook.

8.3 DIABETES SUBTYPES AND CLINICAL PRESENTATION

Diabetes mellitus (DM) is a chronic, progressive disease of the pancreatic beta (β) cells resulting in insulin deficiency and insulin resistance and overt hyperglycemia [55]. Two hallmarks of DM are absolute insulin deficiency and the progressive loss of adequate β cell insulin secretion in the setting of insulin resistance [56] (underlying the two primary types of DM – type 1 [T1DM] and type 2 [T2DM]). A deeper understanding of the pathology underlying DM has led to an updated classification system comprising several subtypes based on clinical presentation of insulin deficiency, insulin resistance, or a combination of both. Subtypes of DM include pre-diabetes (i.e., metabolic syndrome), autoimmune insulin deficiency (T1DM), late-onset type 1 diabetes (i.e., latent autoimmune diabetes in adults [LADA]) [57, 58], ketosis-prone T2DM [59], DM secondary to exocrine pancreatic disorders (e.g., pancreatitis, cystic fibrosis), and monogenic DM (both neonatal and maturity-onset diabetes of the young [MODY]) (Table 8.1) [60]. Adult-onset DM has recently been re-classified as including six categories based on underlying pathophysiology (i.e., insulin deficiency vs. insulin resistance) (Table 8.2), treatment parameters, and clinical outcomes [61]. The following section provides an overview of DM sub-classes with a focus on the clinical presentation of each.

8.3.1 Pre-Diabetes

Pre-diabetes is a term used for individuals who have abnormal carbohydrate metabolism yet who do not meet the criteria for T2DM [56]. Pre-diabetes is defined by the presence of impaired glucose tolerance (IGT) and/or impaired fasting glucose (IFG) and/or glycated hemoglobin (HbA1C) 5.7–6.1% (39–47mmol/mol) [56]. Risk factors associated with pre-diabetes include obesity/central

Table 8.1 Novel diabetes subtype characteristics (adapted from [61])

DM Class	Diagnostic Hallmark(s)	DM Subtype	DM Phenotype
Type 1 DM	Positive Autoimmune Antibodies (GADA)	SAID: Severe Autoimmune Diabetes	(+) GADA, low insulin secretion, poor metabolic control
LADA	Positive Autoimmune Antibodies (GADA)	SAID: Severe Autoimmune Diabetes	(+) GADA, low insulin secretion, poor metabolic control
Type 2 DM	Elevated A1c, Elevated BMI, Increased Age, Elevated HOMA-IR (insulin resistance)	SIDD: Severe Insulin Deficient Diabetes	Low insulin secretion, poor metabolic control, increased risk of retinopathy and neuropathy
		SIRD: Severe Insulin Resistant Diabetes	Insulin resistance, obesity, late onset, increased risk of nephropathy and fatty liver
		MOD: Mild Obesity-Related Diabetes	Obesity, early onset
		MARD: Mild Age-Related Diabetes	Late onset, low risk of complications

Table 8.2 Comparison table: includes presentation differences in T1DM, T2DM, insulin

	Type 1 Diabetes	Pre-Diabetes	Type 2 Diabetes
Pathophysiology	Autoimmune destruction of pancreatic β cells	Impaired β cell function and increased insulin resistance	Progressive loss of β cell function and insulin resistance
Autoantibodies	Present in most cases	Absent	Absent
Endogenous insulin	Decreased or absent	Can be normal, increased, or decreased	Can be normal, increased, or decreased
Ketosis	Common	Rare	Rare, but can occur in ketosis prone T2DM
Age of onset	Childhood or adolescence, can occur in adults (LADA)	Mostly in adults	Mostly in adults
Presentation	Polyphagia, polydipsia, blurred vision, and weight loss; possible diabetic ketoacidosis (DKA)	Will often have no signs or symptoms of diabetes; however, individuals will often exhibit impaired fasting glucose	Hyperglycemia over a long period of time and often coincides with the characteristics of metabolic syndrome (obesity, insulin resistance, hypertension, dyslipidemia)

adiposity (waist circumference >40 in./102 cm in males and >35 in./89 cm in females), dyslipidemia (hypertriglyceridemia >150 mg/dL [1.7 mmol/L], decreased low density lipoprotein [LDL] <40 mg/dL [1.04 mmol/L] in males or <50 mg/dL [1.3 mmol/L] in females), and hypertension (HTN, >130/85 mm/Hg) [56]. Such risk factors are components of the metabolic syndrome that is a constellation of cardiometabolic risk factors. As such, pre-diabetes confers increased risk of cardio-vascular disease (CVD) and progression to T2DM [56].

8.3.2 Type 1 Diabetes (T1DM)

Type 1 DM (T1DM) results from autoimmune destruction of the pancreatic β cells, leading to absolute insulin deficiency and hyperglycemia [56, 62]. Prospective studies in humans have revealed specific islet autoantibodies that predict the onset of T1DM [56]. Autoantibodies associated with T1DM include glutamic acid decarboxylase autoantibodies (GADAs), islet cell autoantibodies (ICAs), insulin autoantibodies (IAAs), and antibodies to islet-specific zinc transporter isoform 8 (ZnT8) [62]. Age upon first detection of autoantibodies, the number of autoantibodies, the specificity of autoantibodies, and the autoantibody titer can help determine the rate of T1DM progression [56]. The "two hit hypothesis" is thought to underlie the pathogenesis of T1DM. This hypothesis posits that both genetic variants and environmental factors contribute to the development of autoantibodies marking T1DM [32]. Genetic variants associated with T1DM are attributed to single nucleotide polymorphisms (SNPs) in the human leukocyte antigen (HLA) region [63].

T1DM accounts for approximately 5% of all DM cases. It occurs in younger individuals (i.e., children and adolescents) and has a higher incidence and prevalence in individuals identifying as non-Hispanic White [64]. Clinical prediction models incorporating immunologic, metabolic, and genetic markers have been developed to facilitate the identification/diagnosis of T1DM [65, 66]. While genetic and autoantibody testing confirms the diagnosis of T1DM, clinical presentation and clinical characteristics typically lead clinicians to test to confirm the diagnosis. Insulin deficiency manifests in patients who present with overt symptoms of hyperglycemia, i.e., polyphagia, polydipsia, polyuria, blurred vision, and weight loss (catabolic state) [56]. Life-threatening complications may result if hyperglycemia and insulin deficiency remain uncorrected (i.e., diabetic keto-acidosis [DKA]) [67]. The COVID-19 pandemic has led to an increase in new-onset T1DM with a more severe clinical presentation, including higher rates of DKA at presentation [68]. Some have postulated that the SARS-CoV-2 induces pancreatic β cell destruction.

8.3.3 Type 2 Diabetes (T2DM)

Type 2 diabetes (T2DM) results from a progressive loss of β cell function, leading to insulin deficiency and worsening insulin resistance [56, 69]. Insulin resistance (IR) is defined as dysregulated insulin signaling and decreased glucose uptake in muscle and adipose tissues. A pro-inflammatory milieu, including hyperinsulinemia, chronic inflammation (i.e., secondary to obesity), and metabolic stress, contributes to IR that underlies the pathogenesis of T2DM [69]. Individuals with insulin resistance and T2DM often exhibit elevated levels of free fatty acids and proinflammatory cytokines [34]. Individuals with insulin resistance and T2DM often exhibit the constellation of factors defining metabolic syndrome and increased CVD risk [70]. Increasing age, obesity, hypertension, a sedentary lifestyle, and poor diet are all associated with metabolic syndrome and T2DM [34, 56, 71]. Importantly, females previously diagnosed with gestational diabetes (GDM) or polycystic ovarian syndrome (PCOS) are at significantly increased risk for developing T2DM [56].

Notably, T2DM is more common among individuals with Black/African American, Indigenous, Hispanic/Latinx, and Asian genetic ancestry [56]. A strong family history of T2DM increases an individual's risk of developing T2DM – particularly among individuals identifying as non-Hispanic Black or Hispanic/LatinX [72]. Accordingly, family history is an important clinical factor that should be elicited for all patients. Prior work demonstrates that 39% of patients with T2DM had at least one parent with the disease [73]. However, the penetrance and expressivity of genes contributing to T2DM confer a relatively small effect size, suggesting that T2DM is a complex genetic condition associated with more than 500 genetic signals [74].

Ahlqvist and others have contributed to classifying the heterogeneous presentation of T2DM into four specific categories: severe insulin-deficient diabetes (SIDD), severe insulin-resistant diabetes (SIRD), mild obesity-related diabetes (MOD), mild age-related diabetes (MARD) [61]. Individuals with SIDD tend to develop T2DM earlier and are at increased risk of retinopathy and neuropathy. MARD is the "mildest" form of T2DM, with the latest age of onset and lowest risk of complications. These subcategories were identified within a large European cohort and replicated in Chinese and Indian populations, demonstrating the generalizability and utility of these metrics

[75, 76]. It is plausible that T2DM subtypes may help individualize pharmacotherapy treatment by targeting the specific T2DM subtype etiopathology.

8.3.4 Latent Autoimmune Diabetes in Adults (LADA)

Latent autoimmune diabetes in adults (LADA) is a slow-progressing autoimmune DM leading to insulin deficiency later in life (often between 40 and 70 years of age). This type of DM has hallmarks of both T1DM (insulin deficiency) and T2DM (insulin resistance) and, in some cases, has been referred to as "Type 1.5 DM" [77]. The presence of the glutamic acid decarboxylase antibodies (GAD Ab) is common, while the presence of IA-2 and insulin autoantibodies is less prevalent [78]. Individuals with LADA present with clinical features similar to T1DM, including normal weight (BMI 18–25), symptoms of severe hyperglycemia (polyphagia, polydipsia, polyuria), and minimal/absent c-peptide levels in the presence of hyperglycemia [79]. Early in the disease course, individuals with LADA have limited β cell function and insulin secretion capacity – a profile that makes oral hypoglycemic agents an effective management strategy. However, insulin therapy is typically required within six months to two years of diagnosis [80]. The diagnosis of LADA is based on three clinical criteria: adult age at onset of DM; the presence of circulating islet autoantibodies (distinguishing LADA from T2DM); and insulin independence at diagnosis (distinguishing LADA from classic T1DM) [80]. Similar to T2DM, individuals with LADA exhibit insulin resistance – suggesting that the etiopathology of LADA involves both metabolic dysfunction and autoimmunity [81]. Further, LADA and T1DM share similar genetic variants in the major histocompatibility complex (MHC) region, *PTPN22*, *SH2B3*, and insulin (INS) [81].

8.3.5 Maturity-Onset Diabetes of the Young (MODY)

Maturity-onset diabetes of the young (MODY) is an autosomal dominant (AD) disease characterized by the onset of hyperglycemia at an early age (<25 years) and defined by impaired insulin secretion with few/no defects in insulin action [56, 82]. Individuals with MODY present with heterogenous characteristics. Thus, traditional DM signs and symptoms may not be reliable in detecting or predicting MODY (PMID: 11575290). Clinical characteristics distinguishing MODY from T2DM include young age of presentation, the absence of obesity, and a family history [82]. Various genetic abnormalities have been associated with MODY. Variants in genes underlying MODY lead to altered cell development, regulation, or function and corresponding different disease sub-types (MODY 1, MODY 2, etc.) [82]. Genes associated with MODY include hepatocyte nuclear factor 4 alpha (*HNF-4a*), glucokinase (*GCK*), hepatocyte nuclear factor-1 (*HNF-1a*), insulin promotor factor – 1 (*I PF-1*), hepatocyte nuclear factor-1 beta (*HNF-1β*), and neuronal differentiation 1 (*NeuroD1*), or beta-2 adrenergic receptor (*BETA* 2) [82]. Variants in these genes result in impaired glucose metabolism, insulin sensitivity, insulin secretion from pancreatic β cells, and dysregulated hepatic gluconeogenesis [82].

8.3.6 MODY 1

Variants in the *HNF-4a* cause MODY 1 [82]. *HNF-4a* is expressed in the liver and the pancreas and regulates the expression *HNF-1a* . Individuals with *HNF-4a* variants may present with a relatively mild form of DM. The precise mechanism remains unclear, yet variants are associated with a reduced insulin secretory response to glucose [83]. Individuals with pathogenic *HNF-4a* variants have progressive loss of insulin secretion that worsens over time, necessitating anti-diabetic treatment. Furthermore, harboring a pathogenic *HNF-4a* variant is associated with defective glucagon secretion (in response to arginine stimulation) and hypoglycemia-induced pancreatic polypeptide secretion, suggesting that *HNF-4a* may have a regulatory role for pancreatic β, α, and pancreatic polypeptide cells [82]. Variants in *HNF-4a* are associated with hepatic effects with deficient triglyceride and apolipoprotein synthesis (AII, CIII, and Lp(a) lipoprotein) [82].

8.3.7 MODY 2

MODY 2 results from heterozygous pathogenic variants in glucokinase (*GCK*), which encodes an enzyme expressed in the pancreas and liver. Glucokinase plays a key role in glucose metabolism functioning as a glucose sensor and regulator in pancreatic β cells. Glucokinase plays a role in hepatic glucose storage in the form of glycogen. Pathogenic *GCK* variants ultimately lead to decreased glucose sensitivity and defective glucose storage. Homozygous mutations result in permanent neonatal DM [83].

8.3.8 MODY 3

Pathogenic variants in *HNF-1a* underlie the most common form of MODY, MODY 3. As *HNF-1a* is regulated by *HNF-4a* , pathogenic variants in either gene produce similar and mild forms of DM. Pathogenic variants in *HNF-1a* have been reported in individuals of all racial and ethnic backgrounds. Diabetes results from a progressive decline in insulin secretion that is thought to stem from β cell dysfunction as opposed to altered insulin activity. The impaired glucagon secretion of MODY 3 can result in impaired renal function and glycosuria [83].

8.3.9 MODY 4

MODY 4 results from a frameshift mutation affecting *IPF-1*. *IPF-1* is a transcription factor that regulates several genes that are critical in pancreas development (glucokinase, islet amyloid polypeptide, glucose transporter 2). As a result, *IPF-1* loss of function results in abnormal β cell development and impaired β cell function, resulting in severe impairment of insulin secretion [83].

8.3.10 MODY 5

MODY 5 results from mutations in the gene encoding *HNF-1β* , a transcription factor that regulates the expression of genes encoding proteins involved in metabolism, glucose transport, and insulin gene expression. Individuals with pathogenic variants in *HNF-1β* exhibit both diabetes and abnormal renal development resulting in renal dysfunction. Internal sex organ anomalies have been reported in females harboring pathogenic *HNF-1β* variants [83].

8.3.11 MODY 6

MODY 6 is one of the rarer forms of MODY, resulting from mutations in *NeuroD1* (Beta2). *NeuroD1* is a transcription factor required for the normal development of pancreatic islets. Pathogenic variants in *NeuroD1* may result in β cell dysfunction, resulting in another subtype of MODY. However, this form of MODY has only been identified in two families [83].

8.3.12 Diabetes Screening, Diagnosis, and Treatment Targets

Clinicians should understand the various sub-types of DM to appropriately identify the underlying cause of DM, working with the patient to develop an individualized treatment plan, and achieve improved short- and long-term outcomes. Taking a detailed patient history, performing a focused physical exam, and using the appropriate screening tests are critical for accurately diagnosing DM and timely initiation of treatment [84].

8.3.13 Diabetes Screening

Universal screening for DM is cost-prohibitive so professional societies have developed consensus guidelines for screening high-risk individuals. Clinicians must consider both non-modifiable DM risk factors (i.e., age, race/ethnicity, genetics, family history) and modifiable risk factors. Modifiable risk factors include being overweight (BMI ≥25, or BMI ≥23 for those of Asian ancestry), cardio-metabolic disease (i.e., hyperlipidemia, HTN, coronary artery disease [CAD], atherosclerotic coronary vascular disease [ASCVD]), and a sedentary lifestyle. The American Diabetes Association (ADA) recommends that all individuals >35 years old be screened for DM. Earlier screening is advocated for individuals who are overweight, have a first-degree relative with DM, are of certain ancestry (Black/African American, Hispanic/Latinx, Indigenous, Asian, Pacific Islander), have a history of HTN (blood pressure ≥140/90 mmHg), CVD, GDM, or PCOS, or exhibit clinical signs of insulin resistance (i.e., acanthosis nigricans). Additional considerations include those with pre-diabetes (i.e., metabolic syndrome) and human immunodeficiency virus (HIV) infection, given the high incidence of DM in these populations [84]. When a screening result is normal, testing should be repeated every three years – except for individuals with pre-diabetes, who merit annual screening [84]. The International Diabetes Federation (IDF) has less stringent screening criteria and recommends screening individuals at high risk of developing T2DM – i.e., >45 years old, positive family history of DM, a history of HTN, and a high waist circumference and/or obesity) [85]. Both organizations underscore the importance of using validated decision tools (i.e., "FINDRISC", "Diabetes Risk Test") to help determine individuals who should be screened for DM [86, 87].

8.3.14 Diagnostic Tests for Diabetes

Diagnostic tests for DM include assays to measure plasma blood glucose, response to glucose load, glucose variability, and serology to identify autoantibodies.

Random and fasting plasma glucose – Measuring plasma glucose is a rapid and inexpensive way to assess plasma glucose levels. Random plasma glucose measurement may occur at any time of the day, regardless of last meal. An elevated random plasma glucose ≥200 mg/dL (>11.1mmol/L) is considered diagnostic for DM. Fasting plasma glucose measures are assessed following an eight-hour fast. A result of 100–125 mg/dL (5.55–6.94mmol/L) is consistent with pre-diabetes, while values ≥126mg/dL (7.0 mmol/L) are diagnostic for DM [84].

Oral glucose tolerance test (OGTT) – An OGTT assesses an individual's fasting (eight hours) response to a standard glucose load (75g) over two hours. The OGTT is a sensitive test for detecting both pre-diabetes (i.e., insulin resistance, metabolic syndrome) and DM. A two-hour plasma glucose measurement of 140–199 mg/dL (7.77–11.05mmol/L) is considered pre-diabetes and a glucose level ≥200 mg/dL (11.1 mmol/L) is diagnostic for DM [88].

Glycated hemoglobin – Hemoglobin A1c (HbA1c) assesses the degree to which erythrocytes have been glycosylated. As erythrocyte lifespan is approximately 120 days, HbA1C indicates the average plasma glucose levels over a two to three month period. A number of large clinical trials (e.g., Diabetes Chronic Complications Trial [DCCT], United Kingdom Prospective Diabetes Study [UKPDS]) demonstrate that HbA1C is a valid and reliable predictor of DM clinical outcomes [89]. Since 2010, the ADA has defined a HbA1C ≥6.5% as diagnostic for diabetes [84]. HbA1c is a point-of-care test that does not require fasting. As such, the utility and ease of testing have made HbA1c the preferred test for diagnosis and monitoring glycemic control. The ADA supports the use of HbA1c for diagnosing pre-diabetes (5.7–6.4%) [84]; however, neither the World Health Organization (WHO) nor the International Diabetes Federation (IDF) support the use of HbA1c for diagnosing pre-diabetes as quality point-of-care testing devices are not available worldwide [85]. For point-of-care testing in the United States, it is important to use a laboratory method certified by the National Glycohemoglobin Standardization Program (NGSP) and standardized to the Diabetes Control and Complications Trial (DCCT) [84].

Discrepancies between HbA1c and fasting glucose warrant prompt further evaluation. Importantly, HbA1c should not be used in individuals with hemoglobinopathies (e.g., sickle cell disease), pregnancy (second and third trimesters), glucose-6-phosphate dehydrogenase (G-6-PD) deficiency, HIV, or individuals on hemodialysis or erythropoietin therapy [90]. In such cases, an alternative test should be employed, such as fasting glucose, OGTT, or fructosamine (glycosylated albumin). Clinical correlations of HbA1c and other measures are provided in Table 8.3 and Table 8.4 [90].

Islet autoantibodies (T1DM, LADA) – The ADA classifies T1DM into three distinct phases based on patient symptoms and severity of hyperglycemia – yet all phases have the presence of autoantibodies at diagnosis [84]. As noted above, several autoantibodies contribute to the pathogenesis of T1DM and the presence of multiple autoantibodies is associated with a higher disease risk T1DM

Table 8.3 Criteria for diagnosing pre-diabetes and diabetes

	Fasting Plasma Glucose	2 Hours Post-75gm Oral Glucose Tolerance Test (OGTT)	A1c
Pre-Diabetes	100–125mg/dl (5.6–6.9mmol/l)	140–199mg/dl (7.8–11mmol/L)	5.7–6.4%
Diabetes	≥126mg/dl (≥7.0mmol/l)	≥200mg/dl (11.1mmol/l)	≥6.5%

Table 8.4 Correlation of fructosamine to A1c (adapted from [91])

HbA1c (%), Mean (Range)	Fructosamine Assay (umol/L)	Mean Blood Glucose Levels Estimated by HbA1c (mg/dl)
5.5 (5.1–5.8)	225.25	111.2
6 (5.5–6.4)	246.83	125.5
7 (6.5–7.5)	297.06	154.2
8 (7.5–8.6)	339.15	182.9
9 (8.6–9.4)	393.61	211.6
10 (9.5–10.5)	444.22	240.3
11 (10.6–11.5)	491.26	269.0
12 (11.5–12.6)	534.83	297.7

Table 8.5 Determination of average target HbA1c level over time (adapted from www.healthquality.va.gov/guidelines/cd/diabetes/index.asp)

Major Comorbidity or Physiologic Age	Microvascular Complications		
	Absent or Mild	Moderate	Advanced
Absent >10–15 years of life expectancy	6.0–7.0%	7.0–8.0%	7.5–8.5%
Present 5–10 years of life expectancy	7.0–8.0%	7.5–8.5%	7.5–8.5%
Marked <5 years of life expectancy	8.0–9.0%	8.0–9.0%	8.0–9.0%

[92]. Both genetic and environmental factors influence the presentation of hyperglycemia (i.e., polyuria, polydipsia, polyphagia, blurred vision), marked hyperglycemia, and individuals having relatives with T1DM [84].

8.3.15 Glycemic Treatment Targets

Per the ADA, glycemic status should be examined at least two times per year in individuals meeting clinical targets and at least quarterly in individuals not meeting clinical targets [93]. Clinicians should use measurements of hemoglobin A1c or time in range using a continuous glucose monitor (CGM) to evaluate glycemic status. Glycemic targets should be individualized based on age, pregnancy status, and whether micro- and macrovascular complications exist [94]. For most patients, A1c levels ≤7% are acceptable if this can be achieved without significant hypoglycemia [93]. The HbA1c target is based on large cohort studies (DCCT and UKPDS) indicating achieving a HbA1c of 6–7% decreases an individual's risk of developing micro- and macrovascular complications (UKPDS) (Table 8.5). Less stringent HbA1c goals (<8%) should be used when the risk of hypoglycemia is high (i.e., individuals with impaired renal function) or the individual has a limited life expectancy [93]. Providers should consider such factors and establish glycemic targets with patients through shared decision-making.

8.3.16 Prevention or Delay of Type 2 Diabetes: Lifestyle Behavior Change/Diabetes Self-Management Education

A robust body of evidence supports the relationship between structured, evidence-based behavior change interventions and the prevention or delay of T2DM [95]. The Diabetes Prevention Program (DPP) was a hallmark study demonstrating that intensive coaching and lifestyle modification in individuals at high risk of developing T2DM resulted in weight loss, improved DM self-management, and delayed onset of T2DM compared to either standard lifestyle intervention plus placebo or standard lifestyle intervention plus pharmacotherapy with metformin [95]. Diabetes incidence was 58% lower in the intensive lifestyle intervention group and 31% lower in the metformin group compared to the placebo. A recent meta-analysis of seven randomized control trials (RCTs) that included 4,090 study participants demonstrated that a Mediterranean diet (i.e., high fiber, low saturated fats) is significantly associated with prevention of T2DM [96]. Similarly, a meta-analysis of 20 longitudinal cohort studies found that interventions to increase physical activity/exercise decrease T2MD risk and prevent progression to T2DM [97]. Thus, evidence cements the use of intensive lifestyle interventions to improve nutrition and physical activity/exercise as cornerstones for all individuals with pre-DM to prevent progression to T2DM and to improve glycemic control for individuals with T2DM.

Behavior change interventions not only slow/prevent the onset of T2DM. Such interventions are also critical for supporting DM self-management behaviors – including healthy eating, glucose monitoring, exercise, social support, adherence to prescribed anti-diabetes medications, and provider engagement, i.e., regular eye exams, influenza vaccines, foot exams, dental exams (Figure 8.1). Diabetes Self-Management Education (DSME) has been shown to improve diabetes behavior change, improve glycemic control, and reduce all-cause mortality [98–100]. Such programs have a structured curriculum developed to support ADA standards for DM care, including patient decision-making, self-care behaviors, problem solving, and engagement with healthcare providers. Many studies have demonstrated that tailored, DSME interventions improve HbA1c in adults with T2DM [101, 102]. A meta-analysis of nine studies involving 1,389 participants from low- and middle-income countries found that structured DSME lowered HbA1c between 0.5–2.6% [103]. Further, programs utilizing weekly meetings with smaller group sizes and peer-to-peer support have a greater beneficial effect on lowering HbA1c [102]. Virtual DSME is promising and has been

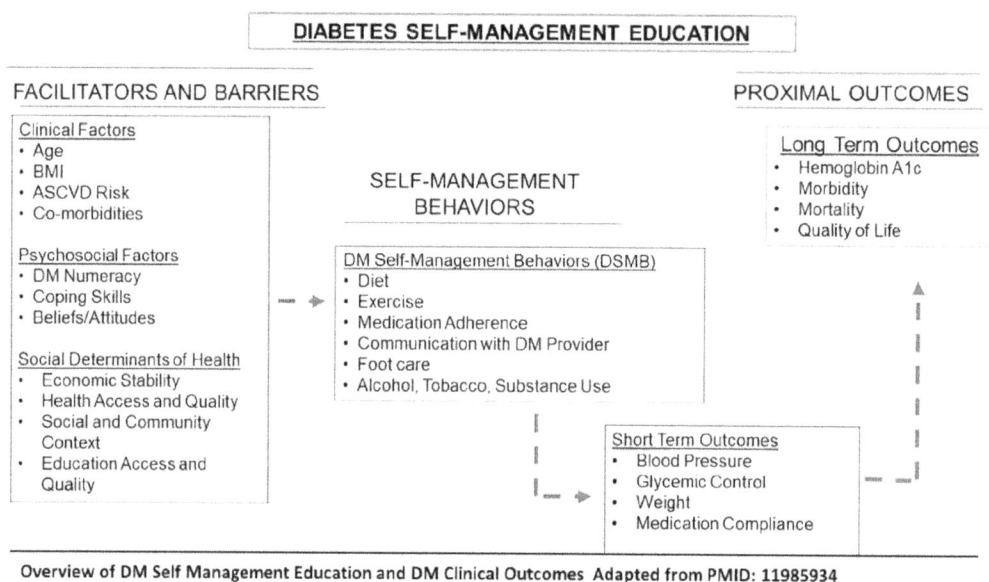

Overview of DM Self Management Education and DM Clinical Outcomes Adapted from PMID: 11985934

Figure 8.1 Overview of DM self-management education and DM clinical outcomes [109]

demonstrated to produce similar HbA1c results compared to traditional in-person formats [104, 105].

Interestingly, the effect of DSME interventions on glycemic control varies across different patient populations. A meta-analysis of eight RCTs revealed that DSME interventions did not significantly improve HbA1c measures in Black people/African Americans with T2DM [106]. However, a separate meta-analysis of 18 RCTs employing culturally tailored DSME interventions for adult Hispanic/Latinx individuals with T2DM produced significantly lower HbA1c levels – but with marked heterogeneity across studies (PMID: 31542186). Such findings indicate that attention to cultural values and beliefs is important when delivering DSME to diverse populations. When possible, DSME should be delivered by a certified diabetes care and education specialist, ensuring appropriate knowledge and training in diabetes management and effective DSME delivery techniques. Further, providers should involve strategies to improve DSME delivery, including engaging in goal-setting with the patient [107] and identifying and addressing language and numeracy barriers [108].

8.3.17 Comprehensive Medical Evaluation and Assessment of Comorbidities

Individuals with DM are at risk of developing both microvascular (nephropathy, neuropathy, retinopathy) and macrovascular complications (CVD, peripheral vascular disease [PVD]), leading to increased morbidity and mortality. Thus, it is important for clinicians to evaluate, prevent, and treat these conditions when managing care for individuals with diabetes (Table 8.6). The most prevalent comorbidities include cardio-metabolic complications, including chronic kidney disease (CKD), HTN, and congestive heart failure (CHF). In a large study of 530,747 patients, cardio-renal-metabolic conditions occurred in more than 80% of the population, with 83% had HTN, 81% hyperlipidemia, 32% CVD, and 20% CKD [110]. While new pharmacotherapeutic agents have been shown to decrease the incidence and progression of cardio-renal-metabolic conditions including sodium-glucose cotransporter-2 (SGLT2) inhibitors and glucagon-like peptide-1 receptor (GLP1R) agonists, preventing and managing these complications continues to be an important component of DM disease management. The effects of pharmacotherapy in reducing DM complications are reviewed in detail in another chapter. This chapter will focus on surveillance and non-pharmacologic treatments demonstrated to be effective in preventing and managing DM complications.

Microvascular complications of diabetes – The microvascular complications of DM affect several systems and include kidney disease (nephropathy), neuropathy, retinopathy, and erectile dysfunction.

Diabetic nephropathy – Chronic kidney disease (CKD) affects ~50% of individuals with T2DM worldwide and is the most costly complication of DM [111]. Diabetic CKD is defined as an elevated

Table 8.6 Components of comprehensive diabetes medical evaluation (adapted from ADA clinical guidelines 2023)

	Diabetes History	Initial Visit	Every Follow-Up Visit	Annual Visit
	DM presentation (e.g. age, symptoms)	X		
	Medication review	X		
	Review hospitalizations	X		
	Family history of DM and autoimmune disorder	X		
	Personal history of complications and common comorbidities	X		X
Past Medical and Family History	HTN/HLD	X		X
	Obesity, NAFLD	X		X
	Macro- and microvascular Complications	X		X
	Presence of hemoglobinopathies or anemias	X		X
	Last dental visit	X		X
	Hypoglycemia	X	X	X
	Last dilated eye exam	X		X
	Specialty visits	X	X	X
	Interval history: change in family/medical history		X	X
Behavior Factors	Behavior factors: nutrition, exercise, sleep, smoking, alcohol, and substance use	X	X	X
Medication HIstory	Medication and vaccination review	X	X	X
Technology Use	Technology use: health apps, glucose monitoring, glucose data	X	X	X
Social Life Assessment	Social support, social determinants of health	X	X	X

urinary albumin/creatinine ratio of ≥30mg/g and/or a reduction in estimated glomerular filtration rate (eGFR: <60ml/min/1.73m2) (PMID: 21693741). Hyperglycemia and poor glycemic control (i.e., elevated HbA1c) are the leading cause of CKD in individuals with T2DM [111]. Treating CKD is expensive due to high rates of hypoglycemia, hospitalization, and transplantation (renal replacement therapy [RRT]) for individuals with end-stage renal disease (ESRD). Screening for CKD should be done annually with prompt nephrology referrals for individuals with an eGFR <45 (i.e., CKD stage IIIb or higher) [112]. Individuals at the greatest risk for CKD include older adults (>65 years) with comorbidities (HTN, hyperlipidemia, obesity) on multiple pharmacologic agents (polypharmacy), as well as BIPOC individuals and those from marginalized and disadvantaged backgrounds [111]. The higher risk of CKD in BIPOC individuals may be due to differences in access to care and/or underlying genetic risk (i.e., variants in apolipoprotein L1 [APOL1]) [113]. Further, individuals with comorbid obesity, HTN, hyperlipidemia, and CVD are at high risk of developing CKD. Accordingly, mitigating CKD risk entails treatment relation to meeting weight, blood pressure, and lipid targets.

Achieving target blood pressure and prescribing renal-protective antihypertensive agents targeting the renin-angiotensin-aldosterone pathway (i.e., angiotensin-converting enzyme inhibitors [ACEi], angiotensinogen receptor blockers [ARBs]) have been repeatedly shown to delay the progression of CKD [114, 115]. Pharmacotherapy with ACEi, ARBs, GLP1-agnoists, and SGLT2 inhibitors has been shown to improve CKD outcomes [116]. Importantly, caution is warranted when prescribing both an ACEi and ARB as several clinical trials highlight the risk of serious adverse events (i.e., hyperkalemia, acute renal injury, increased cardiovascular events) [117, 118].

Achieving individual glycemic targets at the beginning (or early stages) of DM onset and maintaining tight glycemic control are among the most important ways to prevent nephropathy and CKD. Numerous studies indicate that glycemic control decreases an individual's risk of developing renal complications from both T1DM and T2DM [113, 119]. The Diabetes Control and Complications Trial (DCCT) demonstrated that intensive glycemic control (goal HbA1c <6%) resulted in a significantly decreased risk of developing both microalbuminuria (an early sign of nephropathy) and overt proteinuria compared to conventional care (HbA1c = 9%) [120]. A hallmark study by Kussman and colleagues [121] described the progression of nephropathy in individuals with T1DM. Individuals initially presented with microalbuminuria (urine albumin/creatinine ratio <30) approximately 11–23 years after diagnosis that progressed to macroalbuminuria (ratio >300), and subsequent declining kidney function (increasing serum creatinine concentrations, declining eGFR) and finally end-stage renal disease [113].

The combination of DM and CKD places a significant burden on individuals and their families/caregivers. It is essential to recognizing the disease burden and support patients, families, and caregivers to improve health-related quality of life (HR-QoL). Numerous studies demonstrate high levels of distress in individuals with DM. Patients can benefit from supportive interventions that foster active coping strategies, draw on family support, and enhance psychological health [122–124].

Diabetic neuropathy – Neuropathy is a common microvascular complication of DM occurring in ~50% of individuals with DM and is characterized by damage to the peripheral and autonomic nervous systems [125]. The most common form of neuropathy is distal symmetric polyneuropathy. This form of neuropathy is the leading cause of diabetic foot ulcers, and amputations and is a significant cause of falls, pain, and reduced HR-QoL in individuals with diabetes [126]. The global prevalence of DM neuropathy is high and is greater in T2DM compared to T1DM [127]. The ADA recommends screening for diabetic neuropathy at diagnosis and annually for patients with T2DM and five years after diagnosis and then annually for individuals with T1DM [128].

The pattern of nerve damage and symptoms varies depending on the type of neuropathy. Cardiac autonomic neuropathy can lead to weakness, light-headedness, orthostatic hypotension, syncope, orthostatic tachycardia, and bradycardia. Gastrointestinal autonomic dysfunction (gastroparesis) often presents with gastrointestinal discomfort, bloating, postprandial vomiting, and slow gastric absorption, contributing to poor glycemic control, greater glucose variability, and hypoglycemia. Urogenital autonomic neuropathy may result in neurogenic bladder (decreased urinary frequency), as well as sexual dysfunction, including erectile dysfunction and retrograde ejaculation in males and dyspareunia and poor lubrication in females [126].

Peripheral neuropathy can present with a range of subjective symptoms, including numbness, tingling, or burning pain that starts in the feet/toes and progresses proximally to the knees. On physical examination, patients demonstrate decreased sensation (10 g monofilament test) and decreased vibration (128 Hz tuning fork) and proprioception sensation in a "stocking and glove" distribution [126]. A neurology consultation is merited when patients describe atypical symptoms (i.e., acute severe pain, asymmetry of neuropathic symptoms, altered motor symptoms). In such cases, laboratory evaluation (i.e., vitamin B_{12} levels, thyroid function tests, autoimmune panel) is indicated to rule out other potential etiologies causing atypical symptoms.

Chronic hyperglycemia causes initial damage to long sensory neurons and subsequently neuropathy progresses over time. Inflammation, adipogenesis, and lipid synthesis also contribute to nerve damage of neuropathy. As such, metabolic parameters (i.e., obesity, hyperglycemia, hyperlipidemia, HTN) should be appropriately addressed to strive toward meeting treatment goals [126]. Akin to other microvascular complications, the DCCT demonstrated that poor glycemic control increases the risk for developing neuropathy [9]. Thus, tight glycemic control is essential for preventing and slowing the development of microvascular complications. The Action to Control Cardiovascular Risk in Diabetes (ACCORD) trial and the Veterans Affairs Diabetes Trial (VADT) both provide further support for tight glycemic control in preventing neuropathy in individuals with T2DM (PMID: ACCORD and VADT). Current clinical guidelines recommend improving glycemic control as a first-line treatment to prevent and decrease the progression of DM neuropathy (ADA).

As noted above, DSME is an important complement to anti-diabetic medication for enhancing glycemic control. Part of DSME includes equipping patients with strategies for mitigating microvascular complications, including routine, annual diabetes foot care to reduce the incidence of foot ulcers/infections and enable early detection of neuropathy [129]. It is critical to teach patients how to assess their feet for infections, open sores, and wounds, as well underscoring the importance of always wearing appropriate socks (white) and well-fitted footwear (to reduce pressure and abrasions) [130]. Routine (i.e., annual) podiatry visits should be established as needed to provide foot care, assessment, and, when needed, surgical debridement of foot wounds/ulcers [131].

There is no cure for neuropathy, but pharmacologic therapies are available to treat the symptoms (i.e., neuropathic pain). Anticonvulsants, serotonin–noradrenaline reuptake inhibitors (SNRI), and/or tricyclic antidepressants (TCAs) may be prescribed to treat neuropathic pain. Clinical trials have supported the benefit of anticonvulsants (i.e., gabapentin, pregabalin) for neuropathic pain [132]. Of note, gabapentin is significantly less expensive than pregabalin and should be considered for patients when cost is an issue. However, psychotropic medications are associated with a range or adverse effects including confusion and dizziness/syncope that may be exacerbated in older adults taking the medications as part of polypharmacy regimens [126]. Indeed, SNRIs (e.g., duloxetine, venlafaxine) have been shown to improve DM neuropathic pain; however, they are associated with adverse effects, including dizziness, fatigue, nausea, and insomnia [133]. Amitriptyline is the most common TCA prescribed for neuropathic pain [134].

Diabetic retinopathy – Diabetic retinopathy (DR) is among the most common of microvascular complications and is the fifth leading cause of vision impairment and blindness globally [135, 136]. A systematic review estimated the global prevalence of DR to be 22.3%, with the highest prevalence among individuals identifying as Hispanic/Latinx (47.4%) and lower rates in individuals of Middle Eastern (32.9%), Black/African (31%), and European ancestry (23.7%) [135]. Like other microvascular complications, DR results from poor glycemic control. Chronic hyperglycemia initially contributes to the development of microaneurysms, hemorrhages, and hard exudates that progress over time to vision impairment, cataracts, and, in some cases, vitreous hemorrhage and retinal detachment [137]. Hyperglycemia leads to alterations in retinal blood flow and changes in the capillary wall formation. Retinopathy is classified in two stages: non-proliferative diabetic retinopathy and the more advanced stage, proliferative diabetic retinopathy. Macular edema occurs with sub- and intra-retinal fluid accumulation, which increases intraocular pressure, resulting in decreased visual acuity [137]. Correcting hyperglycemia and achieving glycemic targets is the best way to prevent the onset and progression of DR [138].

Early identification of DR (i.e., regular dilated eye exams) and routine surveillance of disease progression have been shown to improve clinical outcomes. As such, many clinical practice guidelines recommend screening for retinopathy within five years of T1DM diagnosis and at the time of T2DM diagnosis with follow-up screening every one to two years (or earlier in the presence of significant DR risk factors) [128]. Notably, individuals with chronic hyperglycemia, nephropathy, hypertension, and dyslipidemia are at increased risk of developing DR and merit aggressive intervention to mitigate DR risk [128].

Several treatment strategies can be employed to treat and delay the progression of DR. Chronic hyperglycemia leads to inflammation, vascular damage, altered blood flow, and the accumulation of advanced glycation end products (AGEs). Most DR treatments target these mechanisms by decreasing inflammation and improving retinal blood flow [137]. A promising class of treatments (anti-vascular endothelial growth factor [VEGF]) decreases vascular permeability and have been shown to improve clinical DR outcomes [139]. Clinical trials of anti-VEGFs (e.g., bevacizumab, ranibuzumab, aflibercept) improve visual acuity and decrease diabetic macular edema (DME), making them first-line therapy for patients with DR and DME [140–142]. If anti-VEGF treatments are not viable (i.e., due to cost, an inability to perform monthly injections, the development of injection-related enophthalmitis), alternatives may include laser monotherapy, non-specific anti-angiogenic treatments, or intravitreal corticosteroids [137].

Macrovascular complications – Atherosclerotic cardiovascular disease (ASCVD), including coronary heart disease (CAD), cerebrovascular disease, CHF, and peripheral heart disease, is the leading cause of mortality in individuals with DM, resulting in high healthcare expenditures [21, 5]. The chronic hyperglycemia of DM produces advanced glycosylated end products, inflammation, and oxidative stress that contribute to arterial plaque formation, endothelial damage, and hypercoagulability. As such, more individuals with DM develop and die from CVD than non-diabetic individuals [143–145]. In addition to chronic hyperglycemia, individuals with T2DM often have additional cardiometabolic risk factors (i.e., metabolic syndrome including obesity, insulin resistance, HTN, and dyslipidemia) that further increase ASCVD risk [146]. Given the significant ASCVD burden, clinicians must focus on preventing and managing ASCVD risk factors, including smoking cessation, weight loss, glycemic control, managing blood pressure, lipids, and protecting renal function [147]. The American College of Cardiology/American Heart Association ASCVD risk calculator is a user-friendly clinical tool that can help patients understand their ten-year risk of a first ASCVD event and guide clinicians in developing a disease management plan [148].

8.3.18 ASCVD Primary Prevention

Lifestyle interventions – Many RCTs have demonstrated the effectiveness of clinical interventions to mitigate ASCVD risk, including intensive lifestyle interventions and weight loss. The "Look AHEAD" (action for health in diabetes) trial evaluated the effect of intensive lifestyle intervention, weight loss, and DSME on adverse ASCVD events (i.e., myocardial infarction [MI], cerebrovascular accident [CVA], congestive heart failure [CHF]) [149]. The "Look AHEAD" intervention failed to reduce cardiac events; however, participants receiving the intervention had greater weight reduction, lower HbA1c, improved fitness, fewer depressive symptoms, improved health-related quality of life (HR-QoL), and decreased microvascular complications (i.e., nephropathy, neuropathy, retinopathy) compared to the control group [150]. Smoking cessation without weight gain has been shown to decrease ASCVD risk in individuals with T2DM [151]. A large cohort study demonstrated that smoking cessation conferred a significantly lower ASCVD risk compared to active smokers. However, the improved ASCVD risk was slightly attenuated by weight gain accompanying smoking cessation, highlighting the importance of weight control in ASCVD risk [152].

Nutritional interventions for individuals with T2DM focusing on weight loss and reduced sodium intake routinely demonstrate improved weight and glycemic control with reduced ASCVD risk. The Diabetes Remission Clinical Trial (DiRECT) examined the effect of low-calorie meal replacement on T2DM remission and found 24% of participants achieved weight loss of >15kg at one year, along with improved glycemic control, diabetes remission, and improved HR-QoL [153]. The Diabetes Intervention Accentuating Diet and Enhancing Metabolism (DIADEM-I) trial found similar results in Middle Eastern and Northern African patients with T2DM [154, 155]. Diets (i.e., Mediterranean diet, the Dietary Approaches to Stop Hypertension [DASH]) emphasizing a plant-based diet low in sodium have been shown to reduce weight, improve glycemic control, and decrease ASCVD risk (i.e., insulin resistance, hypertension, dyslipidemia) and should be encouraged for all individuals with DM [156–158].

Blood pressure control – Current clinical practice guidelines target blood pressure <130/80 mmHg in individuals with DM to prevent end-organ damage (i.e., ASCVD, nephropathy) [147, 159]. Numerous clinical trials have evaluated the effect of reaching target blood pressure on ASCVD events in individuals with DM. The Action to Control Cardiovascular Risk in Diabetes (ACCORD) study failed to demonstrate reduced ASCVD with targeted systolic blood pressure (SBP) <120 mmHg in individuals with DM [160]. However, the Systolic Blood Pressure Intervention Trial (SPRINT) demonstrated decreased ASCVD events with SBP <120 mmHg; however, this study did not include individuals with DM [161]. The Action in Diabetes and Vascular Disease (ADVANCE) study demonstrated reduced ASCVD events with systolic blood pressure <135 mmHg [162]. Similarly, the Strategy of Blood Pressure Intervention in the Elderly Hypertensive Patients (STEP) trial included individuals with DM and demonstrated decreased ASCVD events with SBP <130 mmHg [160] – thus supporting the target SBP <130mmHg cited in many clinical guidelines.

Strategies to achieve BP targets include dietary interventions (i.e., low sodium), physical activity/exercise, and pharmacologic treatment. Blood pressure should be measured at every visit. Pharmacotherapy with an antihypertensive is warranted if BP >130/80 mm/Hg and dual therapy is merited if BP <160/100 mmHg (ADA guidelines). First-line pharmacologic treatment options include angiotensin-converting enzyme inhibitor (ACEi) or angiotensin receptor blocker (ARB). These renal-protective antihypertensive agents are particularly useful for individuals with underlying ASCVD and/or an elevated urine albumin:creatinine ratio (i.e., >30). Combination therapy employing ACEi and ARB should be avoided due to the risk of acute kidney injury and hyperkalemia [163]. Multiple drug therapy is often required to achieve blood pressure targets, and calcium channel blockers and/or a thiazide diuretic may be added if necessary.

Lipid management – Lowering serum cholesterol has been shown to decrease cardiovascular risk in individuals with DM. Multiple trials support the use of statins to lower cholesterol and reduce ASCVD risk in individuals with DM [164, 165]. Current guidelines recommend initiating lifestyle interventions (discussed previously) and initiating moderate-intensity statin therapy in individuals of 20–39 years of age with additional ASCVD risk factors and individuals of 40–75 years of age without ASCVD (ADA). The ADA recommends high-intensity statin therapy for individuals of 40–75 years of age with DM and higher ASCVD risk as well as for patients who fail to achieve low-density lipoprotein (LDL) levels <70 mg/dl (ADA). The ADA also advocates for adding ezetimibe (to inhibit intestinal cholesterol absorption) or a proprotein convertase subtilisin/kexin type 9 (PCSK9) inhibitor (ADA). Elevated triglycerides (hypertriglyceridemia) should also be addressed through dietary and lifestyle intervention (low glycemic diet, weight loss, reduced alcohol intake, physical activity/exercise) [166]. In terms of pharmacotherapy for hypertriglyceridemia, several RCTs have failed to support a role for fenofibrate or niacin in reducing triglyceride levels in DM. However, the Reduction of Cardiovascular Events with Icosapent Ethyl trial (REDUCE-IT) demonstrated a 25% ASCVD event risk reduction in individuals receiving the intervention [167]. As such, icosapent ethyl can be added to statin therapy to reduce triglyceride levels [168].

Non-alcoholic fatty liver disease [169–171] – A common complication of poorly controlled DM is nonalcoholic fatty liver disease (NAFLD). Notably, NAFLD is the leading cause of chronic liver disease in the Western world [171] and occurs in 55–70% of individuals with T2DM [172, 173]. Several conditions are encompassed within the umbrella term NAFLD. The range of liver diseases includes benign fat accumulation (steatosis), fat deposits with inflammation (non-alcoholic steato-hepatitis [NASH]), hepatic fibrosis, cirrhosis, liver failure, and hepatocellular carcinoma (HCC) [170] The pathophysiology underlying the association between NAFLD and T2DM is complex and includes a range of factors including insulin resistance, hyperglycemia, hyperinsulinemia, dyslipidemia (i.e., dysregulation of lipid and triglyceride metabolism) leading to hepatic fat accumulation, and an inflammatory immune response that can lead to liver damage [170, 174]. The presence of NAFLD in the context of T2DM increases an individual's risk of developing cirrhosis, liver failure, and HCC [175].

The ADA recommends screening individuals with T2DM for NAFLD when individuals present with abnormal liver enzymes (i.e., elevated alanine transaminase [ALT], aspartate transferase [AST]) or findings of a fatty liver on ultrasound [176, 177]. Liver biopsy is the gold standard for diagnosing NAFLD; however, this procedure is typically beyond the scope of primary care and requires referral to a specialist [174]. Alternatively, the fibrosis-4 index (FIB-4) calculator can be used in primary care settings to assess the degree of hepatic fibrosis. The FIB-4 yields a calculation based on patient age, platelet count, and serum ALT and ASTAST [178]. When NAFLD is identified, intervention is warranted to promote weight loss, improve/correct dyslipidemia, achieve glycemic targets, avoid excessive alcohol intake, and improve cardio-metabolic health. Some studies suggest that pharmacotherapy with statins can improve outcomes for patients with T2DM and NAFLD and reduce ASCVD risk [179, 180]. Use of GLP1Ra and the thiazolidinedione pioglitazone appear to improve cardio-metabolic risk factors and help improve clinical outcomes in individuals with T2DM and NAFLD [171, 177]. Recent data indicate that SGLT2 inhibitors may also provide therapeutic benefits to patients with T2DM and NAFLD via weight reduction and cardio-renal effects [171, 181].

Hypercoagulability – Aspirin (ASA) use has been shown to reduce ASCVD morbidity and mortality in individuals with prior myocardial infarction or stroke and is recommended in these populations. More recently, ASA (75–162mg/day) has been recommended as a primary means of preventing ASCVD in young individuals (<50 years) with low risk of adverse events (i.e., gastrointestinal bleed, retinal bleed, extracranial bleed) (USPTF). The US Preventative Services Task Force (USPSTF) recommendation draws on recent clinical trials demonstrating reduced ASCVD risk in individuals receiving ASA for primary prevention. The "A Study of Cardiovascular Events in Diabetes" (ASCEND) trial demonstrated that individuals with DM receiving ASA for primary prevention had a 12% reduction in risk of vascular death, myocardial infarction, cerebrovascular accident, or transient ischemic attack (TIA) [182]. Importantly, there is a significant risk of bleeding with ASA. Aspirin is not recommended for primary prevention of ASCVD events in adults >70 years; however, it is advocated as a secondary prevention measure in older individuals [183].

Cognitive dysfunction – Cognitive impairment is a long-term vascular complication of DM [184]. A number of cohort studies identify an association between DM and cognitive decline and dementia [184–189]. The underlying cause of the relationship remains unclear. Notably, cognitive dysfunction is more prevalent among individuals with DM compared to individuals with other ASCVD risk factors (i.e., obesity, hypertension, dyslipidemia), suggesting that inflammation and vascular injury contribute to the pathogenesis of dementia [190–193]. Interestingly, DM status (i.e., having a diagnosis), but not elevated HbA1c, is associated with cognitive decline among middle-aged adults [194]. Such observations suggest that chronic hyperglycemia is not the primary driver of cognitive decline in individuals with DM. Further, an increased incidence of hypoglycemia is associated with accelerated cognitive decline in individuals with DM [195]. A large RCT of individuals with T2DM and self-reported severe hypoglycemia found a significant association with diminished cognitive ability and accelerated cognitive decline [196]. Diabetes status is associated with a range of cognitive dysfunction, including problems with memory, verbal fluency, and executive functioning [197, 198]. The "Study of Longevity in Diabetes" was a large prospective cohort study that compared baseline cognitive function and rates of low cognitive function according to DM status (i.e., T1DM, T2DM, non-diabetic healthy controls). The study found that older adults with T1DM had significantly poorer cognition compared with T2DM counterparts and controls – even after accounting for comorbidities [197]. Further, SDoH contribute to cognitive dysfunction. A recent cross-sectional analysis of the "Healthy Older People Everyday" (HOPE) study identified that SDoH account for 29–57% of variability in cognitive impairment [199]. Studies indicate that older individuals with T2DM who are less educated, living in rural areas, and have limited DM self-management skills (i.e., experience hypoglycemia) are at increased risk of cognitive impairment [200, 201]. Thus, interventions to address such factors early in DM diagnosis may help prevent cognitive decline.

Aggressive DM treatment including achieving target blood sugar, HbA1c, blood pressure, and weight parameters decrease an individual's risk of cognitive decline [202–204]. Older individuals with DM and high cardiometabolic risk (i.e., elevated HbA1c, dyslipidemia, proteinuria) are at significantly greater risk of developing early cognitive dysfunction [205]. Further, treatment with metformin has been shown to slow cognitive decline and decrease dementia risk in older individuals with DM [206]. Interestingly, cognitive decline is associated with poor medication management and decreased DM self-management behavior, suggesting DSME and interventions supporting medication adherence may help decrease the risk of developing cognitive dysfunction [207]. In the setting of established cognitive dysfunction and/or dementia, DM treatment regimens should be simplified and tailored to mitigate hypoglycemic events [208].

Psychosocial health [209] – Individuals with DM often experience both psychological distress, anxiety, and depression – factors that significantly impact DM self-management and the achievement of target glycemic control [209]. Approximately 30% of individuals with DM experience DM-related distress and approximately 20% meet criteria for clinical depression [210, 211]. Comorbid depression increases mortality risk [212]. Currently, the USPSTF recommends universal screening for depression using a validated assessment tool (i.e., Patient Health Questionnaire-9 [PHQ9]) [213, 214]. Further, the ADA recommends screening for DM distress using validated instruments such as the Problem Areas in Diabetes Scale (PADS) and the Diabetes Distress Scale (DDS) [215]. Individuals with DM and a positive screening finding of distress and/or depression should trigger a referral for mental health services/counseling. An approach utilizing both mental health services and DMSE support has been shown to decrease DM distress and improve self-efficacy for DM self-management [216].

8.4 CONCLUSION

Diabetes is a chronic disease characterized by hyperglycemia resulting from decreased β cell function or insulin resistance [55]. Diabetes can be classified into two major types, T1DM and T2DM [56]. T1DM results from the autoimmune destruction of pancreatic β cells whereas T2DM results from loss of β cell function over time and insulin resistance [56]. Pathophysiological findings suggest several sub-types, including pre-diabetes, autoimmune insulin deficiency (T1DM), LADA [57, 58], ketosis prone T2DM [59], DM secondary to exocrine pancreatic disorders, and MODY [60].

To ensure appropriate and timely initiation of treatment, it is important for clinicians to understand the different sub-types of diabetes. Consensus guidelines have been created to screen individuals who are at high risk of DM based on non-modifiable and modifiable risk factors. The ADA recommends screening for all individuals over the age of 35 [84] and the IDF recommends screening individuals over the age of 45 [85]. It is important to use validated decision tools (i.e., "FINDRISC", "Diabetes Risk Test") when screening individuals at risk of DM [86, 87]. Various diagnostic tests can be used to assess for diabetes, including random and fasting plasma glucose levels, OGTT, and HbA1c (refer to Table 8.3, Criteria for Diagnosing Pre-Diabetes and Diabetes). As previously noted, T1DM can be diagnosed with the presence of autoantibodies [84].

To evaluate glycemic status, clinicians should use HbA1c or time in range using a continuous glucose monitor (CGM) [94]. According to the ADA, individuals who meet clinical targets should have their glycemic status evaluated at least twice a year, while those who do not meet clinical targets should have it examined at least quarterly [95] To decrease risk of developing micro- and macrovascular complications, an A1c level <7% is acceptable for most individuals [93]. There is strong evidence to support that behavior change such has weight loss, physical activity, and a healthy diet can delay the onset of progression of T2DM [95]. Clinicians should establish achievable glycemic targets with patients using shared decision-making. To effectively manage diabetes and support self-management, the ADA recommends a multidisciplinary approach using the chronic care model as a guiding framework [27].

REFERENCES

1. Riegel, B., T. Jaarsma, and A. Strömberg, A middle-range theory of self-care of chronic illness. *ANS Adv Nurs Sci*, 2012. **35**(3): pp. 194–204.

2. Grey, M., et al., A revised self- and family management framework. *Nurs Outlook*, 2015. **63**(2): pp. 162–70.

3. ElSayed, N.A., et al., 7Diabetes technology: Standards of care in diabetes-2023. *Diabetes Care*, 2023. **46**(Supplement_1): pp. S111–S127.

4. Sun, H., et al., IDF diabetes Atlas: Global, regional and country-level diabetes prevalence estimates for 2021 and projections for 2045. *Diabetes Res Clin Pract*, 2022. **183**: p. 109119.

5. American Diabetes Association, Economic costs of diabetes in the U.S. in 2017. *Diabetes Care*, 2018. **41**(5): pp. 917–928.

6. Walker, R.J., J.S. Williams, and L.E. Egede, Influence of race, ethnicity and social determinants of health on diabetes outcomes. *Am J Med Sci*, 2016. **351**(4): pp. 366–373.

7. Raghavan, S., et al., Diabetes mellitus-related all-cause and cardiovascular mortality in a national cohort of adults. *J Am Heart Assoc*, 2019. **8**(4): p. e011295.

8. Martinez, M., et al., Glycemic variability and cardiovascular disease in patients with type 2 diabetes. *BMJ Open Diabetes Res Care*, 2021. **9**(1): p. e002032.

9. Nathan, D.M., et al., Diabetes control and complications trial/epidemiology of diabetes interventions and complications study at 30 years: Advances and contributions. *Diabetes*, 2013. **62**(12): pp. 3976–3986.

10. Subramanian, S. and I.B. Hirsch, Intensive diabetes treatment and cardiovascular outcomes in type 1 diabetes mellitus: Implications of the diabetes control and complications trial/epidemiology of diabetes interventions and complications study 30-year follow-up. *Endocrinol Metab Clin North Am*, 2018. **47**(1): pp. 65–79.

11. Stratton, I.M., et al., Association of glycaemia with macrovascular and microvascular complications of type 2 diabetes (UKPDS 35): Prospective observational study. *BMJ*, 2000. **321**(7258): pp. 405–412.

12. An, J., et al., Prevalence and incidence of microvascular and macrovascular complications over 15 years among patients with incident type 2 diabetes. *BMJ Open Diabetes Res Care*, 2021. **9**(1): p. e001847.

13. Wong, T.Y., et al., Diabetic retinopathy. *Nat Rev Dis Primers*, 2016. **2**: p. 16012.

14. Hicks, C.W. and E. Selvin, Epidemiology of peripheral neuropathy and lower extremity disease in diabetes. *Curr Diab Rep*, 2019. **19**(10): p. 86.

15. Pop-Busui, R., et al., Heart failure: An underappreciated complication of diabetes. A consensus report of the American diabetes association. *Diabetes Care*, 2022. **45**(7): pp. 1670–1690.

16. de Boer, I.H., et al., Diabetes management in chronic kidney disease: A consensus report by the American Diabetes Association (ADA) and kidney disease: Improving global outcomes (KDIGO). *Diabetes Care*, 2022. **45**(12): pp. 3075–3090.

17. Defeudis, G., et al., Erectile dysfunction and diabetes: A melting pot of circumstances and treatments. *Diabetes Metab Res Rev*, 2022. **38**(2): p. e3494.

18. Kuo, S., et al., National trends in the achievement of recommended strategies for stroke prevention in U.S. adults with type 2 diabetes, 2001–2018. *Diabetes Care*, 2022. **45**(9): pp. 2003–2011.

19. Ali, M.K., et al., Interpreting global trends in type 2 diabetes complications and mortality. *Diabetologia*, 2022. **65**(1): pp. 3–13.

20. Gregg, E.W., et al., Changes in diabetes-related complications in the United States, 1990–2010. *N Engl J Med*, 2014. **370**(16): pp. 1514–1523.

21. Cheng, Y.J., et al., Trends and disparities in cardiovascular mortality among U.S. adults with and without self-reported diabetes, 1988–2015. *Diabetes Care*, 2018. **41**(11): pp. 2306–2315.

22. Marmot, M., Social determinants of health inequalities. *Lancet*, 2005. **365**(9464): pp. 1099–1104.

23. Canedo, J.R., et al., Racial/ethnic disparities in diabetes quality of care: The role of healthcare access and socioeconomic status. *J Racial Ethn Health Disparities*, 2018. **5**(1): pp. 7–14.

24. Campbell, J.A., et al., Glucose control in diabetes: The impact of racial differences on monitoring and outcomes. *Endocrine*, 2012. **42**(3): pp. 471–482.

25. Egede, L.E., et al., Longitudinal differences in glycemic control by race/ethnicity among veterans with type 2 diabetes. *Med Care*, 2010. **48**(6): pp. 527–533.

26. ElSayed, N.A., et al., 1Improving care and promoting health in populations: Standards of care in diabetes-2023. *Diabetes Care*, 2023. **46** Supplement 1(Supplement_1): pp. S10–S18.

27. Stellefson, M., K. Dipnarine, and C. Stopka, The chronic care model and diabetes management in US primary care settings: A systematic review. *Prev Chronic Dis*, 2013. **10**: p. E26.

28. Agastiya, I.M.C., et al., The impact of telehealth on self-management of patients with type 2 diabetes: A systematic review on interventional studies. *Diabetes Metab Syndr*, 2022. **16**(5): p. 102485.

29. Asmat, K., et al., The effectiveness of patient-centered care vs. usual care in type 2 diabetes self-management: A systematic review and meta-analysis. *Front Public Health*, 2022. **10**: p. 994766.

30. Crowley, M.J., et al., Effect of a comprehensive telehealth intervention vs telemonitoring and care coordination in patients with persistently poor type 2 diabetes control: A randomized clinical trial. *JAMA Intern Med*, 2022. **182**(9): pp. 943–952.

31. Galicia-Garcia, U., et al., Pathophysiology of type 2 diabetes mellitus. *Int J Mol Sci*, 2020. **21**(17): p. 6275.

32. Atkinson, M.A., et al., Organisation of the human pancreas in health and in diabetes. *Diabetologia*, 2020. **63**(10): pp. 1966–1973.

33. Park, S.Y., J.F. Gautier, and S. Chon, Assessment of insulin secretion and insulin resistance in human. *Diabetes Metab J*, 2021. **45**(5): pp. 641–654.

34. Rogers, J. and J. Allen, Understanding the most commonly billed diagnoses in primary care: Type 2 diabetes mellitus. *Nurse Pract*, 2020. **45**(9): pp. 48–54.

35. Talchai, C., et al., Genetic and biochemical pathways of beta-cell failure in type 2 diabetes. *Diabetes Obes Metab*, 2009. **11**(Suppl 4): pp. 38–45.

36. Kahn, B.B., Lilly lecture 1995. Glucose transport: Pivotal step in insulin action. *Diabetes*, 1996. **45**(11): pp. 1644–1654.

37. Haedersdal, S., et al., Revisiting the role of glucagon in health, diabetes mellitus and other metabolic diseases. *Nat Rev Endocrinol*, 2023. **19**: pp. 321–335.

38. Kahn, S.E., R.L. Hull, and K.M. Utzschneider, Mechanisms linking obesity to insulin resistance and type 2 diabetes. *Nature*, 2006. **444**(7121): pp. 840–846.

39. White, M.F., The IRS-signalling system: A network of docking proteins that mediate insulin action. *Mol Cell Biochem*, 1998. **182**(1–2): pp. 3–11.

40. Garvey, W.T., et al., Gene expression of GLUT4 in skeletal muscle from insulin-resistant patients with obesity, IGT, GDM, and NIDDM. *Diabetes*, 1992. **41**(4): pp. 465–475.

41. Boura-Halfon, S. and Y. Zick, Phosphorylation of IRS proteins, insulin action, and insulin resistance. *Am J Physiol Endocrinol Metab*, 2009. **296**(4): pp. E581–591.

42. Shulman, G.I., Cellular mechanisms of insulin resistance. *J Clin Invest*, 2000. **106**(2): pp. 171–176.

43. Witczak, C.A., C.G. Sharoff, and L.J. Goodyear, AMP-activated protein kinase in skeletal muscle: From structure and localization to its role as a master regulator of cellular metabolism. *Cell Mol Life Sci*, 2008. **65**(23): pp. 3737–3755.

44. Eckel, R.H., S.M. Grundy, and P.Z. Zimmet, The metabolic syndrome. *Lancet*, 2005. **365**(9468): pp. 1415–1428.

45. Muoio, D.M. and C.B. Newgard, Mechanisms of disease:Molecular and metabolic mechanisms of insulin resistance and beta-cell failure in type 2 diabetes. *Nat Rev Mol Cell Biol*, 2008. **9**(3): pp. 193–205.

46. Nauck, M.A., et al., GLP-1 receptor agonists in the treatment of type 2 diabetes - State-of-the-art. *Mol Metab*, 2021. **46**: p. 101102.

47. Marathe, C.S., et al., The relationship between plasma GIP and GLP-1 levels in individuals with normal and impaired glucose tolerance. *Acta Diabetol*, 2020. **57**(5): pp. 583–587.

48. Gerich, J.E., Role of the kidney in normal glucose homeostasis and in the hyperglycaemia of diabetes mellitus: Therapeutic implications. *Diabet Med*, 2010. **27**(2): pp. 136–142.

49. Meyer, C., J.M. Dostou, and J.E. Gerich, Role of the human kidney in glucose counterregulation. *Diabetes*, 1999. **48**(5): pp. 943–948.

50. Rahmoune, H., et al., Glucose transporters in human renal proximal tubular cells isolated from the urine of patients with non-insulin-dependent diabetes. *Diabetes*, 2005. **54**(12): pp. 3427–3434.

51. Caban-Martinez, A.J., et al., Objective measurement of carcinogens among dominican republic firefighters using silicone-based wristbands. *J Occup Environ Med*, 2020. **62**(11): pp. e611–e615.

52. Meyer, C., et al., Abnormal renal and hepatic glucose metabolism in type 2 diabetes mellitus. *J Clin Invest*, 1998. **102**(3): pp. 619–624.

53. Brown, E., et al., SGLT2 inhibitors and GLP-1 receptor agonists: Established and emerging indications. *Lancet*, 2021. **398**(10296): pp. 262–276.

54. Cowie, M.R. and M. Fisher, SGLT2 inhibitors: Mechanisms of cardiovascular benefit beyond glycaemic control. *Nat Rev Cardiol*, 2020. **17**(12): pp. 761–772.

55. Wei, J., et al., The influence of different types of diabetes on vascular complications. *J Diabetes Res*, 2022. **2022**: p. 3448618.

56. American Diabetes Association Professional Practice Committee, 2Classification and diagnosis of diabetes: Standards of medical care in diabetes-2022. *Diabetes Care*, 2022. **45**(Suppl 1): pp. S17–S38.

57. Naik, R.G., B.M. Brooks-Worrell, and J.P. Palmer, Latent autoimmune diabetes in adults. *J Clin Endocrinol Metab*, 2009. **94**(12): pp. 4635–4644.

58. Leslie, R.D., R. Williams, and P. Pozzilli, Clinical review: Type 1 diabetes and latent autoimmune diabetes in adults: One end of the rainbow. *J Clin Endocrinol Metab*, 2006. **91**(5): pp. 1654–1659.

59. Vellanki, P. and G.E. Umpierrez, Diabetic ketoacidosis: A common debut of diabetes among African Americans with type 2 diabetes. *Endocr Pract*, 2017. **23**(8): pp. 971–978.

60. Broome, D.T., et al., Approach to the patient with MODY-monogenic diabetes. *J Clin Endocrinol Metab*, 2021. **106**(1): pp. 237–250.

61. Ahlqvist, E., R.B. Prasad, and L. Groop, Subtypes of type 2 diabetes determined from clinical parameters. *Diabetes*, 2020. **69**(10): pp. 2086–2093.

62. Banday, M.Z., A.S. Sameer, and S. Nissar, Pathophysiology of diabetes: An overview. *Avicenna J Med*, 2020. **10**(4): pp. 174–188.

63. Cudworth, A.G. and J.C. Woodrow, Letter: HL-A antigens and diabetes mellitus. *Lancet*, 1974. **2**(7889): p. 1153.

64. Tosur, M. and M.J. Redondo, Heterogeneity of type 1 diabetes: The effect of ethnicity. *Curr Diabetes Rev*, 2018. **14**(3): pp. 266–272.

65. Redondo, M.J., et al., A Type 1 diabetes genetic risk score predicts progression of islet autoimmunity and development of type 1 diabetes in individuals at risk. *Diabetes Care*, 2018. **41**(9): pp. 1887–1894.

66. Xu, P., et al., Prognostic performance of metabolic indexes in predicting onset of type 1 diabetes. *Diabetes Care*, 2010. **33**(12): pp. 2508–2513.

67. Dhatariya, K.K., et al., Diabetic ketoacidosis. *Nat Rev Dis Primers*, 2020. **6**(1): p. 40.

68. Mastromauro, C., et al., Peculiar characteristics of new-onset Type 1 Diabetes during COVID-19 pandemic. *Ital J Pediatr*, 2022. **48**(1): p. 26.

69. Ahmad, E., et al., Type 2 diabetes. *Lancet*, 2022. **400**(10365): pp. 1803–1820.

70. Reaven, G.M., The insulin resistance syndrome: Definition and dietary approaches to treatment. *Annu Rev Nutr*, 2005. **25**: pp. 391–406.

71. Samson, S.L. and A.J. Garber, Metabolic syndrome. *Endocrinol Metab Clin North Am*, 2014. **43**(1): pp. 1–23.

72. Chernausek, S.D., et al., Relationship between parental diabetes and presentation of metabolic and glycemic function in youth with Type 2 diabetes: Baseline findings from the today trial. *Diabetes Care*, 2016. **39**(1): pp. 110–117.

73. Klein, B.E., et al., Parental history of diabetes in a population-based study. *Diabetes Care*, 1996. **19**(8): pp. 827–830.

74. Vujkovic, M., et al., Discovery of 318 new risk loci for type 2 diabetes and related vascular outcomes among 1.4 million participants in a multi-ancestry meta-analysis. *Nat Genet*, 2020. **52**(7): pp. 680–691.

75. Zou, X., et al., Novel subgroups of patients with adult-onset diabetes in Chinese and US populations. *Lancet Diabetes Endocrinol*, 2019. **7**(1): pp. 9–11.

76. Kahkoska, A.R., et al., Validation of distinct type 2 diabetes clusters and their association with diabetes complications in the DEVOTE, LEADER and SUSTAIN-6 cardiovascular outcomes trials. *Diabetes Obes Metab*, 2020. **22**(9): pp. 1537–1547.

77. Gale, E.A., Latent autoimmune diabetes in adults: A guide for the perplexed. *Diabetologia*, 2005. **48**(11): pp. 2195–2199.

78. Palmer, J.P. and I.B. Hirsch, What's in a name: Latent autoimmune diabetes of adults, type 1.5, adult-onset, and type 1 diabetes. *Diabetes Care*, 2003. **26**(2): pp. 536–538.

79. Naik, R.G. and J.P. Palmer, Latent autoimmune diabetes in adults (LADA). *Rev Endocr Metab Disord*, 2003. **4**(3): pp. 233–241.

80. Fourlanos, S., et al., Latent autoimmune diabetes in adults (LADA) should be less latent. *Diabetologia*, 2005. **48**(11): pp. 2206–2212.

81. Rajkumar, V. and S.N. Levine, Latent autoimmune diabetes, in *StatPearls*, 2022, StatPearls Publishing. Copyright © 2022, StatPearls Publishing LLC.: Treasure Island (FL).

82. Fajans, S.S., G.I. Bell, and K.S. Polonsky, Molecular mechanisms and clinical pathophysiology of maturity-onset diabetes of the young. *N Engl J Med*, 2001. **345**(13): pp. 971–980.

83. Gupta, R.K., et al., The MODY1 gene HNF-4alpha regulates selected genes involved in insulin secretion. *J Clin Invest*, 2005. **115**(4): pp. 1006–1015.

84. ElSayed, N.A., et al., 2Classification and diagnosis of diabetes: Standards of care in diabetes-2023. *Diabetes Care*, 2023. **46** Supplement 1(Supplement_1): pp. S19–S40.

85. Magliano, D.J. and E.J. Boyko, *IDF Diabetes Atlas*, 2021. Brussels.

86. Bang, H., et al., Development and validation of a patient self-assessment score for diabetes risk. *Ann Intern Med*, 2009. **151**(11): pp. 775–783.

87. Saaristo, T., et al., National type 2 diabetes prevention programme in Finland: FIN-D2D. *Int J Circumpolar Health*, 2007. **66**(2): pp. 101–112.

88. Meijnikman, A.S., et al., Not performing an OGTT results in significant underdiagnosis of (pre)diabetes in a high risk adult Caucasian population. *Int J Obes (Lond)*, 2017. **41**(11): pp. 1615–1620.

89. Murray, P., G.W. Chune, and V.A. Raghavan, Legacy effects from DCCT and UKPDS: What they mean and implications for future diabetes trials. *Curr Atheroscler Rep*, 2010. **12**(6): pp. 432–439.

90. Radin, M.S., Pitfalls in hemoglobin A1c measurement: When results may be misleading. *J Gen Intern Med*, 2014. **29**(2): pp. 388–94.

91. Kang, D.S., et al., Clinical usefulness of the measurement of serum fructosamine in child-hood diabetes mellitus. *Ann Pediatr Endocrinol Metab*, 2015. **20**(1): pp. 21–26.

92. DiMeglio, L.A., C. Evans-Molina, and R.A. Oram, Type 1 diabetes. *Lancet*, 2018. **391**(10138): pp. 2449–2462.

93. ElSayed, N.A., et al., 6Glycemic targets: Standards of care in diabetes-2023. *Diabetes Care*, 2023. **46**(Supplement_1): pp. S97–S110.

94. Conlin, P.R., et al., Synopsis of the 2017 U.S. Department of Veterans Affairs/U.S. Department of Defense Clinical Practice Guideline: Management of type 2 diabetes mellitus. *Ann Intern Med*, 2017. **167**(9): pp. 655–663.

95. Knowler, W.C., et al., Reduction in the incidence of type 2 diabetes with lifestyle intervention or metformin. *N Engl J Med*, 2002. **346**(6): pp. 393–403.

96. Uusitupa, M., et al., Prevention of type 2 diabetes by lifestyle changes: A systematic review and meta-analysis. *Nutrients*, 2019. **11**(11).

97. Gill, J.M. and A.R. Cooper, Physical activity and prevention of type 2 diabetes mellitus. *Sports Med*, 2008. **38**(10): pp. 807–24.

98. He, X., et al., Diabetes self-management education reduces risk of all-cause mortality in type 2 diabetes patients: A systematic review and meta-analysis. *Endocrine*, 2017. **55**(3): pp. 712–731.

99. Davies, M.J., et al., The DESMOND educational intervention. *Chronic Illn*, 2008. **4**(1): pp. 38–40.

100. Zhao, F.F., et al., Theory-based self-management educational interventions on patients with type 2 diabetes: A systematic review and meta-analysis of randomized controlled trials. *J Adv Nurs*, 2017. **73**(4): pp. 812–833.

101. Bekele, B.B., et al., Effect of diabetes self-management education (DSME) on glycated hemo-globin (HbA1c) level among patients with T2DM: Systematic review and meta-analysis of randomized controlled trials. *Diabetes Metab Syndr*, 2021. **15**(1): pp. 177–185.

102. Azmiardi, A., et al., The effect of peer support in diabetes self-management education on glycemic control in patients with type 2 diabetes: A systematic review and meta-analysis. *Epidemiol Health*, 2021. **43**: p. e2021090.

103. Lamptey, R., et al., Structured diabetes self-management education and glycaemic control in low- and middle-income countries: A systematic review. *Diabet Med*, 2022. **39**(8): p. e14812.

104. Anderson, A., et al., Telehealth interventions to improve diabetes management among Black and hispanic patients: A systematic review and meta-analysis. *J Racial Ethn Health Disparities*, 2022. **9**(6): pp. 2375–2386.

105. Howland, C. and B. Wakefield, Assessing telehealth interventions for physical activity and sedentary behavior self-management in adults with type 2 diabetes mellitus: An integrative review. *Res Nurs Health*, 2021. **44**(1): pp. 92–110.

106. Cunningham, A.T., et al., The effect of diabetes self-management education on HbA1c and quality of life in African-Americans: A systematic review and meta-analysis. *BMC Health Serv Res*, 2018. **18**(1): p. 367.

107. Tamhane, S., et al., Shared decision-making in diabetes care. *Curr Diab Rep*, 2015. **15**(12): p. 112.

108. Stone, R.A., et al., Active care management supported by home telemonitoring in veterans with type 2 diabetes: The DiaTel randomized controlled trial. *Diabetes Care*, 2010. **33**(3): pp. 478–484.

109. Norris, S.L., et al., Increasing diabetes self-management education in community settings. A systematic review. *Am J Prev Med*, 2002. **22**(4 Suppl): pp. 39–66.

110. Arnold, S.V., et al., Burden of cardio-renal-metabolic conditions in adults with type 2 diabetes within the diabetes collaborative registry. *Diabetes Obes Metab*, 2018. **20**(8): pp. 2000–2003.

111. Thomas, M.C., M.E. Cooper, and P. Zimmet, Changing epidemiology of type 2 diabetes mellitus and associated chronic kidney disease. *Nat Rev Nephrol*, 2016. **12**(2): pp. 73–81.

112. Glassock, R.J., Referrals for chronic kidney disease: Real problem or nuisance? *JAMA*, 2010. **303**(12): pp. 1201–1203.

113. Umanath, K. and J.B. Lewis, Update on diabetic nephropathy: Core curriculum 2018. *Am J Kidney Dis*, 2018. **71**(6): pp. 884–895.

114. Brenner, B.M., et al., Effects of losartan on renal and cardiovascular outcomes in patients with type 2 diabetes and nephropathy. *N Engl J Med*, 2001. **345**(12): pp. 861–869.

115. Abbott, K.C. and G.L. Bakris, What have we learned from the current trials? *Med Clin North Am*, 2004. **88**(1): pp. 189–207.

116. Palmer, S.C., et al., Sodium-glucose cotransporter protein-2 (SGLT-2) inhibitors and glucagon-like peptide-1 (GLP-1) receptor agonists for type 2 diabetes: Systematic review and network meta-analysis of randomised controlled trials. *BMJ*, 2021. **372**: p. m4573.

117. Fried, L.F., et al., Combined angiotensin inhibition for the treatment of diabetic nephropathy. *N Engl J Med*, 2013. **369**(20): pp. 1892–903.

118. Rutkowski, B. and L. Tylicki, Nephroprotective action of renin-angiotensin-aldosterone system blockade in chronic kidney disease patients: The landscape after ALTITUDE and VA NEPHRON-D trails. *J Ren Nutr*, 2015. **25**(2): pp. 194–200.

119. Duckworth, W., et al., Glucose control and vascular complications in veterans with type 2 diabetes. *N Engl J Med*, 2009. **360**(2): pp. 129–139.

120. Diabetes, C., et al., The effect of intensive treatment of diabetes on the development and progression of long-term complications in insulin-dependent diabetes mellitus. *N Engl J Med*, 1993. **329**(14): pp. 977–986.

121. Kussman, M.J., H. Goldstein, and R.E. Gleason, The clinical course of diabetic nephropathy. *JAMA*, 1976. **236**(16): pp. 1861–1863.

122. Karlsen, B., B. Oftedal, and E. Bru, The relationship between clinical indicators, coping styles, perceived support and diabetes-related distress among adults with type 2 diabetes. *J Adv Nurs*, 2012. **68**(2): pp. 391–401.

123. Sakraida, T.J. and M.V. Robinson, Mental health and relational self-management experiences of patients with type 2 diabetes and stage 3 chronic kidney disease. *Issues Ment Health Nurs*, 2012. **33**(11): pp. 786–796.

124. Griva, K., et al., Improving outcomes in patients with coexisting multimorbid conditions-the development and evaluation of the combined diabetes and renal control trial (C-DIRECT): Study protocol. *BMJ Open*, 2015. **5**(2): p. e007253.

125. Callaghan, B.C., et al., The importance of rare subtypes in diagnosis and treatment of peripheral neuropathy: A review. *JAMA Neurol*, 2015. **72**(12): pp. 1510–1518.

126. Feldman, E.L., et al., Diabetic neuropathy. *Nat Rev Dis Primers*, 2019. **5**(1): p. 41.

127. Rojas-Carranza, C.A., et al., Diabetes-Related neurological implications and pharmacogenomics. *Curr Pharm Des*, 2018. **24**(15): pp. 1695–1710.

128. American Diabetes Association Professional Practice, C., 12. *Retinopathy, Neuropathy, and Foot Care: Standards of Medical Care in Diabetes*-2022. *Diabetes Care*, 2022. **45**(Suppl 1): pp. S185–S194.

129. Boulton, A.J., Diabetic neuropathy and foot complications. *Handb Clin Neurol*, 2014. **126**: pp. 97–107.

130. Markakis, K., F.L. Bowling, and A.J. Boulton, The diabetic foot in 2015: An overview. *Diabetes Metab Res Rev*, 2016. **32** Suppl 1: pp. 169–178.

131. Singh, N., D.G. Armstrong, and B.A. Lipsky, Preventing foot ulcers in patients with diabetes. *JAMA*, 2005. **293**(2): pp. 217–228.

132. Finnerup, N.B., et al., Pharmacotherapy for neuropathic pain in adults: A systematic review and meta-analysis. *Lancet Neurol*, 2015. **14**(2): pp. 162–173.

133. Raskin, J., et al., Duloxetine versus routine care in the long-term management of diabetic peripheral neuropathic pain. *J Palliat Med*, 2006. **9**(1): pp. 29–40.

134. Finnerup, N.B., R. Kuner, and T.S. Jensen, Neuropathic pain: From mechanisms to treatment. *Physiol Rev*, 2021. **101**(1): pp. 259–301.

135. Teo, Z.L., et al., Global prevalence of diabetic retinopathy and projection of burden through 2045: Systematic review and meta-analysis. *Ophthalmology*, 2021. **128**(11): pp. 1580–1591.

136. Blindness, G.B.D., C. Vision Impairment, and S. Vision Loss Expert Group of the Global Burden of Disease, Causes of blindness and vision impairment in 2020 and trends over 30 years, and prevalence of avoidable blindness in relation to VISION 2020: the Right to Sight: an analysis for the Global Burden of Disease Study. *Lancet Glob Health*, 2021. **9**(2): pp. e144–e160.

137. Wang, W. and A.C.Y. Lo, Diabetic retinopathy: Pathophysiology and treatments. *Int J Mol Sci*, 2018. **19**(6): p. 1816.

138. Malone, J.I., et al., Retinopathy during the first 5 years of type 1 diabetes and subsequent risk of advanced retinopathy. *Diabetes Care*, 2022.

139. Uludag, G., et al., Efficacy and safety of intravitreal anti-VEGF therapy in diabetic retinopathy: What we have learned and what should we learn further? *Expert Opin Biol Ther*, 2022. **22**(10): pp. 1275–1291.

140. Wells, J.A., et al., Aflibercept, bevacizumab, or ranibizumab for diabetic macular edema: Two-Year results from a comparative effectiveness randomized clinical trial. *Ophthalmology*, 2016. **123**(6): pp. 1351–1359.

141. Wells, J.A., et al., Association of baseline visual acuity and retinal thickness with 1-year efficacy of aflibercept, bevacizumab, and ranibizumab for diabetic macular edema. *JAMA Ophthalmol*, 2016. **134**(2): pp. 127–134.

142. Al Qassimi, N., et al., Management of diabetic macular edema: Guidelines from the emirates society of ophthalmology. *Ophthalmol Ther*, 2022. **11**(5): pp. 1937–1950.

143. Joseph, J.J., et al., Comprehensive management of cardiovascular risk factors for adults with type 2 diabetes: A scientific statement from the American Heart Association. *Circulation*, 2022. **145**(9): pp. e722–e759.

144. Domingueti, C.P., et al., Diabetes mellitus: The linkage between oxidative stress, inflammation, hypercoagulability and vascular complications. *J Diabetes Complications*, 2016. **30**(4): pp. 738–745.

145. Gomadam, P., et al., Blood pressure indices and cardiovascular disease mortality in persons with or without diabetes mellitus. *J Hypertens*, 2018. **36**(1): pp. 85–92.

146. Li, W., et al., Incidence and long-term specific mortality trends of metabolic syndrome in the United States. *Front Endocrinol (Lausanne)*, 2022. **13**: p. 1029736.

147. ElSayed, N.A., et al., 10Cardiovascular disease and risk management: Standards of care in diabetes-2023. *Diabetes Care*, 2023. **46**(Supplement_1): pp. S158–S190.

148. Arnett, D.K., et al., 2019 ACC/AHA guideline on the primary prevention of cardiovascular disease: Executive summary: A report of the American College of Cardiology/American Heart Association Task Force on clinical practice guidelines. *Circulation*, 2019. **140**(11): pp. e563–e595.

149. Look, A.R.G., et al., Cardiovascular effects of intensive lifestyle intervention in type 2 diabetes. *N Engl J Med*, 2013. **369**(2): pp. 145–54.

150. Wing, R.R. and A.R.G. Look, Does lifestyle intervention improve health of adults with overweight/obesity and type 2 diabetes? Findings from the look AHEAD randomized trial. *Obesity (Silver Spring)*, 2021. **29**(8): pp. 1246–1258.

151. Walicka, M., et al., Impact of stopping smoking on metabolic parameters in diabetes mellitus: A scoping review. *World J Diabetes*, 2022. **13**(6): pp. 422–433.

152. Liu, G., et al., Smoking cessation and weight change in relation to cardiovascular disease incidence and mortality in people with type 2 diabetes: A population-based cohort study. *Lancet Diabetes Endocrinol*, 2020. **8**(2): pp. 125–133.

153. Lean, M.E., et al., Primary care-led weight management for remission of type 2 diabetes (DiRECT): An open-label, cluster-randomised trial. *Lancet*, 2018. **391**(10120): pp. 541–551.

154. Taheri, S., et al., Effect of intensive lifestyle intervention on bodyweight and glycaemia in early type 2 diabetes (DIADEM-I): An open-label, parallel-group, randomised controlled trial. *Lancet Diabetes Endocrinol*, 2020. **8**(6): pp. 477–489.

155. Zaghloul, H., et al., Clinical and metabolic characteristics of the Diabetes Intervention Accentuating Diet and Enhancing Metabolism (DIADEM-I) randomised clinical trial cohort. *BMJ Open*, 2020. **10**(12): p. e041386.

156. Martinez-Gonzalez, M.A., et al., Benefits of the Mediterranean diet: Insights from the PREDIMED Study. *Prog Cardiovasc Dis*, 2015. **58**(1): pp. 50–60.

157. Zurbau, A., et al., Relation of different fruit and vegetable sources with incident cardiovascular outcomes: A systematic review and meta-analysis of prospective cohort studies. *J Am Heart Assoc*, 2020. **9**(19): p. e017728.

158. Filippou, C., et al., Overview of salt restriction in the Dietary Approaches to Stop Hypertension (DASH) and the Mediterranean diet for blood pressure reduction. *Rev Cardiovasc Med*, 2022. **23**(1): p. 36.

159. de Boer, I.H., et al., Diabetes and hypertension: A position statement by the American diabetes association. *Diabetes Care*, 2017. **40**(9): pp. 1273–1284.

160. Zhang, W., et al., Trial of intensive blood-pressure control in older patients with hypertension. *N Engl J Med*, 2021. **385**(14): pp. 1268–1279.

161. Group, S.R., et al., A randomized trial of intensive versus standard blood-pressure control. *N Engl J Med*, 2015. **373**(22): pp. 2103–2116.

162. Patel, A., et al., Effects of a fixed combination of perindopril and indapamide on macrovascular and microvascular outcomes in patients with type 2 diabetes mellitus (the ADVANCE trial): A randomised controlled trial. *Lancet*, 2007. **370**(9590): pp. 829–840.

163. Villa-Zapata, L., et al., Serum potassium changes due to concomitant ACEI/ARB and spironolactone therapy: A systematic review and meta-analysis. *Am J Health Syst Pharm*, 2021. **78**(24): pp. 2245–2255.

164. Colhoun, H.M., et al., Primary prevention of cardiovascular disease with atorvastatin in type 2 diabetes in the Collaborative Atorvastatin Diabetes Study (CARDS): Multicentre randomised placebo-controlled trial. *Lancet*, 2004. **364**(9435): pp. 685–696.

165. Almourani, R., et al., Diabetes and cardiovascular disease: An update. *Curr Diab Rep*, 2019. **19**(12): p. 161.

166. Elam, M.B., et al., Association of fenofibrate therapy with long-term cardiovascular risk in statin-treated patients with type 2 diabetes. *JAMA Cardiol*, 2017. **2**(4): pp. 370–380.

167. Bhatt, D.L., et al., REDUCE-IT USA: Results from the 3146 patients randomized in the United States. *Circulation*, 2020. **141**(5): pp. 367–375.

168. Bhatt, D.L., et al., Cardiovascular risk reduction with icosapent ethyl for hypertriglyceridemia. *N Engl J Med*, 2019. **380**(1): pp. 11–22.

169. Ferguson, D. and B.N. Finck, Emerging therapeutic approaches for the treatment of NAFLD and type 2 diabetes mellitus. *Nat Rev Endocrinol*, 2021. **17**(8): pp. 484–495.

170. Tanase, D.M., et al., The intricate relationship between Type 2 Diabetes Mellitus (T2DM), Insulin Resistance (IR), and Nonalcoholic Fatty Liver Disease (NAFLD). *J Diabetes Res*, 2020. **2020**: p. 3920196.

171. Ranjbar, G., D.P. Mikhailidis, and A. Sahebkar, Effects of newer antidiabetic drugs on nonalcoholic fatty liver and steatohepatitis: Think out of the box! *Metabolism*, 2019. **101**: p. 154001.

172. Younossi, Z.M., et al., The global epidemiology of NAFLD and NASH in patients with type 2 diabetes: A systematic review and meta-analysis. *J Hepatol*, 2019. **71**(4): pp. 793–801.

173. Lomonaco, R., et al., Advanced liver fibrosis is common in patients with type 2 diabetes followed in the outpatient setting: The need for systematic screening. *Diabetes Care*, 2021. **44**(2): pp. 399–406.

174. Budd, J. and K. Cusi, Role of agents for the treatment of diabetes in the management of nonalcoholic fatty liver disease. *Curr Diab Rep*, 2020. **20**(11): p. 59.

175. Bjorkstrom, K., et al., Risk factors for severe liver disease in patients with type 2 diabetes. *Clin Gastroenterol Hepatol*, 2019. **17**(13): pp. 2769–2775 e4.

176. Handelsman, Y., et al., Early intervention and intensive management of patients with diabetes, cardiorenal, and metabolic diseases. *J Diabetes Complications*, 2023. **37**(2): p. 108389.

177. American Diabetes Association Professional Practice, C., 4Comprehensive medical evaluation and assessment of comorbidities: Standards of medical care in diabetes-2022. *Diabetes Care*, 2022. **45**(Suppl 1): pp. S46–S59.

178. Lee, J., et al., Prognostic accuracy of FIB-4, NAFLD fibrosis score and APRI for NAFLD-related events: A systematic review. *Liver Int*, 2021. **41**(2): pp. 261–270.

179. Doumas, M., et al., The role of statins in the management of nonalcoholic fatty liver disease. *Curr Pharm Des*, 2018. **24**(38): pp. 4587–4592.

180. Athyros, V.G., et al., Statins: An under-appreciated asset for the prevention and the treatment of NAFLD or NASH and the related cardiovascular risk. *Curr Vasc Pharmacol*, 2018. **16**(3): pp. 246–253.

181. Itani, T. and T. Ishihara, *Efficacy of canagliflozin against nonalcoholic fatty liver disease: a prospective cohort study. Obes Sci Pract*, 2018. **4**(5): pp. 477–482.

182. Group, A.S.C., et al., Effects of aspirin for primary prevention in persons with diabetes mellitus. *N Engl J Med*, 2018. **379**(16): pp. 1529–1539.

183. Force, U.S.P.S.T., et al., Aspirin use to prevent cardiovascular disease: US preventive services task force recommendation statement. *JAMA*, 2022. **327**(16): pp. 1577–1584.

184. van Eersel, M.E., et al., The interaction of age and type 2 diabetes on executive function and memory in persons aged 35 years or older. *PLoS One*, 2013. **8**(12): p. e82991.

185. Biessels, G.J., et al., Risk of dementia in diabetes mellitus: A systematic review. *Lancet Neurol*, 2006. **5**(1): pp. 64–74.

186. Cukierman, T., H.C. Gerstein, and J.D. Williamson, Cognitive decline and dementia in diabetes--Systematic overview of prospective observational studies. *Diabetologia*, 2005. **48**(12): pp. 2460–2469.

187. Mayeda, E.R., et al., Type 2 diabetes and 10-year risk of dementia and cognitive impairment among older Mexican Americans. *Diabetes Care*, 2013. **36**(9): pp. 2600–2606.

188. Gorniak, S.L., et al., Cognitive-motor impairment in manual tasks in adults with type 2 diabetes. *OTJR (Thorofare N J)*, 2020. **40**(2): pp. 113–121.

189. Gudala, K., et al., Diabetes mellitus and risk of dementia: A meta-analysis of prospective observational studies. *J Diabetes Investig*, 2013. **4**(6): pp. 640–650.

190. Mallorqui-Bague, N., et al., Type 2 diabetes and cognitive impairment in an older population with overweight or obesity and metabolic syndrome: Baseline cross-sectional analysis of the PREDIMED-plus study. *Sci Rep*, 2018. **8**(1): p. 16128.

191. Geijselaers, S.L.C., et al., The role of hyperglycemia, insulin resistance, and blood pressure in diabetes-associated differences in cognitive performance-the Maastricht study. *Diabetes Care*, 2017. **40**(11): pp. 1537–1547.

192. Albai, O., et al., Risk factors for developing dementia in type 2 diabetes mellitus patients with mild cognitive impairment. *Neuropsychiatric Diseases and Treatment*, 2019. **15**: pp. 167–175.

193. Feinkohl, I., et al., Cardiovascular risk factors and cognitive decline in older people with type 2 diabetes. *Diabetologia*, 2015. **58**(7): pp. 1637–1645.

194. Christman, A.L., et al., Glycated haemoglobin and cognitive decline: The Atherosclerosis Risk in Communities (ARIC) study. *Diabetologia*, 2011. **54**(7): pp. 1645–1652.

195. Sircar, M., A. Bhatia, and M. Munshi, Review of hypoglycemia in the older adult: Clinical implications and management. *Can J Diabetes*, 2016. **40**(1): pp. 66–72.

196. Feinkohl, I., et al., Severe hypoglycemia and cognitive decline in older people with type 2 diabetes: The Edinburgh type 2 diabetes study. *Diabetes Care*, 2014. **37**(2): pp. 507–515.

197. Lacy, M.E., et al., Comparison of cognitive function in older adults with type 1 diabetes, type 2 diabetes, and no diabetes: Results from the Study of Longevity in Diabetes (SOLID). *BMJ Open Diabetes Res Care*, 2022. **10**(2): p. e002557.

198. Callisaya, M.L., et al., Type 2 diabetes mellitus, brain atrophy and cognitive decline in older people: A longitudinal study. *Diabetologia*, 2019. **62**(3): pp. 448–458.

199. Tan, V., C. Chen, and R.A. Merchant, Association of social determinants of health with frailty, cognitive impairment, and self-rated health among older adults. *PLoS One*, 2022. **17**(11): p. e0277290.

200. Xu, W., et al., Cognitive impairment and related factors among middle-aged and elderly patients with type 2 diabetes from a bio-psycho-social perspective. *Diabetes Metab Syndr Obes*, 2021. **14**: pp. 4361–4369.

201. Yerrapragada, D.B., et al., Cognitive dysfunction among adults with type 2 diabetes mellitus in Karnataka, India. *Ochsner J*, 2019. **19**(3): pp. 227–234.

202. Hughes, D., et al., Association of blood pressure lowering with incident dementia or cognitive impairment: A systematic review and meta-analysis. *JAMA*, 2020. **323**(19): pp. 1934–1944.

203. Skinner, J.S., et al., Associations between markers of glucose and insulin function and cognitive function in healthy African American elders. *J Gerontol Geriatr Res*, 2015. **4**(4): p. 23.

204. Zhang, Z., et al., Olfactory dysfunction mediates adiposity in cognitive impairment of type 2 diabetes: insights from clinical and functional neuroimaging studies. *Diabetes Care*, 2019. **42**(7): pp. 1274–1283.

205. Sun, L., et al., Risk factors for cognitive impairment in patients with type 2 diabetes. *J Diabetes Res*, 2020. **2020**: p. 4591938.

206. Samaras, K., et al., Metformin use is associated with slowed cognitive decline and reduced incident dementia in older adults with type 2 diabetes: The Sydney memory and ageing study. *Diabetes Care*, 2020. **43**(11): pp. 2691–2701.

207. Kim, M.J. and C. Fritschi, Relationships between cognitive impairment and self-management in older adults with type 2 diabetes: An integrative review. *Res Gerontol Nurs*, 2021. **14**(2): pp. 104–112.

208. American Diabetes Association Professional Practice Committee, 3Prevention or delay of type 2 diabetes and associated comorbidities: Standards of medical care in diabetes-2022. *Diabetes Care*, 2022. **45**(Suppl 1): pp. S39–S45.

209. Owens-Gary, M.D., et al., The importance of addressing depression and diabetes distress in adults with type 2 diabetes. *J Gen Intern Med*, 2019. **34**(2): pp. 320–324.

210. Perrin, N.E., et al., The prevalence of diabetes-specific emotional distress in people with Type 2 diabetes: A systematic review and meta-analysis. *Diabet Med*, 2017. **34**(11): pp. 1508–1520.

211. Albertorio-Diaz, J.R., et al., Depressive states among adults with diabetes: Findings from the national health and nutrition examination survey, 2007–2012. *Diabetes Res Clin Pract*, 2017. **127**: pp. 80–88.

212. Zhang, X., et al., Depressive symptoms and mortality among persons with and without diabetes. *Am J Epidemiol*, 2005. **161**(7): pp. 652–660.

213. Kroenke, K., R.L. Spitzer, and J.B. Williams, The PHQ-9: Validity of a brief depression severity measure. *J Gen Intern Med*, 2001. **16**(9): pp. 606–613.

214. Siu, A.L., et al., Screening for depression in adults: US preventive services task force recommendation statement. *JAMA*, 2016. **315**(4): pp. 380–387.

215. Schmitt, A., et al., How to assess diabetes distress: Comparison of the Problem Areas in Diabetes Scale (PAID) and the Diabetes Distress Scale (DDS). *Diabet Med*, 2016. **33**(6): pp. 835–843.

216. Zagarins, S.E., et al., Improvement in glycemic control following a diabetes education intervention is associated with change in diabetes distress but not change in depressive symptoms. *J Behav Med*, 2012. **35**(3): pp. 299–304.

9 Lipids and Lipoprotein Metabolism, Dyslipidemias, and Management

Emmanuel Kwaku Ofori

9.1 INTRODUCTION

Lipids are a diverse group of organic compounds that are insoluble in water and soluble in organic solvents, consisting of fatty acids, monoacylglycerols, diacylglycerols, triglycerides, phospholipids, eicosanoids, resolvins, docosanoids, sterols, sterol esters, carotenoids, vitamins A and E, fatty alcohols, hydrocarbons, and wax esters [1, 2]. The storage of energy, their contribution to membrane structure, and signal transduction are among lipids' primary biological roles. Animals rely heavily on lipids, which play an important role in regulating body temperature and serve as the principal energy reserve. They are also essential components of cell membranes and play a role in controlling how molecules enter and leave cells [3]. Lipoproteins are complexes of lipids and proteins that are required for the transport of dietary lipids and endogenously synthesized lipids as well as fat-soluble vitamins in the body. A disruption in the normal control of lipid production has been linked to the development of several metabolic disorders, including obesity, type 2 diabetes, and cardiovascular disease [4]. Lipoprotein metabolism disorders can be either primary (caused by genetic problems) or secondary (induced by other medical conditions or environmental exposures), and they entail either a considerable rise or decrease in certain circulating lipids or lipoproteins.

9.2 FATTY ACIDS

The class of lipids known as fatty acids is comprised of a wide range of molecules. These molecules are distinguished by a series of hydrocarbon groups that are repeated, which is what gives them their hydrophobic quality. These compounds are one of the most fundamental groups of biological lipids since they serve as the primary lipid building blocks that are used in the construction of more complicated lipids [5, 6]. Eicosanoids, fatty alcohols, aldehydes, esters, fatty amides, fatty nitriles, fatty ethers, and hydrocarbons are all examples of this lipid class. Many of the members of this category, in particular the eicosanoids that are produced from polyunsaturated fatty acids (PUFAs), display distinctive biological functions [7]. In the discipline of lipid biochemistry, the study of fatty acids is an essential topic of research due to the diversity and relevance of fatty acids. In addition to being crucial constituents of cellular membranes, fatty acids serve essential functions in the transmission of signals inside cells, the storage of energy, and the control of gene expression [8]. The majority of the other types of lipids are composed of fatty acids that have been esterified. They can be converted into triglycerides by being esterified with glycerol. Either free or linked to albumin, they can be transported through the blood. Fatty acids are the most readily available source of lipid energy, and they supply the body with the fuel it needs to function properly [2]. In addition to this, they serve as the substrate for the production of ketone bodies [9]. Certain fatty acids, such as omega-3 polyunsaturated fatty acids, have been associated with anti-inflammatory effects, and they may offer protection against chronic diseases such as cancer and cardiovascular disease [10]. The fatty acid composition of cell membranes can affect the fluidity and permeability of the membranes, which can in turn affect cellular functions such as transport and receptor signaling. Additional research into the activities and interactions of the various types of fatty acids has the potential to shed light on cellular and physiological processes and could lead to the development of new therapeutic methods for a wide range of disorders.

9.3 GLYCEROLIPIDS

Glycerolipids are a category of lipids that are characterized by the presence of glycerol. The most well-known types of glycerolipids are acylglycerols, which can be broken down into mono-, di-, and triacylglycerols [11]. Triacylglycerols, often known as triglycerides (TGs), are the most common type of glycerolipid and are responsible for the majority of lipids found in seed oils, as well as the majority of the storage fat found in animal tissues [12]. The TGs are numbered in a Fischer projection according to their stereochemical configuration, which places the secondary hydroxyl group to the left of the central prochiral carbon atom. Because sn-2 helps ease the body's absorption of fatty acids in the form of 2-monoacyl-sn-glycerols, the composition of the sn-2 position in TGs is of the utmost significance for the field of nutrition [13]. In seed oils, polyunsaturated fatty acids, also known as PUFAs, are mostly enriched in the sn-2 position, whereas saturated fatty acids,

DOI: 10.1201/9781003384823-9

especially dietary animal fats, are concentrated in the sn-1 and sn-3 positions [14]. Triglycerides, which are major components of very low-density lipoprotein (VLDL) and chylomicrons, play a crucial role in metabolism as energy sources and transporters of dietary fat. Triglycerides also make up a large portion of chylomicrons. They have more than twice the amount of energy per gram than carbs and proteins combined (9 kcal/g). During the process known as lipolysis, which occurs in the intestine, triglycerides are broken down into glycerol and fatty acids with the assistance of lipases and bile secretions. These components are then transported into the cells that line the intestines, which are known as absorptive enterocytes [15].

The chylomicrons are formed when triglycerides are reassembled in the enterocytes from the fragments that remain of them, and then they are bundled with cholesterol and proteins. These are released from the cells, collected by the lymph system, and then carried to the major vessels located close to the heart before being re-mixed with the blood. The chylomicrons can be taken up by a variety of tissues, which then allows the triglycerides to be released and used as a source of energy. Triglycerides can be synthesized and stored in fat cells, as well as liver cells. When the body needs fatty acids as a source of energy, the hormone glucagon sends a signal to the hormone-sensitive lipase that causes the triglycerides to be broken down, which then releases free fatty acids [16]. When triglycerides are broken down, the glycerol component can be turned into glucose for use as brain fuel through a process called gluconeogenesis. This is necessary because the brain is unable to use fatty acids as a source of energy. Triglycerides are unable to freely move through the membranes of cells. Lipoprotein lipases, which are enzymes found on the walls of blood vessels, are responsible for breaking down triglycerides into fatty acids and glycerol [17]. After this process, fatty acids can be taken up by cells using the fatty acid transporter. When it comes to the regulation of metabolism and the formulation of dietary plans for the prevention and treatment of chronic diseases, having a better understanding of the biochemical and physiological roles that glycerolipids play can provide valuable insights.

9.4 GLYCEROPHOSPHOLIPIDS

Glycerophospholipids, which are often referred to as phospholipids (PLs), are an essential component of cell membranes and can be found in a wide variety of foods, as well as oils that have been derived from plants [18]. The type of the polar head group located at the sn-3 position of the glycerol backbone in eukaryotes and prokaryotes, or the sn-1 position in the case of archaebacteria, can be used to further divide these PLs into separate groups [19]. Phosphatidylcholine, phosphatidylethanolamine, and phosphatidylserine are a few examples of the types of glycerophospholipids that can be found in biological membranes [20]. In most cases, the saturated fatty acid, also known as SFA, will be esterified at position 1, whereas the polyunsaturated fatty acid, also known as PUFA, will be esterified at position 2. The PL molecule has a hydrophilic region that is provided by the polar group, which is located at position 3. Position 3 also contains phosphorus and the nitrogenous base or sugar molecule. Some glycerophospholipids in eukaryotic cells, such as phosphatidic acids, are either precursors to or are themselves membrane-derived second messengers [21]. In addition to their role as a major component of cellular membranes and as binding sites for intracellular and intercellular proteins, these glycerophospholipids serve as a primary component of cellular membranes [22]. Important lipid groups including phospholipids and sphingolipids are also synthesized de novo in the body, along with fatty acids and cholesterol. For instance, glycerol-3-phosphate and fatty acids are used to produce phospholipids, while serine and palmitoyl-CoA are required to produce sphingolipids [23].

9.5 SPHINGOLIPIDS

Sphingolipids are a diverse group of substances with a sphingoid base backbone as their unifying structural characteristic. Serine and a long-chain fatty acyl-coenzyme A (CoA) are used to create this backbone from scratch, after which it is transformed into a variety of species, including ceramides, phosphosphingolipids, glycosphingolipids, and others [23, 24]. Sphingosine is the type of sphingoid base that is found most frequently in mammals. A prominent subclass of sphingoid base derivatives, ceramides are characterized by the presence of an amide-linked fatty acid chain. Saturated fatty acids (SFAs) and monounsaturated fatty acids (MUFAs) with chain lengths ranging from 14 to 26 carbon atoms are the types of fatty acids that are typically found in ceramides [25]. The majority of the phosphosphingolipids found in mammals are called sphingomyelins, and they are ceramide phosphocholines. Glycosphingolipids are a varied family of compounds that are made up of one or more sugar residues that are attached to the sphingoid base through the formation of a glycosidic bond [26]. Cerebrosides, gangliosides, and sulfo-glycosphingolipids (sulfatides) are all types of glycosphingolipids that are found in abundance in myelin [27].

9.6 STEROL LIPIDS

Sterols are a class of lipids that all have the same basic structure, which consists of a four-ring core that has been fused, in addition to a hydrocarbon side chain and an alcohol group. Animal fats and the majority of vegetable oils both contain sterols, either in their free form or esterified to other molecules such as fatty acids, glycosides, or ferulic acid. Cholesterol is the most common type of sterol that may be found in animal fats. It is also an essential component of membrane lipids [4, 28]. Cholesterol is essential for the construction and upkeep of cell membranes, and it controls the fluidity of membranes across a wide temperature range. The bulky steroid and the hydrocarbon chain are both embedded in the membrane, whereas the hydroxyl group on cholesterol interacts with the phosphate head of the membrane [29]. In addition to having antioxidant properties, cholesterol is an essential component in the breakdown of fat-soluble vitamins. It also plays a crucial role in the production of bile, which aids in the digestion of fats. It is the primary precursor in the production of numerous steroid hormones (which include the stress hormones cortisol and aldosterone, produced by the adrenal glands, as well as the sex hormones progesterone, the various estrogens, testosterone, and derivatives) [30]. The majority of cholesterol is produced by the body itself, while the remaining small amount comes from the foods we eat. The liver, the spinal cord, and the brain are some examples of tissues that have a high concentration of cholesterol because they either produce more cholesterol or have more abundant tightly packed membranes. Cholesterol is insoluble in blood, and thus, is carried through the circulatory system attached to one of the many different types of lipoprotein. Low-density lipoprotein (LDL) and high-density lipoprotein (HDL), the two primary kinds, are responsible for transporting cholesterol away from and back to the liver. According to the lipid hypothesis, hypercholesterolemia, which refers to unusually high cholesterol levels, and aberrant proportions of LDL and HDL are linked to cardiovascular disease because they promote the development of atheroma in the arteries. Myocardial infarction, stroke, and peripheral vascular disease are all outcomes of this disease process [31]. The term "bad cholesterol" refers to high levels of LDL since it plays a role in this process. On the other hand, high levels of HDL, sometimes known as "good cholesterol", offer some degree of protection. The equilibrium can be restored by engaging in physical activity, maintaining a balanced diet, and, in rare cases, taking medicine. Normal cellular activity in mammalian cells requires cholesterol to be present in the cell membrane. Endocytosis that is mediated by LDL receptors is responsible for the entry of cholesterol into the cell [32]. In most cells and tissues, cholesterol is produced from acetyl CoA via the HMG-CoA reductase route (Figure 9.1). The cholesterol levels that are already present within the body have a direct impact on the synthesis of cholesterol; however, the homeostatic processes that are at play in this process are still partially known. A lower intake of food has the reverse impact, meaning that a greater intake of food results in a net drop in endogenous production, whereas a higher intake of food has the opposite effect.

In recent years, cholesterol has also been shown to have a role in the processes that control cell signaling. The Sterol Regulatory Element Binding Protein (SREBP) 1 and 2 are responsible for the primary regulatory mechanism, which is the sensing of intracellular cholesterol in the endoplasmic reticulum [33]. SREBP can bind to two additional proteins when cholesterol is present. These other proteins are known as SREBP-cleavage activating protein (SCAP) and Insig1. In the Golgi apparatus, SREBP is cleaved by S1P and S2P (site 1/2 protease). After being cleaved, SREBP travels to the nucleus, where it assumes the role of a transcription factor by binding to the sterol regulatory element (SRE) of many genes and thereby stimulating the transcription of those genes. The LDL receptor and the HMG-CoA reductase genes are both transcribed during this process. The former removes circulating LDL from the bloodstream, whereas the latter causes an increase in the body's natural production of cholesterol [34, 35]. The sterols that come from plants are known as phytosterols, and the nature and quantity of phytosterols might change depending on the source of the oil. Steroids, which share the same four-ring core structure as sterols, are also regarded to be a class of sterol lipids according to their composition. Steroids with a carbon number of 18 belong to the estrogen family. Steroids with a carbon number of 19 belong to the androgen family and include testosterone and androsterone. Progestogens, in addition to glucocorticoids and mineralocorticoids, are included in the C21 category of hormones. Cleavage of the B ring in the core structure is a distinguishing feature of secosteroids, like the various forms of vitamin D. Other types

De novo Synthesis: Cholesterol

Acetyl CoA
↓
HMG CoA

HMG CoA Reductase |— Statins
(HMG CoA Inhibitor)
↓
Mevalonate
↓
Squalene
↓
Cholesterol

Bile acids   Steroids   Vitamin D

| Precursor for bile acid & steroid synthesis | Major component of cell membrane | Required for nerve transmission | Precursor for vitamin D synthesis |

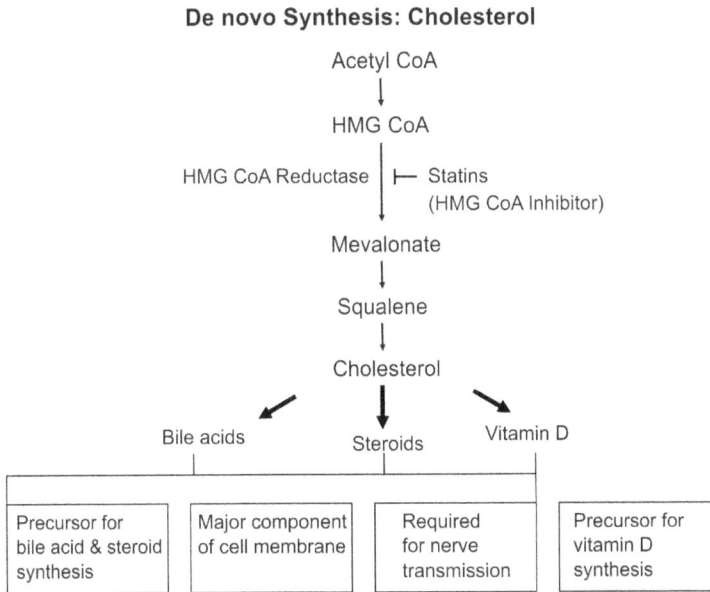

Figure 9.1 De novo synthesis of cholesterol

of sterols include bile acids and the conjugates that are created from them by the body's synthesis process [36, 37].

9.7 PRENOL LIPIDS

Prenol lipids are a type of lipid group that can be produced by synthesizing isopentenyl diphosphate and dimethylallyl diphosphate, both of which contain five carbon atoms as their precursors [7]. Linear alcohols, diphosphates, and other molecules can be included in the category of prenol lipids. These compounds are generated via the serial addition of C5 units. Structures that have 40 carbon atoms or more are referred to as polyterpenes, and they are categorized according to the number of terpene units that they contain. Carotenoids, quinones, hydroquinones, vitamins E and K, and ubiquinones are all examples of prenol lipids. From a mixture of lipid-soluble phenols, vitamin E is the most important lipid group in the prenol lipid category from a nutritional point of view. It is distinguished by an aromatic chromanol head and a side chain that contains 16 carbon atoms [38]. Tocopherols and tocotrienols, both types of vitamin E, come in a set of four isomers: α-, β-, γ-, and δ-tocopherol and tocotrienols. Tocopherols' primary biological role is to prevent the oxidation of polyunsaturated fatty acids (PUFAs). Tocotrienols have a low level of vitamin E activity, yet they function as antioxidants in meals and give stability by preventing oxidation. Tocopherols can be found in fish, nuts and seeds, green leafy vegetables, and vegetable oils, while tocotrienols are abundant in palm oil and rice bran oil. Tocopherols can also be found in rice bran oil and palm oil [39, 40].

9.8 SACCHAROLIPIDS

Those lipids known as saccharolipids have a sugar molecule incorporated into their structure. Saccharolipids have their fatty acids directly attached to a sugar backbone, which is what makes them compatible with the bilayers of membranes. This is not the same as glycerolipids or glycerophospholipids, both of which include a glycerol backbone in their structure. The acylated glucosamine precursors of the lipid A component of the lipopolysaccharides in gram-negative bacteria are the saccharolipids that are the most well known. The normal structure of a lipid A molecule consists of two connected glucosamine molecules, and these glucosamine molecules can have up to seven fatty acyl chains attached to them [6, 41].

9.9 POLYKETIDES

Polyketides are a broad class of chemical compounds that are produced by synthesizing multiple simple precursor molecules, such as acetyl-CoA and malonyl-CoA, in a condensation reaction.

Large enzyme complexes known as polyketide synthases are responsible for assembling these precursor molecules into linear chains. These enzyme complexes are analogous to the fatty acid synthase system in their structure and function. Polyketides are noted for having intricate and fascinating chemical structures, and they can be found in a broad variety of organisms, including bacteria, fungi, plants, and mammals. They are also present in foods. Polyketides come in a wide variety, and many of them have useful biological characteristics, such as antibacterial, antiparasitic, and anticancer characteristics [42, 43]. Polyketides are an important target for drug discovery and development as a result of the wide variety of chemical characteristics that they possess. Other chemical changes in polyketides, such as glycosylation, methylation, hydroxylation, and oxidation, can lead to the production of molecules that are even more complex and diverse, each of which possesses its own set of characteristics [42].

9.10 LIPOPROTEINS

Lipoproteins are soluble complexes of lipids and proteins that are responsible for transporting lipids. This is necessary because lipids are relatively insoluble. In the blood, lipoproteins play an important role in the movement of fat-soluble vitamins, dietary lipids, and lipids that have been synthesized [44]. Lipoproteins are made up of a core that is composed of triglycerides and cholesterol esters, which are encased in a surface monolayer that is composed of phospholipids, free cholesterol, and apolipoproteins [15]. Chylomicrons, very low-density lipoproteins (VLDL), low-density lipoproteins (LDL), and high-density lipoproteins (HDL) are all types of lipoproteins with unique compositions and roles in lipid metabolism. Lipoproteins are distinguished from one another according to the size and composition of their apoprotein content (A, B, C, D, and E), lipid content, and electrophoretic pattern [45]. A heterogeneous collection of lipoprotein particles is produced as a result of the disparities in the types of lipids and apoproteins present, as well as their relative amounts. Because lipids have a lower density than water, the amount and type of lipid that is contained within a lipoprotein particle is the primary factor that determines the particle's overall density. Chylomicrons are the lipoprotein particles that contain the most lipid and, as a result, have the lowest density, whereas HDLs contain the least lipid and, as a result, have the highest density. Lipoprotein particles come in a wide range of sizes, with the largest particles being the ones that contain the most lipids (chylomicrons), and the smallest particles being the ones that are the densest (HDL) (Table 9.1). Lipoprotein metabolism disorders encompass both primary and secondary abnormalities that markedly increase or decrease certain circulating lipids (for example, cholesterol or TGs) or lipoproteins (for example, low-density or high-density lipoproteins). These conditions can contribute to the development of atherosclerosis and other cardiovascular diseases [46].

9.11 APOPROTEINS

These are lipoprotein-associated proteins that are essential for lipoprotein assembly, shape, function, and metabolism (Table 9.1). Apoproteins further activate enzymes that are involved in the metabolism of lipoproteins and act as ligands for cell surface receptors. Apoproteins can also be found on the surface of cells [47]. Apo B is an extremely large protein that serves as the primary structural component of chylomicrons, as well as VLDL, IDL, and LDL [48]. The human intestines are responsible for the production of the smaller Apo B48 protein, while the liver is in charge of making the larger apo B100 protein. Both of these proteins are produced from the same Apo B gene by post-translational modification. The liver and the small intestine are also responsible for the synthesis of apo A, which can be found attached to the majority of HDL particles. In the process of regulating triglyceride-rich lipoproteins, Apo C-2 plays a very significant role. In the process of clearing cholesterol and triglycerides from the body, Apo E is an extremely important player [49].

9.12 HIGH-DENSITY LIPOPROTEIN

The small intestines and the liver are both responsible for the production of high-density lipoprotein particles, which are characterized by an abundance of cholesterol as well as phospholipids and many apolipoproteins. The Apo A-I protein serves as the primary structural component, and individual HDL particles may include numerous copies of this protein. HDL particles are very heterogeneous particles that mediate the transport of cholesterol and other compounds from peripheral tissues to the liver [50]. This is one of the reasons why an increase in circulating HDL may be anti-atherogenic. HDL particles can be classified based on density, size, charge, and the composition of apolipoproteins. The term "good cholesterol" refers to HDL since studies have

Table 9.1 Characteristics of lipoproteins

	CM	VLDL	IDL	LDL	HDL	Lp(a)
Density (g/ml)	<0.930	0.93–1.006	1.006–1.019	1.019–1.063	1.063–1.210	1.050–1.100
Diameter (nm)	80–1200	25–80	25–35	18–25	5–12	~30
Major lipids	TG	TG	TG, C	C	C	C
Major apoproteins	B-48, C, E	B-100, C, E	B-100, E	B-100	A, C, E	B-100, (a)
Origin	Intestines	Liver	Derived from VLDL	Derived from IDL	Intestines & liver	Liver
Electrophoretic mobility	Origin	Pre-beta	Broad beta region	Beta	Alpha	Pre-beta
Components (%) Dry Weight						
Proteins	2	9	12	22	32–50	8
Triglycerides	85	55	30	10	3–7	7
Cholesterol	6	17	38	47	20–32	60-80
Phospholipids	8	19	20	21	27–29	20–30

Table 9.1 shows lipoprotein classes and features. TG is triglycerides, C is cholesterol, CM is chylomicron, VLDL is very low-density lipoprotein, IDL is intermediate density lipoproteins, HDL is high-density lipoproteins, LP is lipoprotein.

shown a correlation between having a high number of big HDL particles and having better health outcomes. On the other hand, having a low total number of big HDL particles is an independent risk factor for the progression of atheromatous disease within the arteries. It is possible that the antioxidant, anti-inflammatory, anti-thrombotic, and anti-apoptotic qualities of HDL particles also play a role in their capacity to reduce atherosclerosis [51, 52].

9.13 CHYLOMICRON

Chylomicrons are big particles that are rich in triglycerides and are secreted by the small intestine. They are essential for the transport of dietary lipids to peripheral tissues, as well as the liver. Every chylomicron particle carries with it an Apo B-48 molecule, which serves as the fundamental structural component. As they travel through the circulatory system from the lymphatic system, chylomicron particles pick up more apoproteins along the way, including Apo A-I to A-V, B-48, C-II, C-III, and E. If you consume a meal that is high in fat, your body will produce large chylomicron particles that contain an increased amount of triglyceride. On the other hand, if you are fasting or consume a meal that is low in fat, your body will produce small chylomicron particles that contain decreased amounts of triglyceride. Similarly, the quantity of cholesterol that is transported in chylomicrons is also subject to change. Chylomicron remnants are produced when muscle and adipose tissue lipoprotein lipase (LPL) removes triglyceride from chylomicrons. This process results in chylomicrons being broken down into smaller particles. These particles are pro-atherogenic and have a higher cholesterol content than average [53, 54].

9.14 VERY LOW-DENSITY LIPOPROTEIN PARTICLES

The liver is responsible for the production of very low-density lipoprotein (VLDL) particles, which have apolipoproteins B-100, C-I, C-II, and C-III in their composition. Apo B-100 is present in each VLDL particle. This protein is responsible for serving as the principal structural component of the VLDL particle. The size of the VLDL particles can alter, and when there is an increase in the production of triglycerides in the liver, the VLDL particles that are released are massive. The removal of triglycerides from VLDL by lipoprotein lipase (LPL) in muscle and adipose tissue results in the production of intermediate-density lipoprotein (IDL) particles. These particles are higher in cholesterol and contribute to the development of atherosclerosis. These IDL particles have been identified as containing apolipoproteins B-100 and E [2, 23].

9.15 LOW-DENSITY LIPOPROTEIN PARTICLES

The catabolism of VLDL and IDL particles produces low-density lipoprotein (LDL) particles. Apo B-100 protein is found in each LDL particle. LDL particles, through the help of apo B, normally transport the vast majority of the body's cholesterol in the extracellular compartment. There is a range of sizes and densities of LDL. The intracellular compartment contains approximately 93% of total body cholesterol. Only 7% of total body cholesterol is found in plasma, where it is carried by LDL (60–70%), HDL (20–30%), and VLDL (1–5%). An increase in LDL levels in the plasma causes the accumulation of cholesterol on the artery walls, which contributes to the development of atherosclerosis. Sometimes, while LDL is circulating in the bloodstream, it is subjected to a chemical change as a result of the action of endogenous chemicals such as free radicals. This results in the production of oxidized LDL (Ox-LDL) and small dense LDL (sdLDL). In addition, the non-enzymatic glycation of LDL, also known as Gly-LDL, causes lipoprotein receptors to recognize it less effectively [55]. There is a correlation between hypertriglyceridemia, low HDL levels, obesity, and type 2 diabetes, all of which contribute to an increase in the amounts of small dense LDL particles, which are more atherogenic than the larger LDL particles [56].

9.16 LIPOPROTEIN (A) PARTICLES

Lipoprotein (a), or Lp(a), is an LDL particle that is disulfide-bonded to Apo B-100. Lp(a) contains an equivalent quantity of both Apo A and B-100 in its composition. The organ that is responsible for producing Apo A is the liver. Because of the size of Apo A, it is conceivable that there is a large degree of variation in the size of Lp(a) particles. This variation could be significant. Plasma levels of Lp(a) can go undetected up to values that are larger than 100 mg/dl, representing a fluctuation of 1,000 times [57]. Individuals whose Apo A proteins have a low molecular weight tend to have higher levels of Lp(a), whereas individuals whose Apo A proteins have a high molecular weight tend to have lower levels. Clearance of Lp(a) does not appear to be much influenced by LDL receptors, although the kidney does appear to play an important part in this process. There is a correlation between a slowed clearance of Lp(a) and higher levels of kidney disease [58]. Apo A acts as an inhibitor of fibrinolysis and stimulates the absorption of lipoproteins by macrophages, both of which contribute to an increased risk of atherosclerosis in patients whose levels of Apo A are raised [59]. In addition, Lp(a) is the principal lipoprotein transporter of oxidized phospholipids, which are associated with an increased risk of atherosclerosis [60]. There is a considerable hereditary component to the levels of Lp(a). Between 20% to 30% of people of Caucasian descent have levels that point to a potential danger to their cardiovascular system. The Lp(a) normal ranges of black people are approximately two and a half times higher than those of white people and Asian people [60, 61].

9.17 LIPID TRANSPORT METABOLISM

The digestion, synthesis, and transport of lipids throughout the body are all part of the complicated process of lipid metabolism. The exogenous pathway, the endogenous pathway, and the reverse cholesterol transport metabolism all influence lipid and lipoprotein transport.

9.17.1 Exogenous Lipoprotein Pathway

The exogenous lipoprotein route leads to the effective transport of dietary triglycerides, also known as fatty acids, to muscle and adipose tissue, where they can be used for energy and stored [62, 63]. Triglycerides are first broken down in the oral cavity by lingual lipases, which are produced by glands in the tongue. The digestive process is carried out by stomach-produced enzymes. Peristalsis has a crucial function as one of the contributing components in the emulsification of dietary fat and fat-soluble vitamins, which takes place mostly in the stomach. After passing through the duodenum as minute lipid droplets, crude emulsions of lipids continue to be formed and the lipids undergo significant alterations in their chemical composition and their physical state as a result of their interaction with the bile and the pancreatic juice. In the duodenum, the process of emulsification, in addition to hydrolysis and micellization, continues to prepare for absorption. Triacylglycerol (TAG), often known as triglycerides (TG), is the most prevalent type of fat in the diet, accounting for 90–95% of the total amount of energy that is produced from fat in the diet. Phospholipids (PLs), sterols (such as cholesterol), and a wide variety of other lipids (such as fat-soluble vitamins) are all considered to be types of dietary fats [15]. Phosphatidylcholine (PC), which is primarily derived from bile but can also be obtained from food, is the primary phospholipid found in the lumen of the digestive tract [64]. Cholesterol, which comes primarily from animal sources, and sitosterol, which comes primarily from plants, are the most common sterols found in food. Once fatty acids and monoglycerides are absorbed, they are re-esterified into triglycerides and bundled into chylomicrons. About half of the cholesterol that is present in the intestine is absorbed, while the other half is eliminated through the stool. Only about 10–15% of dietary cholesterol is found in the cholesteryl ester form; the rest of the cholesterol comes in the form of free sterol [65]. This latter component needs to be digested by cholesterol esterase to liberate free cholesterol, which may then be absorbed. Because cholesterol has very low solubility in water, it must first be encapsulated in bile salt micelles before it can be absorbed.

Chylomicrons (CM) are a type of lipoprotein that are generated in enterocytes. They are involved in the movement of dietary (exogenous) lipids from the intestine to the lymphatic system and then into circulation via the pathway that is responsible for the metabolism of exogenous lipids. This particular CM is transported to the peripheral tissues (typically the muscle and adipose tissues), where it delivers cholesterol esters (CE) and triglycerides (TG), both of which are generated by the re-esterification of free fatty acids. The lipoprotein core contains TAG, cholesteryl esters, and fat-soluble vitamins, while the lipoprotein surface contains a monolayer of PLs (mainly phosphatidylcholine), free cholesterol, and proteins. The enormous, hydrophobic, non-exchangeable protein known as Apo B48 is an essential component in the chylomicron's structural makeup. Other proteins that are associated with nascent chylomicrons include Apo A-I, Apo AIV, and Apo Cs. These proteins are made in enterocytes, which are the cells that produce chylomicrons. The quantity of lipids that are transported during the condition of postprandial digestion is many times more than that which is transported during the state of fasting. During the postprandial state, there is an increase in the size of the particles, which results in an increased transfer of fat even though similar levels of Apo B48 are present [66]. A diet high in fat also boosts the expression of Apo A-IV, which acts as a surface component for Apo B48 particles in the enterocyte [67]. Chylomicrons that are manufactured in the intestine are released into the lymph and transported to systemic circulation via the thoracic duct. This improves the supply of nutrients to adipose and muscular tissue, which are both necessary for the storage and utilization of energy [68]. Lipoprotein lipase (LPL) is the enzyme responsible for the release of free fatty acids, which then either proceed through the process of beta-oxidation to become sources of energy or are stored as fat in the adipose tissue. Apo C2 and Apo E are acquired by CM from HDL in the lymphatic system. Apo C2 is necessary for the activation of LPL, whereas Apo E is necessary for the identification of CM residues by particular receptors in the liver (Figure 9.2). Both of these proteins are produced by the liver. Apo C2, which is carried on chylomicrons, activates LPL, which leads to the hydrolysis of the triglycerides contained in chylomicrons, which in turn leads to the generation of free fatty acids [69]. These free fatty acids are then taken up by muscle cells and adipocytes and used for either the production of energy or the storage of energy. Some of the free fatty acids that are liberated when the CM triglycerides are hydrolyzed into free fatty acids bind to albumin and are then able to be transferred to other tissues. Mutations in LPL, Apo C-II, and Apo A-V can cause familial chylomicronemia syndrome, which manifests as severe hypertriglyceridemia [70]. Apo C-III is known to limit LPL activity, and mutations in this gene that cause a loss of function have been linked to increases in LPL activity, as well as reductions in plasma triglyceride levels. Similarly, the activity of LPL is controlled by angiopoietin-like proteins 3 and 4, which specifically target LPL for inactivation. Plasma triglyceride levels tend to drop when there is a mutation in angiopoietin-like proteins 3 and 4 that causes the proteins to lose their function [71]. Because of the hydrolysis of the triglycerides that are carried in the chylomicrons, the size of the chylomicrons significantly decreases. This leads to the creation of chylomicron remnants, which are rich in cholesteryl esters and contain Apo E. Phospholipids and apolipoproteins (Apo A and C) on the surface of the chylomicrons are transferred to other lipoproteins, most significantly HDL, when the chylomicrons shrink in size. When Apo C-II moves from chylomicrons to HDL, the ability of LPL to continue breaking down triglycerides is reduced. The liver is the principal organ responsible for the removal of chylomicrons from the blood circulation. The Apo E that is present on the chylomicron remnants binds to the LDL receptor, as well as other hepatic receptors such as LRP-1 and syndecan-4, which causes the hepatocytes to take up the complete particle. Polymorphisms in Apo E, such as those found in the Apo E2 isoform, can lead to reduced chylomicron remnant clearance, as well as elevations in plasma cholesterol and triglyceride levels (a condition known as familial dysbetalipoproteinemia) [72].

9.17.2 Endogenous Lipoprotein Pathway

Triglycerides and cholesterol are both synthesized in the liver, where they are then packaged in the form of a VLDL particle that also contains apo B100 [62]. The process of adding apo C and E to the VLDL particle (which was obtained from HDL) is quite similar to the procedure that is detailed in exogenous lipid transport. In peripheral tissues, the activation of lipoprotein lipase

Exogenous Lipid Transport

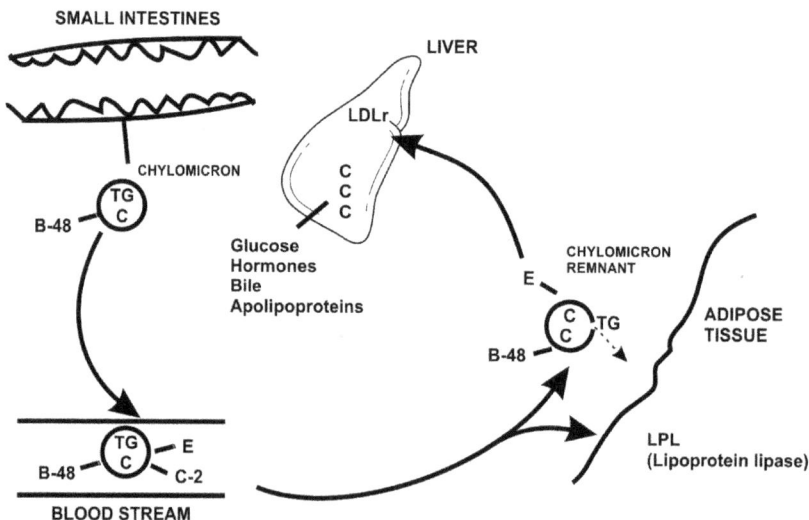

Figure 9.2 Exogenous lipid and lipoprotein transport. TG is triglyceride, C is cholesterol

(LPL) is caused by Apo C. After this step, the triglycerides that were being transported by VLDL particles are digested by LPL, which results in the release of fatty acids into the cell. The process of removing triglycerides from VLDL particles leads to the creation of VLDL remnants (IDL), which are richer in cholesteryl esters than the original VLDL particles. The liver is responsible for removing VLDL remnant particles from circulation by binding Apo E. This process is analogous to the elimination of chylomicron remnant particles. In contrast to chylomicron remnants, of which the great majority are swiftly removed from the circulation by the liver, only a portion of VLDL remnant particles is eliminated (about 50%). Hepatic lipase breaks down the lingering triglycerides in the VLDL remnant particles, which results in the production of LDL particles. The vast majority of triglycerides have been removed from LDL particles, and exchangeable apolipoproteins have been transported from the VLDL residual particles to other lipoproteins. As a result, LDL particles primarily consist of cholesteryl esters and Apo B-100 (Figure 9.3). Since the number of hepatic LDL receptors is the primary regulator of both the rate of LDL clearance and the rate of LDL generation, the number of hepatic LDL receptors is also the primary predictor of plasma LDL levels. When the activity of the LDL receptor is high, the conversion of VLDL remnants to LDL is reduced, whereas when the activity of the LDL receptor is low, the conversion of VLDL remnants to LDL is increased (which results in higher LDL production). LDL receptors in the liver are responsible for clearing around 70% of the circulating LDL, while extrahepatic tissues are responsible for taking up the remaining 30%. Therefore, the number of LDL receptors in the liver is an important factor in the regulation of the levels of LDL in the plasma.

9.17.3 Reverse Cholesterol Transport

Reverse cholesterol transport is the process by which cholesterol in peripheral tissues is moved from the plasma membranes of peripheral cells to the liver and intestines with the assistance of HDL [73]. This pathway brings cholesterol that has accumulated in the body's tissues back to the liver so that it can be eliminated in the bile. The formation of nascent HDL takes place in the liver and the small intestine. It takes a few different processes for HDL particles to develop into their mature state. The production of Apo A-I, which is HDL's primary structural protein, is the first stage in the process. Apo A-1 is responsible for acquiring cholesterol and phospholipids that are effluxed from hepatocytes and enterocytes. Antigen-binding cassette 1 (ABCA1) is a protein that mediates the efflux of cholesterol and phospholipids [74]. During the process of lipolysis, more

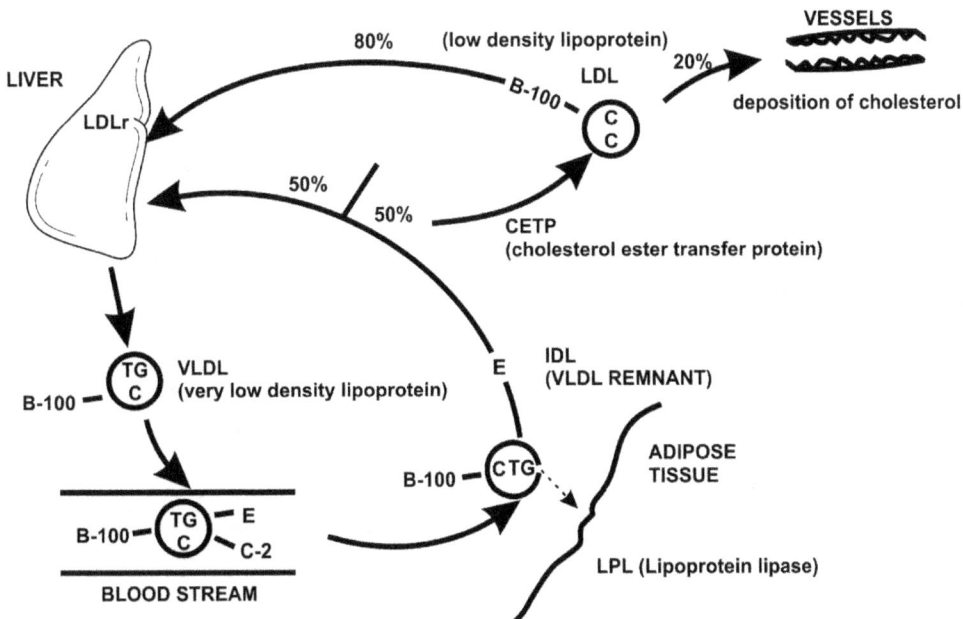

Figure 9.3 Endogenous lipid and lipoprotein transport. TG is triglyceride, C is cholesterol

apoproteins and lipids are transferred from the surfaces of other lipoproteins to HDL as it accumulates an increasing number of cholesterol esters (CE). This causes HDL to grow more spherical. Patients with loss-of-function mutations in ABCA1 have very low HDL levels and experience a fast breakdown of Apo A-I because they are unable to add lipids to the newly generated Apo A-I [75, 76]. Low HDL levels are commonly observed in patients with high plasma triglyceride levels due to impaired triglyceride-rich lipoprotein metabolism. This is likely due to the transfer of cholesterol and phospholipids from chylomicrons and very low-density lipoproteins to newly formed HDL [77].

Two primary routes are utilized in the process of transporting HDL cholesterol to the hepatocytes. Scavenger receptor class B1 (SR-B1) is a cell surface receptor that mediates the selective transfer of CE from HDL and subsequent dissociation from the HDL particle [78]. HDL-cholesterol can be preferentially picked up by the liver via SR-B1. Endocytosis that is mediated by the LDL receptor is subsequently used to remove the cholesterols from the circulation. After this, the HDL particle is no longer inhibited in its ability to acquire more cholesterol from the body's periphery. Alternately, cholesterol can be transferred from HDL to VLDL and chylomicron remnants by a protein called cholesterol ester transfer protein (CETP) [32], which is then absorbed by the liver (Figure 9.4).

9.18 PRIMARY HYPERLIPIDEMIA

A collection of physiologically connected plasma lipid and lipoprotein abnormalities is referred to as dyslipidemia. Dyslipidemia is frequently the first sign that anything is wrong with lipid metabolism. These abnormalities include low levels of HDL, and high levels of LDL, total cholesterol, and triglyceride (TG) [79, 80]. Dyslipidemia also includes an increase in the phenotype of LDL particles that are small and dense, a rise in VLDL that is rich in triglycerides, and an increase in both LDL and VLDL together (mixed dyslipidemia) [81]. Quantitative changes, on the other hand, are referred to as hyperlipidemias or hypolipidemias, depending on whether there is an increase or a reduction in the concentration of lipoproteins in the plasma.

There are two types of hyperlipoproteinemias: primary and secondary. Primary hyperlipoproteinemias are caused by genetic problems, while secondary hyperlipoproteinemias are caused by various conditions, such as diabetes, hepatopathy, renal failure, alcoholism, and endocrinopathy [82, 83]. Some forms of hyperlipoproteinemia have been linked to the disease atherosclerosis, as well as obesity [84]. The difficulty presented by the classification of lipoprotein diseases is to reconcile conventional and historical paradigms with newly emerging scientific discoveries. This is especially difficult because clinical patterns and the effects of those patterns are almost always the result of complex interactions between genes and the environment. Following a fast of 12 hours, a

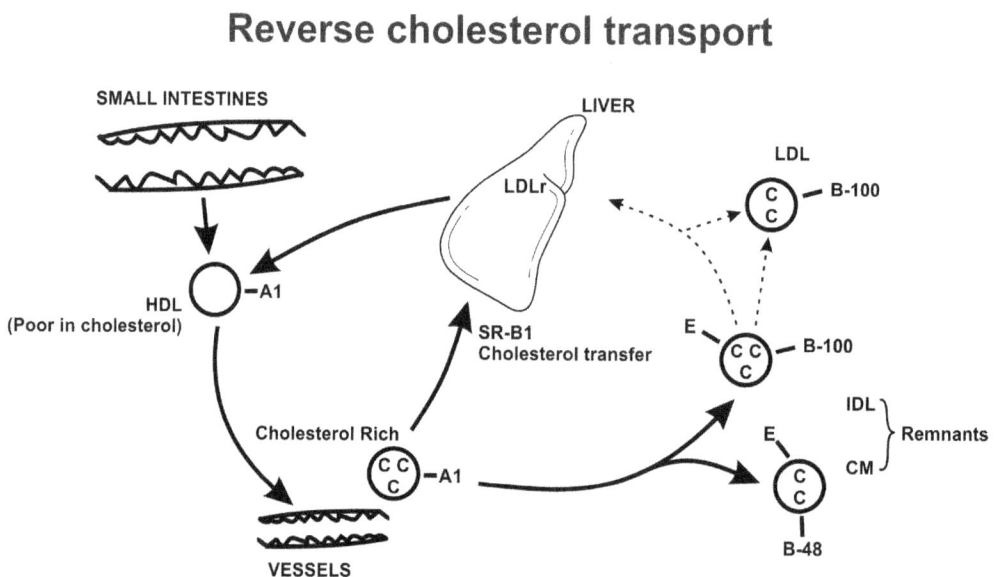

Figure 9.4 Reverse cholesterol transport. C is cholesterol

measurement of total cholesterol, HDL, and TG is performed as part of the routine clinical evaluation of lipoprotein metabolism. The absence of standardization renders non-fasting samples inappropriate for diagnostic categorization. However, non-fasting samples may be useful for improved detection of people who have an increased risk of CVD.

In addition, patients who have significantly elevated levels of TGs are more likely to be at risk of acute pancreatitis [85]. The Friedewald equation can be used to compute LDL cholesterol from the fasting values; however, there is a limitation to this calculation in that its reliability decreases as TG levels climb beyond around 4.5 mmol/L. Analyses of cholesterol and triglycerides are the simplest methods available for identifying hyperlipoproteinemia. Because the quantity of these lipids changes from one lipoprotein family to another, cholesterol and triglycerides also provide some information regarding the type of hyperlipoproteinemia that the individual is suffering from [86].

The types of hyperlipidemia roughly correspond to certain types of hyperlipoproteinemia. Lipoprotein fractions are studied and analyzed to provide a clinical picture that is helpful in the diagnosis and treatment of dyslipidemias. While CM, VLDL, and their remnant families are rich in triglycerides, LDL is rich in cholesterol. Conditions that have elevated concentrations of oxidized LDL particles, particularly "small dense LDL" (sdLDL) particles, have been linked to the formation of atheroma in the arterial walls [87]. Atheromas are complicated lesions that comprise biological components, collagen, and lipids in addition to other substances.

The presence of unesterified cholesterol and cholesteryl esters in the lesion is the primary factor that contributes to the lesion's growth [88]. LDL, IDL, VLDL, and Lp(a) species are all examples of atherogenic lipoproteins. These lipoproteins all include the B100 apolipoprotein (Apo B100) [89]. Atherogenic properties are also exhibited by chylomicron remnants that carry apoB48. All of these can become oxidized due to the presence of reactive oxygen species in the tissues, in addition to lipoxygenases that are released by macrophages in atheromas. Impairment of endothelial cell-mediated vasodilation is caused by modifications in lipoproteins such as oxidized lipoproteins, which also encourage the endothelium to release monocyte chemoattractant protein 1 (MCP1) and adhesion molecules, which recruit monocytes to the lesion [90]. The production of foam cells can also be attributed to the oxidation of lipoproteins, which induces the endocytosis of those lipoproteins via scavenger receptors on macrophages and smooth muscle cells [75].

The classification of primary hyperlipidemia is done using Fredrickson's approach, which is based on the observed pattern of lipoprotein abnormalities [91]. It does not appear that any sickness could be responsible for the irregularity. The majority of the time, it is brought on by mistakes in metabolism that have been traced back to a familial (or inherited) foundation. The high lipid fraction can be either cholesterol or triglycerides, or it can be both.

Chylomicron syndrome, also known as familial chylomicronemia, falls under the category of type I hyperlipidemia and is inherited in an autosomal recessive manner [92]. It affects one in every one million persons. Lipoprotein lipase or its activator, apo C-2, must be lacking for this condition to manifest itself. A higher level of plasma chylomicron (CM) and total cholesterol is a result of this disorder. Onset occurs during childhood and is characterized by hepatomegaly, eruptive xanthomata, and stomach discomfort. A diet low in fat should be prescribed for management. To temporarily replenish apo C-2, fresh plasma should be administered. To verify a diagnosis of familial lipoprotein lipase deficiency, a test called a plasma lipoprotein lipase (LPL) test can be performed after an infusion of heparin. This procedure is necessary because heparin causes the enzyme to be released from endothelial sites. Plasma concentrations of LDL activators can also

Table 9.2 Classification of primary dyslipidemia

Phenotype	Primary Lipid Elevation	Lipoprotein Fraction	Occurrence
I	TG	Chylomicron	Rare
IIa	C	LDL	Common
IIb	TG, C	LDL, VLDL	Most common
III	TG, C	IDL	Rare
IV	TG	VLDL	Common
V	TG	Chylomicron, VLDL	Rare

Table 9.2 shows lipoprotein phenotype classification by Fredrickson. TG is triglycerides, C is cholesterol, VLDL is very low-density lipoprotein, and IDL is intermediate-density lipoproteins.

be measured to investigate the possibility of an Apo C-2 deficiency. When a primary disorder is suspected, it is important to evaluate the patient's family members as well.

High plasma cholesterol concentrations are characteristic of familial hypercholesterolemia [93]. These high concentrations are prevalent from an early age and are unrelated to the presence of environmental factors. It is the most common primary hyperlipidemia. It is passed down in an autosomal dominant manner. Although distinct mutations can affect the processes of LDL production, transport, and ligand binding, the result is always the same. This primary disorder is most commonly brought on by a mutation in the apo B gene, which lowers the avidity of LDL for its receptor and is the principal contributor to the condition [94]. In every instance, there is a problem with the absorption and catabolism of LDL, which results in an elevated concentration of LDL in the plasma. Homozygous patients commonly show in early infancy, typically before the age of 4 years, with yellow-orange elevated cutaneous plaques on the eyelids (i.e. xanthelasmas) and tendinous xanthomas that are notably noticed over the Achilles tendon area [95]. Additionally, a total cholesterol level that is higher than 7.5 mmol/L and an LDL level that is higher than 4.5 mmol/L are usually observed. Heterozygotes only have 50% of the usual receptor activity and are 20 times more likely to develop coronary artery disease than the general population [96]. Homozygotes are extremely uncommon. There are no receptors, and the plasma levels can reach above 20 mmol/L. According to Frederickson's classification, this disorder is also known as familial type IIA hyperlipoproteinemia; however, some patients may have a phenotype that is more consistent with type IIB hyperlipidemia.

Familial combined hyperlipidemia (FCHL) is associated with the presence of an excessive amount of VLDL in plasma [97]. The condition rarely appears in children as it typically manifests itself after the onset of puberty. Classification can be challenging due to the murky nature of the inheritance process, even within the same family. The overproduction of VLDL particles by the livers of individuals affected by FCHL as a means of compensating for an underlying defective peripheral uptake of LDL-derived cholesterol is a notion that has gained widespread acceptance as a possible explanation for the elevated levels of VLDL found in FCHL [95]. In patients who come from the same family, the risk of developing coronary artery disease is higher. If there is a history of hyperlipidemia in the family, particularly if various members of the family display different lipoprotein phenotypes, then the diagnosis of FCHL should be considered a possibility. Frederickson's phenotypes IIA, IIB, and IV can be observed in this situation respectively. There is an increase in the concentration of TG and VLDL in the plasma. Plasma HDL levels are frequently reduced. The disorder can be treated with dietary changes and, on occasion, with medications that reduce lipid levels.

Familial dysbetalipoproteinemia is sometimes referred to as type III hyperlipoproteinemia or broad beta hyperlipidemia [98]. When serum lipoproteins are taken through electrophoresis, the presence of remnant particles leads to the appearance of broadband that extends between the pre-β (VLDL) and β (LDL) positions. Apo E is polymorphic and has three alleles (E-2, E-3, and E-4) that can result in one of six potential phenotypes. These phenotypes are as follows: E-2/2, E-3/3, E-4/4, E-2/3, E-2/4, and E-3/4. The E-3/3 isoform (iso-protein) is the most prevalent one, and it is the one that allows for the most effective elimination of chylomicron remnants and IDL [98, 99]. The liver can have reduced uptake when affected by familial dysbetalipoproteinemia because this condition is linked to the E2/E2 phenotype. In this case, the patient has a higher frequency of the E2 allele, specifically the E-2/2 and E-2/3 variants, which are not acknowledged by the residual receptor to a significant degree. This causes increases in the amounts of CM remnant and IDL in the blood, which ultimately results in the broad-beta electrophoretic pattern being seen.

In patients with familial hypertriglyceridemia, also referred to as type IV hyperlipidemia, triglyceride levels are extremely increased, whereas HDL levels are significantly lowered. The precise genetic cause of the illness cannot be determined at this time. On the other hand, it is believed that this main condition results from excessive production of VLDL particles and/or impaired metabolism of these particles. This kind of heredity is autosomal dominant [100].

Another less prevalent variant of familial hypertriglyceridemia is familial mixed hypertriglyceridemia, also known as type V hyperlipidemia, with an estimated prevalence of 1 in 600 people. The disorder is characterized by high plasma levels of both chylomicrons and VLDL particles; as a result, it brings together under one disorder the lipid phenotypes that are seen in types I and IV hyperlipidemia [72, 101].

Plasma levels of high-density lipoprotein (HDL) are significantly elevated in people who have a familial form of hyperalphalipoproteinemia. There is also a little rise in the amount of cholesterol in the plasma. There has been a significant decline in the prevalence of coronary heart disease in patients with this condition. The elevated levels of plasma cholesterol seldom call for any kind of medical therapy.

9.19 SECONDARY HYPERLIPIDEMIA

The presence of secondary hyperlipidemia is a complication of other disorders. This particular form of hyperlipidemia is treatable by addressing the underlying cause of the condition. When dealing with hyperlipidemia, it is important to rule out conditions such as diabetes mellitus (DM), hypothyroidism, and nephrotic syndrome (NS). Clinical research has shown that diabetes is linked to several metabolic risk factors, including obesity, hypertension, and dyslipidemia [102]. Dyslipidemia in DM is primarily identified by an increase in triglyceride-rich lipoproteins, a decrease in HDL-C, and a consistently or slightly increased number of tiny and dense LDL-C particles [103]. This can be explained by the action of insulin in the liver, which stimulates the production of VLDL. Because it speeds up the production of triglycerides, alcohol is one of the leading causes of hypertriglyceridemia. Atherogenic dyslipidemia is characterized by the triad of high levels of TG, low levels of HDL, and LDL particles that are both small and dense. The expression of the LDL receptor is boosted by thyroid hormones. As a consequence of this, LDL plasmatic clearance is reduced when hormone levels are low in the case of primary hypothyroidism [104]. When someone has hypothyroidism, their intestinal absorption of cholesterol is increased, with a decrease in both the levels of the cholesterol ester transfer protein in the plasma and its activity [105]. Levels of lipoprotein lipase, hepatic lipase, and the activity of plasma lipase are reduced when hypothyroidism is present.

9.20 INVESTIGATION OF HYPERLIPIDEMIAS

Alterations in nutrition, posture, and stress can all affect the patterns of lipoproteins and the concentration of lipids in plasma. Therefore, it is of the utmost importance to stick to established protocols in the investigation of hyperlipidemias. Individuals should stick to their typical diet and maintain the same weight for the two weeks leading up to their blood lipids test. Abuse of alcohol should be avoided because it leads to an increase in the body's production of triglycerides [106]. If the therapy is not being monitored, the patient should not be given medication that could influence plasma lipids (oral contraceptives, and heparin therapy are all examples of treatments that could affect lipids). It is well established that acute viral infections also contribute to an increase in the HDL concentrations found in the blood [107]. It is necessary for the patient to abstain from food and liquid intake for at least 12 hours and not to be receiving any lipid infusions. The standardized posture, which involves as little venostasis as possible (for example, sitting for 10 minutes), is the one that is used. It is preferable to use coagulated blood (with the serum that results from it). The blood sample ought to be brought to the laboratory as soon as possible so that it can be analyzed. The concentration of glucose in the blood can help determine whether or not someone has DM. Liver function tests are diagnostic of liver diseases such as cholestasis, whereas measuring the quantities of protein in the urine and albumin in the plasma can identify nephrotic syndrome (NS). In addition, tests of thyroid function are carried out to look into the possibility of thyroid malfunction. Because the levels of lipids in the blood might vary significantly from one person to the next, it is not possible to rely on the results of just one set of measurements and hence it is prudent to re-test a patient's blood lipids at regular intervals over a few months. Specialist lipid assay testing could be of assistance in defining the abnormalities. Because many individuals with type III hyperlipoproteinemia have the apo E2/E2 genotype, the apo E genotype can help make a diagnosis of the condition. In patients with chylomicron syndrome, tests for plasma lipoprotein lipase and apo C-2 might be helpful. Studies of LDL receptor DNA can help determine whether or not a patient has familial hypercholesterolemia [83, 100].

9.21 HYPOALPHALIPOPROTEINEMIA

The most common inherited cause of low HDL levels is Tangier disease, which is caused by abnormalities in the ABCA1 transporter [108]. This transporter is responsible for transferring excess cellular cholesterol to HDL. Because of this situation, the amount of HDL in the circulation is significantly lowered. Mutations in the LCAT gene are connected with the creation of an aberrant lipoprotein particle known as Lipoprotein-X, which can lead to disorders of the renal system and the liver [109]. These mutations also result in low HDL-C levels. Hypobetalipoproteinemia is characterized by a partial lack of apoB, which leads to extremely low levels of CM, VLDL, and IDL in the blood [72]. This condition can also affect the liver. Abetalipoproteinemia, on the other hand, is characterized by the absence of lipoproteins in the plasma. Patients who suffer from protein-energy malnutrition (also known as kwashiorkor), malabsorption syndromes, or end-stage parenchymal liver disease are more likely to have secondary hypolipidemia.

9.22 MANAGEMENT OF HYPERLIPIDEMIA

Modifications to one's food and way of life are the initial stages in the treatment of hyperlipidemia for patients of any age category. These non-pharmacological techniques involve making precise adjustments to multiple aspects of day-to-day living, most notably one's nutrition and level of physical activity. In addition, for obese individuals, it is recommended that they lose weight. In children who have particular forms of dyslipidemia or in those who are unable to obtain an appropriate therapeutic response with prolonged lifestyle alterations, pharmacotherapy may be administered as an adjuvant therapy to lifestyle modification as a means of treating dyslipidemia.

The first and most important step in the treatment of any hyperlipidemia is dietary therapy. This method typically yields positive results (after three to six months) and has the fewest problems [110]. When dealing with endogenous hypertriglyceridemia, it is essential to limit carbohydrate consumption. Reducing the amount of fat consumed in the diet is necessary when dealing with exogenously increased triglycerides. Reducing one's consumption of saturated (animal) fat as well as cholesterol from one's diet is the treatment for hypercholesterolemia. It is of the utmost importance to discuss daily calorie intake and limitations with a dietitian or nutritionist to ensure optimal results.

For patients over the age of 5 years, engaging in regular physical exercise means consistently participating in moderate or strenuous physical activity for 30–60 minutes per day. Walking quickly or playing games that require tossing and catching are examples of moderately strenuous physical activities. On the other hand, vigorous activity might include things like jogging, biking, jumping rope, playing basketball or football, or engaging in martial arts, all of which entail running at some point. Young children, including infants and preschoolers, should be allowed to engage in as much physically stimulating play as they choose, provided it is safe and supervised by an adult.

When a child has a severe form of hypercholesterolemia or when comprehensive lifestyle adjustment for six months does not result in substantial reductions in LDL-C levels, pharmaceutical intervention becomes a necessary additional therapy option [111]. The cholesterol or triglyceride fractions in the blood are the primary focus of treatment with lipid-lowering medications. Statins, also known as HMG-CoA reductase inhibitors, are the drugs of choice for the initial course of treatment for high levels of LDL cholesterol [112]. These lipid-lowering medications are very effective, are well received by patients, and have a low incidence of undesirable side effects and high levels of safety. They inhibit the activity of the enzyme (HMG-CoA reductase) that controls the rate at which cholesterol is produced. Niacin is a type of vitamin B that, when taken in larger amounts, is capable of reducing lipid levels. There is still a lot of mystery surrounding the actual mechanism of action; however, current research suggests that it may inhibit VLDL synthesis. Niacin has been shown to boost HDL levels while simultaneously lowering LDL and VLDL levels when administered in quantities of 1,000 mg or more [113]. Cholesterol absorption inhibitors, also known as cholestyramine, colestipol, colesevelam, and ezetimibe, are drugs that prevent cholesterol from being absorbed in the digestive tract. They accomplish this goal by interfering with the process of cholesterol micellar solubilization and further blocking the trafficking of cholesterol into enterocytes [114]. The most significant disadvantages associated with the consumption of these inhibitors are gastrointestinal side effects, such as constipation, bloating, heartburn, and nausea. It is usual practice to make use of these in combination with statin therapy to achieve larger LDL reductions or in cases in which statins are not well tolerated. Fibrates, such as gemfibrozil and fenofibrate, achieve their therapeutic effects through the activation of nuclear transcription factors [115]. As a consequence, there is a reduction in the amount of VLDL formation, as well as an improvement in the amount of VLDL clearance; hence, these medications are particularly useful for the treatment of excessive triglyceride levels. Patients who have mixed abnormalities of VLDL and LDL can be treated with medications in combination with statins; however, this therapy is associated with an increased risk of significant muscle breakdown.

REFERENCES

1. Cox, R.A. and M.R. García-Palmieri, Cholesterol, triglycerides, and associated lipoproteins. In: Walker H.K., Hall W.D., Hurst J.W., eds. *Clinical Methods: The History, Physical, and Laboratory Examinations*. 3rd ed. Boston: Butterworths; 1990. pp. 153–160.

2. Ference, B.A., J.J. Kastelein, and A.L. Catapano, Lipids and lipoproteins in 2020. *JAMA*, 2020. **324**(6): pp. 595–596.

3. Maxfield, F.R. and I. Tabas, Role of cholesterol and lipid organization in disease. *Nature*, 2005. **438**(7068): pp. 612–621.

4. Natesan, V. and S.-J. Kim, Lipid metabolism, disorders and therapeutic drugs–review. *Biomolecules & Therapeutics*, 2021. **29**(6): p. 596.

5. Sud, M., et al., Lmsd: Lipid maps structure database. *Nucleic Acids Research*, 2007. **35**(suppl_1): pp. D527–D532.

6. Fahy, E., et al., Update of the LIPID MAPS comprehensive classification system for lipids1. *Journal of Lipid Research*, 2009. **50**(Supplement): pp. S9–S14.

7. Fahy, E., et al., Lipid classification, structures and tools. *Biochimica et Biophysica Acta (BBA)-Molecular and Cell Biology of Lipids*, 2011. **1811**(11): pp. 637–647.

8. Holthuis, J.C. and A.K. Menon, Lipid landscapes and pipelines in membrane homeostasis. *Nature*, 2014. **510**(7503): pp. 48–57.

9. Saasa, V., et al., Blood ketone bodies and breath acetone analysis and their correlations in type 2 diabetes mellitus. *Diagnostics*, 2019. **9**(4): p. 224.

10. Saini, R.K. and Y.-S. Keum, Omega-3 and omega-6 polyunsaturated fatty acids: Dietary sources, metabolism, and significance—A review. *Life Sciences*, 2018. **203**: pp. 255–267.

11. Craven, R.J. and R.W. Lencki, Polymorphism of acylglycerols: A stereochemical perspective. *Chemical Reviews*, 2013. **113**(10): pp. 7402–7420.

12. Shamsi, I.H., B.H. Shamsi, and L. Jiang, Biochemistry of fatty acids, in *Technological Innovations in Major World Oil Crops, Volume 2: Perspectives*. 2011, Springer. pp. 123–150.

13. Broadhurst, C., Balanced intakes of natural triglycerides for optimum nutrition: An evolutionary and phytochemical perspective. *Medical Hypotheses*, 1997. **49**(3): pp. 247–261.

14. May, C.Y. and K. Nesaretnam, Research advancements in palm oil nutrition. *European Journal of Lipid Science and Technology*, 2014. **116**(10): pp. 1301–1315.

15. Iqbal, J. and M.M. Hussain, Intestinal lipid absorption. *American Journal of Physiology-Endocrinology and Metabolism*, 2009. **296**(6): pp. E1183–E1194.

16. Goodman, B.E., Insights into digestion and absorption of major nutrients in humans. *Advances in Physiology Education*, 2010. **34**(2): pp. 44–53.

17. Loli, H., et al., Lipases in medicine: An overview. *Mini Reviews in Medicinal Chemistry*, 2015. **15**(14): pp. 1209–1216.

18. Küllenberg, D., et al., Health effects of dietary phospholipids. *Lipids in Health and Disease*, 2012. **11**: pp. 1–16.

19. Kinney, A.J., Phospholipid head groups, in *Lipid Metabolism in Plants*. 2018, CRC Press. pp. 259–284.

20. Calzada, E., O. Onguka, and S.M. Claypool, Phosphatidylethanolamine metabolism in health and disease. *International Review of Cell and Molecular Biology*, 2016. **321**: pp. 29–88.

21. Mato, J.M., Lipid Components of Cellular Membranes, in *Phospholipid Metabolism in Cellular Signaling*. 2018, CRC Press. pp. 1–8.

22. Hermansson, M., K. Hokynar, and P. Somerharju, Mechanisms of glycerophospholipid homeostasis in mammalian cells. *Progress in Lipid Research*, 2011. **50**(3): pp. 240–257.

23. Chandel, N.S., Lipid metabolism. *Cold Spring Harbor Perspectives in Biology*, 2021. **13**(9): p. a040576.

24. Lahiri, S. and A.H. Futerman, The metabolism and function of sphingolipids and glycosphingolipids. *Cellular and Molecular Life Sciences*, 2007. **64**: pp. 2270–2284.

25. Fanani, M.L. and B. Maggio, The many faces (and phases) of ceramide and sphingomyelin I–single lipids. *Biophysical Reviews*, 2017. **9**: pp. 589–600.

26. D'Angelo, G., et al., Glycosphingolipids: Synthesis and functions. *The FEBS Journal*, 2013. **280**(24): pp. 6338–6353.

27. Kulkarni, S.S., Synthesis of glycosphingolipids. *Glycochemical Synthesis: Strategies and Applications*, 2016: pp. 293–326.

28. Santos, C.R. and A. Schulze, Lipid metabolism in cancer. *The FEBS Journal*, 2012. **279**(15): pp. 2610–2623.

29. Ohvo-Rekilä, H., et al., Cholesterol interactions with phospholipids in membranes. *Progress in Lipid Research*, 2002. **41**(1): pp. 66–97.

30. Bacila, I.-A., C. Elder, and N. Krone, Update on adrenal steroid hormone biosynthesis and clinical implications. *Archives of Disease in Childhood*, 2019. **104**(12): pp. 1223–1228.

31. Dai, X., et al., Genetics of coronary artery disease and myocardial infarction. *World Journal of Cardiology*, 2016. **8**(1): p. 1.

32. Charlton-Menys, V. and P. Durrington, Human cholesterol metabolism and therapeutic molecules. *Experimental Physiology*, 2008. **93**(1): pp. 27–42.

33. Lian, C.-Y., et al., High fat diet-triggered non-alcoholic fatty liver disease: A review of proposed mechanisms. *Chemico-Biological Interactions*, 2020. **330**: p. 109199.

34. Raghow, R., et al., SREBPs: The crossroads of physiological and pathological lipid homeostasis. *Trends in Endocrinology & Metabolism*, 2008. **19**(2): pp. 65–73.

35. Daemen, S., M. Kutmon, and C.T. Evelo, A pathway approach to investigate the function and regulation of SREBPs. *Genes & Nutrition*, 2013. **8**(3): pp. 289–300.

36. Guengerich, F.P., et al., Recent structural insights into cytochrome P450 function. *Trends in Pharmacological Sciences*, 2016. **37**(8): pp. 625–640.

37. Miller, W.L. and R.J. Auchus, The molecular biology, biochemistry, and physiology of human steroidogenesis and its disorders. *Endocrine Reviews*, 2011. **32**(1): pp. 81–151.

38. Ratnayake, W.N. and C. Galli, Fat and fatty acid terminology, methods of analysis and fat digestion and metabolism. *Annals of Nutrition & Metabolism*, 2009. **55**(1/3): pp. 8–43.

39. Schneider, C., Chemistry and biology of vitamin E. *Molecular Nutrition & Food Research*, 2005. **49**(1): pp. 7–30.

40. Zaaboul, F. and Y. Liu, Vitamin E in foodstuff: Nutritional, analytical, and food technology aspects. *Comprehensive Reviews in Food Science and Food Safety*, 2022. **21**(2): pp. 964–998.

41. Bou Khalil, M., et al., Lipidomics era: Accomplishments and challenges. *Mass Spectrometry Reviews*, 2010. **29**(6): pp. 877–929.

42. Wang, J., et al., Biosynthesis of aromatic polyketides in microorganisms using type II polyketide synthases. *Microbial Cell Factories*, 2020. **19**: pp. 1–11.

43. Yu, O. and J.M. Jez, Nature's assembly line: Biosynthesis of simple phenylpropanoids and polyketides. *The Plant Journal*, 2008. **54**(4): pp. 750–762.

44. Zhang, Y., T. Zhang, Y. Liang, L. Jiang, and X. Sui, Dietary Bioactive Lipids: A review on absorption, metabolism, and health properties. *Journal of Agricultural and Food Chemistry*, 2021. **69**(32): pp. 8929–8943.

45. German, J.B., J.T. Smilowitz, and A.M. Zivkovic, Lipoproteins: When size really matters. *Current Opinion in Colloid & Interface Science*, 2006. **11**(2–3): pp. 171–183.

46. Berberich, A.J. and R.A. Hegele, A modern approach to dyslipidemia. *Endocrine Reviews*, 2022. **43**(4): pp. 611–653.

47. Jonas, A. and M.C. Phillips, Lipoprotein structure, in *Biochemistry of Lipids, Lipoproteins and Membranes*, 2008, Elsevier. pp. 485–506.

48. Haas, M.E., A.D. Attie, and S.B. Biddinger, The regulation of ApoB metabolism by insulin. *Trends in Endocrinology & Metabolism*, 2013. **24**(8): pp. 391–397.

49. Whitfield, A.J., et al., Lipid disorders and mutations in the APOB gene. *Clinical Chemistry*, 2004. **50**(10): pp. 1725–1732.

50. Khera, A.V. and D.J. Rader, Future therapeutic directions in reverse cholesterol transport. *Current Atherosclerosis Reports*, 2010. **12**: pp. 73–81.

51. Casula, M., et al., HDL in atherosclerotic cardiovascular disease: In search of a role. *Cells*, 2021. **10**(8): p. 1869.

52. Ali, K.M., et al., Cardiovascular disease risk reduction by raising HDL cholesterol–current therapies and future opportunities. *British Journal of Pharmacology*, 2012. **167**(6): pp. 1177–1194.

53. Li, Y., et al., Lipoprotein lipase: from gene to atherosclerosis. *Atherosclerosis*, 2014. **237**(2): pp. 597–608.

54. Kumari, A., et al., The importance of lipoprotein lipase regulation in atherosclerosis. *Biomedicines*, 2021. **9**(7): p. 782.

55. Aldanganova, K.K., The importance of modified lipoproteins in diabetes mellitus. *International Student's Journal of Medicine*, 2015. **1**(2): pp. 39–44.

56. Subramanian, S. and A. Chait, Hypertriglyceridemia secondary to obesity and diabetes. *Biochimica et Biophysica Acta (BBA)-Molecular and Cell Biology of Lipids*, 2012. **1821**(5): pp. 819–825.

57. Marcovina, S.M. and M.L. Koschinsky, Lipoprotein (a) as a risk factor for coronary artery disease. *The American Journal of Cardiology*, 1998. **82**(12): pp. 57U–66U.

58. Weiner, D.E. and M.J. Sarnak, Managing dyslipidemia in chronic kidney disease. *Journal of General Internal Medicine*, 2004. **19**(10): pp. 1045–1052.

59. Rehberger Likozar, A., M. Zavrtanik, and M. Šebeštjen, Lipoprotein (a) in atherosclerosis: from pathophysiology to clinical relevance and treatment options. *Annals of Medicine*, 2020. **52**(5): pp. 162–177.

60. Koutsogianni, A.D., et al., Oxidized phospholipids and lipoprotein (a): An update. *European Journal of Clinical Investigation*, 2022. **52**(4): p. e13710.

61. Carnethon, M.R., et al., Cardiovascular health in African Americans: A scientific statement from the American Heart Association. *Circulation*, 2017. **136**(21): pp. e393–e423.

62. Ginsberg, H.N., Lipoprotein metabolism and its relationship to atherosclerosis. *Medical Clinics of North America*, 1994. **78**(1): pp. 1–20.

63. Lambert, J.E. and E.J. Parks, Postprandial metabolism of meal triglyceride in humans. *Biochimica et Biophysica Acta (BBA)-Molecular and Cell Biology of Lipids*, 2012. **1821**(5): pp. 721–726.

64. Ehehalt, R., et al., Phosphatidylcholine as a constituent in the colonic mucosal barrier—Physiological and clinical relevance. *Biochimica et Biophysica Acta (BBA)-Molecular and Cell Biology of Lipids*, 2010. **1801**(9): pp. 983–993.

65. Lu, K., M.-H. Lee, and S.B. Patel, Dietary cholesterol absorption; more than just bile. *Trends in Endocrinology & Metabolism*, 2001. **12**(7): pp. 314–320.

66. Otokozawa, S., et al., Fasting and postprandial apolipoprotein B-48 levels in healthy, obese, and hyperlipidemic subjects. *Metabolism*, 2009. **58**(11): pp. 1536–1542.

67. Tomkin, G.H. and D. Owens, The chylomicron: Relationship to atherosclerosis. *International Journal of Vascular Medicine*, 2012. **2012**: p. 784536.

68. MacFarlane, N.G., Digestion and absorption. *Anaesthesia & Intensive Care Medicine*, 2018. **19**(3): pp. 125–127.

69. Dash, S., et al., New insights into the regulation of chylomicron production. *Annual Review of Nutrition*, 2015. **35**: pp. 265–294.

70. Baass, A., et al., Familial chylomicronemia syndrome: An under-recognized cause of severe hypertriglyceridaemia. *Journal of Internal Medicine*, 2020. **287**(4): pp. 340–348.

71. Miida, T. and S. Hirayama, Impacts of angiopoietin-like proteins on lipoprotein metabolism and cardiovascular events. *Current Opinion in Lipidology*, 2010. **21**(1): pp. 70–75.

72. Ramasamy, I., Update on the molecular biology of dyslipidemias. *Clinica Chimica Acta*, 2016. **454**: pp. 143–185.

73. Trajkovska, K.T. and S. Topuzovska, High-density lipoprotein metabolism and reverse cholesterol transport: Strategies for raising HDL cholesterol. *Anatolian Journal of Cardiology*, 2017. **18**(2): p. 149.

74. Liu, Y. and C. Tang, Regulation of ABCA1 functions by signaling pathways. *Biochimica et Biophysica Acta (BBA)-Molecular and Cell Biology of Lipids*, 2012. **1821**(3): pp. 522–529.

75. Rosenson, R.S., et al., Dysfunctional HDL and atherosclerotic cardiovascular disease. *Nature Reviews Cardiology*, 2016. **13**(1): pp. 48–60.

76. Wu, L. and K.G. Parhofer, Diabetic dyslipidemia. *Metabolism*, 2014. **63**(12): pp. 1469–1479.

77. Brown, W.V., High-density lipoprotein and transport of cholesterol and triglyceride in blood. *Journal of Clinical Lipidology*, 2007. **1**(1): pp. 7–19.

78. Shen, W.-J., S. Azhar, and F.B. Kraemer, SR-B1: a unique multifunctional receptor for cholesterol influx and efflux. *Annual Review of Physiology*, 2018. **80**: pp. 95–116.

79. Lin, C.-F., et al., Epidemiology of dyslipidemia in the Asia Pacific region. *International Journal of Gerontology*, 2018. **12**(1): pp. 2–6.

80. Ofori, E.K., et al., Dyslipidaemia is common among patients with type 2 diabetes: A cross-sectional study at Tema Port Clinic. *BMC Research Notes*, 2019. **12**(1): pp. 1–5.

81. Packard, C.J., J. Boren, and M.-R. Taskinen, Causes and consequences of hypertriglyceridemia. *Frontiers in Endocrinology*, 2020. **11**: p. 252.

82. Garg, A. and V. Simha, Update on dyslipidemia. *The Journal of Clinical Endocrinology & Metabolism*, 2007. **92**(5): pp. 1581–1589.

83. De Costa, G. and A. Park, Hyperlipidaemia. *Medicine*, 2017. **45**(9): pp. 579–582.

84. Kahn, B.B. and J.S. Flier, Obesity and insulin resistance. *The Journal of Clinical Investigation*, 2000. **106**(4): pp. 473–481.

85. Amblee, A., et al., Acute pancreatitis in patients with severe hypertriglyceridemia in a multiethnic minority population. *Endocrine Practice*, 2018. **24**(5): pp. 429–437.

86. Terlemez, S., et al., Insulin resistance in children with familial hyperlipidemia. *Journal of Pediatric Endocrinology and Metabolism*, 2018. **31**(12): pp. 1349–1354.

87. Castillo-Núñez, Y., E. Morales-Villegas, and C.A. Aguilar-Salinas, Triglyceride-rich lipoproteins: Their role in atherosclerosis. *Revista de investigación clínica*, 2022. **74**(2): pp. 61–70.

88. Chistiakov, D.A., et al., Mechanisms of foam cell formation in atherosclerosis. *Journal of Molecular Medicine*, 2017. **95**(11): pp. 1153–1165.

89. Olofsson, S.O. and J. Boren, Apolipoprotein B: A clinically important apolipoprotein which assembles atherogenic lipoproteins and promotes the development of atherosclerosis. *Journal of Internal Medicine*, 2005. **258**(5): pp. 395–410.

90. Jiang, H., et al., Mechanisms of oxidized LDL-mediated endothelial dysfunction and its consequences for the development of atherosclerosis. *Frontiers in Cardiovascular Medicine*, 2022. **9**: p. 925923.

91. Fredrickson, D.S., R.I. Levy, and R.S. Lees, Fat transport in lipoproteins—An integrated approach to mechanisms and disorders. *New England Journal of Medicine*, 1967. **276**(3): pp. 148–156.

92. Dron, J.S., and R.A. Hegele, Genetics of lipid and lipoprotein disorders and traits. *Current Genetic Medicine Reports*, 2016. **4**(3): pp. 130–141.

93. Benito-Vicente, A., et al., Familial hypercholesterolemia: The most frequent cholesterol metabolism disorder caused disease. *International Journal of Molecular Sciences*, 2018. **19**(11): p. 3426.

94. Fahed, A.C. and G.M. Nemer, Familial hypercholesterolemia: The lipids or the genes? *Nutrition & Metabolism*, 2011. **8**(1): pp. 1–12.

95. Ballout, R.A. and A.T. Remaley, Pediatric dyslipidemias: Lipoprotein metabolism disorders in children, in *Biochemical and Molecular Basis of Pediatric Disease*, 2021, Elsevier. pp. 965–1022.

96. Youngblom, E., M. Pariani, and J.W. Knowles, *Familial hypercholesterolemia*. 2016.

97. Gaddi, A., et al., Practical guidelines for familial combined hyperlipidemia diagnosis: An update. *Vascular Health and Risk Management*, 2007. **3**(6): pp. 877–886.

98. Koopal, C., A.D. Marais, and F.L. Visseren, Familial dysbetalipoproteinemia: An underdiagnosed lipid disorder. *Current Opinion in Endocrinology, Diabetes and Obesity*, 2017. **24**(2): pp. 133–139.

99. Boot, C.S., A. Luvai, and R.D. Neely, The clinical and laboratory investigation of dysbetalipo-proteinemia. *Critical Reviews in Clinical Laboratory Sciences*, 2020. **57**(7): pp. 458–469.

100. Brahm, A. and R.A. Hegele, Hypertriglyceridemia. *Nutrients*, 2013. **5**(3): pp. 981–1001.

101. Gotoda, T., et al., Diagnosis and management of type I and type V hyperlipoproteinemia. *Journal of Atherosclerosis and Thrombosis*, 2012. **19**(1): pp. 1–12.

102. Shin, J.A., et al., Metabolic syndrome as a predictor of type 2 diabetes, and its clinical inter-pretations and usefulness. *Journal of Diabetes Investigation*, 2013. **4**(4): pp. 334–343.

103. Sugden, M. and M. Holness, Pathophysiology of diabetic dyslipidemia: Implications for ath-erogenesis and treatment. *Clinical Lipidology*, 2011. **6**(4): pp. 401–411.

104. Mavromati, M. and F.R. Jornayvaz, Hypothyroidism-associated dyslipidemia: Potential molecular mechanisms leading to NAFLD. *International Journal of Molecular Sciences*, 2021. **22**(23): p. 12797.

105. Dullaart, R., et al., The activity of cholesteryl ester transfer protein is decreased in hypothy-roidism: A possible contribution to alterations in high-density lipoproteins. *European Journal of Clinical Investigation*, 1990. **20**(6): pp. 581–587.

106. Klop, B., A.T. do Rego, and M.C. Cabezas, Alcohol and plasma triglycerides. *Current Opinion in Lipidology*, 2013. **24**(4): pp. 321–326.

107. Masana, L., et al., Low HDL and high triglycerides predict COVID-19 severity. *Scientific Reports*, 2021. **11**(1): p. 7217.

108. Puntoni, M., et al., Tangier disease: Epidemiology, pathophysiology, and management. *American Journal of Cardiovascular Drugs*, 2012. **12**: pp. 303–311.

109. Ossoli, A., et al., Lipoprotein X causes renal disease in LCAT deficiency. *PLoS One*, 2016. **11**(2): p. e0150083.

110. Agarwala, A., et al., Dietary management of dyslipidemia and the impact of dietary patterns on lipid disorders. *Progress in Cardiovascular Diseases*, 2022. **75**: pp. 49–58.

111. Harada-Shiba, M., et al., Guidance for pediatric familial hypercholesterolemia 2017. *Journal of Atherosclerosis and Thrombosis*, 2018. **25**(6): pp. 539–553.

112. Faltaos, D.W., et al., Use of an indirect effect model to describe the LDL cholesterol-lowering effect by statins in hypercholesterolaemic patients. *Fundamental & Clinical Pharmacology*, 2006. **20**(3): pp. 321–330.

113. Sinthupoom, N., et al., Nicotinic acid and derivatives as multifunctional pharmacophores for medical applications. *European Food Research and Technology*, 2015. **240**: pp. 1–17.

114. Bays, H., Cholesterol Absorption Inhibitors (Ezetimibe) and Bile Acid Binding Resins (Colesevelam HCl) as Therapy for Dyslipidemia in Patients with Diabetes Mellitus, in *Lipoproteins in Diabetes Mellitus*. 2013, Springer. pp. 415–433.

115. Fazio, S. and M.F. Linton, The role of fibrates in managing hyperlipidemia: Mechanisms of action and clinical efficacy. *Current Atherosclerosis Reports*, 2004. **6**(2): pp. 148–157.

10 Mineral Metabolism and Metabolic Bone Diseases

Shradha Devi Dwivedi, Divya Sahu, Lokendra Singh Rathor,
Deependra Singh, and Manju Rawat Singh

10.1 INTRODUCTION

Mineral metabolism is the process by which the body regulates the levels of minerals, like phosphorus, calcium, magnesium, and salt, in the blood and tissues. These minerals are necessary for a number of processes, including bone development, nerve conduction, muscle contraction, and enzyme functioning. Hormones, food consumption, renal function, and other factors all have an impact on how minerals are metabolized. The main mineral metabolism regulator and repository for calcium and phosphate is the bone. Osteocytes, osteoblasts, and osteoclasts are the key bone remodeling cells that maintain the balance of bone mass. Hence, any dysfunctions of bone homeostasis affect bone and mineral metabolism. However, a variety of factors, including poor diet, changes in the microbiota, and aging, can affect the homeostasis of bones and minerals [1]. Other systemic diseases or hormonal imbalances frequently endanger the equilibrium of the bones. Disorders like diabetes or renal insufficiency affect bone formation and resorption, followed by alterations in the production of bone hormones. These events compromise bone health, leading to fractures and complications. Many of these conditions aggravate inflammatory reactions that worsen bone loss and resorption, leading to metabolic bone diseases.

Metabolic bone disease (MBD) encompasses an assorted group of diseases that diffusely influence anomalies in bone turnover and mineral metabolism [2]. Rheumatoid osteodystrophy, Paget's disease, rickets, osteoporosis, and osteomalacia are a few of the major MBDs. Numerous problems, including fractures, deformities, discomfort, and a lower quality of life, can result from these disorders. Promoting bone health and preventing the onset of metabolic bone disease requires maintaining optimal amounts of calcium, phosphorus, and vitamin D, as well as taking care of any underlying hormonal or medical disorders [3].

The underlying reason, the severity of the symptoms, and the patient's general health all play a role in the diagnosis and treatment of metabolic bone diseases. A sufficient diet of calcium and vitamin D, regular exercise, abstaining from tobacco use and excessive alcohol use, and monitoring bone density and blood tests are some broad strategies that can help prevent or treat metabolic bone diseases. Several blood and urinary molecules have been identified as markers of bone metabolic activity over the past ten years of research and development, providing estimates of the rates and directions of the biological processes regulating bone turnover [4]. Bone turnover markers (BTMs) are generally subdivided into two categories: bone formation/resorption and osteoclastogenesis biomarkers that can be determined via commercial testing. The bone alkaline phosphatase (BSAP), N-terminal propeptide (PINP), osteocalcin (OC), and C-terminal propeptide of type-I procollagen (PICP) are markers of bone formation that result from osteoblastic activity. The breakdown of type-I collagen produces markers of bone resorption and osteoclastogenesis, such as the intermolecular crosslinks deoxypyridinoline (DPD), pyridinoline (PYD), the C-terminal telopeptide (CTX), the tartrate-resistant acid phosphate 5b isoform (TRAP-5b), N-terminal telopeptide (NTX), and type I collagen fragments produced by matrix metalloproteases (MMP) or ICTP, and the receptor activator of nuclear factor NF-κB ligand (RANKL), an osteoclast regulatory protein produced by osteoblasts, osteocytes, and immune system cells. This chapter attempts to provide an overview of the causative factors of mineral metabolic bone disorders, the various types of MBDs (osteoporosis, rickets and osteomalacia, hyperparathyroidism, hypophosphatasia, renal osteodystrophy, hypoparathyroidism, hyperthyroidism, hypothyroidism, scurvy, and acromegaly), and different available treatment strategies (commercial and novel).

10.2 METABOLIC BONE DISEASES AND THEIR CAUSATIVE FACTORS

Metabolic bone diseases (MBDs) are a group of disorders that affect the normal mineralization, growth, density, strength, and structure of bones. Several causative factors can contribute to the development of MBD depending on the specific conditions [5]. However, here are some general factors that can play a role in mineral metabolism and contribute to metabolic bone diseases: genetics, organ dysfunction and mitochondrial dysfunction, abnormalities in the levels of minerals like calcium (Ca^{2+}) or phosphorus (P^{2+}), vitamin D, or an abnormality of bone structure. Some

DOI: 10.1201/9781003384823-10

factors that can worsen osteoporosis include decreased estrogen in women, a family history of the condition, small bones, poor diet, excessive alcohol use, and smoking [6].

Two of the most significant minerals involved in bone metabolism are Ca^{2+} and P^{2+}. In contrast to P^{2+}, which is necessary for the production of the hydroxyapatite crystals that give bone its strength, Ca^{2+} is essential for the mineralization of bone. An imbalance of Ca^{2+} and P^{2+} in the body can cause anomalies in mineral metabolism and bone turnover, which can result in MBD. Another essential nutrient, vitamin D, is crucial for the metabolism of minerals and bone health. In addition to being essential for the control of parathyroid hormone (PTH), which aids in maintaining the body's Ca^{2+} balance, vitamin D is also important in the absorption of Ca^{2+} and P^{2+} from food [7]. A vitamin D deficit can result in decreased Ca^{2+} absorption, increased PTH secretion, and bone loss, as well as the emergence of MBD. The body's mineral balance is crucially maintained by hormones. Hormonal abnormalities can cause decreased bone density and an increased risk of fractures, such as lower estrogen levels in postmenopausal women or lower PTH output. Kidneys play a crucial part in controlling the balance of minerals in the body by eliminating waste products and ensuring correct levels of calcium and phosphate in the body. Renal osteodystrophy and other similar disorders can result from poor mineral metabolism in chronic kidney disease (CKD) [8].

MBD also arises due to some specific genetic abnormalities that impair mineral metabolism. Examples include familial hypophosphatemia, a hereditary illness characterized by low levels of phosphate in the blood, and osteogenesis imperfecta, a genetic ailment that affects collagen formation and bone strength. Certain drugs or medical procedures may influence the metabolism of minerals and increase the risk of MBD. For instance, long-term corticosteroid use raises the risk of osteoporosis and bone loss. Additionally, chemotherapy and hormonal therapies for cancer might have a negative impact on bone health. The risk of MBD can rise as a result of certain lifestyle choices, which can affect mineral metabolism. These include a sedentary lifestyle, binge drinking, smoking, and inadequate nutrition. It is crucial to remember that the underlying causes of metabolic bone diseases can be multifactorial, which means that a number of different factors may interact and play a role in the emergence of these conditions. Additionally, depending on the exact metabolic bone disease under consideration, the specific components might change [9].

10.3 TYPES OF METABOLIC BONE DISEASES

A variety of diseases marked by anomalies in bone metabolism fall under the umbrella term of metabolic bone diseases (Figure 10.1). These illnesses can result in weaker bones, a higher risk of fractures, and other consequences. Metabolic bone disease is classified into

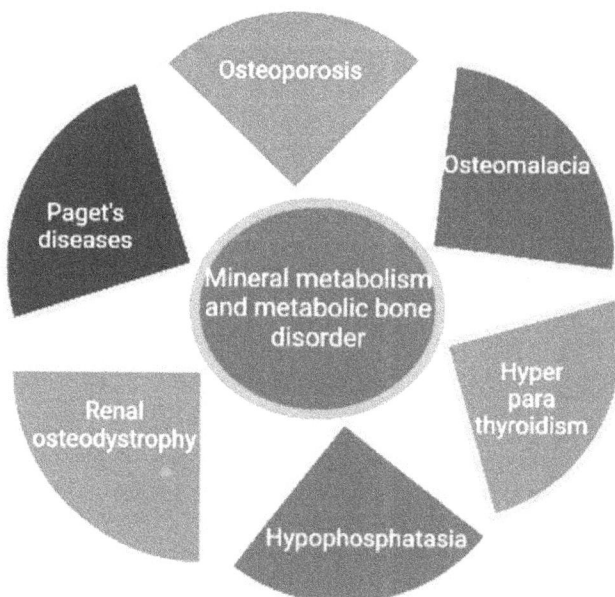

Figure 10.1 Types of metabolic bone diseases

numerous kinds, including fibrous dysplasia, osteoporosis, renal osteodystrophy, osteomalacia, Hyperparathyroidism, Paget's disease of bone, and rickets.

10.3.1 Osteoporosis

Osteoporosis is a common MBD characterized by decreased bone density and degradation of bone tissue, resulting in increased bone fragility and a higher risk of fracture. It primarily affects elderly people, particularly postmenopausal women; however, men can also acquire osteoporosis. Osteoporosis, also known as the "silent disease", may not manifest symptoms until a fracture occurs. Fractures most usually damage the spine, hip, wrist, or other bones, and even mild falls or bumps can result in severe osteoporosis [10].

Hormonal variables play an important part in the pathophysiology of osteoporosis. When estrogen levels fall in women following menopause, bone loss speeds up. Estrogen helps control bone remodeling and has a protective effect on bone. The rate of bone resorption rises when estrogen levels are decreased. Loss of bone mass in men may also be influenced by age-related declines in testosterone levels [11]. Osteoporosis is significantly increased by aging. Age-related declines in bone remodeling efficiency result in a shift in the ratio of increasing bone resorption to decreased bone synthesis. The slow loss of bone density and strength due to aging is facilitated by this age-related bone loss. In order to maintain healthy bones, calcium and vitamin D are necessary. Reduced Ca^{2+} availability for bone mineralization can be brought on by insufficient dietary Ca^{2+} and vitamin D consumption, poor absorption, or low vitamin D levels. PTH is secreted as a coping mechanism, encouraging bone resorption to release calcium into the bloodstream. Bone loss can become more pronounced when PTH is elevated chronically [12].

10.3.2 Osteomalacia

Osteomalacia is a weakening of the bones caused mostly by a lack of vitamin D or defective vitamin D metabolism. It causes bone pain, muscle weakness, and an increased risk of fractures by reducing bone mineralization. Both children (as rickets) and adults can develop osteomalacia. Because of the lower levels of active vitamin D (calcitriol), osteomalacia affects how well calcium is absorbed from the intestines. Hypocalcemia (low calcium levels in the bloodstream) is the result of this. To stimulate calcium release from the bones, greater calcium reabsorption in the kidneys, and enhanced vitamin D activation in the kidneys, the parathyroid glands secrete PTH [13].

PTH levels that are too high encourage bone resorption, which causes bone tissue to break down and release calcium into the circulation. The increased bone resorption will continue if the underlying cause of osteomalacia, such as a vitamin D deficiency, is not treated, leading to further bone loss and thinning. Increased bone remodeling is brought on by osteomalacia in an effort to strengthen the weaker bone. Both osteoclasts (involved in bone resorption) and osteoblasts (involved in bone production), are activated as a result of the enhanced bone turnover [14]. However, because of the faults in mineralization, the newly produced bone is insufficiently mineralized, continuing the cycle of weakening bone.

10.3.3 Paget's Disease

Paget's disease is a long-term condition characterized by aberrant bone remodeling. It causes excessive bone breakdown and production, resulting in structurally deformed and weaker bone. The spine, pelvis, skull, and long bones are frequently damaged. Paget's disease can result in bone discomfort, abnormalities, fractures, and other problems [15].

In Paget's disease, bone resorption first increases, leading to an excessive disintegration of bone tissue. Osteoclasts become overactive and larger than normal, leading to enhanced bone resorption. The increased osteoclastic activity can lead to the formation of irregularly shaped, disorganized bone. New bone is formed as a defense against the accelerated bone resorption. The freshly produced bone, however, exhibits aberrant structural development and disorganized architecture [16].

The osteoblasts, responsible for bone formation, attempt to lay down new bone, but the process is inefficient and leads to the characteristic thickened, enlarged, and weakened bone seen in Paget's disease. An imbalance between bone resorption and bone production underlies the pathophysiology of Paget's disease. The disease's hallmark bone abnormalities, increased bone fragility, and risk of fractures are caused by bone resorption, despite the fact that both processes are elevated. The severity and clinical manifestations of Paget's disease can vary greatly from person to person, and symptoms, including bone pain, deformities, fractures, and consequences like osteoarthritis or nerve compression, may be present or absent altogether [17].

10.3.4 Renal Osteodystrophy

Renal osteodystrophy is a type of bone alteration that occurs as a result of CKD. In CKD, poor renal function results in decreased P^{2+} excretion and decreased vitamin D activation. As a result, serum P^{2+} levels rise while levels of active vitamin D (calcitriol) fall. Phosphate levels in the blood can cause osteocytes to secrete fibroblast growth factor 23 (FGF-23). Depending on the underlying processes, renal osteodystrophy can result in either high-turnover or low-turnover bone disease. Vitamin D (25-hydroxyvitamin D) is converted by the kidneys into its active form, calcitriol (1, 25-dihydroxyvitamin D). Reduced renal function in CKD leads to decreased calcitriol production. Calcitriol is required for Ca^{2+} absorption from the intestine, as well as bone mineralization. Insufficient calcitriol causes decreased intestinal Ca^{2+} absorption and hypocalcemia. The parathyroid glands secrete more PTH in response to low Ca^{2+} levels and elevated P^{2+} and FGF-23 levels [18]. PTH regulates calcium and phosphate balance in the bones, kidneys, and intestines. In renal osteodystrophy, however, high PTH levels are frequently insufficient to maintain normal Ca^{2+} and P^{2+} levels, resulting in secondary hyperparathyroidism. Increased osteoclast activity and bone resorption are caused by the persistent elevation of PTH levels, which accelerates bone resorption. Bone development is also compromised as a result of vitamin D deficiency-related poor mineralization. MBD is brought on by these imbalances between bone resorption and production, which cause aberrant bone turnover [19].

Overall, altered bone turnover, secondary hyperparathyroidism, disordered mineral metabolism, and reduced vitamin D activation are all part of the pathogenesis of renal osteodystrophy. Numerous abnormalities of the bone are caused by these processes, including osteomalacia (softening of the bones as a result of poor mineralization), osteitis fibrosa cystica (increased bone resorption and fibrosis), and a dynamic bone disease (reduced bone turnover). The underlying etiology, duration, and stage of chronic kidney disease can all affect the severity and type of renal osteodystrophy.

10.3.5 Hyperparathyroidism

Hyperparathyroidism is a disorder in which the parathyroid glands create an excess of PTH, which regulates calcium levels in the body. PTH elevations can cause greater bone resorption, resulting in weaker bones. A benign tumor in one or more parathyroid glands is the most prevalent cause of primary hyperparathyroidism [20].

10.3.6 Hypophosphatasia

Hypophosphatasia is a rare hereditary condition characterized by insufficient alkaline phosphatase activity. This enzyme is required for the mineralization of bones. Hypophosphatasia can cause skeletal deformities and decreased bone growth in children and osteomalacia in adults [21].

10.4 TREATMENT STRATEGIES

Numerous therapies have been developed for the most effective management of MBD, which depends on the specific condition being addressed. There are two groups of treatment approaches. Treatment-based techniques are covered in one class, while delivery-based ones are covered in the second. Chemical, enzymatic, gene, and hormone-based therapies are examples of treatment-based techniques, and they can be supplied in the proper ways using both traditional and novel delivery systems. Vesicular, particle, self-assembled, and cellular carriers are frequently used in novel systems. For the local treatment of RA, targeted therapies delivering medications, enzymes, oligonucleotides, genes, and/or peptides to the sick region are particularly desirable.

10.4.1 Treatment-Based Approaches

10.4.1.1 Essential Nutrients

Although Ca^{2+} appears to have some favorable benefits on bone mineral density (BMD), there is debate over whether it is effective in preventing fractures caused by MBD. A meta-analysis by Shea et al. found that calcium supplementation very modestly increased BMD compared to a placebo. The total percentage change from the starting point was 2.05%. Similar results from a trial involving 1,471 healthy postmenopausal women were reported by Tai et al. Total BMD improved with Ca^{2+} supplementation, with a 1.2% difference between the calcium and placebo groups after five years [22]. According to a meta-analysis by Tang et al., Ca^{2+} supplementation was linked to a 12% lower incidence of fractures (relative risk [RR], 0.88; 95% confidence interval [CI], 0.83–0.95) [23]. According to several studies, Ca^{2+} lowers the risk of vertebral fractures but has no effect on non-vertebral fractures. However, some research indicated that calcium had little impact on osteoporotic fractures. The efficacy may be constrained by long-term compliance.

Recent research has concentrated on the interaction between Ca^{2+} and vitamin D. A meta-analysis revealed a significant 15% decrease in the overall osteoporotic fractures summary relative risk estimations. However, Kahwati et al. found through a systematic review that this combination was not linked to a lower incidence of total fractures (one RCT, n = 36,282; absolute risk difference [ARD], 0.35%; 95% CI, 1.02% to 0.31%) or hip fractures (two RCTs, n = 36,727; ARD from the larger trial, 0.14%; 95% CI, 0.34%) [24].

In three randomized controlled trials (RCTs), individuals who received vitamin K_2 (Menatetrenone) had higher lumbar BMD, with percentage changes ranging from −0.5% to 1.74%. Menatetrenone can prevent both vertebral and non-vertebral fractures, according to a meta-analysis of RCTs of postmenopausal women and patients using oral steroids for kidney disease (OR favoring vitamin K2 in vertebral fractures, 0.40 [95% CI, 0.25–0.65]; OR in non-vertebral fractures, 0.19 [95% CI, 0.11–0.35]). Menatetrenone, according to Shiraki et al., can mostly prevent vertebral fractures over the course of two years (10.9% at 12 months in the vitamin K2 group versus 30.3% in the control group) [25]. Menatetrenone could reduce the incidence of vertebral fracture in patients with at least five vertebral fractures at enrollment by 39% (20.3% in the calcium plus vitamin K2 group vs. 33% in the calcium-only group, p = 0.029), according to a significant phase IV RCT conducted in Japan for osteoporotic fractures. Menatetrenone monotherapy can somewhat raise the lumbar spine BMD, and it mostly lowers the incidence of vertebral fractures, according to a recent review by Iwamoto et al. [26].

10.4.1.2 Hormone-Based Therapies

The parathyroid gland releases PTH, an 84-amino-acid polypeptide, primarily in reaction to low blood Ca^{2+} levels. The hormone modifies serum phosphate and Ca^{2+} levels. PTH binding to osteoblasts causes them to express more RANKL. PTH thus indirectly promotes osteoclast differentiation and activity. As a result, PTH increases the release of Ca^{2+} during bone resorption. Thus, PTH is crucial for bone remodeling. The biologically active portion of the skeleton is called teriparatide (PTH1-34), which is made up of the first 34 N-terminal amino acids of PTH. It is widely established that administering PTH1-34 continuously has a catabolic effect while doing so intermittently has an anabolic effect on bone. Abaloparatide (PTHrP1-34) is a PTH-related protein analogue that shares a similarity with PTH1-34 and has been linked to humoral hypercalcemia of malignancy. Both PTH-receptor 1 and the PTHrP-specific receptor are involved in PTHrP1-34's actions. A number of abaloparatide clinical trials have lately been reported. Increases in lumbar spine BMD were comparable 24 weeks after beginning treatment involving 80 g of daily abaloparatide and 20 g of daily teriparatide (6.7% and 5.5%, respectively) in a multicenter, international, double-blind placebo experiment involving 222 postmenopausal women with osteoporosis. Abaloparatide and teriparatide, in that order, enhanced femoral neck BMD by 3.1% and 1.1%, respectively. Additionally, total hip BMD increased more significantly (2.6% vs. 0.5%) following abaloparatide treatment than after teriparatide treatment .

Since postmenopausal osteoporosis was first identified in 1940, estrogen insufficiency in postmenopausal women has been acknowledged as a potential risk factor for the impairment of bone production [6]. Based on increases in both bone resorption and formation markers, it has been hypothesized that bone remodeling is expedited during menopause. Therefore, in contrast to the initial theory, it appears that increased bone resorption rather than reduced bone formation is what primarily contributes to bone loss in the context of a shortage of estrogen. Cellular targets of sex steroid action in vivo have been identified as a result of the recent development of mice models that use the Cre/LoxP system to delete the estrogen receptor in particular cell types. According to Almeida et al., ablation of estrogen receptors (ERs) in mesenchymal progenitors or from osteoblast progenitors (using Prx1- or Osx1-Cre) resulted in a reduction in cortical bone mass and periosteal bone apposition [27]. The potentiation of Wnt/-catenin signaling, which boosts the proliferation and differentiation of periosteal osteoblast progenitor cells, was responsible for these results. On the other hand, bone bulk and architecture were unaffected by ER loss in osteoblasts and osteocytes expressing Col1a1- or Dmp1-Cre [93, 94]. The OPG/RANKL system is one of estrogen's most significant downstream mediators, even though its effect on osteoblast lineage has not yet been fully understood. For the bone resorption process, calcitonin is a primary choice. Selective estrogen receptor modulator (SERM) medications like raloxifene can be prescribed to prevent bone loss in postmenopausal women. Calcitonin is a peptide hormone secreted by the parafollicular cells of the thyroid gland. It binds to the osteoporosis membrane receptor and reduces their motility and bone resorption ability. Calcitonin prevents osteoclast precursors from maturing and also has a pain relief effect [24]

10.4.1.3 Gene Therapy

Gene therapy has potential in the treatment of osteoporosis. Small interfering RNA (siRNA) therapy has shown tremendous potential for the treatment of osteoporosis. A siRNA-mediated knockdown of a nuclear factor of active T cells (NFATc1), a transcription factor involved in osteoclast formation, can inhibit LPS-induced osteoclast generation in murine monocyte RAW264.7 cells. A knockdown of PPAR-γ or adiponectin receptor 1 in osteoblastic cells from a liposome-based siRNA transfection prevented the down-regulation of mRNA expression of Runx-related transcription factor 2 (Runx2) [28]. siRNA delivery targeting of RANK to both RAW264.7 and primary bone marrow cell cultures produced a short-term repression of RANK expression without off-target effects, and significantly inhibited both osteoclast formation and bone resorption [29]. One of gene therapy's most significant benefits is the ability to express the protein as needed, whether locally and focally or more widely. Notably, gene therapy opens the door to protein creation within cells. As a result, this makes therapeutic routes possible. It is a safe and effective approach that could have a significant impact on today's incurable diseases [30].

10.4.1.4 Chemical Treatment

Nitrogen-containing BPs (N-BPs) and the human monoclonal antibody denosumab are very effective in slowing this bone decay. Bisphosphonate drugs help reduce bone loss and improve bone density. Examples include alendronate, risedronate, and ibandronate. Newer antiresorptives include cathepsin K inhibitors, which act on the cysteine protease cathepsin K, highly expressed in osteoclasts and essential for the digestion of cartilage and bone collagenous matrix. Additionally, another class used in osteoporosis therapy is represented by selective estrogen receptor modulators (SERMs) and tissue-selective estrogen complexes (TSECs) [31].

Anti-resorptive drugs, which suppress bone resorption, include calcitonin, estrogen and selective estrogen receptor modulators (SERMs), bisphosphonates (BPs), and anti-RANKL antibody. Anabolic drugs, which enhance bone formation, include parathyroid hormone (PTH) and sclerostin inhibitors. Additionally, stem cell therapies for osteoporosis have been receiving increased attention in recent years.

10.4.1.5 Other Treatments

Teriparatide is a form of parathyroid hormone (PTH) that stimulates bone formation and can be used in severe osteoporosis cases. If the condition is caused by a parathyroid tumor (primary hyperparathyroidism), surgical removal of the tumor may be necessary. For the treatment of hypercalcemia, adequate hydration with intravenous fluids may be required to help flush out excess calcium from the bloodstream. (Diuretics or bisphosphonates may be prescribed to lower calcium levels.) Addressing the underlying condition responsible for hypercalcemia is crucial. It is important to consult a healthcare professional, such as an endocrinologist or a rheumatologist, for a thorough evaluation and personalized treatment plan based on the specific condition and individual needs. Hormone replacement therapy (HRT) is used for postmenopausal women; hormone replacement therapy may be considered to alleviate symptoms of menopause, including bone loss. Some lifestyle modifications are also applicable, such as regular exercise (weight-bearing exercises, resistance training, and activities that promote balance can help strengthen bones), a balanced diet (consuming a diet rich in calcium, vitamin D, and other essential nutrients is important for bone health), smoking cessation (smoking can negatively affect bone health, so quitting smoking is beneficial), and limiting alcohol intake (excessive alcohol consumption can impair bone formation and increase the risk of fractures).

There are several treatment strategies for metabolic bone diseases and disorders of mineral metabolism. These strategies vary depending on the specific condition being treated. For example, for osteoporosis and osteomalacia, calcium and vitamin D supplementation is imperative. Bisphosphonates may also be given to increase bone mass. In premature neonates with metabolic bone disease (MBD), management includes adequate calcium, phosphorous, and vitamin D supplementation, along with optimum nutrition and physical activity. Diagnosis of metabolic bone diseases is made through analysis of metabolic bone blood chemistries as well as radiologic studies such as dual energy X-ray absorptiometry (DXA) scans, bone scans, and X-rays .

10.5 DELIVERY-BASED APPROACHES

Various lipid-based nano-delivery systems are used in treating the bone mineral metabolism and bone-deforming diseases, such as liposome tranferosome, noisome, tocosome, spingosome, ufosome, etc. Liposomes can deliver drugs directly to the area where they work and keep them there for a long time without causing harm. Conventional liposomes typically have significant concentrations of non-bioactive lipids such as cholesterol and phospholipids, which do not naturally promote bone regeneration. Additionally, liposomes can be used in a variety of ways to transport scaffolds or genes to the damaged bone in order to encourage bone regeneration. The negative consequences of medication delivery that occurs off-target are avoided by using liposomes to deliver various pharmaceuticals and targeting agents to the bone in a cell-specific targeted manner. They can integrate numerous medications and distribute them through different pathways in a regulated release pattern with improved bioavailability and fewer side effects [32]. The delivery-based approaches for the mineral metabolism and metabolic bone diseases are shown in Table 10.1.

Table 10.1   Delivery-based approaches used for various mineral bone diseases

Disease's Name	Delivery System	Formulation	Outcomes	References
Delayed fracture	Liposomes	Salvianic acid-loaded bone-targeting liposome formulation (SAA-BTL)	SAA-BTL significantly improves fracture callus formation and micro-architecture with accelerated mineralization rate in callus	[33]
Osteoarthritis	Liposomes	Adenosine	Adenosine A2A receptor suppresses OA via increases in M1 macrophage infiltration in the joint synovium	[34]
	Polymeric nanoparticles	CrmA-HA- Chitosan nanoparticles	HA/CS/pCrmA nanoparticles on synoviocytes in OA, decreased MMP–3 and MMP–13 gene expression levels	[35]
	Dendrimers	PAMAM/IGF-1	Through reversible electrostatic interaction mechanism with anionic cartilage tissue to improve tissue binding, penetration, and residence time	[36]
		Clodronate	Depletion of synovial lining cells which reduced production of biochemicals and prevention of cartilage damage, synovial hyperplasia, and proteoglycans loss; reduction in joint inflammation, joint swelling, and osteophyte	[37]
	Nanoparticles	Etoricoxib-loaded bio-adhesive hybridized polylactic acid-based nanoparticles	Formulation-enhanced ALP activity and increased calcium ion deposition and binding	[38]
	Polymeric nanoparticles	Curcuminoid-HA-CNPs	NPs interact with tissues and reflect biochemicals which change the structural properties of the cartilage ECM and synovial fluid	[39]

	Micelles	MRC-PPL/Psoralidin	Overexpressed matrix metalloproteinases-13 (MMP-13) are characteristic markers in osteoarthritis (OA) treatment	[40]
	Nanoparticles	Fish oil protein (FP), gold nanoparticles-dipalmitoyl phosphatidylcholine (GNP)	FP increased the hydrophilicity of GNP, while encapsulation of FP-GNP within liposomes increased the hydrophobicity	[41]
	Micelles	HA-PEG/KGN	Formulation is prepared by co-valent cross-linking	[36]
	Polymeric nanoparticles	Etoricoxib/PLGA-PEG-PLGA	Inhibited the expression of inflammation mediators and chondro-protective effect to celecoxib through down-regulating matrix degrading enzymes matrix metalloproteinase-13 (MMP-13) and a disintegrin and metalloproteinase with thrombospondin motifs (ADAMTS-5)	[42]
	Nanoparticles	Berberine chloride-loaded chitosan nanoparticles	Formulation is prepared by ion-crosslinking mechanism	[43]
Osteolysis	Microspheres	Bisphosphonate Loaded Microspheres	Chitosan microspheres gave first order release while PLGA microspheres gave zero order release	[44]
	Liposomes	Curcumin-loaded liposome (Cur-LP)	Cur-LPs have great potential for the clinical treatment of inflammatory osteolysis by modulating macrophage polarization and secretion of inflammatory factors	[45]
	Nanoparticles	Melatonin assuages titanium nanoparticles	Butyrate alleviated osteolysis via activating its receptor GPR109A, and suppressing the activation of NLRP3 infammasome triggered by Ti-particles	[46]
	Nanoparticles	Polyether-ether-ketone ZnO NPs	ZnO NPs attenuated polymer wear particle-induced inflammation via regulation of the MEK-ERK-COX-2 axis and reduced bone tissue damage caused by particle-induced inflammatory osteolysis	[47]
	Liposomes	RANKL-directed siRNAs loaded in cationic liposome RPR209120/DOPE	Formulation inhibitS RANKL expression by small interfering RNAs (Rkl-siRNAs) combined with cationic liposome RPR209120/DOPE to treat osteosarcoma	[48]

Bone diseases (including osteoporosis, osteoarthritis, and bone cancer)	Lipid nanoparticles	Calcium phosphate-coated lipid nanoparticles	CaP-coated NPs have a higher uptake by osteosarcoma cells	[49]
Osteoporosis	Dendrimers	PEGylated carboxylic acid-modified polyamidoamine dendrimers	Fluorescein isothiocyanate-labeled PEG(5)-Asp-PAMAM predominantly accumulated on eroded and quiescent surfaces	[50]
	Nanoparticles	Silica nanoparticle functionalized with ALN modified PEG	Fluorescein isothiocyanate-labeled PEG(5)-Asp-PAMAM predominantly accumulated on eroded and quiescent surfaces	[51]
	Nanoparticles	Iron oxide nanoparticles	BTNPs target surface of bone and reduces bone loss	[52]
	Liposomes	ZEB1 gene-loaded liposome	Reversal of low level of ZEB1/Notch signaling	[53]
	Nanoparticles	siRNA and osteostatin-loaded mesoporous silica nanoparticles	siRNA and osteostatin-loaded nanoparticles increase the bone microarchitecture and augment expression of osteogenic allied genes.	[51]
Femur fracture	Exosomes	BMSC-Exosome-Aptamer Complex	miRNA, lncRNA, and proteins carried by exosomes generated from cells related to bone may serve as possible bone markers to assess and identify disorders connected to bone	[54]
Osteoporotic diseases (Paget's disease, Legg Calve Perthes disease, osteogenesis imperfecta)	Gold nanoparticles	Alendronate and pamidronate functionalized gold nanoparticles	Bisphosphonate functionalized gold nanoparticles reduce osteoporotic symptoms	[55]
Osteochondral defect	Hydrogel	Semi-solid hydrogel carrier drug with MSC	Synergistic effect in area of bone defects	[56]
Hyperparathyroidism	Carbon nanoparticles	Suspension of carbon nanoparticles	Cure secondary hyperparathyroidism in uremic patients	[57]
Bone deformation	Exosome with hydrogel	HA-based hydrogels encapsulated with MSCs-exosome	Prepared hydrogel through crosslinking mechanism shows mechanical properties in bone regeneration	[58]
Osteoporosis	Serum	Serum micro-RNAs noninvasive biomarkers expression	miRNA-23a-3p and miRNA-124-3p increase osteoblastogenesis and osteoclastogenesis	[59]

Abbreviations: MRC: MMP-13 responsive/Coll-II 1 chain-binding peptide–CollB; ALN: alendronate; HA: hyaluronic acid; PEG: poly (ethylene glycol); HA/CS-CrmA: hyaluronic acid-chitosan nanoparticles containing plasmid DNA encoding CrmA; RANKL: receptor activator of nuclear factor κB ligand; ZnO NPs: zinc oxide nanoparticles; BTNPs: bone-targeting iron oxide nanoparticles; siRNA: small interfering RNA; ZEB1: zinc-finger transcription factor

10.6 CONCLUSION

Mineral metabolism and subsequent metabolic bone disorders have been treated based on different treatment strategies. All treatment accentuates the significance of fast recognition of these diseases, understanding their pathophysiology consequences, and scheduling interventions to protect from complications. In recent years, innovative nano-delivery approaches to allow drugs to reach a particular site in the body with non-toxicity, biocompatibility, stability, and bioavailability have succeeded over conventional therapy. These treatment strategies and delivery-based approaches could be a major breakthrough in future for mineral metabolism and metabolic bone disorder.

REFERENCES

1. H.M. Kronenberg, Bone and mineral metabolism: Where are we, where are we going, and how will we get there? *J. Clin. Endocrinol. Metab.* 101 (2016) 795–798. https://doi.org/10.1210/jc.2015-3607.

2. M.L. Ojeda, F. Nogales, O. Carreras, E. Pajuelo, M. del C. Gallego-López, I. Romero-Herrera, B. Begines, J. Moreno-Fernández, J. Díaz-Castro, A. Alcudia, Different effects of low selenite and selenium-nanoparticle supplementation on adipose tissue function and insulin secretion in adolescent male rats, *Nutrients.* 14 (2022). https://doi.org/10.3390/nu14173571.

3. J.C. Fleet, R. Replogle, D.E. Salt, Systems genetics of mineral metabolism, *J. Nutr.* 141 (2011) 520–525. https://doi.org/10.3945/jn.110.128736.

4. T. Cavalier-Smith, Higher classification and phylogeny of Euglenozoa, *Eur. J. Protistol.* 56 (2016) 250–276. https://doi.org/10.1016/j.ejop.2016.09.003.

5. N. Charoenngam, A. Nasr, A. Shirvani, M.F. Holick, Hereditary metabolic bone diseases: A review of pathogenesis, diagnosis and management, *Genes (Basel).* 13 (2022). https://doi.org/10.3390/genes13101880.

6. V. Natesan, S.J. Kim, Metabolic bone diseases and new drug developments, *Biomol. Ther.* 30 (2022) 309–319. https://doi.org/10.4062/biomolther.2022.007.

7. S.K. Boddu, V.K.T. Venkata, Hypophosphatemia and metabolic bone disease associated with the use of elemental formula: Case report and review, *J. Neonatol.* 36 (2022) 58–62. https://doi.org/10.1177/09732179211065383.

8. W. Gunaratne, D. Dissanayake, K. Jayaratne, N.P. Premawardhana, S. Siribaddana, A case series of distal renal tubular acidosis, Southeast Asian ovalocytosis and metabolic bone disease, *BMC Nephrol.* 21 (2020) 1–10. https://doi.org/10.1186/s12882-020-01959-7.

9. F.M. Hannan, P.J. Newey, M.P. Whyte, R. V. Thakker, Genetic approaches to metabolic bone diseases, *Br. J. Clin. Pharmacol.* 85 (2019) 1147–1160. https://doi.org/10.1111/bcp.13803.

10. T. Sozen, L. Ozisik, N. Calik Basaran, An overview and management of osteoporosis, *Eur. J. Rheumatol.* 4 (2017) 46–56. https://doi.org/10.5152/eurjrheum.2016.048.

11. I. Akkawi, H. Zmerly, Osteoporosis : Current concepts, *Joints* 6(2) (2018) 122–127.

12. N. Salari, H. Ghasemi, L. Mohammadi, M. hasan Behzadi, E. Rabieenia, S. Shohaimi, M. Mohammadi, The global prevalence of osteoporosis in the world: A comprehensive systematic review and meta-analysis, *J. Orthop. Surg. Res.* 16 (2021). https://doi.org/10.1186/s13018-021-02772-0.

13. S. Minisola, L. Colangelo, J. Pepe, D. Diacinti, C. Cipriani, S.D. Rao, Osteomalacia and vitamin D status: A clinical update 2020, *JBMR Plus.* 5 (2021) 1–6. https://doi.org/10.1002/jbm4.10447.

14. L. Cianferotti, Osteomalacia is not a single disease, *Int. J. Mol. Sci.* 23 (2022). https://doi.org/10.3390/ijms232314896.

15. S.P. Tuck, J. Walker, Adult Paget's disease of bone, *Clin. Med. J. R. Coll. Physicians London.* 20 (2020) 568–571. https://doi.org/10.7861/clinmed.20.6.page.

16. S.H. Ralston, L. Corral-Gudino, C. Cooper, R.M. Francis, W.D. Fraser, L. Gennari, N. Guañabens, M.K. Javaid, R. Layfield, T.W. O'Neill, R.G.G. Russell, M.D. Stone, K. Simpson, D. Wilkinson, R. Wills, M.C. Zillikens, S.P. Tuck, Diagnosis and management of Paget's disease of bone in adults: A clinical guideline, *J. Bone Miner. Res.* 34 (2019) 579–604. https://doi.org/10.1002/jbmr.3657.

17. I. Kravets, Paget's disease of bone: Diagnosis and treatment, *Am. J. Med.* 131 (2018) 1298–1303. https://doi.org/10.1016/j.amjmed.2018.04.028.

18. P.D. Miller, Chronic kidney disease and the skeleton, *Bone Res.* 2 (2015). https://doi.org/10.1038/boneres.2014.44.

19. G. Eknoyan, S.M. Moe, Renal osteodystrophy: A historical review of its origins and conceptual evolution, *Bone Reports.* 17 (2022) 101641. https://doi.org/10.1016/j.bonr.2022.101641.

20. A.C. Bianco, Hypothyrodisis, Encycl. *Clin. Neuropsychol.* 390 (2011) 1290–1290. https://doi.org/10.1007/978-0-387-79948-3_3710.

21. A. Bangura, L. Wright, T. Shuler, Hypophosphatasia: Current literature for pathophysiology, clinical manifestations, diagnosis, and treatment, *Cureus.* 12 (2020) 1–6. https://doi.org/10.7759/cureus.8594.

22. V. Tai, W. Leung, A. Grey, I.R. Reid, M.J. Bolland, Calcium intake and bone mineral density: Systematic review and meta-analysis, *BMJ.* 351 (2015) 1–14. https://doi.org/10.1136/bmj.h4183.

23. C.M. Weaver, D.D. Alexander, C.J. Boushey, B. Dawson-Hughes, J.M. Lappe, M.S. LeBoff, S. Liu, A.C. Looker, T.C. Wallace, D.D. Wang, Calcium plus vitamin D supplementation and risk of fractures: An updated meta-analysis from the National Osteoporosis Foundation, *Osteoporos. Int.* 27 (2016) 367–376. https://doi.org/10.1007/s00198-015-3386-5.

24. Y. Ukon, T. Makino, J. Kodama, H. Tsukazaki, D. Tateiwa, H. Yoshikawa, T. Kaito, Molecular-based treatment strategies for osteoporosis: A literature review, *Int. J. Mol. Sci.* 20 (2019) 1–24. https://doi.org/10.3390/ijms20102557.

25. M. Shiraki, Y. Shiraki, C. Aoki, M. Miura, Vitamin K2 (menatetrenone) effectively prevents fractures and sustains lumbar bone mineral density in osteoporosis, *J. Bone Miner. Res.* 15 (2000) 515–521. https://doi.org/10.1359/jbmr.2000.15.3.515.

26. J. Iwamoto, Vitamin K2 therapy for postmenopausal osteoporosis, *Nutrients.* 6 (2014) 1971–1980. https://doi.org/10.3390/nu6051971.

27. M. Almeida, S. Iyer, M. Martin-Millan, S.M. Bartell, L. Han, E. Ambrogini, M. Onal, J. Xiong, R.S. Weinstein, R.L. Jilka, C.A. O'Brien, S.C. Manolagas, Estrogen receptor-α signaling in osteoblast progenitors stimulates cortical bone accrual, *J. Clin. Invest.* 123 (2013) 394–404. https://doi.org/10.1172/JCI65910.

28. Y. Wang, D.W. Grainger, Developing siRNA therapies to address osteoporosis, *Ther. Deliv.* 4 (2013) 1239–1246. https://doi.org/10.4155/tde.13.85.

29. J. Li, G. Feng, H. He, H. Wang, J. Tang, A. Han, X. Mu, W. Zhu, Development of software enabling Chinese medicine-based precision treatment for osteoporosis at the gene and pathway levels, *Chinese Med. (United Kingdom).* 17 (2022) 1–20. https://doi.org/10.1186/s13020-022-00596-6.

30. E.R. Balmayor, M. van Griensven, Gene therapy for bone engineering, *Front. Bioeng. Biotechnol.* 3 (2015) 1–7. https://doi.org/10.3389/fbioe.2015.00009.

31. G. Chindamo, S. Sapino, E. Peira, D. Chirio, M.C. Gonzalez, M. Gallarate, Bone diseases: Current approach and future perspectives in drug delivery systems for bone targeted therapeutics, *Nanomaterials.* 10 (2020). https://doi.org/10.3390/nano10050875.

32. A.C. Burduşel, E. Andronescu, Lipid nanoparticles and liposomes for bone diseases treatment, *Biomedicines.* 10 (2022). https://doi.org/10.3390/biomedicines10123158.

33. Y. Liu, Z. Jia, M.P. Akhter, X. Gao, X. Wang, X. Wang, G. Zhao, X. Wei, Y. Zhou, X. Wang, C.W. Hartman, E. V. Fehringer, L. Cui, D. Wang, *Bone-targeting liposome formulation of Salvianic acid A accelerates the healing of delayed fracture Union in Mice,* Elsevier Inc, 2018. https://doi.org/10.1016/j.nano.2018.07.011.

34. C. Corciulo, C.M. Castro, T. Coughlin, S. Jacob, Z. Li, D. Fenyö, D.B. Rifkin, O.D. Kennedy, B.N. Cronstein, Intraarticular injection of liposomal adenosine reduces cartilage damage in established murine and rat models of osteoarthritis, *Sci. Rep.* 10 (2020) 1–16. https://doi.org/10.1038/s41598-020-68302-w.

35. P.H. Zhou, B. Qiu, R.H. Deng, H.J. Li, X.F. Xu, X.F. Shang, Chondroprotective effects of hyaluronic acid-chitosan nanoparticles containing plasmid DNA encoding cytokine response modifier A in a rat knee osteoarthritis model, *Cell. Physiol. Biochem.* 47 (2018) 1207–1216. https://doi.org/10.1159/000490217.

36. M.L. Kang, S.Y. Jeong, G. Il Im, Hyaluronic acid hydrogel functionalized with self-assembled micelles of amphiphilic PEGylated Kartogenin for the treatment of osteoarthritis, *Tissue Eng. - Part A.* 23 (2017) 630–639. https://doi.org/10.1089/ten.tea.2016.0524.

37. A.R. Sun, X. Wu, B. Liu, Y. Chen, C.W. Armitage, A. Kollipara, R. Crawford, K.W. Beagley, X. Mao, Y. Xiao, I. Prasadam, Pro-resolving lipid mediator ameliorates obesity induced osteoarthritis by regulating synovial macrophage polarisation, *Sci. Rep.* 9 (2019) 1–13. https://doi.org/10.1038/s41598-018-36909-9.

38. A.H. Salama, A.A. Abdelkhalek, N.A. Elkasabgy, Etoricoxib-loaded bio-adhesive hybridized polylactic acid-based nanoparticles as an intra-articular injection for the treatment of osteoarthritis, *Int. J. Pharm.* 578 (2020) 119081. https://doi.org/10.1016/j.ijpharm.2020.119081.

39. J. Wang, X. Wang, Y. Cao, T. Huang, D.X. Song, H.R. Tao, Therapeutic potential of hyaluronic acid/chitosan nanoparticles for the delivery of curcuminoid in knee osteoarthritis and an in vitro evaluation in chondrocytes, *Int. J. Mol. Med.* 42 (2018) 2604–2614. https://doi.org/10.3892/ijmm.2018.3817.

40. C. Kang, E. Jung, H. Hyeon, S. Seon, D. Lee, Acid-activatable polymeric curcumin nanoparticles as therapeutic agents for osteoarthritis, *Nanomedicine Nanotechnology, Biol. Med.* 23 (2020) 102104. https://doi.org/10.1016/j.nano.2019.102104.

41. A. Sarkar, E. Carvalho, A.A. D'Souza, R. Banerjee, Liposome-encapsulated fish oil protein-tagged gold nanoparticles for intra-articular therapy in osteoarthritis, *Nanomedicine.* 14 (2019) 871–887. https://doi.org/10.2217/nnm-2018-0221.

42. P. Liu, L. Gu, L. Ren, J. Chen, T. Li, X. Wang, J. Yang, C. Chen, L. Sun, Intra-articular injection of etoricoxib-loaded PLGA-PEG-PLGA triblock copolymeric nanoparticles attenuates osteoarthritis progression, *Am. J. Transl. Res.* 11 (2019) 6775–6789. http://www.ncbi.nlm.nih.gov/pubmed/31814887%0Ahttp://www.pubmedcentral.nih.gov/articlerender.fcgi?artid=PMC6895527.

43. Y. Zhou, S.Q. Liu, H. Peng, L. Yu, B. He, Q. Zhao, In vivo anti-apoptosis activity of novel berberine-loaded chitosan nanoparticles effectively ameliorates osteoarthritis, *Int. Immunopharmacol.* 28 (2015) 34–43. https://doi.org/10.1016/j.intimp.2015.05.014.

44. S. Samdancioglu, S. Calis, M. Sumnu, A.A. Hincal, Formulation and in vitro evaluation of bisphosphonate loaded microspheres for implantation in osteolysis, *Drug Dev. Ind. Pharm.* 32 (2006) 473–481. https://doi.org/10.1080/03639040500528871.

45. S. Huang, D. Xu, L. Zhang, L. Hao, Y. Jia, X. Zhang, T. Cheng, J. Chen, Therapeutic effects of curcumin liposomes and nanocrystals on inflammatory osteolysis: In vitro and in vivo comparative study, *Pharmacol. Res.* 192 (2023) 106778. https://doi.org/10.1016/j.phrs.2023.106778.

46. Y. Wu, F. He, C. Zhang, Q. Zhang, X. Su, X. Zhu, A. Liu, W. Shi, W. Lin, Z. Jin, H. Yang, J. Lin, Melatonin alleviates titanium nanoparticles induced osteolysis via activation of butyrate/GPR109A signaling pathway, *J. Nanobiotechnology.* 19 (2021) 1–16. https://doi.org/10.1186/s12951-021-00915-3.

47. X. Meng, W. Zhang, Z. Lyu, T. Long, Y. Wang, ZnO nanoparticles attenuate polymer-wear-particle induced inflammatory osteolysis by regulating the MEK-ERK-COX-2 axis, *J. Orthop. Transl.* 34 (2022) 1–10. https://doi.org/10.1016/j.jot.2022.04.001.

48. J. Rousseau, V. Escriou, F. Lamoureux, R. Brion, J. Chesneau, S. Battaglia, J. Amiaud, D. Scherman, D. Heymann, F. Rédini, V. Trichet, Formulated siRNAs targeting Rankl prevent osteolysis and enhance chemotherapeutic response in osteosarcoma models, *J. Bone Miner. Res.* 26 (2011) 2452–2462. https://doi.org/10.1002/jbmr.455.

49. S. Sapino, G. Chindamo, D. Chirio, M. Manzoli, E. Peira, C. Riganti, M. Gallarate, Calcium phosphate-coated lipid nanoparticles as a potential tool in bone diseases therapy, *Nanomaterials.* 11 (2021). https://doi.org/10.3390/nano11112983.

50. S. Yamashita, H. Katsumi, N. Hibino, Y. Isobe, Y. Yagi, K. Kusamori, T. Sakane, A. Yamamoto, Development of PEGylated carboxylic acid-modified polyamidoamine dendrimers as bone-targeting carriers for the treatment of bone diseases, *J. Control. Release.* 262 (2017) 10–17. https://doi.org/10.1016/j.jconrel.2017.07.018.

51. P. Mora-Raimundo, D. Lozano, M. Benito, F. Mulero, M. Manzano, M. Vallet-Regí, Osteoporosis remission and new bone formation with mesoporous silica nanoparticles, *Adv. Sci.* 8 (2021) 1–14. https://doi.org/10.1002/advs.202101107.

52. L. Zheng, Z. Zhuang, Y. Li, T. Shi, K. Fu, W. Yan, L. Zhang, P. Wang, L. Li, Q. Jiang, Bone targeting antioxidative nano-iron oxide for treating postmenopausal osteoporosis, *Bioact. Mater.* 14 (2022) 250–261. https://doi.org/10.1016/j.bioactmat.2021.11.012.

53. R. Fu, W.C. Lv, Y. Xu, M.Y. Gong, X.J. Chen, N. Jiang, Y. Xu, Q.Q. Yao, L. Di, T. Lu, L.M. Wang, R. Mo, Z.Q. Wu, Endothelial ZEB1 promotes angiogenesis-dependent bone formation and reverses osteoporosis, *Nat. Commun.* 11 (2020) 1–16. https://doi.org/10.1038/s41467-019-14076-3.

54. J. Huang, Y. Xu, Y. Wang, Z. Su, T. Li, S. Wu, Y. Mao, S. Zhang, X. Weng, Y. Yuan, Advances in the study of exosomes as drug delivery systems for bone-related diseases, *Pharmaceutics.* 15 (2023) 1–20. https://doi.org/10.3390/pharmaceutics15010220.

55. C.M. Conners, V.R. Bhethanabotla, V.K. Gupta, Concentration-dependent effects of alendronate and pamidronate functionalized gold nanoparticles on osteoclast and osteoblast viability, *J. Biomed. Mater. Res. - Part B Appl. Biomater.* 105 (2017) 21–29. https://doi.org/10.1002/jbm.b.33527.

56. L. Bai, G. Tao, M. Feng, Y. Xie, S. Cai, S. Peng, J. Xiao, Hydrogel drug delivery systems for bone regeneration, *Pharmaceutics.* 15 (2023). https://doi.org/10.3390/pharmaceutics15051334.

57. Q. Liu, Y. Gan, J. Wu, X. Li, Application of carbon nanoparticles suspension injection in uremic patients with secondary hyperparathyroidism underwent total parathyroidectomy: 2 case report and literature review, *J. Cent. South Univ. Medical Sci.* 42 (2017) 865–868. https://doi.org/10.11817/j.issn.1672-7347.2017.07.021.

58. H. Deng, J. Wang, R. An, Hyaluronic acid-based hydrogels: As an exosome delivery system in bone regeneration, *Front. Pharmacol.* 14 (2023) 1–15. https://doi.org/10.3389/fphar.2023.1131001.

59. M.P. Yavropoulou, V. Vaios, P. Makras, P. Georgianos, A. Batas, D. Tsalikakis, A. Tzallas, G. Ntritsos, S. Roumeliotis, T. Eleftheriadis, V. Liakopoulos, Expression of circulating micrornas linked to bone metabolism in chronic kidney disease-mineral and bone disorder, *Biomedicines.* 8 (2020) 1–15. https://doi.org/10.3390/biomedicines8120601.

11 The Biochemical Basis of Renal Diseases

Elikem Kwami Kumahor

11.1 OVERVIEW OF THE ANATOMY AND PHYSIOLOGY OF THE KIDNEY

11.1.1 Gross Anatomy

The kidneys, which are two bean-shaped organs, are situated in the lower back (retroperitoneum). The normal dimensions of an adult kidney are 11–12 cm in length, 5–7 cm in width, and 2.5–3 cm in thickness. When compared to the right kidney, the left one is slightly bigger. Male kidneys weigh between 150 and 200 grammes, while female kidneys weigh between 120 and 135 grammes [1]. The kidney is surrounded by a capsule and adipose tissue [2]. The kidney is divided into several lobes. The pyramid and its cortical tissues comprise a lobe [3]. The dark outer continuous layer of the kidney is known as the cortex and is mainly composed of glomeruli, as well as proximal and distal convoluted tubules. The inner portion is paler and subdivided into renal pyramids and it is mainly composed of the descending limb, the ascending limb, the collecting ducts, and associated blood vessels. The renal pyramids extend into the renal pelvis forming papillae [4]

11.1.2 Embryology

The embryonal kidney develops together with the urinary tract and reproductive system from a progenitor structure known as the urogenital ridge. The embryological development of the kidney starts in the fourth week with the development of the nephrogenic cord. The metanephric kidney acts as a functional excretory unit as early as the eleventh week but nephrogenesis is not complete until week 32 [5]. The metanephric duct can excrete urine into the amniotic fluid by the third month of fetal development [6].

11.1.3 Blood Supply

The kidney receives about 20% of the cardiac output via the renal artery [7]. After multiple branches, the terminal portion of each renal artery ultimately forms the afferent arteriole, which grows into the highly specialized capillary bed known as the glomerulus. The capillaries merge again, forming the efferent arterioles. Other efferent arterioles from other glomeruli merge to form a capillary plexus and vasa recta (which is an elongated blood vessel). The vasa recta and capillary plexuses together pass around the remaining nephron, providing oxygen and nutrients, as well as removing ions and molecules that were reabsorbed by the nephrons. The efferent arteriole subsequently combines with renal venules to form the renal veins, which then merge into the inferior vena cava [8]. Renal blood flow is tightly regulated through complex mechanisms intrinsic to the kidney. The glomerular perfusion pressure is maintained at 45 mmHg across a wide systemic pressure range of 90–200 mm Hg [9].

11.1.4 Nephron

Nephron is the term for the fundamental structural and functional unit that makes up the kidney [10]. There are around one million nephrons in each human kidney [11]. A renal corpuscle, also known as a glomerulus, is found at the center of each nephron. This renal corpuscle is attached to a convoluted tube that ultimately empties into a collecting duct. The tubular component of the nephron is made up of a proximal convoluted tubule and a distal convoluted tubule that are joined to one another by a loop of Henle [12].

11.1.5 Glomerulus

The glomerulus consists of a highly vascular glomerular tuft contained within a globoid epithelial sac called the Bowman's capsule [13]. The glomerular tuft forms plasma ultra-filtrate. The space bound by the Bowman's capsule receives the ultra-filtrate and transmits it to the uriniferous tubule [14]. Physiologically, the glomerulus has a three-layer filtration barrier. The first layer is formed by the endothelial cells of the capillaries, which are fenestrated. The middle layer is the basement membrane (of the capillaries), which is composed of glycoproteins and proteoglycans. The third layer is composed of epithelial cells called podocytes, which have foot processes (pedicles) whose surface is negatively charged [13]. These layers work in concert to generate a selective barrier to prevent the leakage of proteins. The selectivity of this barrier is based on the size of the molecule and the charge on the molecule. Molecules larger than 70 kDa are generally not filtered

DOI: 10.1201/9781003384823-11

(i.e. albumin). Also, positively charged molecules are filtered to a greater extent than negatively charged macromolecules when it comes to the filtration process [15].

11.1.6 Renal Tubules

The renal tubule begins with the Bowman's capsule, which receives the ultra-filtrate from the glomerulus, then continues as the proximal convoluted tubule, progressing toward the renal medulla. The cuboidal or columnar cells that line the proximal tubule have a brush border of microvilli that improves their surface area for the absorption of molecules [12]. Nearly 80% of the ultra-filtrate is absorbed by the proximal tubule, which is responsible for this process [9]. The proximal tubule continues into the descending thin loop of Henle, passing through a U-shaped loop to form the thin and thick ascending limb [12]. The loop of Henle's primary function is to produce concentrated urine. The juxta-glomerular apparatus, which secretes renin, is located near the beginning of the thick ascending limb, although the distal convoluted tubule does not begin until much later [16]. The reabsorption of sodium occurs in the distal convoluted tubule under the effect of aldosterone, while the reabsorption of water occurs in the distal convoluted tubule under the influence of ADH [17]. The collecting duct, which plays a role in the reabsorption of water and sodium while also contributing to the excretion of hydrogen ions, is formed by the connection of an average of six distal tubules [18].

11.1.7 Functions of the Kidney

The kidney's main function is the excretion of some metabolic waste substances; however, the kidney performs several other functions. These include the following.

11.1.7.1 Filtration

The kidney filters out the plasma, allowing excess metabolites like hydrogen ions, electrolytes, water, and metabolic waste substance to be excreted in the ultra-filtrate. Dysfunction in the filtration function of the kidney results in the accumulation of metabolic waste, leading to uremic syndrome and renal failure.

11.1.7.2 Resorption

Essential metabolites, such as glucose, amino acids, electrolytes, and proteins, are reabsorbed by the renal tubules to prevent them from being flushed out in the ultra-filtrate.

11.1.7.3 Homeostasis

The kidney regulates extracellular volume by regulating water balance. It is also important for maintaining normal levels of acids and bases, blood pressure, and electrolytes.

11.1.7.4 Metabolism

The kidney is responsible for the synthesis of a few metabolites, including glutathione, glycogen (via glycogenesis), and ammonia.

11.1.7.5 Endocrine

The kidney is a crucial endocrine organ that triggers vitamin D production and also produces erythropoietin and renin.

11.2 GLOMERULAR FUNCTION TESTS

As previously described, the glomerulus is responsible for filtering blood to form the ultra-filtrate. The glomerular filtration rate provides an objective method for determining how efficiently the kidney filters are functioning. The glomerular filtration rate (GFR) is the volume of plasma that is filtered by the glomerulus per unit of time. This rate is measured in liters per minute [19]. Clinically, GFR can be measured directly using renal clearance; however, it is currently common practice to estimate GFR using various formulas.

Glomerular function can be assessed using:

1. Serum creatinine concentrations (as a sole indicator)

2. Measure GFR using creatinine clearance

3. Estimated GFR using creatinine or cystatin C

Table 11.1   Markers of glomerular filtration rate

EXOGENOUS MARKERS	ENDOGENOUS MARKERS
Non-Radioactive	Creatinine
Inulin	Cystatin C
Iohexol	Urea
Radioactive	Retinol-binding protein (RBP)
^{51}Cr EDTA	α_2-microglobulin
^{99m}Tc-DTPA	α_1-microglobulin
	β-trace protein

11.2.1 Renal Clearance

The rate at which a substance is eliminated from the blood plasma by the kidneys and passed into the urine is known as its renal clearance [20]. It is used as a method of measuring GFR. The ideal marker for measuring renal clearance must have the following properties: it must be stable in the plasma, it must be physiologically inert, it must be freely filtered at the glomerulus, it must not be secreted by the tubules, it must not be absorbed by the tubules, it must not be synthesized by the kidneys, and it must not be metabolized by the kidneys. Several endogenous and exogenous markers have been used to measure GFR (Table 11.1).

The inulin clearance test is considered to be the gold standard for determining GFR; however, because it is technically difficult and time-consuming, it is only used for research [21].

11.2.2 Creatinine Clearance

Utilizing creatinine clearance as a method for calculating GFR is a practically applicable approach. The breakdown of the high-energy molecule creatine, which is metabolized by both muscle and the brain, results in the production of creatinine as the waste product [22]. Because skeletal muscle continuously releases creatinine into the blood at a relatively constant concentration, serum creatinine concentration is directly proportional to skeletal muscle mass [23]. A kinetic variant of the Jaffe process is used to test serum creatinine. This procedure involves the reaction of creatinine with picric acid at alkaline pH, which results in the formation of a yellow-orange complex [24]. Creatinine can be freely filtered at the glomerulus, and it is not reabsorbed by the tubules; however, proximal tubules are responsible for the excretion of a minor amount of creatinine [25]. Since filtered creatinine is almost equal to creatinine excreted in the urine, the formula for creatinine clearance can be summarized as:

$$\text{Creatinine clearance}\left(\text{GFR}\right) = \frac{U_{cr} \, XV}{P_{cr} \, XT}$$

Where

U_{cr} is urine creatinine concentration

P_{cr} is plasma creatinine concentration

V is urine volume in mls

T is the time of urine collection in minutes

The unit for creatinine clearance is in mls/min.

Creatinine clearance is about 10–20% higher than GFR; however, this is not practically significant [26]. Urine is often collected for 24 hours, and plasma samples are typically extracted at one specific point in time throughout that timeframe. Both urine and serum creatinine concentrations are assayed and applied to the formula to calculate the creatinine clearance.

11.2.3 Serum Creatinine as an Indicator of Glomerular Function

Creatinine can be used alone as an indicator of GFR. Plasma creatinine concentration and GFR have a strong inverse relationship [27]; see Figure 11.1.

A valuable diagnostic tool for early renal impairment is serum creatinine when serial measurements are followed in a patient. Increasing serum creatinine concentrations is always a red flag for renal impairment [27].

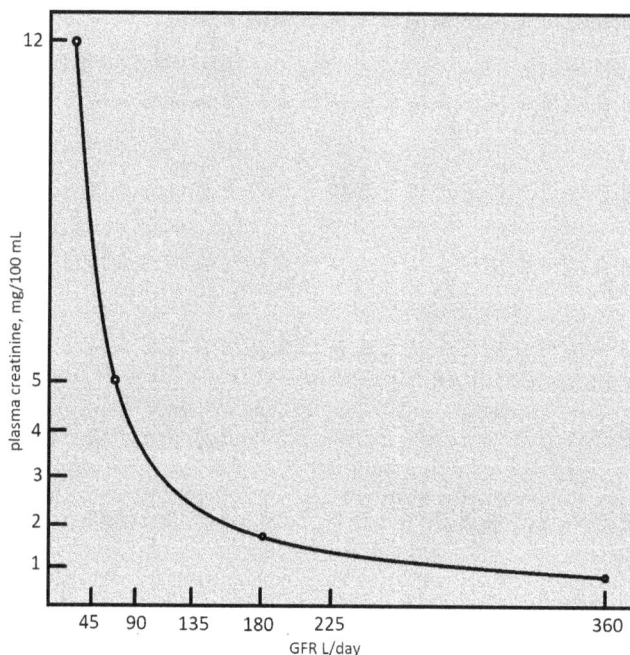

Figure 11.1   Relation between plasma creatinine and GFR

11.2.4 Estimated GFR

GFR is an important clinical parameter for assessing renal function, especially in patients with chronic disease. However, measuring GFR accurately using creatinine clearance is technically cumbersome and introduces several sources of error and variation. Various formulas have been devised to estimate GFR, offering a close agreement to measured GFR. GFR can be calculated based on serum creatinine (and/or cystatin C), together with other variables like age, sex, weight, and race (Table 11.2).

11.3 TUBULAR FUNCTION TESTS

The renal tubules are responsible for the resorption of water, electrolytes, and other molecules from the ultra-filtrate. This allows the kidney to concentrate or dilute urine, as well as maintain acid–base balance.

11.3.1 Proximal Tubular Function Tests

Several parameters may indicate renal tubular dysfunction. These include the following.

Glycosuria: Glycosuria in the presence of normal blood glucose is termed renal glycosuria and indicates a specific tubular defect. It is benign in most cases but may need to be followed up, especially if it occurs persistently [32].

Table 11.2   Equations for estimating GFR

COCKROFT-GAULT FORMULA [28]

 eGFR = (140 − age) × body weight/plasma creatinine × 72 (× 0.85 if female)

MDRD (Modified Diet in Renal Disease)[29]

eGFR = 175×(Scr)$^{-1.154}$ × (Age)$^{-0.203}$ × 0.742 [if female] × 1.212 [if Black]

CKD-EPI [30]

eGFR = 141 × min(Scr/κ, 1)$^{\alpha}$ × max(Scr/κ, 1)$^{-1.209}$ × 0.993^{Age} × 1.018 [if female] × 1.159 [if Black]

κ = 0.7 (females) or 0.9 (males); α = −0.329 (females) or −0.411 (males)

SCHWART (PEDIATRIC) [31]

eGFR = 41.3 × (ht(cm)/Scr (umol/L)) or 0.45 × (ht(cm)/Scr(mg/dL))

Aminoaciduria: Normally amino acids are more or less completely reabsorbed in the proximal tubule. Aminoaciduria may mean a specific tubular defect, for example, cystinuria or more commonly acquired renal tubular damage [33].

Tubular proteinuria: Tubular proteinuria is characterized by the presence of beta (β)-2-microglobulin and alpha (α)-1-microglobulin, two tiny proteins that are typically reabsorbed by tubular cells after being filtered at the glomeruli. High levels of these proteins in the urine are a reliable predictor of kidney injury from nephrotoxins like heavy metals [34].

11.3.2 Distal Tubular Function Tests

The concentrating and acidifying functions of the tubules can be tested clinically.

1. Water Deprivation Test

Primary urine is finally concentrated from an osmolality of 300 to about 1,400 mOsm/kg H2O. It can be concentrated to 1,800 mOsm/kg in states of severe water deficiency (dehydration). The ability of the tubules to concentrate urine can be tested using the water deprivation test.

Procedure

The bladder is emptied on going to bed at night. During the night, no fluid intake is allowed. The first morning sample of urine passed thereafter should have an osmolality of at least 700 mOsm/kg of water. If the overnight water deprivation test produced less than 700 mOsm/kg or is equivocal, fluids are further withheld for 24 hours, with urine osmolality being measured hourly. Only dry foods such as sandwiches, biscuits, and toast are allowed. The procedure should be stopped immediately after urine osmolality rises to >800 mOSm/kg H20. This is an unpleasant test and should be done under close clinical monitoring. Urine osmolality that remains lower than 700 mOsm/kg H20 indicates significant tubular damage or diabetes insipidus.

2. Urine Acidifying Test

The primary urine is also normally acidified from pH 7.4 to pH 6.0. Metabolic acidosis is induced by the oral administration of NH_4Cl. Urine samples are collected hourly for the following 8 hours. One sample's pH should drop to 5.3 or lower if the kidneys are functioning normally; if they are not, a hereditary disorder called renal tubular acidosis is to blame for the failure of H+ secretion in the distal tubule, leading to metabolic acidosis. NH_4Cl is metabolized in the body to ammonia and HCl, the latter constituting the acid load. The NH_3 is metabolized by the liver to urea. The test should therefore not be carried out on a patient who is already acidotic or who has liver disease.

11.4 PROTEINURIA

The protein load presented to the kidney is about 10 kg each day. However, only 1g of protein passes through the glomerulus. Out of this, only 150 mg of protein is lost by a healthy kidney each day and this is because the glomerulus is a selective barrier that can retain proteins with a molecular weight greater than albumin (i.e. 66kDa) [35]. Proteinuria can be attributed to increased filtered load, increased circulation of low molecular weight proteins, and lower resorptive ability (Table 11.3). All three of these factors contribute to increased protein loss. Physiologically, the main protein lost by the kidney in urine is albumin. Tamm-Horsfall glycoprotein and other small proteins released by tubular cells are also excreted in the urine. Clinically significant (pathological) proteinuria is >300 mg/day [35]. This is routinely detected through urine dipstick tests. The gold standard method for detecting proteinuria is measuring the 24-hour urinary protein, but current best-practice guidelines prefer using the urinary albumin creatinine ratio to estimate urinary protein concentration. Physiologically, proteinuria may be due to fever, strenuous exercise, and posture (orthostatic) [36].

11.4.1 Laboratory Investigation of Proteinuria

Positive protein on the dipstick should be repeated and confirmed by 24-hour urine protein or urinary albumin creatinine or urinary protein creatinine ratio on a fresh first morning specimen collected in a standard sterile urine container. Confirmed proteinuria should be supported with formal renal function tests (serum: urea, creatinine, and electrolytes). Further tests to investigate significant proteinuria include urinalysis, microscopy, urine culture, renal radiology, ultrasound,

Table 11.3   Causes of Proteinuria

1. Overflow Proteinuria

Because of the abundance of low molecular weight proteins in the plasma <70 kDa

Bence Jones protein (44kDa) in multiple myeloma

Albumin (66.5kDa) following intravenous albumin infusion

Amylase (45kDa) in acute pancreatitis

Hemoglobin (68kDa) following intravascular hemolysis

Lysozyme (15kDa) in monocytic and myelomonocytic leukaemias

Myoglobin (17kDa) following muscle damage in crush injuries

2. Glomerular Proteinuria

Glomerulonephritis (all forms)

Diabetic nephropathy

Hypertensive renal disease

Pregnancy

Pre-eclampsia/eclampsia

Congestive heart failure

3. Tubular Proteinuria

Failure of tubular cells to reabsorb these LMW proteins, e.g. B2 macroglobulin and lysozyme

Tubular damage from heavy metals

Acute tubular necrosis

Chronic nephritis

Pyelonephritis

Renal tubular defect (Fanconi's)

Renal transplantation

4. Post-renal Proteinuria

Distal to the kidney, proteins enter the urine tract

Pyelonephritis

Renal calculi

Cystitis

Urethritis

Transplantation of the ureters into the bowel

renal biopsy, and histopathology. Urine electrophoresis can also be used to identify and quantify proteins present, e.g. Bence Jones proteins in multiple myeloma.

11.5 BIOCHEMICAL TESTS IN URINALYSIS

Urinalysis (also known as urine routine examination) is a commonly performed test in the clinical laboratory. It consists of a gross examination of the urine, urine biochemistry using a reagent dipstick, and urine microscopy.

11.5.1 An Overall Inspection of the Urine

This pertains to the urine's physical characteristics, including its color, smell, and visual appearance (Table 11.4). Normal urine is colorless and has a straw-yellow (amber) hue; the strength of this color typically roughly correlates to the concentration (density) of the urine. Normal urine is not cloudy. It is usual for urine to appear cloudy when there are leukocytes and bacteria present, which indicates an infection of the urinary system. Cloudiness could also be an indication of sample contamination with vaginal discharge in women or the presence of sperm in males, or it could be an indication that the sample was not maintained properly.

11.5.2 Urine Biochemistry

Biochemical tests routinely performed on urine include leucocyte esterase, urobilinogen, nitrite specific gravity, pH, blood, bilirubin, protein, glucose, and ketones. These tests are usually incorporated on a reagent strip (dipstick) as a panel of tests.

Table 11.4   Physical characteristics (color) of urine

Color	Cause	Comments
Light yellow to colorless	Normal after drinking more water; polyuria; diabetes mellitus and diabetes insipidus	Increased 24-hour urine output in polyuria; urine with glucose in diabetic mellitus
Dark yellow	Concentrated sample Use of riboflavin (vitamin B_2)	Consistent with a first-thing-in-the-morning sample or a post-workout sample
Orange	Bilirubin, urobilin (which has a yellow-orange color and is produced when urobilinogen is photo-oxidized), drugs (nitrofurantoin), and biliverdin. The carotenes that come from food	It is possible to determine the presence of bilirubin and urobilinogen by utilizing a test strip (but not after photo-oxidation)
Pink/red/brown	Blood present, methemoglobin is brown (indicating that hemoglobin oxidation has occurred due to the acidic pH of the urine), presence of hemoproteins (myoglobin, hemoglobin porphyrins) but a negative result from a chemical blood test Medications (e.g. rifampicin) Beetroot, a type of food	Erythrocytes, hemoglobin, and myoglobin all respond when they come into contact with a blood test strip, which indicates a positive result. Distinguishable by the appearance of the urine (which is typically cloudy when there is blood present) or serum (which may be red in intravascular hemolysis but not in myoglobinuria); or by specialized tests (such as the presence of myoglobin in the urine or a complement fixation reaction)
Black/brown	Bilirubin, urological tea, melanoma, alkaptonuria	Analysis of blood chemicals was negative
Blue/green	Pseudomonas infection, drug use (methylene blue, amitryptiline), and inherited deficiencies in amino acid metabolism	

11.5.3 Specific Gravity (Density)

This expresses the density ratio between the urine sample and distilled water. The specific gravity (SG) range is 1.015 to 1.025. The SG reflects renal tubular function (i.e. the secretion and absorption of ions and water). Isothenuria is the loss of reaction of urine SG to changes in urine intake.

11.5.4 pH

The pH of urine indicates the acidity or alkalinity of urine. A healthy person has a wide range of urine pH from 4.5 to 8. Urine pH usually reflects the acid–base status of the patient; therefore, urine pH will be acidic in patients with acidosis and will be alkaline in patients with alkalosis. The inability of urine pH to reflect the patient's acid–base status may indicate renal tubular acidosis [37]. A vegan diet may also produce alkaline urine because of low protein (amino acid content) [38]. Urine with a pH of 7.0 or higher indicates an infection of the urinary tract that was caused by bacteria that produce urease, such as Klebsiella.

11.5.5 Leucocyte and Nitrite

The primary goal of this test is to confirm or disprove the presence of a urinary tract infection. A positive leucocyte esterase on the urine dipstick indicates a bacterial urinary tract infection. This enzyme is found in granulocytes (WBCs). A positive test necessitates a urine culture to identify bacteria. The nitrite test takes advantage of the fact that certain bacteria can convert nitrate into nitrite. Nitrite-producing bacteria include *E. coli* and *Proteus* sp. [39].

11.5.6 Protein

The dipstick strip test for protein is specific for albumin (and less sensitive to other proteins). It is sensitive to 200 mg–300 mg/L of albumin in the urine. The principle for the determination of urine protein is the "protein error of indicators". This causes a reagent to change color in the presence of albumin in the urine. A positive urine protein test indicates glomerular damage, causing albumin to leak into urine. This may be an indication of early renal disease. False positives may be caused by strongly alkaline urine, which may occur in some UTIs. A false negative may be due to another pre-renal and tubular proteinuria where the protein is not albumin, including Bence Jones proteins (free light chains). Also, microalbuminuria (albumin 30–150 mg/L) may be missed by conventional protein dipstick tests.

11.5.7 Glucose

The principle for detecting urinary glucose is based on glucose oxidase, which is specific to glucose. Glucose is normally absent in urine but may be detected in patients with renal glycosuria (a benign condition in which the renal threshold for glucose excretion is reduced), diabetes mellitus, pregnancy, and renal tubular damage/dysfunction.

11.5.8 Ketones

Ketone bodies include β-hydroxybutyrate, acetoacetic acid, and acetone. These are usually absent in urine. Detection of ketones in the urine is based on the nitroprusside reaction that reacts strongest with aceto-acetatic acid, followed by acetone; β-hydroxybutyric acid does not react at all. However 80% of urinary ketones are β-hydroxybutyrate, hence the tendency of the dipstick method to underestimate the severity of ketosis [40]. A positive ketone test on a urine dipstick may indicate starvation, diabetic ketoacidosis, or alcoholic ketoacidosis.

11.5.9 Blood/Hemoglobin

Intact RBCs or lysed RBCs may produce a positive result. The principle of this test is based on the pseudo-peroxidase property of hemoglobin. A positive test must be confirmed with microscopy to distinguish hematuria from hemoglobinuria (as a result of hemolysis). Common causes of positive blood on a dipstick include schistosomiasis, renal calculi, tumors of the bladder and prostate, urinary tract infections, and hemolysis.

11.5.10 Bilirubin and Urobilinogen

Normally, the amount of urobilinogen in urine is too small to be detected. In conditions of hepatic jaundice, however, greater amounts of both conjugated bilirubin and urobilinogen may appear in urine, which reflects the inability of the damaged liver cells to properly metabolize and excrete bilirubin and urobilinogen. Positive bilirubin and urobilinogen indicate hepatocellular dysfunction [41].

11.5.11 Urine Microscopy

Microscopic examination of urine sediments usually follows biochemical tests and is especially indicated when the biochemistry results are pathological. Collecting accurate samples and processing them promptly are both extremely crucial since cells and cylinders deteriorate very quickly, particularly in hypotonic and alkaline urine. After collecting the urine, the sediment should be treated within an hour. When a person is healthy, their urine sediment may contain a variety of differently shaped objects (Table 11.5). These also include a small amount of erythrocytes (<5/μl), leukocytes (<10/μl), some epithelial cells (mainly squamous epithelium), hyaline cylinders, or various crystals [42].

11.6 ACUTE KIDNEY INJURY (AKI)

A rise in serum creatinine levels that occurs suddenly or a decrease in urine production that occurs suddenly are both signs of acute kidney injury [43], which is distinguished by a sudden decline in renal function, as well as the retention of urea, creatinine, and other metabolic byproducts [44]. Changes in the plasma creatinine concentration and the amount of urine produced can be used to provide an estimate of the severity of the injury. The diagnostic criteria for acute kidney injury are shown in Table 11.6.

Those at greater risk for acute kidney injury include elderly patients; those with preexisting CKD, sepsis, diabetes, heart disease, those taking nephrotoxic drugs, particularly in the context of hypovolemia; and those who have been given x-ray contrast agents. The etiological classification of acute kidney injury (AKI) includes pre-renal, renal, and post-renal.

11.6.1 Pre-renal AKI

A decrease in renal blood flow is caused by pre-renal factors, which are connected with systemic hemodynamic insufficiency (hypovolemia or hypotension) [45]. This insufficiency can lead to acute kidney injury. If pre-renal AKI is not treated promptly, with adequate renal perfusion being

Table 11.5   Urine cells and sediments

Erythrocytes (RBCs)	>5 red cells/µl is abnormal. Can originate from any point across the urinary tract. Isomorphic red cells are very similar to circulating red cells, and their presence may indicate bleeding from an external or internal source. Red cells that are dysmorphic have an irregular size and form. Dysmorphism can occur for several reasons, including changes in pH, osmolality, and protein, as well as due to tube transit, and although they may suggest bleeding from the glomerulus, judgment is subjective.
Leucocytes (WBCs)	An unspun specimen that has more than ten white cells per microliter is considered abnormal. A urinary tract infection, glomerulonephritis, tubulointerstitial nephritis, rejection of a kidney transplant, or cancer could be the cause.
Squamous epithelial cell	Frequently observed, but not pathological.
Bacteria and yeast	Bacteria or yeast + leucocyturia indicates urinary tract infection.
Parasites	E.g. *Trichomonas vaginalis, Schistosoma hematobium*.
Casts	Casts are entities that are generated in the lumen of distal tubules and have a cylindrical shape. They originate from the combination of cells and a protein called Tamm-Horsfall. • The presence of a hyaline cast in normal urine. • The presence of a red cell cast is indicative of an inflammatory condition taking place in the glomerulus, such as glomerulonephritis. • Pyelonephritis, interstitial nephritis, and glomerulonephritis are diseases that can cause a white cell cast. The granular cast is a byproduct of damaged tubular cells and can be seen in patients with any chronic renal disease.
Crystals	Crystals are frequent in urine that is old or cold, and their presence may not indicate a pathological condition. They play a crucial role in the formation of stones. • Uric acid has been linked to tumor lysis syndrome and uric acid stones. • Calcium oxalate, which can cause kidney stones, eating a diet heavy in oxalates, and ethylene glycol poisoning. • Cystine – seen in cystinuria.

restored, it can develop into intrinsic kidney damage, also known as acute tubular necrosis. Burns, hemorrhaging, diarrhea, post-operative fluid loss and blood loss, septic shock, and abrupt heart failure are some of the causes of this condition. The tubular function is usually retained in pre-renal acute kidney injury, and stimulation of the renin–angiotensin–aldosterone system and vasopressin production leads to small amounts of concentrated urine with a low salt concentration [46].

Biochemical indicators of pre-renal AKI include increased urea in disproportion to creatinine. Other biochemical features of pre-renal AKI include hyperkalemia and metabolic acidosis due

Table 11.6   Diagnostic criteria for acute kidney injury

Diagnostic criteria for AKI

• Increase in blood creatinine by > or = 0.3 mg/dL (26.5 umol/L) within 48 hours; or
• Increase in blood creatinine to > or = 1.5 times baseline, known or presumed to have occurred in the past seven days; or
• Urine volume <0.5 mL/kg/h for 6 hours

AKI Staging

AKI Stage I	• An increase in blood creatinine ≥0.3 mg/dL (26.5 umol/L); • An increase in blood creatinine that is 1.5–1.9 times higher than the initial value; • A decrease in urine volume of less than 0.5 mL/kg/h over 6–12 hours
AKI Stage II	• Increase in blood creatinine to 2.0–2.9 times from baseline; or • Urine volume <0.5 mL/kg/h for > or = 12 hours
AKI Stage III	• Increase in blood creatinine to 3.0 times from baseline; or • Blood creatinine >4.0 mg/dL (>354 mmol/L); or • Initiation of kidney replacement therapy; or • Decrease in eGFR to <35 mL/min/1.73m2 in patients <18 years; or • Urine volume <0.3 mL/kg/h for 24 hours; or • Anuria for >12 hours

to decreased excretion of hydrogen and potassium ions. The anion gap is elevated due to the retention of sulfates and phosphates. Urinalysis occasionally shows the presence of hyaline casts. Restoring fluid volume quickly, and, in some cases, using a vasoactive agent to raise blood pressure and, in turn, renal blood flow, are central to the management of pre-renal acute kidney injury.

11.6.2 Intrinsic Acute Kidney Injury

Intrinsic acute kidney injury may follow pre-renal causes or may be caused by nephrotoxic drugs, renal ischemia, intrinsic renal diseases, and systemic diseases that affect the kidneys. The term acute tubular necrosis (ATN) is used when AKI follows pre-renal causes or renal ischemia. In ATN, there is observed injury to the renal tubules leading to the production of dilute urine (in contrast with pre-renal AKI). Biochemical features in intrinsic renal disease include hyponatremia, hyperkalemia, metabolic acidosis, hyperphosphatemia, hypocalcemia (with raised PTH), hypermagnesemia, proteinuria, and dark urine (due to the presence of heme pigments) [47]. The natural history of ATN follows an oliguric phase, a diuretic phase, and a recovery phase.

Nutritional support, with certain restrictions placed on the amount of protein that can be consumed, as well as the prevention of metabolic complications such as hyperkalemia, acidosis, and infections, are all part of the management of AKI. These conservative techniques include rigorous regulation of sodium and water intake to preserve normovolemia. Some patients may require renal replacement therapy, e.g. hemodialysis. Some indications of renal injury include uremic encephalopathy, pulmonary edema, severe hyperkalemia (potassium >7.0 mmol/L), or severe acidosis (bicarbonate <12 mmol/L, H+ >70 nmol/L). Monitoring of creatinine, urea, electrolytes, and bicarbonate is essential during renal dialysis. Fluids and electrolytes must be adequately replaced to compensate for excessive losses. Dialysis must be continued until GFR has sufficiently recovered for plasma concentrations of creatinine to start falling.

11.6.3 Post-renal AKI

Acute kidney injury may arise from the back pressure of urine caused by blockages in the urinary tract. The result is a reduction in the effective filtration pressure at the glomerulus. Causes include renal stones, blood clots in the urinary tract, bladder outlet obstruction from tumors, benign prostate enlargement, and prostate carcinomas. Recently, AKI has been specifically described as a syndrome that includes hepato-renal, cardio-renal, nephrotoxic, perioperative, and sepsis-associated AKI [48].

11.6.4 Novel Biomarkers for Diagnosing AKI

Creatinine has been used for many decades as the biomarker for assessing kidney function; however, it is slow to react to acute kidney injury and may take 24 to 40 hours to increase in response to kidney injury. New biomarkers have emerged that can identify the earliest changes seen in AKI. Many of these biomarkers are still in the phase of human clinical trials to ascertain their efficacy.

11.6.5 Blood Cystatin C

Cystatin C is a chemical that is continually created by all nucleated cells in the human body. It is found throughout the body. It is a reliable biomarker of kidney function, particularly glomerular filtration. Even though cystatin C may be less sensitive in diagnosing acute kidney injury compared to creatinine, it appears that it can serve to identify a subset of individuals with AKI who are at a higher risk of adverse outcomes [49]. This has been demonstrated by some studies. Therefore, it is superior to serum creatinine in terms of its predictive value. Cystatin C has also been demonstrated to predict renal recovery earlier than AKI, which could result in a shorter hospital stay for the patient [50]. Cystatin C may be helpful in the monitoring of acute kidney injury in individuals who have non-steady states of creatinine, such as rhabdomyolysis, in which creatinine concentrations may be unpredictable.

11.6.6 Kidney Injury Molecule 1 (KIM 1)

Acute kidney injury causes an upregulation of the receptor known as KIM 1, which is found in renal epithelial cells. It is not normally found in the proximal tubular cells of healthy individuals. It has been observed in the urine of individuals who have renal tubular necrosis and is expressed in high concentrations in renal biopsies taken from people who have AKI [51].

11.6.7 Neutrophil Gelatinase-Associated Lipocalin (NGAL)

NGAL also known as lipocalin 2 is a protein that increases rapidly in kidney injury. It appears in the urine when there are early changes associated with acute kidney injury hours to days before other biomarkers. Both urine and plasma NGAL levels have been shown to be excellent predictors of AKI in a prospective study among children undergoing elective cardiac surgery [52]. Despite showing promise as a biomarker for AKI, NGAL has shown low accuracy and variability [53].

11.6.8 Urinary Insulin-Like Growth Factor Binding Protein 7 (IGFBP7) and Tissue Inhibitor of Metalloproteinases 2 (TIMP2)

TIMP2 and IGFBP7, both mostly produced in the distal and proximal tubules, are cell-cycle regulators with the ability to induce cell-cycle arrest [54]. They are sensitive biomarkers of acute kidney damage; however, their clinical utility is currently being studied.

11.7 CHRONIC KIDNEY DISEASE (CKD)

A lower estimated glomerular filtration rate (GFR), proteinuria, hematuria, and/or renal structural abnormalities that have lasted for more than 90 days are the hallmarks of chronic kidney disease (CKD). The prevalence of CKD ranges from 11% to 13% across the globe, with the majority of cases occurring at stage 3. Despite this, all stages of CKD are linked with morbidity, premature mortality, and a deterioration in quality of life [55]. Chronic kidney disease is typically an end-stage complication of diabetes mellitus, hypertension, glomerulonephritis, autoimmune disease, obstructive uropathy, polycystic disease, renal artery stenosis, infections, tubular dysfunction, and the use of nephrotoxic medications. Chronic kidney disease can also be caused by obstructive uropathy, polycystic disease, and renal artery stenosis. Reduced renal reserve, renal insufficiency, and end-stage uremia are the three main categories that can be used to classify the functional adaptation mechanisms that are present in CKD patients [56]. The KDIGO guidelines for CKD and albuminemia classifications are shown in Tables 11.7 and 11.8, respectively.

11.7.1 Biochemical Features of Chronic Kidney Disease

In CKD, there is an initial polyuric phase characterized by increased urine output as a result of a decreased number of functional nephrons and decreased excretion of urea, which leads to osmotic diuresis in functional nephrons [44]. Tubular damage results in decreased resorption of water and solutes, worsening the polyuria. The polyuric phase eventually ends in the oliguric phase, in which >75% of nephrons are damaged, GFR falls significantly, and there is a steep rise in plasma creatinine, urea, and potassium concentrations [57].

11.7.1.1 Uremia

Uremia is a clinical syndrome associated with CKD caused by the accumulation of uremic toxins, including urea, creatinine, cyanate, polyols, phenols, and middle molecules (cystatin c, PTH, atrial natriuretic peptide, and IL-6) [58]. Progressive weakness and weariness, lack of appetite with

Table 11.7 The KDIGO guidelines for CKD classification based on GFR

GFR categories (ml/min/ 1.73 m2)	G1	Normal or high	> or = 90
	G2	Slight decline	60–89
	G3a	Minimal to moderate decline	45–59
	G3b	Decreases ranging from moderate to severe	30–44
	G4	Drastically reduced	15–29
	G5	Failure of the kidneys	<15

Table 11.8 CKD classification based on albuminuria

Persistent albuminuria categories		
A1	A2	A3
Normal to slightly higher than normal	Increased to a moderate degree	Dramatically increased
<30 mg/g	30–300 mg/g	>300 mg/g
<3 mg/mmol	3–30 mg/mmol	>30 mg/mmol

subsequent nausea and vomiting, muscle wasting, tremors, altered mental function, rapid but shallow breathing, and metabolic acidosis are all classic symptoms of uremia. Uremia is a sign that renal replacement therapy is necessary [59].

11.7.1.2 Hyperphosphatemia and Hypocalcemia

High plasma concentrations of inorganic phosphates are a result of impaired renal tubular function and impaired activation of vitamin D [60]. Impaired activation leads to hypocalcemia, which results in increased parathyroid hormone levels. Increased PTH leads to increased bone decalcification, as well as increased alkaline phosphatase activity [61].

11.7.1.3 Hyperuricemia

Plasma uric acid levels rise in parallel with urea levels; however, the development of gout is rare [62].

11.7.1.4 Hypermagnesemia

High plasma magnesium levels occur as a result of impaired renal secretion in CKD [63].

11.7.1.5 Normocytic Normochromic Anemia

CKD patients develop normocytic normochromic anemia as a result of erythropoietin deficiency. Erythropoietin is a hormone produced by the peritubular cortex in the cortex of the kidneys in response to low oxygen tension and anemia (from hemolysis or hemorrhage) [64]. The ability of the kidney to produce erythropoietin is markedly impaired in CKD. Other factors that worsen anemia in CKD include impaired platelet function secondary to uremia, GI bleeding from uremic gastritis, functional iron deficiency, folate and vitamin B12 deficiency, infection, and chronic inflammation [65].

11.7.1.6 Dyslipidemia

Patients with CKD show an increased cardiovascular risk as a result of increased triglycerides, increased low-density lipoprotein (LDL) cholesterol, and reduced high-density lipoprotein (HDL) cholesterol [66].

11.7.1.7 Others

Chronic renal failure has been linked to the presence of aberrant endocrine function, including hyperprolactinemia, insulin resistance, low plasma testosterone levels, and abnormal thyroid function.

REFERENCES

1. Soriano RM, Penfold D, Leslie SW. Anatomy, abdomen and pelvis, kidneys. *StatPearls* [Internet]. 2022 Jul 25; Available from: https://www.ncbi.nlm.nih.gov/books/NBK482385/.

2. Rayner H, Thomas M, Milford D. Kidney anatomy and physiology. In: *Understanding Kidney Diseases*. Springer International Publishing; 2016. pp. 1–10.

3. Zhang JL, Rusinek H, Chandarana H, Lee VS. Functional MRI of the kidneys. *Journal of Magnetic Resonance Imaging* [Internet]. 2013 Feb;37(2):282. Available from: https://www.ncbi.nlm.nih.gov/pmc/articles/PMC3558841/.

4. McBride JM. Embryology, anatomy, and histology of the kidney. *Kidney* [Internet]. 2016 [cited 2023 Mar 17];1–18. Available from: https://link.springer.com/chapter/10.1007/978-1-4939-3286-3_1.

5. Uetani N, Bouchard M. Plumbing in the embryo: Developmental defects of the urinary tracts. *Clinical Genetics* [Internet]. 2009 Apr 1 [cited 2023 Mar 17];75(4):307–17. Available from: https://onlinelibrary.wiley.com/doi/full/10.1111/j.1399-0004.2009.01175.x.

6. Kreidberg JA. Podocyte differentiation and glomerulogenesis. *Journal of the American Society of Nephrology* [Internet]. 2003 Mar 1;14(3):806–14. Available from: https://journals.lww.com/jasn/Fulltext/2003/03000/Podocyte_Differentiation_and_Glomerulogenesis.31.aspx.

7. Kopitko C, Medve L, Gondos T. Pathophysiology of renal blood supply. *New Medicine*. 2016 Jan 4;20(1):27–9.

8. Marsh DJ, Postnov DD, Sosnovtseva OV., Holstein-Rathlou NH. The nephron-arterial network and its interactions. *American Journal of Physiology-Renal Physiology*. 2019 May 1;316(5):F769–84.

9. Eaton D, Pooler J. *Vander's Renal Physiology* [Internet]. 2009 Available from: https://www.academia.edu/download/61179202/Douglas_C._Eaton_-_Vanders_Renal_Physiology_-_7th20191110-43386-wrjs6o.pdf.

10. Zhuo JL, Li XC. Proximal nephron. In: *Comprehensive Physiology*. Wiley; 2013. pp. 1079–123.

11. Bertram JF, Douglas-Denton RN, Diouf B, Hughson MD, Hoy WE. Human nephron number: Implications for health and disease. *Pediatric Nephrology*. 2011 Sep;26(9):1529–33.

12. Madrazo-Ibarra A, Vaitla P. Histology, nephron. *StatPearls* [Internet]. 2021 Nov 21 [cited 2023 Mar 20]; Available from: https://www.ncbi.nlm.nih.gov/books/NBK554411/.

13. Falkson SR, Bordoni B. Anatomy, abdomen and pelvis, bowman capsule. *StatPearls* [Internet]. 2022 Aug 8 [cited 2023 Mar 20]; Available from: https://www.ncbi.nlm.nih.gov/books/NBK554474/.

14. Pollak MR, Quaggin SE, Hoenig MP, Dworkin LD. The glomerulus: The sphere of influence. *Clinical Journal of the American Society of Nephrology*. 2014 Aug 7;9(8):1461–9.

15. Haraldsson B, Nyström J, Deen WM. Properties of the glomerular barrier and mechanisms of proteinuria. *Physiological Reviews*. 2008 Apr;88(2):451–87.

16. McCormick JA, Ellison DH. Distal convoluted tubule. *Comprehensive Physiology*. 2015 Jan;5(1):45–98.

17. Subramanya AR, Ellison DH. Distal convoluted tubule. *Clinical Journal of the American Society of Nephrology*. 2014 Dec 5;9(12):2147–63.

18. McMahon AP. Development of the Mammalian kidney. *Curr Top Dev Biol*. 2016 Dec 1;117:31–64.

19. Topf JM, Inker LA. *Measurement of Glomerular Filtration Rate. Nephrology Secrets*: Fourth Edition. 2019;22–9. Elsevier.

20. Stevens LA, Shastri S, Levey AS. *Assessment of Renal Function. Comprehensive Clinical Nephrology*: Fourth Edition. 2010 Nov 8;31–8.

21. Mian AN, Schwartz GJ. Tests of kidney function in children. *Pediatric Critical Care: Expert Consult Premium Edition*. 2011 Apr 14;998–1008.

22. Koeppen BM, Stanton BA. Glomerular filtration and renal blood flow. *Renal Physiology*. 2013;27–43.

23. Guignard JP, Sulyok E. Renal morphogenesis and development of renal function. *Avery's Diseases of the Newborn*. 2011 Sep 21;1165–75.

24. Toora BD, Rajagopal G. Measurement of creatinine by Jaffe's reaction – Determination of concentration of sodium hydroxide required for maximum color development in standard, urine and protein free filtrate of serum. *Indian Journal of Experimental Biology*. 2002 Mar;40(3):352–4.

25. Bagshaw SM, Bellomo R. Kidney function tests and urinalysis in acute renal failure. *Critical Care Nephrology*. 2009;251–9.

26. Prowle JR, Forni LG. *Functional Biomarkers. Critical Care Nephrology*: Third Edition. 2019;141–145.e1.

27. Toffaletti JG. Relationships and clinical utility of creatinine, cystatin C, eGFRs, GFRs, and clearances. *The Journal of Applied Laboratory Medicine* [Internet]. 2017 Nov 1 [cited 2023 Mar 24];2(3):413–22. Available from: https://pubmed.ncbi.nlm.nih.gov/33636846/.

28. Cockcroft D, Nephron HG, 1976 undefined. Prediction of creatinine clearance from serum creatinine. karger.com [Internet]. 1976 [cited 2023 Mar 24]. Available from: https://www.karger.com/Article/Abstract/180580.

29. Levey AS, Coresh J, Greene T, Stevens LA, Zhang Y, Hendriksen S, et al. Using standardized serum creatinine values in the modification of diet in renal disease study equation for estimating glomerular filtration rate. *Annals of Internal Medicine*. 2006 Aug 15;145(4):247–54.

30. van den Brand JAJG, van Boekel GAJ, Willems HL, Kiemeney LALM, den Heijer M, Wetzels JFM. Introduction of the CKD-EPI equation to estimate glomerular filtration rate in a Caucasian population. *Nephrology Dialysis Transplantation* [Internet]. 2011 Oct 1 [cited 2023 Mar 24];26(10):3176–81. Available from: https://academic.oup.com/ndt/article/26/10/3176/1901121.

31. Schwartz G, Haycock G, Pediatrics CEJ, 1976 undefined. A simple estimate of glomerular filtration rate in children derived from body length and plasma creatinine. publications.aap.org [Internet]. 1976 [cited 2023 Mar 24]. Available from: https://publications.aap.org/pediatrics/article-abstract/58/2/259/78787.

32. Alsahli M, Gerich JE. Renal glucose metabolism in normal physiological conditions and in diabetes. *Diabetes Research and Clinical Practice*. 2017 Nov 1;133:1–9.

33. Zelikovic, I, Servais, A. Aminoaciduria and glycosuria in children. In: Emma, F., Goldstein, S., Bagga, A., Bates, C.M., Shroff, R. (eds) *Pediatric Nephrology* 2021; 1–29. Springer, Berlin, Heidelberg.

34. Vaidya VS, Ferguson MA, Bonventre JV. Biomarkers of acute kidney injury. *Annual Review of Pharmacology and Toxicology*. 2008;48:463–93.

35. Waller K V., Ward KM, Mahan JD, Wismatt DK. Current concepts in proteinuria. *Clinical Chemistry* [Internet]. 1989 [cited 2023 Mar 24];35(5):755–65. Available from: https://pubmed.ncbi.nlm.nih.gov/2656000/.

36. Bellinghieri G, Savica V, Santoro D. Renal alterations during exercise. *Journal of Renal Nutrition*. 2008 Jan;18(1):158–64.

37. Unwin RJ, Capasso G. The renal tubular acidoses. *Journal of the Royal Society of Medicine*. 2001 May;94(5):221–5.

38. Müller A, Zimmermann-Klemd AM, Lederer AK, Hannibal L, Kowarschik S, Huber R, et al. A vegan diet is associated with a significant reduction in dietary acid load: Post hoc analysis of a randomized controlled trial in healthy individuals. *International Journal of Environmental Research and Public Health*. 2021 Sep 23;18(19):1–12.

39. Schaffer JN, Pearson MM. Proteus mirabilis and urinary tract infections. *Microbiology Spectrum*. 2015 Oct;3(5):1–66.

40. Kuru B, Sever M, Aksay E, Dogan T, Yalcin N, Eren ES, *et al.* Comparing finger-stick β-hydroxybutyrate with dipstick urine tests in the detection of ketone bodies. *Turkish Journal of Emergency Medicine*. 2014 Jun;14(2):47–52.

41. Foley KF, Wasserman J. Are unexpected positive dipstick urine bilirubin results clinically significant? A retrospective review. *Laboratory Medicine*. 2014;45(1):59–61.

42. Echeverry G, Hortin GL, Rai AJ. Introduction to urinalysis: Historical perspectives and clinical application. *Methods in Molecular Biology*. 2010;641:1–12.

43. Makris K, Spanou L. Acute kidney injury: Definition, pathophysiology and clinical phenotypes. *Clinical Biochemist Reviews*. 2016 May;37(2):85–98.

44. Basile DP, Anderson MD, Sutton TA. Pathophysiology of acute kidney injury. *Comprehensive Physiology*. 2012 Apr;2(2):1303–53.

45. Zarjou A, Agarwal A. Sepsis and acute kidney injury. *Journal of the American Society of Nephrology* [Internet]. 2011 Jun [cited 2023 Mar 27];22(6):999–1006. Available from: https://journals.lww.com/jasn/Fulltext/2011/06000/Sepsis_and_Acute_Kidney_Injury.7.aspx.

46. Sparks MA, Crowley SD, Gurley SB, Mirotsou M, Coffman TM. Classical renin-Angiotensin system in kidney physiology. *Comprehensive Physiology*. 2014 Jul;4(3):1201–28.

47. Ostermann M, Philips BJ, Forni LG. Clinical review: Biomarkers of acute kidney injury: Where are we now? *Critical Care*. 2012;16(5):233.

48. El-Khoury JM, Hoenig MP, Jones GRD, Lamb EJ, Parikh CR, Tolan N V, et al. AACC guidance document on laboratory investigation of acute kidney injury. [cited 2023 Mar 15]; Available from: https://academic.oup.com/jalm/article/6/5/1316/6272705.

49. Spahillari A, Parikh C, Sint K, … JKAJ of, 2012 undefined. Serum cystatin C–versus creatinine-based definitions of acute kidney injury following cardiac surgery: A prospective cohort study. 2012 [cited 2023 Mar 15]; Available from: https://www.sciencedirect.com/science/article/pii/S0272638612008566.

50. Gharaibeh KA, Hamadah AM, El-Zoghby ZM, Lieske JC, Larson TS, Leung N. Cystatin C predicts renal recovery earlier than creatinine among patients with acute kidney injury. *Kidney International Reports* 2018 Mar 1;3(2):337–42.

51. Ichimura T, Bonventre J, Bailly V, … HWJ of B, 1998 undefined. Kidney injury molecule-1 (KIM-1), a putative epithelial cell adhesion molecule containing a novel immunoglobulin domain, is up-regulated in renal cells after. ASBMB [Internet]. [cited 2023 Mar 15]; Available from: https://www.jbc.org/article/S0021-9258(17)47182-1/abstract.

52. Mishra J, Dent C, Tarabishi R, Mitsnefes MM, Ma Q, Kelly C, et al. Neutrophil gelatinase-associated lipocalin (NGAL) as a biomarker for acute renal injury after cardiac surgery. *Lancet*. 2005 Apr 2;365(9466):1231–8.

53. Devarajan P. Biomarkers for the early detection of acute kidney injury. *Current Opinion in Pediatrics*. 2011 Apr;23(2):194–200.

54. Gunnerson KJ, Shaw AD, Chawla LS, Bihorac A, Al-Khafaji A, Kashani K, et al. TIMP2•IGFBP7 biomarker panel accurately predicts acute kidney injury in high-risk surgical patients. *Journal of Trauma and Acute Care Surgery*. 2016 Feb;80(2):243–9.

55. Hill NR, Fatoba ST, Oke JL, Hirst JA, O'Callaghan CA, Lasserson DS, et al. Global prevalence of chronic kidney disease – A systematic review and meta-analysis. *PLoS One*. 2016 Jul 1;11(7).

56. Crook M. *Clinical Chemistry & Metabolic Medicine*. Google Scholar [Internet]. [cited 2023 Mar 15]. Available from: https://scholar.google.com/scholar?hl=en&as_sdt=0%2C5&q=16.%09Crook+M.+Clinical+chemistry+%26+metabolic+medicine.+8th+ed.+London%3A+Hodder+Arnold%3B+2012%3B+48&btnG=.

57. Shahbaz H, Gupta M. *Creatinine Clearance*. 2022 Jul 25 [cited 2023 Mar 27]. Available from: https://www.ncbi.nlm.nih.gov/books/NBK544228/.

58. Nigam SK, Bush KT. Uremic syndrome of chronic kidney disease: Altered remote sensing and signaling HHS Public Access. *Nature Reviews Nephrology*. 2019;15(5):301–16.

59. Joannidis M, Forni LG. Clinical review: Timing of renal replacement therapy. *Critical Care*. 2011;15(3):223.

60. Fukumoto S. Phosphate metabolism and vitamin D. *BoneKEy Reports*. 2014;3:497.

61. Tariq S, Tariq S, Lone KP, Khaliq S. Alkaline phosphatase is a predictor of Bone Mineral Density in postmenopausal females. *Pakistan Journal of Medical Sciences* [Internet]. 2019 May 1 [cited 2023 Mar 27];35(3):749. Available from: https://www.ncbi.nlm.nih.gov/pmc/articles/PMC6572960/.

62. Johnson RJ, Nakagawa T, Jalal D, Sánchez-Lozada LG, Kang DH, Ritz E. Uric acid and chronic kidney disease: Which is chasing which? *Nephrology Dialysis Transplantation* [Internet]. 2013 Sep [cited 2023 Mar 27];28(9):2221. Available from: https://www.ncbi.nlm.nih.gov/pmc/articles/PMC4318947/.

63. Cascella M, Vaqar S. Hypermagnesemia. *Nutrition Reviews* [Internet]. 2022 Nov 7 [cited 2023 Mar 27];26(1):12–5. Available from: https://www.ncbi.nlm.nih.gov/books/NBK549811/.

64. Bunn HF. Erythropoietin. *Cold Spring Harb Perspect Med* [Internet]. 2013 Mar 1 [cited 2023 Mar 15];3(3):a011619. Available from: http://perspectivesinmedicine.cshlp.org/content/3/3/a011619.full.

65. Rifai N. Tietz textbook of clinical chemistry and molecular diagnostics-e-book [Internet]. 2017 [cited 2023 Mar 15]. Available from: https://books.google.com/books?hl=en&lr=&id=3mRgDwAAQBAJ&oi=fnd&pg=PP1&dq=18.%09Rifai+N.+Tietz+textbook+of+clinical+chemistry+and+molecular+diagnostics+6th+ed-e-book.+Elsevier+Health+Sciences%3B+2018%3B+1283&ots=bNOtpgtv_-&sig=OwOhb25xXeJo_j5K-C5-Hvvj2JY.

66. Rysz J, Gluba-Brzózka A, Rysz-Górzyńska M, Franczyk B. The role and function of HDL in patients with chronic kidney disease and the risk of cardiovascular disease. *International Journal of Molecular Sciences* [Internet]. 2020 Jan 2 [cited 2023 Mar 27];21(2). Available from: https://www.ncbi.nlm.nih.gov/pmc/articles/PMC7014265/.

12 Clinical Management of Renal Diseases

Shivani Jani, Hitesh Katariya, and Bhupendra Prajapati

12.1 INTRODUCTION TO RENAL DISEASES

The term "renal disease" refers to a diverse range of conditions that affect the structure and operation of the kidneys. It is now understood that even slight variations in kidney shape and function can increase the risk of mortality and problems in different organ systems, both of which arise much more commonly than renal failure. Renal disease is a major public health issue on a global scale. Kidney failure is becoming more common in all the countries of the world, with poor consequences and high costs. Even more people have chronic renal disease in its initial stages. There is growing evidence, accumulated over the past few decades, that renal disease's negative effects, including renal failure, heart disease, and early death, can be avoided or postponed. Laboratory testing can identify renal disease in its early stages. Early treatment is useful in delaying the development of renal failure. Starting treatment for cardiac risk markers at an early point of kidney disease would be beneficial in lowering heart disease occurrences both prior to and following the beginning of renal failure. Regrettably, the opportunities for prophylaxis are squandered because renal disease is not well diagnosed and is inadequately treated worldwide (1). One of the causes of this is the lack of consensus over the diagnosis and categorization of the stages of chronic renal disease progression. Relying on laboratory assessment of the intensity of kidney disease, the correlation of renal function level with comorbidities, segmentation of the chances of acute renal failure, and the onset of cardiovascular disease, a clinically appropriate classification would be created.

The right interpretation and application of the renal disease indicators and stages, early illness detection, and coordination between primary-care physicians and medical specialists are necessary for the best handling of patients suffering from kidney disease. The National Kidney Foundation Kidney Disease Outcomes Quality Initiative (NKF KDOQI) has described chronic kidney disease (CKD), a term that can refer to a variety of conditions, including chronic renal disease and insufficiency, and chronic renal failure. Better comprehension is achieved by individuals, relatives, healthcare professionals, and the general public when "kidney" is used instead of "renal". "Chronic" is defined as lasting longer than three months, whereas "acute" is defined as lasting less than three months. Acute kidney injury (AKI) is a subset of acute kidney illnesses and disorders (AKD) marked by rapid alterations in kidney function over the course of one week. AKI can cause CKD, and CKD raises the risk of AKI, so there is a complicated link between the two conditions (2). There are two types of renal failures: acute and chronic.

12.1.1 Acute Renal Failure (ARF)

Glomerular filtration reduces suddenly (over hours to days) and is typically reversible in ARF syndrome. Kidney Disease: Improving Global Outcomes (KDIGO) criteria state that AKI can be identified by any combination of the following: (1) a rise in creatinine of 0.3 mg/dL within 48 hours, (2) a rise in creatinine of 1.5 times the baseline during the previous 7 days, or (3) a decrease in urine output of less than 0.5 mL/kg/hour for 6 hours. ARF has recently been superseded by the terminology "acute kidney injury" (AKI), which encompasses the complete clinical range from a slight rise in blood creatinine to explicit renal failure.

12.1.2 Chronic Renal Failure (CRF)

A sustained deterioration of kidney function, also known as chronic renal failure (CRF) or chronic kidney disease (CKD), is indicated by either a computed glomerular filtration rate (GFR) under 60 ml per min/1.73 m² or excessively increased blood creatinine over longer than three months. Dialysis or kidney transplantation may be necessary as a result of the increasing loss of renal function. End-stage renal disease (ESRD) is the term used when a patient requires renal replacement treatment (3).

12.1.3 Classification of CKD

The CKD classification scheme was developed in the United States and quickly spread worldwide. Table 12.1 displays the updated version adopted by the United Kingdom. It is dependent on the GFR, as well as whether or not renal impairment is present. The latter is generally characterized as the continuous prevalence of proteinuria (especially microalbuminuria), hematuria, or anatomical

DOI: 10.1201/9781003384823-12

Table 12.1 Classification of chronic kidney disease (5)

Stage	Description	GFR (ml/min/1.73 m^2)	Affected population (%)
1	Renal injury present with normal or increased GFR	>90	1.8
2	Renal injury present and moderately decreased GFR	60–89	3.2
3A	GFR slightly reduced	45–59	6.3
3B	GFR slightly reduced	30–44	1.4
4	Severe reduction in GFR	15–29	0.4
5	Worsened renal disease	<15	0.2

kidney disease (as determined by imaging or histology). To prove chronicity, the lower GFR and/or damage must have been persistent for more than 90 days. It should be noted that stages 1 and 2 involve renal injury, but stages 3–5 only require a lower GFR (4).

12.2 ETIOLOGY

12.2.1 Renal Failure Etiopathogenesis

12.2.1.1 Acute Renal Failure

1. Prerenal (about 60%): Cyclosporine, hypotension, volume shrinkage (e.g., sepsis, hemorrhage), serious organ failure, like heart malfunction or liver malfunction, and medications like non-steroidal anti-inflammatory agents, angiotensin receptor blockers (ARBs), and angiotensin-converting enzyme (ACE) inhibitors.

2. Intrarenal (about 35%): Arteriolar insults, acute interstitial nephritis, fat emboli, connective tissue diseases, intrarenal accumulation (observed in tumor-lysis disorder, elevated uric acid output, and numerous myeloma proteins), and rhabdomyolysis.

3. Postrenal (about 5%): Extrinsic constriction (prostatic hypertrophy, carcinoma), intrinsic blockage (clot, calculus, tumor, stricture), and impaired function.

12.2.1.2 Chronic Renal Failure

1. The most common cause of ESRD is diabetes mellitus, particularly type 2 diabetes mellitus with the second most common cause being hypertension

2. Renal polycystic disorders, disorders of renal arteries, and glomerulonephritis have all been associated with ESRD.

3. Other recognized causes include nephrolithiasis and chronic blockage of the urinary system.

4. The disorder known as vesicoureteral reflux, which causes urine to flow back up into the kidneys and recurring pyelonephritis have also been observed to be linked with ESRD (6).

12.3 EPIDEMIOLOGY

AKI has been reported to occur in as high as 37% of treated patients in intensive care centers, 2% to 5% of patients throughout hospitalization, and 4% to 15% of patients following cardiovascular operations. AKI has been predicted to affect 209 in every million individuals annually, with 36% of those affected needing kidney replacement treatment. Uncertainty surrounds the prevalence and incidence of CRF in the United States. Nearly 2 million Americans, according to the National Health and Nutrition Examination Survey, have blood creatinine levels of 2 mg/dl or higher. It is well recognized that men are more likely to develop CRF than women. Over 100,000 people in the United States develop ESRD each year. Race affects ESRD rates differently. Black people experience three to four times the prevalence and incidence of ESRD than white people (6).

12.4 PATHOPHYSIOLOGY

A series of events that take place following an acute shock in the context of acute renal collapse, as well as progressively over time in the event of chronic kidney illnesses (Figure 12.1), can be used to describe the pathophysiology of kidney failure.

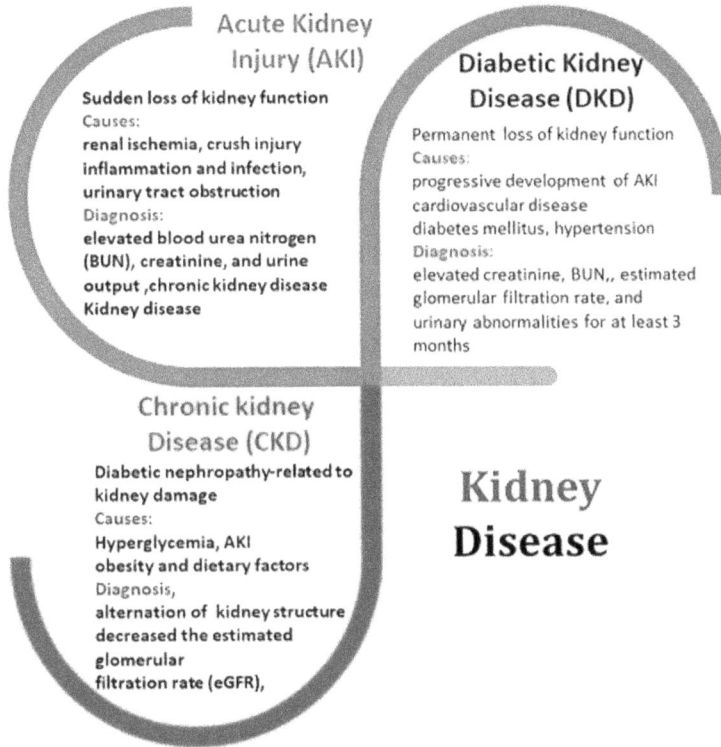

Figure 12.1 Overview of the entire kidney disease along with its diversified symptoms (8).

(Adapted from Yun CW, Lee SH. Potential and therapeutic efficacy of cell-based therapy using mesenchymal stem cells for acute/chronic kidney disease. International journal of molecular sciences. 2019; 20(7):1619.)

AKI can be broadly divided into three categories.

1. Prerenal azotemia: a reduction in renal blood circulation, in severe cirrhosis, cardiac arrest, and sepsis. Prerenal AKI develops as a result of perhaps an absolute decrease in extracellular fluid capacity or a decrease in circulating capacity leading to an inadequate maintenance of overall fluid balance.. Normal kidney auto-regulatory mechanisms dilate afferent arterioles and constrict efferent arterioles to maintain intra-capillary tension during the early phase. Renal adaptation mechanisms fall short in severe prerenal circumstances, hiding the decline in GFR and the rise in blood urea nitrogen (BUN) and creatinine concentrations.

2. Renal azotemia is an example of an intrinsic ailment that affects the renal parenchyma. Internal disorders can further be split into those that affect the vasculature, glomeruli, and/or tubule-interstitium.

3. Postrenal azotemia, that is, blocking of the passage of urine.

Specific starting mechanisms are mostly connected to the pathophysiology of CRF. Time-adaptive physiology plays a part, causing corrective hyperfiltration and hypertrophy of the residual functional nephrons. As the insult progresses, histopathologic alterations, such as glomerular architectural distortion, aberrant podocyte activity, and interruption of filtration resulting in sclerosis, occur in a series of steps. (7)

The following are some pertinent history and physical exam results linked to renal failure:

History:

a. A detailed medical history of the present disease

b. Medical history includes type 1 diabetes and hypertension

c. A history of renal illness in the family

d. A history of renal function

e. Medications, particularly the initiation date, the dosage of nephrotoxic substances, and nonsteroidal anti-inflammatory drugs (NSAIDs)

f. Any operation that involves the application of a contrast substance (7).

Physical examination:

a. Check hemodynamic factors such as weight, heart rate, and blood pressure (BP)

b. Look for lung crackles, edema, jugular venous distention, S3 gallop, and volume status

c. Skin: look for any uremic frost or diffuse rash

d. Watch out for uremia symptoms: seizures, pericardial friction rub, asterixis, lethargy, peripheral neuropathies

e. Examine the abdomen for distention of the bladder and any suprapubic fullness.

12.4.1 CKD's Clinical Manifestations

Since CKD is typically asymptomatic and up to 90% of renal function can be impaired before symptoms appear, it is crucial to monitor people at risk annually. Indeed, CKD patients may not have any symptoms until they are at stage 5 of the disease. General warning symptoms of CKD include, although are not restricted to: hematuria, nocturia, hypertension, restless legs, pruritus, sluggishness, dyspnea, nausea and/or vomiting, malaise, and anorexia.

12.4.2 Advantages of Early Detection

- There is a strong correlation between a decrease in estimated glomerular filtration rate (eGFR) and the progression of chronic kidney disease (CKD), leading to an increased susceptibility to adverse events such as cardiovascular disease and death.

- Increasing levels of albumin in urine correspond directly with an accelerated rate of development to ESKD and elevated heart disease risk.

- The risk of progression and cardiovascular can be lowered by up to 50% through early intervention, which includes lowering blood pressure and using ACE inhibitors or angiotensin renin blockers. This may also enhance quality of life.

- Iatrogenic AKI risk can be decreased through early identification.

- To lessen the growing burden of CKD, testing for the condition is crucial and beneficial since it enables early detection and therapy.

- CKD testing should not be done on everyone; instead, it should be aimed at people who are more likely to develop the disease.

- A urine albumin to creatinine ratio (ACR) test, a blood measurement for serum creatinine to determine glomerular filtration rate (GFR), as well as a kidney health checkup where blood pressure assessment is done, should all be performed as part of CKD testing.

- Every one to two years, people with CKD risk factors should have a kidney health checkup (9).

12.5 INVESTIGATIONAL TESTS FOR CKD

12.5.1 Glomerular Filtration Rate

The best overall assessment of kidney function is generally agreed to be GFR. However GFR measurements are very uncomfortable and usually results in errors due to non-compliance from patients. Using prediction formulas, the GFR may be calculated or estimated (eGFR) from serum creatinine. Furthermore, eGFR is a more accurate indicator of CKD than only serum creatinine. If the serum creatinine rises above the maximum normal level, 50% or more of the kidney's function can be compromised. Serious loss of renal function is not necessarily excluded by normal serum creatinine values (10).

12.5.1.1 Determination of eGFR

For people under the age of 18, eGFR is typically provided (with the Chronic kidney disease-epidemiology collaboration, CKD-EPI equation) when requests for serum creatinine are made. The

CKD-EPI equation has been demonstrated to have more accuracy and precision relative to other equations, making it the technique of choice for calculating eGFR. When calculating eGFR to diagnose CKD, the Cockcroft-Gault formula is no longer advised. Further research into lowered eGFR is only necessary if eGFR is less than 60 mL/min/1.73m^2. A retest should be carried out within 7 days if eGFR is 60 mL/min/1.73m^2, taking into account clinical circumstances in which eGFR results can be incorrect and/or deceptive; alternatively, this could indicate a case of acute kidney injury.

Clinical circumstances in which eGFR values might be inaccurate or misleading include sudden kidney function alterations (e.g., AKI), dialysis patients, recent ingestion of cooked meat (reassessment should be carried out if the person has fasted or has purposefully avoided eating cooked meat within 4 hours of the blood sample being taken), extraordinary dietary intake, such as a high-protein diet or the use of creatinine probiotics, body size extremes, skeletal muscular disorders, paralysis, amputees (eGFR may be higher), lots of muscle mass, young people under the age of 18, severe liver disease, eGFR readings greater than 90 mL/min/1.73m^2, medicines that affect how much creatinine is excreted, such as trimethoprim and fenofibrate, being pregnant, variability in the lab, or physiological processes, which can cause slight fluctuations in eGFR.

It is unknown whether eGFR is reliable during pregnancy. It is not advised to use eGFR to evaluate renal function in pregnant women. The preferred test for assessing kidney function in pregnant women should continue to be serum creatinine (11).

12.5.1.2 Drug Dosage and eGFR

- Some medications should be taken at lower doses if the kidneys are not functioning properly.

- Cockcroft-Gault values of creatinine clearance (CrCl mL/min) are frequently used by manufacturers to determine the renal dosage recommendations for drugs.

- eGFR, which is commonly accessible on laboratory reports, offers a reliable estimation of renal drug clearance.

- In addition to consulting the authorized information about the product, body size must be taken into account when using eGFR for drug dosing.

- Therapeutic drug surveillance or a reliable drug effect marker must be used to personalize dosing for medications with a smaller dose therapeutic index.

- It may be preferable to determine an eGFR that is not standardized to 1.73m^2 BSA for drug medicating in very large or very small individuals (12).

12.5.2 Ratio of Albumin to Creatinine in Urine (ACR)

An important indicator of kidney damage and an elevated risk of renal and cardiovascular disorders is an inordinate amount of proteins in the urine. Albumin makes up the majority of these proteins (albuminuria), but they also include lysozyme, beta-2 microglobulin, insulin, and low molecular weight immunoglobulin. It is uncommon for someone to have increased non-albumin protein excretion without also having increased albumin excretion. In population research, urine ACR successfully forecasts renal and cardiovascular risks. In intervention trials, a decrease in urine ACR indicates renoprotective benefits. A high urine ACR is a more frequent indicator of CKD than a low eGFR.

12.5.2.1 Ways to Detect Albuminuria

Urinary ACR assessment using the first morning void samples is the recommended technique for determining albuminuria in those with diabetes and those without the disease. In cases where a fresh void sample is not feasible or practicable, a random spot urine sample for urine ACR is permissible. Urinary protein discharge follows a rhythmic cycle and appears to be at its highest in the afternoon. As a result, ACR tests are most accurate when conducted in the early hours of the morning. To confirm albuminuria recurrence, a positive ACR test on an initial void sample should be redone. Whenever a minimum of two out of every three ACR findings are positive, albuminuria is considered to be present. If the albuminuria continues for at minimum three months, CKD is evident (14).

The use of a urine protein dipstick is no longer advised due to subpar specificity and sensitivity. The protein–creatinine ratio (PCR) is less sensitive than urine ACR for detecting clinically significant albuminuria in lower concentrations. Other factors that are known to elevate excretion of urine albumin besides CKD are urinary tract disease, eating a lot of protein, acute febrile sickness, congestive heart failure, menstruation, genital discharge, drugs (specifically NSAIDs), as well as strenuous exercise during the previous 24 hours.

For CKD, the following diagnostic assessment tests are always recommended: ultrasonography of the kidneys, repeats of the serum urea, electrolytes, creatinine, eGFR, and albumin assays (within a week), referral to the AKI management strategy if the eGFR declines further, a complete blood count, CRP, and ESR, urine ACR (ideally during the initial morning void to reduce the impact of postural changes on albumin excretion; however, if that is not possible, any urine is fine), fasting glucose and lipids, and urine microscopy to check for crystallized or cast red blood cells (15).

12.6 MANAGEMENT OF RENAL DISEASES

The management of renal diseases is divided into various plans based on the conditions of the diseases and the results obtained from the lab tests.

12.6.1 Yellow Clinical Action Plan

This plan is applicable when eGFR ≥60 mL/min/1.73m^2, with microalbuminuria or eGFR 45–59 mL/min/1.73m^2 and normoalbuminuria. The management goals are investigations to identify the root reason, slowing the spread of renal disease, evaluation of total cardiovascular risk, and refraining from using drugs that are nephrotoxic or deplete body fluids.

Management strategy:

Reviewing frequency should be every year. Clinical evaluation of blood pressure, weight, and smoking should be carried out. Laboratory evaluation includes the following tests: urine ACR, eGFR, biochemical profile with urea, creatinine, and electrolytes, HbA1c (for diabetics), and fasting lipids. Assessing the absolute cardiovascular risk, lowering blood pressure, lifestyle changes, lowering cholesterol, controlling blood sugar, avoiding nephrotoxic drugs, and treating chronic kidney disease holistically are all recommended (16).

12.6.2 Orange Clinical Action Plan

This plan is applicable when eGFR 30–59 mL/min/1.73m^2, with microalbuminuria or eGFR 30–44 mL/min/1.73m^2 and normoalbuminuria. The particular management goals follow the goals of the yellow action plan in addition to goals like diagnosis and treatment of problems early on, modification of medicine dosages to reflect renal function, and appropriately referring patients to a nephrologist as necessary.

Management strategy:

Reviewing frequency should be almost every three to six months. Clinical action is the same as in the yellow action plan. Laboratory evaluation includes urea, creatinine, and electrolytes, urine ACR, eGFR and biochemical profile, HbA1c (for people with diabetes), a full blood count, calcium and phosphate levels, fasting lipids, and parathyroid hormone (biannually or annually if eGFR is 45 mL/min/1.73m^2). Other recommendations include assessment of absolute heart disease risk, lowering blood pressure, lifestyle changes, lowering cholesterol, assessing the likelihood of atherosclerotic events, considering antiplatelet therapy in accordance with current cardiovascular recommendations, glycemic management, avoiding nephrotoxic drugs or fluid depletion, and adjusting doses to appropriate levels based on kidney function, checking for common problems, and, where necessary, appropriately referring patients to nephrologists. These recommendations amount to a comprehensive approach to managing CKD.

12.6.3 Red Clinical Action Plan

This plan is applicable when macroalbuminuria, irrespective of eGFR, is found or eGFR <30 mL/min/1.73m^2, irrespective of albuminuria, is found. The management goals include those of the yellow and orange action plans, as well as a few new goals, such as, if necessary, getting ready for kidney replacement treatment and, if necessary, getting ready for supporting care other than dialysis.

Management strategy:

The reviewing now needs to be carried out every one to three months. Also, the clinical assessment includes edema, along with other criteria from the yellow and orange action plans. Laboratory assessment is also the same as in the yellow and orange action plans; only a few new points are added, like discussing treatment options such as dialysis, kidney transplant, and non-dialysis supportive care (17).

12.6.4 Whole-of-Practice Strategy for Managing CKD

A whole-of-practice strategy combining the general practitioner (GP), the preliminary healthcare nurse, and practice personnel maximizes the chance of recommended practice care taking place in the management of CKD. The selection of a clinical lead, clinical management, accurate CKD coding, and e-health deployment all have an effect on the results. A whole-of-practice perspective becomes even more crucial in providing the best care when kidney function falls and difficulties and comorbidities increase. Doctors play a critical role in organizing the support offered by everyone else and assuring that it remains centered on the patient's personal goals and interests. They do this by maintaining continuous contact with the patient and their loved ones.

The GP might occasionally need to represent the patient's interests when speaking with other specialists. Additionally, he or she is in charge of the patient's ongoing basic care, which might also entail helping the patient manage his or her kidney disease and other long-term medical conditions, collaborating with the patient to create a management strategy that promotes and supports compliance with the diet and medication plan, reacting suitably to fresh symptoms, checking for new issues and comorbidities, offering suggestions and strategies for illness prevention and health promotion, offering the necessary vaccines, and offering help resolving psychosocial problems (18). Figure 12.2 shows the areas in the management of chronic kidney disease and the treatment selection plan.

Primary care nurses are important in identifying those at danger of CKD. They collaborate with general practitioners to provide best-practice treatment to individuals with CKD. They also help in assisting CKD patients with self-management techniques, promoting customized, patient-centered care planning, providing motivational counseling, which supports behavior change, and providing the CKD patient with continual education and support (19).

12.6.5 Patient-Led Behavior Modification

Enabling patients to take the initiative in adopting behavior improvements that will improve their health results is a beneficial technique in the management of chronic diseases. Behavior change is a challenging process. Health practitioners should consider providing health coaching to patients to help them reflect on lifestyle and behavioral choices that will work for them in controlling their disease. The "phases of behavior adjustment" paradigm, which describe the steps people take to recognize necessary changes and incorporate them into their life, is helpful to consider: precontemplation or ignorance, contemplation, action, preparation, maintenance, conclusion, advocacy, and transcendence. It is important to strongly encourage patients to participate in their care.

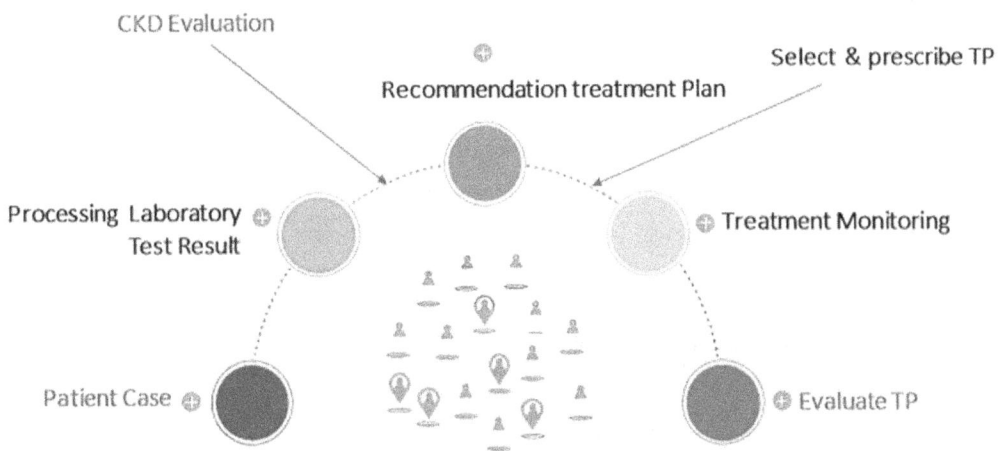

Figure 12.2 Management of CKD and Treatment Selection (14).

Adapted from Ali SI, Jung SW, Bilal HS, Lee SH, Hussain J, Afzal M, Hussain M, Ali T, Chung T, Lee S. Clinical decision support system based on hybrid knowledge modeling: a case study of chronic kidney disease-mineral and bone disorder treatment. International Journal of Environmental Research and Public Health. 2021; 19(1):226.

14.6.6 Lifestyle Changes

Living a healthier lifestyle must always be the primary line of management for those with CKD. Incorporating lifestyle adjustments (relating to alcohol, smoking, physical activity, and nutrition) can improve results for people with CKD and slow the disease's progression. A crucial framework for tackling lifestyle difficulties is provided by the five As: agree/advice, ask, arrange, assist, assess.

14.6.6.1 Obesity

The risk of CKD is doubled for people with obesity (BMI ≥30) compared to those with a healthy weight. Waist circumference is essential, but central obesity is much more significant than generalized obesity. People who are obese may be more prone to developing albuminuria (20).

14.6.6.2 Smoking

Compared with non-smokers, people who smoke have a 40% to 105% higher risk of developing CKD (based on their pack-year record). Kidney disease has been linked to smoking. People with diabetes who smoke are much more prone to albuminuria, and smoking speeds up the course of diabetic nephropathy, leading to kidney failure.

14.6.6.3 Physical Activity

The general health and wellbeing advantages of physical activity are substantial. Beyond its positive effects on overall health, physical activity has been shown to help manage a number of chronic diseases, according to mounting research. Better CKD results are linked to improved levels of cardiorespiratory fitness, increased physical activity, and less time spent sitting still. For the majority of people, gradually increasing physical activity is probably safer than staying sedentary, though hazards should be considered individually. Table 12.2 describes the measures for patients suffering from CKD and also the parameters that need to be changed after a diagnosis of CKD (21).

Table 12.2 Objectives for healthy living for those with CKD (21)

Parameter	Target	Approximate drop in systolic blood pressure
Smoking	Utilizing counseling or nicotine substitution treatment, or other medications, smoking can be stopped.	–
Nutrition	Be sure to eat a variety of foods, such as the Dietary Approaches to Stop Hypertension (DASH) diet, which is high in fruits, vegetables, whole-grain cereals, sources of protein, livestock, fish, eggs, nuts and seeds, legumes and beans, and low-fat dairy products. • Keep your daily salt intake to 6 g (or 100 mmol) or less. • Eat fewer foods that are high in saturated and trans fats. • Consume foods with added sugars in moderation.	4–7 mm Hg of sodium restriction (for a daily salt intake reduction of 6g). DASH diet: 5.5 mm Hg for normal blood pressure; 11.4 mmHg for high blood pressure.
Alcohol	Limit daily alcohol intake to two standard drinks.	3 mm Hg (a 67% decrease from the daily baseline of 3–6 drinks).
Physical activity	Be active most days of the week, ideally every day. Get in 150–300 minutes of reasonable intensity exercise, 75–150 minutes of strenuous intensity exercise, or an equivalent mix of both each week. Perform muscle-building exercises at least twice a week.	3–5 mm Hg
Obesity	Reduce your energy consumption to keep your weight in check. A BMI of 25 kg/m² or less indicates ideal weight. Waist circumference of 80 cm for women and 94 cm for men should be considered ideal.	4.4 mm Hg

14.6.6.4 *Nutrition*

Individuals with CKD must be encouraged to consume a balanced and sufficient diet in accordance with their energy needs and the dietary recommendations provided by regulatory agencies. People with CKD who are overweight or obese should be urged to lose weight under the supervision of a certified practicing dietician (22).

12.7 MANAGEMENT OF CKD IN ADDITION TO OTHER CHRONIC ILLNESSES

CKD rarely develops on its own. It is likely that patients with CKD will also be diagnosed with one or more additional chronic illnesses in a basic care context. CKD and other prevalent chronic illnesses like diabetes and cardiac disease share many therapeutic objectives and management techniques. Improved patient results will emerge from treating the patient as a whole and addressing chronic conditions jointly.

12.7.1 Heart Disease and CKD

Significant albuminuria and decreased eGFR are separate risk factors for cardiovascular disease (CVD). Diabetes is less of a risk factor for CVD than CKD. A substantial risk marker for cardiac diseases and death is CKD, even in the early stages. The chance of death from cardiovascular causes can be nearly 20 times higher for patients with CKD than the likelihood of needing dialysis or a transplant. An assessment of total cardiovascular risk quantifies the likelihood that a person will have a cardiovascular ailment within a specific time frame. Instead of focusing solely on a specific risk factor (like cholesterol levels), the assessment considers the mix of risk variables and their intensity.. Absolute cardiovascular risk-based clinical decisions can result in better health outcomes and prove helpful in educating and motivating patients.

Individuals over the age of 45 must have their cardiovascular concerns evaluated. Additionally, individuals without cardiovascular disease already present or not already recognized as having a higher risk of developing CVD should have a checkup (23).

12.7.2 CKD and Diabetes

Every second person with type 2 diabetes who attends their primary-care provider will also have CKD. Approximately 40% of CKD cases can be attributed to diabetes, making it a serious risk factor for the disease. All stages of CKD (cardiovascular results, dialysis prognosis, and post-transplant longevity) are worsened when diabetes is present. The primary indicator of heart disease risk in diabetes is kidney dysfunction. The development of chronic kidney disease in patients with diabetes can be slowed down or stopped through early diagnosis and the right treatments. In persons with type 1 or type 2 diabetes, adequate blood glucose regulation dramatically lowers the chance of developing microalbuminuria, macroalbuminuria, and/or blatant nephropathy.. In CKD, some drugs might have to be stopped or their dosage may have to be lowered. It is crucial to keep in mind that having CKD essentially increases the chance of hypoglycemia when thinking about diabetes treatment alternatives. Complex mechanisms including both endogenous and exogenous insulin clearance underlie this. As eGFR decreases, hypoglycemia occurs more frequently, necessitating possible prescription adjustments.

12.7.3 CKD and Hypertension

Both the cause and a consequence of CKD, hypertension can be challenging to manage. Uncontrolled hypertension increases the chance of coronary heart disease, stroke, and kidney disease progression. Consideration of hypertension as a component of absolute cardiovascular danger is necessary. Striving for a reduced blood pressure goal (systolic BP less than 120 mmHg) in CKD patients that are at an elevated CVD risk may enhance outcomes, according to some new research and clinical guidelines. In some people who are at an extremely high risk of cardiovascular disease, striving toward a systolic blood pressure of less than 120 mmHg may be prudent. Lower blood pressure goals must be weighed against a higher risk of adverse effects, such as hypotension resulting in more falls, vertigo, abnormal electrolytes, and more AKI episodes (24).

One of the most crucial objectives in the treatment of CKD is to lower blood pressure to below target levels. Changes in lifestyle should always be encouraged because they can significantly lower blood pressure. Blood pressure-reducing medication for CKD patients should start with either an ACE inhibitor or an ARB. Combining ACE inhibitor and ARB treatment is not advised. It is advised to use the highest dosage of either an ACE inhibitor or an ARB.

When an ACE inhibitor or ARB is started as a therapy, the GFR may drop and potassium levels may rise. Any ACE inhibitor, spironolactone, or ARB should be terminated if the blood potassium level is higher than 6 mmol/L after dose decrease, diuretic treatment, and dietary potassium limitation. Most persons with CKD require many medications (typically three or more) to appropriately control their hypertension. Based on cardiovascular reasons and comorbidities, extra antihypertensive medications can be selected. Unless there is an elevated risk of bleeding, evaluate the likelihood of atherosclerotic episodes and consider treatment with an antiplatelet medication. Think of sleep apnea as a contributing factor to resistant hypertension. As compared to office BP readings, 24-hour ambulatory blood pressure monitoring (ABPM) and home blood pressure monitoring (HBPM) have indeed been shown to be better indications of target organ damage, heart mortality, and morbidity. Additionally, using ABPM or HBPM can help with the identification of hidden hypertension, overtreatment (hypotension), and tracking the effectiveness of antihypertensive medication (18). When HBPM and education are used together, adherence may rise and ultimate blood pressure control may improve. When practical, HBPM should be taken into account to help in the diagnosis and treatment of hypertension.

12.7.4 Considerations for Medications in CKD

It is critical to assess medications that are excreted in the urine and avoid use of nephrotoxic drugs in CKD patients. Once the GFR drops below 60 mL/min/1.73m^2, dosage adjustments or drug discontinuation are typically necessary. The Medicare item numbers that promote collaboration between general practitioners and pharmacists are Home Medicines Assessments and Residential Medication Reconciliation Assessments. Correct coding is required for CKD. The practice software can be useful when thinking about medications. Encourage patients to inform other medical professionals of their kidney health and make sure they are conscious that suffering from CKD can impact medication prescriptions. If GFR is between 30 and 60 mL/min/1.73 m^2, metformin can be used with caution; if GFR is below 30 mL/min/1.73 m^2, it should not be used. It should be momentarily stopped whenever there is a shift in kidney function or when the patient is unwell. Although it can increase creatinine, trimethoprim has no impact on GFR. The often-recommended medications that might have to be discontinued or whose dosage should be reduced in CKD include, but are not restricted to, acarbose, colchicine, allopurinol, apixaban, antivirals, apixaban, benzodiazepines, etc. Commonly given medicines that can harm renal function in CKD include aminoglycosides, gadolinium, NSAIDs and COX-2 inhibitors, calcineurin inhibitors, lithium, and radiographic contrast agents (25).

12.7.5 Acute Kidney Injury

A prevalent syndrome that is independently and substantially linked to higher morbidity and death, especially in hospitalized patients, is AKI. Continuous monitoring is essential because CKD raises the probability of AKI; moreover, an incident of AKI raises the possibility that CKD will later develop. A rapid rise in serum creatinine or persistent oliguria can both be used to diagnose AKI. AKI can be prevented by identifying those who are more likely to develop it and addressing possibly modifiable exposures. This is something that practitioners are uniquely positioned to do. Potential risk factors for AKI include cancer, diabetes, anemia, diabetes, heart disease, lung illness, other chronic diseases, old age, and being female. Modifiable kidney damage includes hypovolemia, infection, major illness, circulatory crisis, burns, and trauma. Other causes include drugs, radiocontrast chemicals, poisonous animals (such as snakes and spiders), heatwaves, and critical sickness (26).

12.7.5.1 AKI Management and Prevention Strategy

Identifying those who are at danger is the first step. Everyone with CKD stage 3 to 5 has an elevated chance of developing AKI. Reduce utilization of NSAIDs and other possibly nephrotoxic medicine in CKD patients. ARB, diuretics, and ACE inhibitors may need to be temporarily stopped in patients who have acute illnesses that are causing hypovolemia or hypotension. AKI can be diagnosed if the serum creatinine levels rise by 26.5 µmol/l or more within 48 hours, or if they have risen by 1.5 times the baseline over the previous 7 days, or if there is a significant decrease in urine output relative to normal output. Removing dangers during the earliest stages of the illness is the first step to be performed during an AKI incident. A specialist should be asked early on for a comprehensive fluid evaluation and medication review for all individuals at risk when an acute sickness arises. After an episode of AKI, annual kidney health checks must be carried out for the following three years. Training and self-management should be taught to lower the risk of future exposures (27).

12.7.6 Kidney Stones

One of the most prevalent conditions affecting the urinary tract is kidney stone disease. Age, family history, and being an Indigenous person all raise the risk of developing a kidney stone. The likelihood of developing a second kidney stone each year after having one is between 5% and 10%. Within five years, the risk of developing a second kidney stone decreases to about 30–50% for those who have already experienced one. An overall chemistry screening that includes serum uric acid, parathyroid status, calcium or stone evaluation (when available), or 24-hour urine quantity and chemistries (including calcium, uric acid, citrate, oxalate) are the main focus of early evaluation and monitoring in adults and can all be used to identify kidney stones. Calcium stones already present are usually impossible to dissolve. Reversing the anomalies found in the preliminary workup is the aim of therapy. Changes in nutrition, fluid intake, and medication use may all be essential. Before beginning medication therapy, consult a certified practicing dietitian about a three- to six-month study of diet and hydration adjustments. Increased fluid consumption during the day, increased dietary potassium, increased dietary phytate (e.g., nuts and beans), maintenance of normal calcium absorption, and decreased ingestion of oxalate, sucrose, animal protein, fructose, and supplemental calcium are dietary changes that can help reduce the likelihood of developing calcium oxalate stones. A urologist typically participates in the emergency department's acute treatment of a stone incident. An alpha blocker drug such as prazosin or tamsulosin should be used in the treatment of a stone incident when the stone is confirmed to be of a diameter capable of being freely passed (5 mm) (28).

12.7.7 Kidney Cysts

Simple kidney cysts are typically benign and do not require any more testing. Simple cysts are frequently asymptomatic and they are quite common (not hereditary). Simple cysts can develop as people age. They may be connected to underlying CKD. The kidneys are not damaged by them. Only numerous cysts, bilateral recurrent cysts, cysts with complicated internal structures or solid components, difficulty distinguishing cysts from blockage, a past record of malignancy, or cyst-related symptoms would necessitate further assessment and research. A set of chronic kidney illnesses known as polycystic kidney disease (PKD) cause the production of many cysts in the kidney. The most prevalent hereditary kidney disease is PKD. PKD frequently leads to CKD.

If there are at least three cysts on the ultrasound and the age of the patient is between 15 and 39 years, PKD may be suspected. If the patient's age is between 40 to 59 years and if there are at least two cysts in each kidney shown on the ultrasound, a checkup must be carried out. For patients aged above 60 years, having at least four cysts in each kidney can lead to PKD (29).

12.8 MANAGEMENT OF PROGRESSIVE CKD

Suitable consultation with a nephrologist is linked to favorable outcomes, including a decreased percentage of advancement to ESKD, decreased death rates, and lowered necessity and duration of hospitalization. Referral to nephrology is advised in cases with eGFR 30 mL/min/1.73m^2 (stage 4 or 5 CKD of either etiology), chronic substantial albuminuria (urine ACR ≥30 mg/mmol), prolonged eGFR decline of at least 25% over the course of 12 months, or sustained eGFR decline of at least 15 mL/min/1.73m^2 per year. Referral is not required when the eGFR is stable and greater than 30 mL/min/1.73m^2, ACR in urine is less than 30 mg/mmol (with absence of hematuria), and blood pressure is regulated.

Regular blood biochemistry and histology, urine ACR and urine imaging for red cell structure and deposits, present and previous blood pressure, and ureteral ultrasound are tests that are advised prior to referral (30).

12.8.1 Solutions for Stage 5 CKD Treatment

The characteristics of stage 5 CKD and the available treatment choices should be adequately explained to individuals and their relatives or caretakers so they can make an educated decision about how to manage their disease. It is highly advised that patients, families, and healthcare professionals all participate in the decision-making process. An online decision assistance tool like "My Kidneys My Choice" is a great option for supporting this. A program called Renal Supportive Care (RSC) is integrated into routine renal care at every stage of the therapeutic process. RSC is given in addition to regular renal care, not as a substitute for it, for individuals undergoing renal replacement treatment (dialysis or transplant). To assist patients suffering from CKD and ESKD to live as fully as possible, RSC uses an interdisciplinary strategy that combines the abilities of renal care and palliative treatment. This is accomplished through assisting patients as they cope with their advanced disease and effectively regulating their symptoms. Table 12.3 contains a list of treatments available for kidney care (31).

12.8.2 Cooperative Decision-Making

This enables the patient and the practitioner to jointly engage in making a health-related choice. It involves talking about the patient's options, the advantages and disadvantages of each, and taking the patient's beliefs, preferences, and situation into account. It is not a one-time conversation, but a continuous procedure that can be utilized to direct choices in relation to screening, inquiries, and appropriate therapies. The benefits include: it takes into account the values and preferences of the patient; it improves patient involvement; and it increases patient education. Although collaborative decision-taking can proceed without aids, a variety of decision assistance tools are now available. There are five questions that can help clinicians with collaborative decision-making (33).

Table 12.3   A basic comparison of available treatments for CKD (32)

Procedure	Forms	Involves	Lifestyle results and effects
Comprehensive conservative kidney care	• No transplant or dialysis. • Managed locally. • Assisted by renal supporting care or palliative care groups.	• Control of nutrition and medication. • Careful preparation. • Monitoring symptoms and treating without dialysis.	• In most cases, a transplant or dialysis procedure will result in a shorter life expectancy. • In older patients with multiple comorbidities, dialysis therapy might not be linked with survivability or a performance advantage over non-dialysis supportive therapy. • The management of symptoms (without dialysis) may enhance quality of life.
Home hemodialysis	Daytime, three to five treatments each week, lasting 4–6 hours. 8 hours during the night, three to five evenings per week.	• Artificial filter used to purify the blood. • Fistula surgery at least three months before use.	• Three months on average for training. • An adaptable daily schedule. The same as above, with improved health outcomes coming from longer dialysis sessions.
Home peritoneal dialysis (PD)	Continuous ambulatory peritoneal dialysis (CAPD).	At least four daytime bags were manually swapped.	• Requires a PD catheter. • Easy, light, and transportable. • A one-week course. • Risk of infection: one every two years. • Ability to work and travel freely. • A high standard of living. • Lasts typically 2–5 years.
Transplant	Deceased donor. Healthy donor.	• Surgery. • Immunosuppressants taken for life. • You might have to wait 3–7 years for a dead donor. • A suitable living donor.	• Liberty to work and travel after stabilizing renal function. • No extra limitations are necessary other than maintaining a healthy diet. • High prevalence of infections and malignancies; high survival rates.
Center-based hemodialysis	• Three times each week; hospital or satellite facility. • 4–6 hours individualized. • On occasion, clinics provide overnight care.	• Artificial filter used to purify the blood. • Fistula surgery at least three months before use.	• Strict protocol. • A rigid diet. • Need for transportation to a hospital or satellite facility. • No training is necessary. • Risk of infection (worse results than home-based peritoneal dialysis or home hemodialysis).

1. What will occur if we wait and watch?

2. What tests or treatments are available?

3. What are the advantages and disadvantages of these choices?

4. Do the advantages outweigh the costs/disadvantages??

5. Does the patient have sufficient knowledge to make a decision?

12.8.2.1 Planned Care in Advance

This could be a combination of any acts that lead to end-of-life planning. Advance care preparation is different from choosing a dialysis treatment and can be done while the treatment remains "active". All capable patients of 65 years of age and older and all capable patients, regardless of age, who meet any or all of the preceding requirements should begin advance care planning. This would apply when the treating physician believes that pre-existing illnesses will shorten life expectancy or the patient has multiple or more debilitating comorbid conditions, a diminished functional status, persistent malnourishment, or a low standard of living. Comorbidities, variations in physical status, life span, and wellness goals must all be addressed individually while caring for older adults with CKD. Underdiagnosis of CKD is brought on by reliance on creatinine alone. Age-adjusted eGFR increases diagnostic precision. Even if an eGFR of less than 60 mL/min/1.73 m^2 is typical in the elderly, it is nonetheless indicative of much higher risks of negative clinical consequences and cannot be regarded as natural or age-appropriate. The choice of treatment has a greater impact on lifestyle than on morbidity or mortality. In older patients with several comorbidities, dialysis treatment might not be linked to a survival benefit in comparison to supportive care that is not dialysis-related (34).

12.8.2.2 Suitable Referral

Elderly patients can be successfully maintained in primary care if they have a consistent eGFR greater than 30mL/min/1.73m^2, microalbuminuria, and regulated blood pressure. The reduction in eGFR can be unpredictable and may vary depending on age, acute events, and other circumstances. Management problems should be addressed with an expert by letter, email, or telephone in circumstances in which it might not be essential for the individual with CKD to be visited by the specialist. A plan for the regularity of screening should be developed for patients with an eGFR of less than 30mL/min/1.73m^2.

12.8.2.3 Management of Cardiovascular Risk

As cardiovascular disease deaths are more frequent than ESKD deaths among patients with CKD at all ages, cardiovascular risk should be monitored utilizing pharmaceutical and lifestyle management techniques (if necessary) based on the patient's level of risk and clinical assessment. Rather than lowering blood pressure to a target level, the purpose of treatment is to increase the patient's cognitive capability, life quality, and ability to avoid injury from falls (such as postural hypotension).

12.8.2.4 Concerns Relating to Medications

With advancing age, there is typically a decreased tolerance of side effects and an increased chance of adverse outcomes. Many medications should be taken at lower doses in elderly patients with decreased eGFR. Elderly people who take many medications run a higher risk of falling, becoming confused, and functional deterioration. The Medicare item numbers that promote collaboration between general practitioners and pharmacists are Home Medicines Assessments and Senior Medication Management Assessments (35).

12.9 GENERAL ISSUES IN CKD

It has been demonstrated that early detection and treatment can slow the progress of CKD and associated consequences. It is crucial to monitor treatment goals and carry out routine checks for the recognized consequences of CKD.

12.9.1 Acidosis

People who have an eGFR below 30 mL/min/1.73 m^2 are more likely to experience metabolic acidosis. Reduced renal acid output, combined with a decrease in bicarbonate synthesis, is the primary contributing cause. Acidosis causes increased protein breakdown and bone demineralization, both of which may increase morbidity.

In patients with acidosis, sodium bicarbonate supplementation (SodiBic 840 mg capsule) could be considered. A typical initial dose would be one capsule taken on an as-needed or daily basis, with the dose being adjusted to maintain the HCO_3 levels above 22 mmol/L. Although higher doses are possible, they increase the risk of excess fluid. A higher sodium intake may result in worse blood pressure control (36).

12.9.2 Anemia

Reduced kidney synthesis of erythropoietin is a factor in CKD-related anemia. Less iron is absorbed. When the GFR falls below 60 mL/min/1.73m², CKD-related anemia typically begins to manifest. With declining GFR, anemia is more common. Additional types of anemia must be considered and ruled out. If B12 and folate concentrations are low, they should be tested and increased. In persons with CKD, iron insufficiency is a frequent cause of anemia. If an iron shortage is found, possible reasons should be ruled out, especially gastrointestinal loss of blood. A trial of intravenous iron should be explored before starting an ESA to keep ferritin levels above 100 g/L and TSAT levels above 20%. If hypothyroidism is present, thyroid-stimulating hormone must be evaluated and treated. Greater hyperparathyroidism and widespread inflammation may both be responsible for anemia and erythropoietin treatment resistance.

12.9.3 Albuminuria

A major prognostic factor for CKD is albuminuria. The complexity of the kidney damage and the chance of ESKD progression are correlated with the level of albuminuria. Taking an ACE blocker or ARB medication can considerably lower the quantity of albuminuria. As first-line therapies, ACE inhibitors or ARBs can be used to manage the condition. Oral salt consumption can be reduced to reduce salt production. Spironolactone can be taken with caution and only as directed by a physician; serum potassium levels should be regularly checked (37).

12.9.4 Mental Deterioration

It is critical to evaluate cognition in persons with CKD. Cognitive dysfunction is prevalent in CKD patients and the prevalence rises with the severity of the disease. When considering ESKD, cognitive dysfunction is crucial since it will affect the types of treatments chosen and decisions made about future treatment. The prevalence of CKD may have an impact on executive functioning, global thinking, attention, and memory, and contributes to the decrease in the physical and mental abilities of older people. In people over 70, the risk of physical disability, cognitive impairment, and frailty can quadruple.. Many facets of CKD management are impacted by cognition. Primary-care evaluations should the following take into account: assessment for cognition in CKD; mini-mental state examination (MMSE); security; adherence to medication; a review of the drugs being taken; delirium risk; relationship to depression; problems with self-care; and involvement in care.

12.9.5 Depression

One in five individuals with CKD and one in three dialysis patients experience depression.

Depression negatively impacts CKD patients' death rates, hospitalization rates, adherence to medicine and treatment, diet, and overall life quality. Treatment of depression symptoms in CKD patients may lead to better health outcomes. Regularly screen for depression and maintain a sufficient degree of clinical attention. People with CKD frequently have modifiable reasons for depression, including sleeplessness, drug side effects, and insufficient dialysis, which should be taken into account and ruled out. Non-pharmacological interventions (such as education, dialectical behavior therapy, and exercise programs) and antidepressant medications are used to treat persistent depressed symptoms. In patients with CKD, the safety of selective serotonin reuptake inhibitors (SSRIs) has been demonstrated. Depression and anxiety frequently interfere with a patient's ability to use self-management techniques for their chronic medical condition or conditions. Consider including a recommendation to a psychologist in the general practice psychological healthcare strategy to provide the patient with psychological assistance (38).

12.9.6 Food Protein

Restricting protein intake has been demonstrated to slightly decrease the progression of CKD. The negative effects of dietary restriction often outweigh the advantages of protein restriction. Many individuals with more severe CKD suffer from anorexia and could develop protein malnutrition. A certified practicing dietitian can analyze the patient's nutrition to manage the condition.

12.9.7 Hematuria

The most frequent causes of hematuria include non-glomerular disorders such as menstruation contamination and urological disorders such as urinary tract infections (UTIs), renal kidney stones, prostatic disease, and urinary malignancies. Investigate any apparent (or macroscopic) hematuria right away. Glomerular hematuria is the term for hematuria brought on by kidney disease. Investigation is required if the hematuria is persistent or is observed in association with other signs of renal injury. Isolated hematuria in people under the age of 40 is typically caused by a mild glomerulonephritis with a low potential for advancement. Use dipsticks instead of urine microscopy for hematuria since they are more accurate and precise. Whenever there is a qualitative score of a positive (1+ or more), continue to evaluate. A positive result should not be verified using urine microscopy. Urine microscopy, however, might be helpful in separating glomerular hematuria from other sources. If two out of three reagent strip results are affirmative, continuous invisible (microscopic) hematuria in the absence of albuminuria can be distinguished from temporary hematuria (39).

12.9.8 Hyperkalemia

Potassium (K+) elimination in the urine is hampered by CKD. Spironolactone use or the usage of ACE antagonists and ARBs for the treatment of hypertension can both cause an increase in potassium levels. Potassium levels that are persistently higher than 6.0 mmol/L should be controlled. Cardiac arrhythmias are more likely in those with hyperkalemia, especially when potassium levels are above 6.5 mmol/L (40).

12.10 CONCLUSION

The prevalence of renal failure is increasing globally, encompassing all nations, and is accompanied by significant adverse outcomes and substantial financial burdens. A larger proportion of individuals experience the early stages of chronic renal disease. There is a mounting body of research, amassed over the course of recent decades, suggesting that the adverse consequences associated with renal illness, such as renal failure, heart disease, and premature mortality, can be mitigated or delayed. Renal disease can be detected in its early stages by laboratory testing. The timely initiation of treatment has been found to be beneficial in slowing down the progression of renal failure. Initiating treatment for cardiac risk factors during the early stages of renal disease would Initiating treatment for cardiac risk factors at an early stage of kidney illness may have a positive impact on reducing the incidence of heart disease, both before and after the onset of renal failure. The steps delineated in this chapter, as well as the management criteria described, can be utilised by nephrologists in conjunction with the clinical recommendations presented to them. Furthermore, it is recommended that greater focus be placed on these aspects.

ABBREVIATIONS

ABPM:	Ambulatory blood pressure monitoring
AKD:	Acute kidney disease
AKI:	Acute kidney injury
ARF:	Acute renal failure
BSA:	Body surface area
BUN:	Blood urea nitrogen
CAPD:	Continuous ambulatory peritoneal dialysis
CKD:	Chronic kidney disease
CRF:	Chronic renal failure
CVD:	Cardiovascular disease
DASH:	Dietary Approaches to Stop Hypertension
ESRD:	End-stage renal disease
GFR:	Glomerular filtration rate
GP:	General practitioner
HBPM:	Home blood pressure monitoring
KDIGO:	Kidney Disease: Improving Global Outcomes
NHANES:	National Health and Nutrition Examination Survey
NKF KDOQI:	National Kidney Foundation Kidney Disease Outcomes Quality Initiative
PKD:	Polycystic kidney disease

REFERENCES

1. Dhaun N, Bellamy CO, Cattran DC, Kluth DC. Utility of renal biopsy in the clinical management of renal disease. *Kidney International.* 2014; 85(5):1039–1048.

2. Agochukwu N, Shuch B. Clinical management of renal cell carcinoma with venous tumor thrombus. *World Journal of Urology.* 2014; 32:581–589.

3. Nelson CP, Sanda MG. Contemporary diagnosis and management of renal angiomyolipoma. *The Journal of Urology.* 2002; 168(4):1315–1325.

4. Sakhaee K, Gonzalez GB. Update on Renal Osteodystrophy: Pathogenesis Clinical Management. *The American Journal of the Medical Sciences.* 1999; 317(4):251–260.

5. Methven S, MacGregor MS. Clinical management of chronic kidney disease. *Clinical Medicine.* 2009; 9(3):269–272.

6. Kopple JD, Massry SG, editors. *Kopple and Massry's Nutritional Management of Renal Disease.* 2nd ed. Lippincott Williams & Wilkins; 2004; 11–20.

7. Davenport A, Anker SD, Mebazaa A, Palazzuoli A, Vescovo G, Bellomo R, Ponikowski P, Anand I, Aspromonte N, Bagshaw S, Berl T. ADQI 7: the clinical management of the Cardio-Renal syndromes: work group statements from the 7th ADQI consensus conference. *Nephrology Dialysis Transplantation.* 2010; 25(7):2077–2089.

8. Yun CW, Lee SH. Potential and therapeutic efficacy of cell-based therapy using mesenchymal stem cells for acute/chronic kidney disease. *International Journal of Molecular Sciences.* 2019; 20(7):1619.

9. Coresh J, Selvin E, Stevens LA, Manzi J, Kusek JW, Eggers P, Van Lente F, Levey AS. Prevalence of chronic kidney disease in the United States. *JAMA.* 2007; 298(17):2038–2047.

10. Go AS, Chertow GM, Fan D, McCulloch CE, Hsu CY. Chronic kidney disease and the risks of death, cardiovascular events, and hospitalization. *New England Journal of Medicine.* 2004; 351(13):1296–1305.

11. Kidney Disease Outcomes Quality Initiative. Clinical practice guidelines for chronic kidney disease: Evaluation, classification and stratification. *Am J Kidney Dis* 2002; 39(Suppl 1): S46–75.

12. Scottish Intercollegiate Guideline Network. *Diagnosis and Management of Chronic Kidney Disease. A National Clinical Guideline. SIGN Guideline 103.* Edinburgh: SIGN, 2008. https://www.seqc.es/download/gpc/62/3729/1043258133/1073968/cms/sign-diagnosis-and-management-of-chronic-kidney-disease_guideline.

14. Ali SI, Jung SW, Bilal HS, Lee SH, Hussain J, Afzal M, Hussain M, Ali T, Chung T, Lee S. Clinical decision support system based on hybrid knowledge modeling: A case study of chronic kidney disease-mineral and bone disorder treatment. *International Journal of Environmental Research and Public Health.* 2021; 19(1):226.

15. Lamb EJ, Tomson CR, Roderick PJ. Estimating kidney function in adults using formulae. *Annals of Clinical Biochemistry.* 2005; 42(5):321–345.

16. Jafar TH, Stark PC, Schmid CH, Landa M, Maschio G, De Jong PE, De Zeeuw D, Shahinfar S, Toto R, Levey AS, AIPRD Study Group. Progression of chronic kidney disease: The role of blood pressure control, proteinuria, and angiotensin-converting enzyme inhibition: A patient-level meta-analysis. *Annals of Internal Medicine.* 2003; 139(4):244–252.

17. Cavanaugh C, Perazella MA. Urine sediment examination in the diagnosis and management of kidney disease: Core curriculum 2019. *American Journal of Kidney Diseases*. 2019; 73(2):258–272.

18. Cheung AK, Chang TI, Cushman WC, Furth SL, Hou FF, Ix JH, Knoll GA, Muntner P, Pecoits-Filho R, Sarnak MJ, Tobe SW. Executive summary of the KDIGO 2021 clinical practice guideline for the management of blood pressure in chronic kidney disease. *Kidney International*. 2021; 99(3):559–569.

19. Navaneethan SD, Zoungas S, Caramori ML, Chan JC, Heerspink HJ, Hurst C, Liew A, Michos ED, Olowu WA, Sadusky T, Tandon N. Diabetes management in chronic kidney disease: Synopsis of the 2020 KDIGO clinical practice guideline. *Annals of Internal Medicine*. 2021; 174(3):385–394.

20. Lameire NH, Levin A, Kellum JA, Cheung M, Jadoul M, Winkelmayer WC, Stevens PE, Caskey FJ, Farmer CK, Fuentes AF, Fukagawa M. Harmonizing acute and chronic kidney disease definition and classification: Report of a Kidney Disease: Improving Global Outcomes (KDIGO) Consensus Conference. *Kidney International*. 2021; 100(3):516–526.

21. Vaidya SR, Aeddula NR. Chronic renal failure. In *StatPearls* [Internet]. StatPearls Publishing. 2021. https://www.ncbi.nlm.nih.gov/books/NBK535404/.

22. Matsuzawa R. Renal rehabilitation as a management strategy for physical frailty in CKD. *Renal Replacement Therapy*. 2022; 8(1):2–9.

23. Hamer RA, El Nahas AM. The burden of chronic kidney disease. *BMJ*. 2006; 332(7541):563–564.

24. Canaud B, Tong L, Tentori F, Akiba T, Karaboyas A, Gillespie B, Akizawa T, Pisoni RL, Bommer J, Port FK. Clinical practices and outcomes in elderly hemodialysis patients: Results from the Dialysis Outcomes and Practice Patterns Study (DOPPS). *Clinical Journal of the American Society of Nephrology*. 2011; 6(7):1651–1662.

25. Farrington K, Covic A, Aucella F, Clyne N, De Vos L, Findlay A, Fouque D, Grodzicki T, Iyasere O, Jager KJ, Joosten H. Clinical Practice Guideline on management of older patients with chronic kidney disease stage 3b or higher (eGFR< 45 mL/min/1.73 m2). *Nephrology Dialysis Transplantation*. 2016; 31(suppl_2):1–66.

26. Yamagata K, Hoshino J, Sugiyama H, Hanafusa N, Shibagaki Y, Komatsu Y, Konta T, Fujii N, Kanda E, Sofue T, Ishizuka K. Clinical practice guideline for renal rehabilitation: Systematic reviews and recommendations of exercise therapies in patients with kidney diseases. *Renal Replacement Therapy*. 2019; 5(1):1–9.

27. Wagner EH. Chronic disease management: What will it take to improve care for chronic illness? *Effective Clinical Practice*. 1998; 1(1):2–4.

28. Grady PA, Gough LL. Self-management: A comprehensive approach to management of chronic conditions. *American Journal of Public Health*. 2014; 104(8):25–31.

29. National Institute for Health and Care Excellence. *Chronic Kidney Disease: Assessment and Management NICE Guideline [NG203]*. 2021. https://www.nice.org.uk/guidance/ng203.

30. Lentine KL, Kasiske BL, Levey AS, Adams PL, Alberú J, Bakr MA, Gallon L, Garvey CA, Guleria S, Li PK, Segev DL. Summary of kidney disease: Improving Global Outcomes (KDIGO) clinical practice guideline on the evaluation and care of living kidney donors. *Transplantation*. 2017; 101(8):1783.

31. Rahman M, Shad F, Smith MC. Acute kidney injury: A guide to diagnosis and management. *American Family Physician*. 2012; 86(7):631–639.

32. McFetridge ML, Del Borgo MP, Aguilar MI, Ricardo SD. The use of hydrogels for cell-based treatment of chronic kidney disease. *Clinical Science*. 2018; 132(17):1977–1994.

33. Bilal HS, Amin MB, Hussain J, Ali SI, Hussain S, Sadiq M, Razzaq MA, Abbas A, Choi C, Lee S. On computing critical factors based healthy behavior index for behavior assessment. *International Journal of Medical Informatics*. 2020; 141:104181.

34. Awdishu L, Coates CR, Lyddane A, Tran K, Daniels CE, Lee J, El-Kareh R. The impact of real-time alerting on appropriate prescribing in kidney disease: A cluster randomized controlled trial. *Journal of the American Medical Informatics Association*. 2016; 23(3):609–616.

35. Shemeikka T, Bastholm-Rahmner P, Elinder CG, Vég A, Törnqvist E, Cornelius B, Korkmaz S. A health record integrated clinical decision support system to support prescriptions of pharmaceutical drugs in patients with reduced renal function: Design, development and proof of concept. *International Journal of Medical Informatics*. 2015; 84(6):387–395.

36. Pirnejad H, Amiri P, Niazkhani Z, Shiva A, Makhdoomi K, Abkhiz S, van der Sijs H, Bal R. Preventing potential drug-drug interactions through alerting decision support systems: A clinical context-based methodology. *International Journal of Medical Informatics*. 2019; 127:18–26.

37. Management of Chronic Kidney Disease, Guidelines for Clinical Care Ambulatory. *Michigan Medicine*, University of Michigan. https://www.med.umich.edu/1info/FHP/practiceguides/kidney/CKD.

38. *Clinical Practice Guidelines, Clinical K/DOQI Practice Guidelines for Chronic Kidney Disease: Evaluation, Classification and Stratification*. National Kidney Foundation. 2002, https://www.kidney.org/sites/default/files/docs/ckd_evaluation_classification_stratification.

39. *Chronic Kidney Disease (CKD) Management in Primary Care, Guidance and Clinical Tips to Help Detect, Manage and Refer Patients in Your Practice with CKD*. Kidney Health Australia, 4th Edition 2020. https://kidney.org.au/health-professionals/ckd-management-handbook.

40. *Chronic Kidney Disease (CKD), Clinical Practice Recommendations for Primary Care Physicians and Healthcare Providers, Divisions of Nephrology & Hypertension and General Internal Medicine*. Henry Ford Health System, 6th Edition, 2011. https://www.asn-online.org/education/training/fellows/HFHS_CKD_V6.

13 Metabolic Dysregulation in Cardiovascular Diseases

A Beat on Cardiometabolic Diseases

Patrick Diaba-Nuhoho and Michael Amponsah-Offeh

13.1 INTRODUCTION

Cardiometabolic diseases (CMDs) are a group of conditions that include cardiovascular diseases (CVDs), and metabolic disorders such as heart failure, atherosclerosis, stroke, and diabetes [1]. They are among the leading causes of death and disability globally, especially in low- and middle-income countries, where they account for at least 60% of all deaths [2]. CVDs contributed to 20.5 million of all global deaths in 2021 [3]. As a prevalent metabolic disorder, cardiometabolic syndrome is characterized by a cluster of interrelated risk factors, such as obesity, insulin resistance, hyperglycemia, hypertension, dyslipidemia, and inflammation [1, 4]. In addition to the complex interplay of environmental, social, political, and commercial determinants of health, cardiometabolic diseases are influenced by genetic and biological factors. Although some of these factors, such as smoking, physical inactivity, and unhealthy diet, are modifiable risk factors that can be prevented or controlled, other factors, such as age, sex, ethnicity, and family history, are non-modifiable risk factors that cannot be easily changed [1]. The global burden of CMDs is expected to increase further due to population aging, urbanization, globalization, and lifestyle changes. However, the burden of cardiometabolic diseases varies across regions and countries, reflecting differences in population characteristics, health systems, and policies [2].

Owing to its maladaptive cardiovascular, renal, metabolic, and inflammatory dysregulation, cardiometabolic syndrome has been recognized as a disease entity by the World Health Organization (WHO) and the American Society of Endocrinology [5]. Although CMDs share common pathophysiological mechanisms, such as endothelial dysfunction, inflammation, fibrosis, and end-organ damage, the prevention and management of CMDs pose major challenges for health systems worldwide [6, 7]. This can be attributed to limited effective therapeutic strategies as a result of the complexity and epidemiologic transitions (changes in disease patterns) of CMDs [7]. Thus, understanding the disease mechanisms and common pathways of the various CMDs will pave the way for the development of effective interventions that can address the multiple determinants and risk factors of CMDs at different levels: individual, community, national, and global. This chapter provides an overview of metabolic dysfunction in CVDs with a focus on two rapidly increasing CMDs: heart failure with preserved ejection fraction and atherosclerosis.

13.2 METABOLISM AND CARDIOVASCULAR FUNCTION

Metabolism is a complex set of chemical processes of converting nutrients into energy and biomolecules that are essential for cellular functions and the maintenance of life within living organisms [8]. Metabolism is regulated by several hormones, such as insulin, glucagon, and catecholamines. Insulin stimulates glucose uptake and storage in muscle and adipose tissue, while glucagon stimulates the breakdown of glycogen in the liver and muscle. Catecholamines, including epinephrine and norepinephrine, are released from the adrenal gland and stimulate the release of glucose from the liver and adipose tissue [8–10]. Dysregulation of these hormones can lead to metabolic dysfunction and insulin resistance, which are major risk factors for CVD. The cardiovascular system plays an important role in the maintenance of metabolic homeostasis via the delivery of oxygen, nutrients, and hormones throughout the body [10].

The metabolic and cardiovascular systems are tightly linked, as the heart requires a constant supply of energy to support its contractile activity and electrical stability. The mitochondrial adenosine triphosphate (ATP) production mainly determines the extent of cardiac performance [10–12]. Although myocardial (cardiac) metabolism is normally aerobic, the oxygen reserve that is bound to myoglobin in the cardiomyocytes (cardiac cells) is very minimal. This means that to maintain a sufficient amount of mitochondrial ATP (energy) production, a continuous supply of oxygen through the vascular system (e.g. coronary vessel) is required [12]. Although various sources of carbon are utilized by the heart for ATP production, the mitochondrial oxidation of free fatty acids primarily supplies 60–90% of cardiac energy under healthy conditions. The remaining 10–40% is supplied by glucose and lactate [11]. Thus, the heart is a highly metabolic organ, and cardiac metabolism is tightly regulated to maintain contractile function. However, the metabolic flexibility of the heart is crucial for adapting to physiological conditions (such as exercise) and

DOI: 10.1201/9781003384823-13

pathological conditions (such as heart failure, diabetes, and atherosclerosis). Dysregulation of cardiac metabolism is associated with the onset of cardiometabolic diseases, which are characterized by impaired contractile function, decreased cardiac output, and impaired vascular function [11, 12].

The complementary interplay between metabolism and cardiovascular function is closely interlinked in such a manner that dysregulation of one can lead to dysfunction of the other. In addition to the complex and multifactorial mechanisms underlying this association, metabolic dysfunction is a key risk factor for CVDs [4].

13.3 HEART FAILURE WITH PRESERVED EJECTION FRACTION

Heart failure with preserved ejection fraction (HFpEF) is a clinical syndrome characterized by either elevated natriuretic peptide (NP) levels or other evidence of congestion, in addition to symptoms of heart failure with a normal or preserved left ventricular ejection fraction (EF) of ≥50% [13]. HFpEF currently represents half of all patients with heart failure and is a major cause of morbidity and mortality throughout the industrialized world. Due to increases in aging, obesity, hypertension, physical inactivity, and associated cardiometabolic disorders, there is a continuous rapid increase in the incidence and prevalence of HFpEF [14]. Although there are no gender-specific differences in the incidence of HFpEF, there is a higher prevalence of HFpEF in women compared to men [13, 15]. The number of HFpEF hospitalizations in women is double that of men. Additionally, there are racial and ethnic disparities in the prevalence of HFpEF. The Atherosclerosis Risk in Communities (ARIC) study of heart failure-related hospitalizations in four communities in the United States between 2005 and 2014 showed that average event rates for first HFpEF hospitalization were higher in black than in white individuals [16]. Despite its high prevalence, there is still a limited understanding of the pathophysiology and availability of effective treatment of HFpEF.

13.3.1 HFpEF-Mediated Organ Damage

HFpEF is a complex syndrome that affects multiple organs and systems. In addition to cardiovascular complications, HFpEF can lead to systemic organ damage and dysfunction. Thus, identification of HFpEF-mediated organ damage has significant implications for the prognosis and management of patients with this condition.

As the name implies, a dominant target of HFpEF is the heart, resulting in cardiac dysfunction. This is characterized by impairments in cardiac structure and function, leading to myocardial stiffness, fibrosis, and hypertrophy [17]. The presence of increased myocardial stiffness and changes in the left ventricular relaxation significantly contribute to an increase in left ventricular filling pressures [18]. Atrial fibrillation, which may be thought of as a "biomarker" of underlying left atrial myopathy and an indicator of more advanced HFpEF, frequently results from the remodeling and dysfunction of the left atrium over time as a result of chronic, sustained, or intermittent elevation in left ventricular filling pressures in HFpEF [13].

HFpEF is associated with stiffening of the aorta, which in turn elevates arterial blood pressure amplification and decreases aortic compliance [14]. In HFpEF, the endothelium becomes dysfunctional due to several factors, such as diabetes, obesity, hypertension, coronary artery disease, atherosclerosis, and chronic inflammation [19]. These factors cause oxidative stress, inflammation, and reduced production of nitric oxide, which is a vasodilator that relaxes the blood vessels [20]. As a result, the blood vessels become stiff, narrow, and leaky, leading to increased resistance and pressure in the circulation [14, 19]. Endothelial dysfunction and stiffening of the aorta contribute to aortic remodeling, which is characterized by the deposition and accumulation of collagen fibers (fibrosis), as well as the gradual fragmentation and degradation of the elastin fibers in the aortic wall [18].

HFpEF is associated with pulmonary congestion, which can lead to pulmonary hypertension, interstitial lung disease, and respiratory failure [21]. Elevation of the left-sided heart pressures may lead to pulmonary congestion, while systemic inflammation and oxidative stress may contribute to lung injury and fibrosis [22]. Recent studies have suggested that pulmonary function tests, such as forced expiratory volume in 1 second (FEV1) and diffusion capacity of the lungs for carbon monoxide (DLCO), may be useful for identifying patients with HFpEF-related lung damage [23, 24].

Kidney dysfunction is a common comorbidity in patients with HFpEF. Renal dysfunction in HFpEF is characterized by a reduction in glomerular filtration rate and an increase in urine albumin excretion, and has been linked to worse outcomes [8]. Reduced renal perfusion, increased renal venous pressure, and activation of the renin–angiotensin–aldosterone system may contribute to kidney dysfunction in HFpEF [14]. Along with systemic inflammation, oxidative stress, and endothelial dysfunction may play a key role in the development of kidney damage in HFpEF. Recent studies have suggested that novel biomarkers, such as cystatin C and neutrophil gelatin-ase-associated lipocalin (NGAL), may be useful in the early detection of kidney dysfunction in HFpEF [25].

In sum, HFpEF is a complex syndrome that can lead to organ damage beyond the cardiovascular system. Kidney dysfunction, liver dysfunction, and cognitive and pulmonary dysfunction are common in patients with HFpEF and have been associated with worse outcomes.

13.3.2 Metabolic Plasticity in HFpEF

Although metabolic impairment is a common hallmark of the onset and progression of heart failure, the role of metabolic remodeling in HFpEF pathophysiology is still not well understood. This can be associated with the complex interaction of several diseases and the scarcity of preclinical models to elucidate underlying mechanisms and test therapies in HFpEF. The heart utilizes a variety of metabolic substrates, such as triglycerides, non-esterified fatty acids, carbohydrates, and ketone bodies to meet the high energy demands of the cardiac cycle. The metabolic flexibility of the heart reflects its capacity to quickly switch between substrates in response to needs and availability. Thus, cardiac energy metabolism, particularly fatty acid oxidation, seems to play a significant role in the etiology of heart disease [26]. The alteration in fatty acid metabolism in heart failure remains controversial, with some studies showing increased reliance on fatty acid oxidation and reduced glucose uptake in the early stages [27]. On the other hand, similar to observations in animal models of heart failure, decreased fatty acid and elevated glucose metabolism were observed in patients with advanced myocardial remodeling [28].

Notwithstanding the alterations in fatty acid metabolism, heart failure is characterized by systemic neurohumoral activation and increased lipolysis, which leads to an excess of fatty acids that causes further dysfunction of the mitochondria. The impaired coupling of substrate availability and cardiac metabolism, as observed in other metabolic disorders, such as obesity and diabetes, both of which are frequent comorbidities in HFpEF and may possibly be associated with dysregulated fatty acid oxidation, represents a potential mechanism linking both heart failure with reduced ejection fraction (HFrEF) and HFpEF [26]. The extent of impairment in the left ventricular ejection fraction in HFpEF patients was observed to be negatively correlated with circulating free fatty acid levels [29]. Obesity promotes a systemic fatty acid overflow from adipose tissue that is redirected to peripheral organs, including the heart, and is very common in HFpEF patients. This leads to myocardial accumulation of diglycerides and ceramides due to an imbalance between cardiac fatty acid absorption and fatty acid oxidation, which decouples their oxidative phosphorylation and subsequently promotes mitochondrial dysfunction and the generation of reactive oxygen species (ROS). [14]. Human HFpEF has been associated with elevated myocardial triglyceride levels, and the degree of myocardial steatosis is significantly and independently correlated with impaired diastolic strain rate and decreased exercise capacity in HFpEF patients [30]. A higher risk of HFpEF development is associated with higher plasma fatty acid levels [31]. However, the oxidation of fatty acids in heart failure is dependent on the specific scenario and context, with metabolic comorbidities appearing to be linked with an increase in fatty acid (FA) oxidation, while hypertension or ischemia often leads to a reduction in FA oxidation during heart failure [26, 27].

Moreover, HFpEF individuals exhibit distinctive metabolomic markers, which include elevated oxidative stress, inflammation, and fibrosis, as well as abnormal nitric oxide signaling. These markers are indicative of endothelial dysfunction and a pro-inflammatory state, both of which are characteristic of HFpEF. In addition to impaired lipid metabolism, metabolic inflexibility is rooted in compromised mitochondrial metabolism in three crucial tissues (heart, skeletal muscle, and fat) [26]. Increased glycolysis is associated with reduced mitochondrial oxidative metabolism. However, this phenomenon is not necessarily accompanied by higher glucose uptake via the pyruvate dehydrogenase complex, which causes a decoupling of glycolysis and pyruvate oxidation [32]. Abnormalities in mitochondrial oxidative metabolism may result in a decrease in the production and reserves of high-energy phosphates, leading to a resting myocardial ATP level that is 20–40% lower than normal and reduced amounts of phosphocreatine (PCr) stores [14]. Through a decrease in exercise-induced cardiac output, oxygen uptake, and relaxation, a 27% decrease in the PCr/ATP ratio was observed in HFpEF patients compared to controls [33].

Additionally, the role of ketones in cardiac metabolism is quite significant in the insulin-resistant state linked to HFpEF. Augmenting the levels of ketones in a murine model of HFpEF mitigated inflammasome activation, thereby counteracting inflammation-induced mitochondrial dysfunction [34]. Consequently, the serum concentrations of ketone bodies, namely acetoacetate,

2-hydroxybutyrate, and 3-hydroxybutyrate, were observed to be lower in HFrEF patients compared to those with HFpEF and non-HF controls [35]. Ketones possess the ability to inhibit glucose and fatty acid oxidation, ultimately leading to a greater production of ATP for each unit of oxygen expended. This characteristic serves to make them a particularly efficient source of energy. Thus, the increase in ketone oxidation noted in HFpEF may signify an adaptive response that serves to reduce the disease burden [14, 26].

13.3.3 Diagnosis of HFpEF

The accurate diagnosis and management of HFpEF necessitates a thorough and all-encompassing methodology that incorporates a meticulous analysis of the patient's symptoms, medical background, physical examination, and diagnostic assessments. The integration of cutting-edge imaging modalities, biomarkers, invasive hemodynamic monitoring, and a collaborative multi-disciplinary approach potentially enhance the precision and efficacy of the diagnosis and treatment of HFpEF.

Experiencing shortness of breath during physical activity and reduced ability to exercise is one of the most prevalent indications of HFpEF. For this reason, it is essential to obtain a comprehensive medical history that emphasizes any changes in exercise capacity over time and current exercise tolerance [36]. Despite the fact that shortness of breath during physical activity is a very sensitive measure in detecting HF, it only has a specificity of 50% in identifying a cardiac cause [37]. Therefore, the clinical history should concentrate on all possible non-cardiac causes of shortness of breath, including lung disease. In addition, the comprehensive clinical assessment/history should focus on other HFpEF-associated comorbidities, such as hypertension, diabetes, obesity, atrial fibrillation, and coronary artery and chronic kidney disease [36]. Thus, clinical assessment of blood pressure, indications of volume overload (such as raised jugular venous pressure, peripheral oedema), radial pulse rhythm and rate, as well as body mass and build weight index, remains key in the diagnosis of HFpEF [13, 38]. Addressing these underlying conditions can help improve the management of HFpEF.

Moreover, initial laboratory blood assessment ought to encompass natriuretic peptides (NP), complete blood count, ferritin, and transferrin saturation in order to rule out anemia, which could trigger breathlessness symptoms [36]. It is imperative to evaluate the renal function profile, encompassing urea, creatinine, electrolytes, and estimated glomerular filtration rate (eGFR), alongside hemoglobin A1c (HbA1c). Additionally, liver function tests, thyroid function tests, and lipid profiles are instrumental in gauging the likelihood of metabolic syndrome. Normal NP levels in HFpEF patients can lead to false negative results in diagnosing heart failure, as approximately 20% of HFpEF patients have normal NP levels due to the mechanism of NP release [36, 37]. Elevated left ventricular (LV) diastolic wall stress triggers the release of natriuretic peptides. It should be noted that the LV diastolic wall stress displays an inverse relationship with the wall thickness. Therefore, in instances of mild left ventricular hypertrophy (LVH), which is frequently observed in HFpEF, the impact of diastolic LV wall stress may be attenuated, and the release of NPs could be limited [36]. In addition, assessment of peripheral blood biomarkers provides substantiation of inflammatory states in HFpEF, although it is challenging to decipher which specific organ(s) is afflicted. These biomarkers (such as C-reactive protein, tumor necrosis factor (TNF), tumor necrosis factor receptor (TNFR), interleukin 1 beta (IL-1β), interleukin 6 (IL-6), interleukin 10 (IL-10), monocytes, macrophages and T cells) are primarily utilized for stratifying HFpEF patients into low-risk versus high-risk cohorts and are frequently observed in HFrEF [14].

Furthermore, non-invasive imaging techniques such as echocardiography (ECHO) and magnetic resonance (MRI) can be employed for the evaluation of structural/functional cardiac abnormalities. These techniques have the potential to be a valuable tool in the assessment of ambient or chronic markers of congestion. This includes the identification of increases in the E/e' ratio (E wave divided by e' velocities), left atrial enlargement, reduced left atrial reservoir strain, increases in estimated pulmonary artery pressures, and distention of the inferior vena cava, which are present in HFpEF [13]. Although these non-invasive techniques provide useful information that can be strongly associated with unfavorable HFpEF outcomes, their use does not prove to be beneficial in the exclusion of HFpEF. This is partly due to the insensitivity of estimations and the observation that LV filling pressures are normal at rest and only increase during exercise in roughly one-third of patients with HFpEF [13].

Therefore, exercise testing is crucial in determining the presence or absence of HFpEF in these patients. The gold standard method for diagnosis involves a comprehensive evaluation of hemodynamics during right heart catheterization, encompassing both rest and exercise. This approach is aligned with the newly established universal criteria, which mandate the presence of objective indications of congestion. Specifically, confirmation of the diagnosis is achieved through detection of an escalation in pulmonary capillary wedge pressure (PCWP) during supine exercise, with a threshold of $\geq$15 mm Hg at rest and $\geq$25 mm Hg during exercise at end expiration [13, 38].

In view of the challenges and scarcity of tests that can definitively establish the diagnosis of HFpEF, the use of clinical scoring systems (H$_2$FPEF and HFA-PEFF) may be useful in facilitating the diagnostic assessment of suspected HFpEF. The H$_2$FPEF score (shown in Figure 15.1) has been created and tested based on a gold-standard frame of reference that includes invasive exercise hemodynamic measurements. It is regarded as a more pragmatic system that can be utilized by clinicians [38]. In contrast, the HFA-PEFF (Heart Failure Association Pre-test assessment, Echocardiography and natriuretic peptide, Functional testing, Final etiology) score was formulated through the combined expertise of specialists and is more complex, with the ability to assess hemodynamic parameters as shown in Figure 13.1 [13]. Both the scoring systems, H$_2$FPEF and HFA-PEFF, possess the potential to facilitate clinicians in the identification of HFpEF. Nevertheless, there are certain limitations. Inconsistencies between the HFA-PEFF and H$_2$FPEF scoring frameworks, as well as a considerable proportion of individuals being categorized as "intermediate" (without a definitive diagnosis), emphasize the significance of additional testing as outlined above [13, 38].

13.3.4 Therapeutic Interventions for HFpEF

The current treatment and management of HFpEF centers around several strategies with a key emphasis on risk stratification and the management of comorbidities, such as hypertension, diabetes mellitus, obesity, atrial fibrillation, coronary artery disease, chronic kidney disease, and obstructive sleep apnea. This can be achieved through pharmacological interventions, such as the use of loop diuretic agents, sodium-glucose transporter-2 inhibitors (SGLT2is), mineralocorticoid antagonists (MRAs), angiotensin receptor–neprilysin inhibitors (ARNIs), and angiotensin receptor blockers (ARBs). In addition, non-pharmacological approaches including exercise and weight loss, as well as the implementation of wireless, implantable pulmonary artery monitors, are utilized [38]. The objectives of treatment for individuals diagnosed with HFpEF are to ameliorate symptoms, enhance overall functional capacity, and mitigate the likelihood of hospitalization.

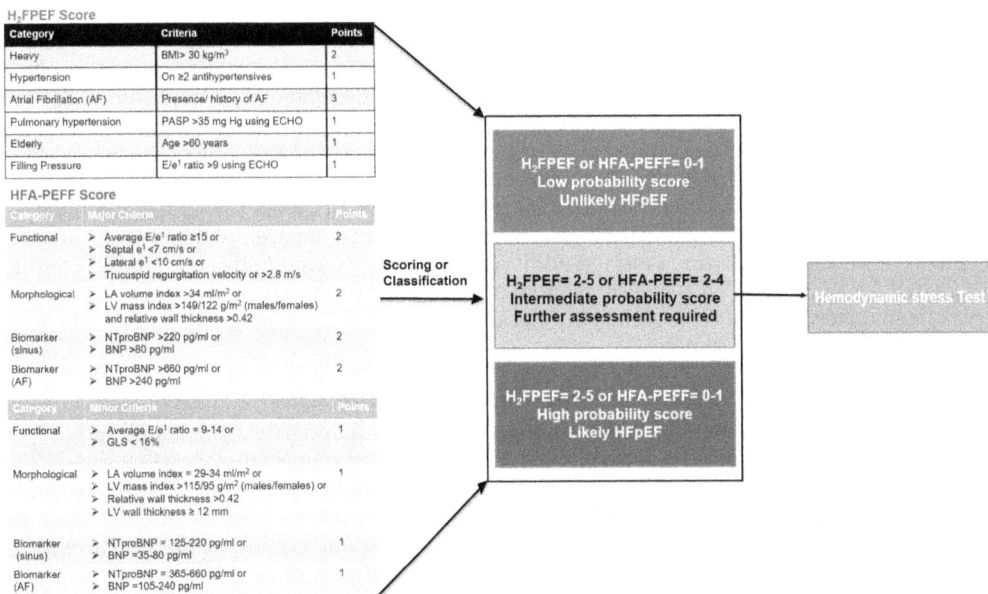

Figure 13.1 Diagnostic scoring systems for HFpEF. AF = atrial fibrillation; LA = left atrial; LV = left ventricle; BMI = body mass index; PASP = pulmonary arterial systolic pressure; BNP = brain natriuretic peptide; NT-proBNP = N-terminal pro b-type natriuretic peptide

13.3.4.1 Pharmacological Strategies

HFpEF patients with confirmed volume overload should be provided with a diuretic therapy. Treatment should be initiated using loop diuretics, with the type and dosage contingent on the severity of volume overload. In the event that a patient demonstrates resistance to diuretic therapy, sequential nephron blockade may be accomplished through the utilization of thiazide/thiazide-like diuretics and/or MRAs. The recommendation to include the latter in the management of HFpEF is based on the 2022 American Heart Association Heart Failure (AHA HF) guidelines, in which it features as a class 2b-level recommendation [36, 39]. However, the prudent implementation of diuretic agents is necessary in order to manage congestion and ameliorate symptoms.

The SGLT2 inhibitors were initially designed to enhance glucose management in patients suffering from type 2 diabetes mellitus (T2DM). However, recent findings have shown that these inhibitors offer significant cardiovascular advantages to individuals with or without T2DM. This is particularly pronounced in individuals with heart failure, as the use of SGLT2 inhibitors has been found to significantly decrease the likelihood of hospitalization for HF and cardiovascular mortality, regardless of their ejection fraction subgroups. The DELIVER (Dapagliflozin Evaluation to Improve the Lives of Patients with Preserved Ejection Fraction Heart Failure) [40] and EMPEROR-Preserved (Empagliflozin Outcome Trial in Patients with Chronic Heart Failure with Preserved Ejection Fraction) [41] trials were conducted to assess the impact of dapagliflozin and empagliflozin, respectively, on clinical outcomes among individuals with HF and LVEF $\geq$40%. The findings from both trials demonstrated a considerable reduction in hospitalization for HF. Furthermore, a meta-analysis indicated a potential reduction in cardiovascular mortality with SGLT2is in individuals with HFmrEF/HFpEF [42]. The use of SGLT2is also led to improvements in health status, as observed in both trials, with the most significant benefits observed in those with baseline symptomatic impairment. Moreover, the PRESERVED-HF (Dapagliflozin in Preserved Ejection Fraction Heart Failure) trial provided additional evidence of the positive impact of SGLT2is on health status and quality of life among individuals with HFpEF [43]. Thus, it is recommended that administration of SGLT2i is commenced for all HFpEF patients without any contraindications [13, 38].

The implementation of MRAs yields a marked enhancement in measures of diastolic function among those afflicted with HFpEF. Spironolactone may confer a reduction in the likelihood of hospitalizations for HF in certain select subpopulations of HFpEF patients. Nevertheless, careful monitoring of both potassium levels and renal function is imperative to curtail the risk of hyperkalemia and worsening kidney function [13, 38]. While there is currently no evidence to support the notion that MRAs contribute to an improved quality of life or increased exercise tolerance for those with HFpEF, the vast majority of individuals who suffer from this condition will still reap the benefits of MRAs due to their ability to provide balanced diuresis through sequential nephron blockade, control hypertension, and reduce the frequency of HF-related hospitalizations [38].

Sacubitril acts as a neprilysin inhibitor, targeting an enzyme accountable for the deactivation of various vasoactive peptides (such as natriuretic peptides, bradykinin) that contribute to both the initiation and development of heart failure. Inhibition of neprilysin, however, increases angiotensin levels, which may offset the vasodilatory effect of sacubitril unless that is also inhibited [38]. As a result, combination with valsartan is necessary. When compared with valsartan alone, sacubitril/valsartan provides only modest additional benefits in individuals with HFpEF. Despite the fact that ARNI therapy leads to less frequent occurrences of serum creatinine elevations and hyperkalemia, there is a higher likelihood of hypotension and angioedema with ARNIs, although these occurrences are rare [38, 44].

13.3.4.2 Non-pharmacological approaches

The association between both obesity and physical inactivity and poorer health status and unfavorable prognosis is strong in the context of HFpEF. Studies suggest that weight reduction (achieved through caloric restriction or bariatric surgery) can have a positive impact on the occurrence of heart failure events and physical activity capacity [45]. In addition, exercise training has been shown to enhance aerobic capacity and improve the quality of life in individuals with HFpEF. Furthermore, moderate intensity training has been found to be equivalent to higher intensities [13, 46]. Also, it is imperative to adhere to the recommendations provided by the 2019 ACC/AHA Guideline on the Primary Prevention of Cardiovascular Disease. This involves the implementation of a comprehensive lifestyle intervention program, which includes a structured regimen of regular self-monitoring of food intake, physical activity, and weight. The recommendation is to increase physical activity, preferably in the form of aerobic physical activity (such as brisk walking, as this constitutes a beneficial yet inexpensive way to be physically active), for a minimum of 150 minutes per week (equivalent to at least 30 minutes per day for most days of the week) as the initial measure for weight loss [38, 47, 48].

Furthermore, due to the critical role of volume management in the therapeutic approach to HFpEF, numerous devices have been devised to effectively monitor filling pressures and provide guidance for the management of diuretic agents. The utilization of pulmonary artery pressure monitoring has been shown to be advantageous in the management of HFpEF, as evidenced by the results of the CHAMPION (CardioMEMS Heart Sensor Allows Monitoring of Pressure to Improve Outcomes in NYHA Class III Heart Failure Patients) trial [49]. During the 18-month follow-up period, there was a noteworthy decrease in HF hospitalization rates of 50% compared to standard care. The overall number needed to treat (NNT) to prevent one HF hospitalization was 2 [13, 49]. Although, this trial had some methodological concerns of bias, these findings demonstrate the potential benefits of utilizing pulmonary artery pressure monitoring in the treatment of HFpEF. Alternative device targeted interventions for HFpEF, including but not limited to the analysis of blood volume, the utilization of interatrial shunting devices, splanchnic nerve ablation, and cardiac contractility modulation, are currently undergoing evaluation. These interventions have yet to be fully comprehended and necessitate further investigation. It is noteworthy that these procedures should only be considered within the confines of clinical trials [38].

13.4 ATHEROSCLEROSIS

Atherosclerosis is a lifelong process dependent on genetic and nongenetic factors [50]. Other known risk factors of atherosclerosis, such as smoking, diabetes, hypertension, hyperlipidemia, and inflammation, further lead to metabolic dysregulation [50]. However, atherosclerosis as a chronic disease is initiated in the vascular wall due to chronic inflammation and the interaction of the known risk factors [51]. In early life, atherosclerosis has been observed as fatty streak formation in human fetal arteries of hypercholesterolemic mothers [52]. Over time, the formation of a fatty streak in the arterial wall leads to worldwide morbidity and mortality in diseases such as myocardial infarction, stroke, and peripheral artery disease [51]. Interestingly, recent advances have implicated the role of microRNA, intestinal flora, clonal hematopoiesis, neutrophil extracellular traps, and the immune system in the pathogenesis of atherosclerosis [53–57]. Here we focus on the pathophysiological contributions of lipids to atherosclerosis, its diagnosis, and therapy.

13.4.1 Pathophysiology of Atherosclerosis: A Focus on Lipid Metabolism

Atherosclerosis as a disease process involves the accumulation of lipids, inflammation, and fibrosis in the arterial walls [58, 59]. The arterial wall, a trilaminar structure consisting of the outer layer (adventitia), the middle layer (tunica media), and the inner layer (intima), is well organized (see Figure 13.2). These layers contain nerve endings, mast cells, microvessels, smooth muscle cells, elastin, collagens, and macromolecules that become dysregulated in the presence of increased risk factors for atherosclerosis [51]. Lipid accumulation arising from dyslipidemia increases the levels of low-density lipoprotein cholesterol (LDL-C) and triglycerides (TG) in the bloodstream, further accumulating in the arterial walls, particularly in areas where there is endothelial dysfunction or injury [58, 59]. During endothelial dysfunction, dyslipidemia impairs the function of the endothelium, which is the inner lining of the arteries, and further reduces the production of nitric oxide, a molecule that helps to regulate vascular tone and protect against inflammation and oxidative stress [20]. Both clinical and genetic evidence have established LDL-C as a major cause of atherosclerotic cardiovascular disease while drugs that target the lowering of LDL-C have proved efficacious in lowering their cardiovascular risks [60].

13.4.2 Initiation and Fatty Streak Formation in the Vessel Wall

The changing trend in the dynamics of atherosclerosis, which was once thought of as a mere accumulation of lipids in the vessel wall and is now viewed as a more complex chronic inflammatory disease, has advanced our understanding of its disease progression [61]. The investigation of both molecular and cellular pathways in experimental studies has provided valuable insights into the progression of atherosclerosis, contributing to the advancement of translational research by uncovering unique mechanistic understandings.. The accumulation of low-density lipoprotein (LDL) in the intima starts the initiation of the early phase of lesion and fatty streak formation. A disturbance in blood flow triggered by the LDL accumulation induces shear stress and mechanical stimuli that trigger pathways, reducing expression levels of endothelial nitric oxide synthase

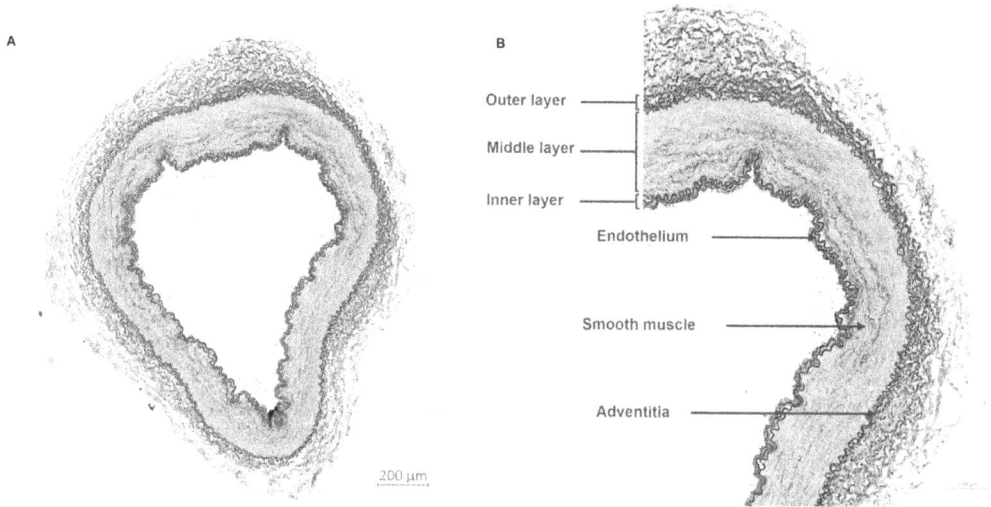

Figure 13.2 A cross staining of an internal mammary artery using Elastica van Gieson stain (A and B)

(eNOS). A further imbalance between oxidative stress and antioxidants increases production of reactive oxygen species due to the activation of endothelial cells, causing lipoprotein particle modifications, oxidized LDL (ox-LDL). This leads to the retention and accumulation of subendo-thelial atherogenic apolipoprotein B-containing LDL, remnants of very low-density lipoprotein (VLDL), and chylomicrons (CM), rendering the LDL proinflammatory and immunogenic [51, 62]. Monocytes that exhibit classical proinflammatory characteristics are recruited into the intima, binding to adhesion molecules on activated endothelial cells, with chemokines facilitating their migration into the arterial wall. In the intima, monocytes develop into resident macrophages expressing scavenger receptors that allow them to bind ox-LDL and, ultimately, change pheno-typically to become foam cells (Figure 13.3), resulting in the release of proinflammatory cells and the formation of fatty lesions. Accumulation of leukocytes in the intima causes the migration of T-lymphocytes, smooth muscle cells, platelets, and platelet-derived growth factors (PDGF) into the intima [51].

With the recruitment of inflammatory cells to the intima, activated endothelial cells express leukocyte adhesion molecules that capture blood monocytes. After inflammatory activation, monocytes express scavenger receptors becoming resident macrophages, leading to the uptake of modified LDL (ox-LDL). Cholesterol loading leads to the formation of foam cells and eventually to a matured lipid-laden macrophage and contributes to fatty deposits in the arterial wall character-ized by the entry of leukocytes into the smooth muscle cells and T-cell migration, resulting in the release of PDGF and platelet aggregation.

13.4.3 Atherosclerosis Progression: Plaque Formation

Dyslipidemia is a major risk factor for cardiometabolic disease. It is characterized by an imbal-ance of the lipid profile, with elevated levels of LDL, VLDL, CM, and TG, and reduced levels of high-density lipoprotein (HDL) [63, 64]. Over time, the accumulation of lipids, a characteristic of the atherosclerotic plaque, in the arterial wall is infiltrated by immune cells like macrophages, mast cells, T cells, and dendritic cells. [65]. The accumulation of lipids and fatty lesions facilitates the progression of atherosclerotic plaques. Vascular smooth muscle cells have been implicated in atherosclerosis, giving rise to foam cells that resemble macrophages [66]. At atherogenic sites in the intima, it has been established that smooth muscle cells migrate from the media to these sites and participate in the formation of atherosclerotic plaque by becoming macrophage-like cells, senescent and apoptotic, producing extracellular matrix molecules that promote inflammation [66]. Lipid accumulation increases as the extracellular matrix molecules entrap lipoproteins in the intima, leading to the proliferation and infiltration of inflammatory leukocytes and the forma-tion of atherosclerotic plaque through their persistent presence [67]. T-lymphocytes localize in the lesion, differentiating into T_H1 and T_H2 cells. T_H1 cells produce inflammatory cells and promote

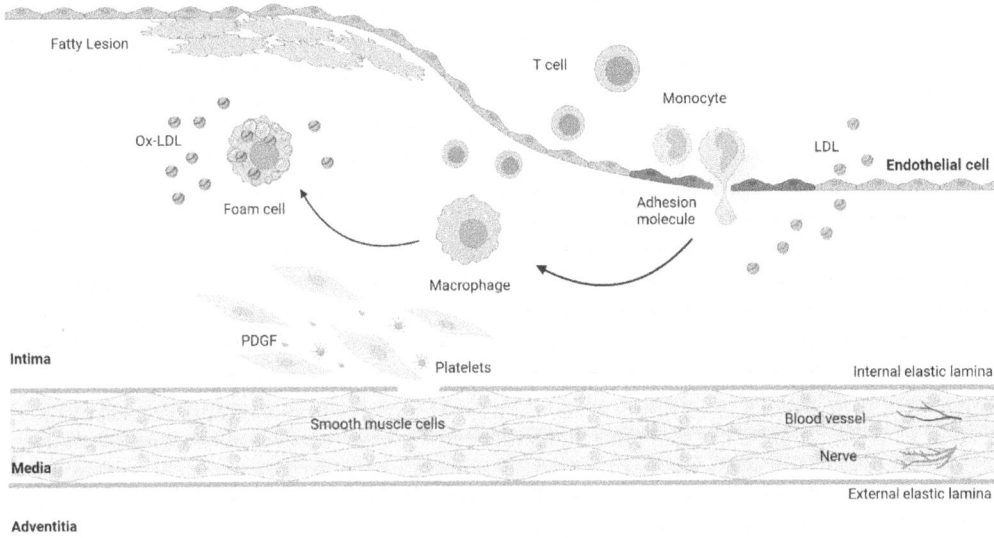

Figure 13.3 Schematic representation of the initiation and fatty lesion formation in the vessel wall

atherosclerosis, while T_H2 cells release cytokines like IL-10, and T_{reg} cells that secrete transforming growth factor β (TGF-β) that can limit inflammation and smooth muscle cell proliferation and promote interstitial collagen synthesis [51, 68]. Drains from atherosclerotic plaques that reach lymph nodes can serve as antigens for T and B cells and can be modulated by locally produced cytokines. For instance, interleukin 17 (IL-17) helps plaques lie dormant in a mouse model of atherosclerosis that had T cells with enhanced expression of TGF-β, such that IL-17 could drain lymph nodes and expand collagen-rich fibrous caps [69]. In advanced atherosclerosis, interaction between the adventitia, the media, and the intima activates smooth muscle cells and recruits B and T cells that promote lymphocyte activation and autoreactive antigens and antibodies against LDL particle lesions [70]. A necrotic lipid-rich core begins to form as macrophage and smooth muscle cells undergo programmed cell death with increased expression of interleukin-1β. Further defective efferocytosis in advanced atherosclerosis drives necrotic core formation, triggering plaque rupture and thrombotic cardiovascular events and complications [71–73].

13.4.4 Diagnosis

Diagnostic techniques (Figure 13.4) such as blood markers, stress testing, computed tomography (CT), and nuclear scanning, which are non-invasive, and coronary arteriography, an invasive selective procedure, allow for cardiovascular disease risk assessment and the determination of therapy targets [51]. While CT angiography, ultrasonography, and magnetic resonance imaging (MRI) are non-invasive, both CT angiography and ultrasonography enable differentiation of some plaque components and MRI allows quantification of endothelial permeability and dysfunction in cardiovascular diseases [51, 74]. While intravascular ultrasonography and optical coherence tomography involve an invasive method and exposure to radiation, they are excellent for plaque burden, composition, and detailed visualization of internal morphology [51]. Tools for indirect plaque visualization, such as positron emission tomography (PET) and invasive angiography, present useful techniques for evaluating plaque metabolism and characterizing high-risk features of atherosclerotic plaque prone to rupture [51, 75]. Recently, the use of gene and protein markers and other trace elements has been reviewed as a method for diagnosing patients presenting with early atherosclerosis [76]. Though medical imaging techniques provide a definitive diagnosis for the

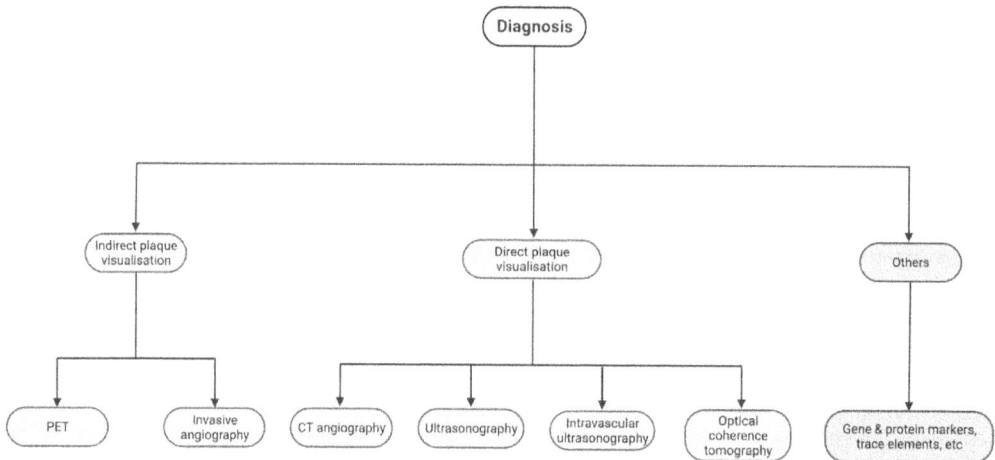

Figure 13.4 Atherosclerosis diagnostic tests. PET indicates positron emission tomography and CT, computed tomography. Created with BioRender.com

management of clinical symptoms, lipid-lowing medications such as statins and other interventions can be used to improve lipid profiles and reduce the risk of cardiovascular disease.

13.4.5 Therapy

Therapy in LDL pathways using inhibitors, such as statins, a 3-hydroxy-3-methylglutaryl coenzyme A (HMG-CoA) reductase, has shown promising outcomes in reducing CVD [77]. Despite the use of statins, a revolutionary drug in the medical field, many patients treated with them still have cardiovascular risk burdens and LDL levels above recommended guidelines [78, 79]. Interestingly, clinical trials focused on new biological targets, such as proprotein convertase subtilisin/kexin type 9 (PCSK9), Niemann-Pick C1-like protein 1, and others (see Table 13.1), are suggested to reduce LDL levels compared to high-dose statin therapy [59] and targeting PCSK9 is promising in alleviating oxidation, inflammation, and atherosclerosis [80]. Furthermore, lifestyle modifications, such as a healthy diet, regular exercise, and smoking cessation, can be useful in improving lipid profiles and reducing the risk of cardiovascular disease.

Table 13.1 Clinical trials of drug targets reducing LDL cholesterol levels

Drug Target	Mechanism	NCT Number
Proprotein convertase subtilisin/kexin type 9 (PCSK9)	Monoclonal antibody to PCSK9; anti-PCSK9 small binding protein; interfering RNA targeting PCSK9	NCT04790513; NCT04798430; NCT04929249; NCT02508896
Apo inhibitors	Antisense oligonucleotides targeting Lipoprotein (a); ApoA-1; Apo-B; and Apo-CIII	NCT04023552; NCT03473223; NCT00794664; NCT02658175
Angiopoietin-like protein 3 (ANGPTL3)	Monoclonal antibody or antisense oligonucleotide targeting ANGPTL3	NCT04233918; NCT02709850
Diacylglycerol acyltransferase 1 (DGAT1)	Small molecule inhibition of DGAT1	NCT01474434
Microsomal triglyceride transfer protein (MTP)	Inhibition of MTP	NCT02145468
Niemann-Pick C1-like protein 1 (NPC1L1)	Inhibition of intestinal cholesterol transporter NPC1L1	NCT00202878
ATP citrate lyase	Inhibition of ATP citrate lyase	NCT03067441

Abbreviations: ANGPTL3, angiopoietin-like protein 3; ApoA-1, apolipoprotein a1; Apo-B, apolipoprotein b; Apo-CIII, apolipoprotein cIII; ATP, adenosine triphosphate; DGAT1, diacylglycerol acyltransferase 1; MTP, microsomal triglyceride transfer protein; NPC1L1, niemann-Pick C1-like protein 1; PCSK9, proprotein convertase subtilisin/kexin type 9.

13.5 CONCLUSIONS

Cardiometabolic diseases are a significant public health concern, with a substantial burden in terms of morbidity, mortality, and healthcare costs. Major mechanisms involved in the development of cardiometabolic disease include: dyslipidemia, insulin resistance, inflammation, oxidative stress, endothelial dysfunction, as well as abnormal glucose metabolism and adipose tissue function. Understanding these mechanisms and training future clinicians in cardiometabolic disease research is essential for improving patient outcomes and addressing the growing prevalence of these complex conditions. The diagnosis of CMDs requires a comprehensive approach that takes into account the patient's symptoms, medical history, physical examination, and diagnostic tests. The use of advanced imaging techniques, biomarkers, invasive hemodynamic monitoring, and a multi-disciplinary approach can all help improve the accuracy of the diagnosis and management of CMDs. Despite the availability of effective therapies, a therapeutic gap exists globally, which is influenced by several factors, including access to care, inadequate resources, poor patient adherence, and inadequate provider education and training. Addressing these challenges is critical to improving the management of cardiometabolic diseases and reducing their burden on public health.

Overall, metabolic dysregulation is an important contributor to cardiovascular disease, and recent studies have shed light on its underlying mechanisms and potential interventions. However, more research is required to fully understand this complex condition and its overall impact on cardiovascular diseases.

REFERENCES

1. Amin AM. The metabolic signatures of cardiometabolic diseases: Does the shared metabotype offer new therapeutic targets? *Lifestyle Medicine.* 2021;2:1–20.

2. Miranda JJ, Barrientos-Gutiérrez T, Corvalan C, Hyder AA, Lazo-Porras M, Oni T, et al. Understanding the rise of cardiometabolic diseases in low- and middle-income countries. 2019;25:1667–1679.

3. Megan L, Nicole D, Henry D, Valentin F, Johnson CO, LeGrand KE, et al. Global burden of cardiovascular diseases and risks collaboration, 1990–2021. *J Am Coll Cardiol.* 2022;80:2372–425.

4. Sattar N, Gill JMR, Alazawi W. Improving prevention strategies for cardiometabolic disease. *Nat Med.* 2020;26:320–5.

5. Castro JP, El-Atat FA, McFarlane SI, Aneja A, Sowers JR. Cardiometabolic syndrome: Pathophysiology and treatment. *Curr Hypertens Rep.* 2003;5:393–401.

6. Boutagy NE, Singh AK, Sessa WC. Targeting the vasculature in cardiometabolic disease. *J Clin Invest.* 2022;132:e148556.

7. Schmidt HHHW, Menche J. The regulatory network architecture of cardiometabolic diseases. *Nat Genet.* 2022;54:2–3.

8. Nava ASL de, Raja A. Physiology, metabolism. In *StatPearls [Internet].* 2022 StatPearls Publishing.

9. Judge A, Dodd MS. Metabolism. *Essays Biochem.* 2020;64:607.

10. Pulinilkunnil T, Kienesberger P, Nagendran J. Editorial: Novel concepts in cardiac energy metabolism: From biology to disease. *Front Cardiovasc Med.* 2019;6:97.

11. Lopaschuk GD, Karwi QG, Tian R, Wende AR, Abel ED. Cardiac energy metabolism in heart failure. *Circ Res.* 2021;128:1487.

12. Kolwicz SC, Purohit S, Tian R. Cardiac metabolism and its interactions with contraction, growth, and survival of cardiomyocytes. *Circ Res.* 2013;113:603–16.

13. Borlaug BA, Sharma K, Shah SJ, Ho JE. Heart failure with preserved ejection fraction: JACC scientific statement. *J Am Coll Cardiol.* 2023;81:1810–1834.

14. Mishra S, Kass DA. Cellular and molecular pathobiology of heart failure with preserved ejection fraction. *Nat Rev Cardiol.* 2021;18:400.

15. Dunlay SM, Roger VL, Redfield MM. Epidemiology of heart failure with preserved ejection fraction. *Nat Rev Cardiol.* 2017;14:591–602.

16. Chang PP, Wruck LM, Shahar E, Rossi JS, Loehr LR, Russell SD, et al. Trends in hospitalizations and survival of acute decompensated heart failure in four US communities (2005–2014). *Circulation.* 2018;138:12–24.

17. Schiattarella GG, Altamirano F, Tong D, French KM, Villalobos E, Kim SY, et al. Nitrosative stress drives heart failure with preserved ejection fraction. *Nature.* 2019;568:351.

18. Failer T, Amponsah-Offeh M, Neuwirth A, Kourtzelis I, Subramanian P, Mirtschink P, et al. Developmental endothelial locus-1 protects from hypertension-induced cardiovascular remodeling via immunomodulation. *J Clin Invest.* 2022;132(6):1–26.

19. Cuijpers I, Simmonds SJ, van Bilsen M, Czarnowska E, González Miqueo A, Heymans S, et al. Microvascular and lymphatic dysfunction in HFpEF and its associated comorbidities. *Basic Res Cardiol.* 2020;115:39.

20. Amponsah-Offeh M, Diaba-Nuhoho P, Speier S, Morawietz H. Oxidative stress, Antioxidants and hypertension. *Antioxidants.* 2023;12:281.

21. Lam CSP, Roger VL, Rodeheffer RJ, Borlaug BA, Enders FT, Redfield MM. Pulmonary hypertension in heart failure with preserved ejection fraction: A community-based study. *J Am Coll Cardiol.* 2009;53:1119.

22. Huston JH, Shah SJ. Understanding the pathobiology of pulmonary hypertension due to left heart disease. *Circ Res.* 2022;130:1382–403.

23. Ramalho SHR, Claggett BL, Washko GR, Estepar RSJ, Chang PP, Kitzman DW, et al. Association of pulmonary function with late-life cardiac function and heart failure risk: The ARIC study. *J Am Heart Assoc.* 2022;11:23990.

24. Borlaug BA, Olson TP. The lungs in heart failure: Not an innocent bystander∗. *JACC Hear Fail.* 2016;4:450–2.

25. Mullens W, Damman K, Testani JM, Martens P, Mueller C, Lassus J, et al. Evaluation of kidney function throughout the heart failure trajectory – A position statement from the Heart Failure Association of the European Society of Cardiology. *Eur J Heart Fail.* 2020;22:584–603.

26. del Campo A, Perez G, Castro PF, Parra V, Verdejo HE. Mitochondrial function, dynamics and quality control in the pathophysiology of HFpEF. *Biochim Biophys Acta - Mol Basis Dis.* 2021;1867:166208.

27. Fillmore N, Mori J, Lopaschuk GD. Mitochondrial fatty acid oxidation alterations in heart failure, ischaemic heart disease and diabetic cardiomyopathy. *Br J Pharmacol.* 2014;171:2080–90.

28. Dávila-Román VG, Vedala G, Herrero P, De Las Fuentes L, Rogers JG, Kelly DP, et al. Altered myocardial fatty acid and glucose metabolism in idiopathic dilated cardiomyopathy. *J Am Coll Cardiol*. 2002;40:271–7.

29. Zhu N, Jiang W, Wang Y, Wu Y, Chen H, Zhao X. Plasma levels of free fatty acid differ in patients with left ventricular preserved, mid-range, and reduced ejection fraction. *BMC Cardiovasc Disord*. 2018;18:1–8.

30. Mahmod M, Pal N, Rayner J, Holloway C, Raman B, Dass S, et al. The interplay between metabolic alterations, diastolic strain rate and exercise capacity in mild heart failure with preserved ejection fraction: A cardiovascular magnetic resonance study. *J Cardiovasc Magn Reson*. 2018;20(1):1–10.

31. Djoussé L, Benkeser D, Arnold A, Kizer JR, Zieman SJ, Lemaitre RN, et al. Plasma free fatty acids and risk of heart failure: The Cardiovascular Health Study. *Circ Heart Fail*. 2013;6:964–9.

32. Lei B, Lionetti V, Young ME, Chandler MP, D'Agostino C, Kang E, et al. Paradoxical down-regulation of the glucose oxidation pathway despite enhanced flux in severe heart failure. *J Mol Cell Cardiol*. 2004;36:567–76.

33. Phan TT, Abozguia K, Nallur Shivu G, Mahadevan G, Ahmed I, Williams L, et al. Heart failure with preserved ejection fraction is characterized by dynamic impairment of active relaxation and contraction of the left ventricle on exercise and associated with myocardial energy deficiency. *J Am Coll Cardiol*. 2009;54:402–9.

34. Deng Y, Xie M, Li Q, Xu X, Ou W, Zhang Y, et al. Targeting Mitochondria-Inflammation Circuit by β-Hydroxybutyrate Mitigates HFpEF. *Circ Res*. 2021;128:232–45.

35. Zordoky BN, Sung MM, Ezekowitz J, Mandal R, Han B, Bjorndahl TC, et al. Metabolomic fingerprint of heart failure with preserved ejection fraction. *PLoS One*. 2015;10:e0124844.

36. Jasinska-Piadlo A, Campbell P. Management of patients with heart failure and preserved ejection fraction. *Heart*. 2023;109(11):874–883.

37. McDonagh TA, Metra M, Adamo M, Baumbach A, Böhm M, Burri H, et al. 2021 ESC Guidelines for the diagnosis and treatment of acute and chronic heart failureDeveloped by the Task Force for the diagnosis and treatment of acute and chronic heart failure of the European Society of Cardiology (ESC) With the special contribution of the Heart Failure Association (HFA) of the ESC. *Eur Heart J*. 2021;42:3599–726.

38. Kittleson MM, Panjrath GS, Amancherla K, Davis LL, Deswal A, Dixon DL, et al. 2023 ACC expert consensus decision pathway on management of heart failure with preserved ejection fraction: A report of the American College of Cardiology solution set oversight committee. *J Am Coll Cardiol*. 2023;81:1835–78.

39. Heidenreich PA, Bozkurt B, Aguilar D, Allen LA, Byun JJ, Colvin MM, et al. 2022 AHA/ACC/HFSA guideline for the management of heart failure: A report of the American College of Cardiology/American Heart Association Joint Committee on clinical practice guidelines. *Circulation*. 2022;145:E895–1032.

40. Solomon SD, McMurray JJV, Claggett B, de Boer RA, DeMets D, Hernandez AF, et al. Dapagliflozin in heart failure with mildly reduced or preserved ejection fraction. *N Engl J Med*. 2022;387:1089–98.

41. Anker SD, Butler J, Filippatos G, Ferreira JP, Bocchi E, Böhm M, et al. Empagliflozin in heart failure with a preserved ejection fraction. *N Engl J Med*. 2021;385:1451–61.

42. Vaduganathan M, Docherty KF, Claggett BL, Jhund PS, de Boer RA, Hernandez AF, et al. SGLT-2 inhibitors in patients with heart failure: A comprehensive meta-analysis of five randomised controlled trials. *Lancet*. 2022;400:757–67.

43. Nassif ME, Windsor SL, Borlaug BA, Kitzman DW, Shah SJ, Tang F, et al. The SGLT2 inhibitor dapagliflozin in heart failure with preserved ejection fraction: A multicenter randomized trial. *Nat Med*. 2021;27:1954–60.

44. Solomon SD, McMurray JJV, Anand IS, Ge J, Lam CSP, Maggioni AP, et al. Angiotensin–Neprilysin inhibition in heart failure with preserved ejection fraction. *N Engl J Med*. 2019;381:1609–20.

45. Rider OJ, Francis JM, Ali MK, Petersen SE, Robinson M, Robson MD, et al. Beneficial cardiovascular effects of bariatric surgical and dietary weight loss in obesity. *J Am Coll Cardiol*. 2009;54:718–26.

46. Mueller S, Winzer EB, Duvinage A, Gevaert AB, Edelmann F, Haller B, et al. Effect of high-intensity interval training, moderate continuous training, or guideline-based physical activity advice on peak oxygen consumption in patients with heart failure with preserved ejection fraction: A randomized clinical trial. *JAMA*. 2021;325:542–51.

47. Arnett DK, Roger Blumenthal C-CS, Michelle Albert C-CA, Buroker AB, Zachary Goldberger D, Hahn EJ, et al. 2019 ACC/AHA guideline on the primary prevention of cardiovascular disease: A report of the American College of Cardiology/American Heart Association task force on clinical practice guidelines. *J Am Coll Cardiol*. 2019;74:e177–232.

48. Diaba-Nuhoho P, Ofori EK, Asare-Anane H, Oppong SY, Boamah I, Blackhurst D. Impact of exercise intensity on oxidative stress and selected metabolic markers in young adults in Ghana. *BMC Res Notes*. 2018;11(1):1–7.

49. Adamson PB, Abraham WT, Bourge RC, Costanzo MR, Hasan A, Yadav C, et al. Wireless pulmonary artery pressure monitoring guides management to reduce decompensation in heart failure with preserved ejection fraction. *Circ Hear Fail*. 2014;7:935–44.

50. Lechner K, McKenzie AL, Krankel N, Von Schacky C, Worm N, Nixdorff U, et al. High-risk atherosclerosis and metabolic phenotype: The roles of ectopic adiposity, atherogenic dyslipidemia, and inflammation. *Metab Syndr Relat Disord*. 2020;18:176–85.

51. Libby P, Buring JE, Badimon L, Hansson GK, Deanfield J, Bittencourt MS, et al. Atherosclerosis. *Nat Rev Dis Prim*. 2019;5:56.

52. Palinski W, Napoli C. Pathophysiological events during pregnancy influence the development of atherosclerosis in humans. *Trends Cardiovasc Med*. 1999;9:205–14.

53. Doring Y, Soehnlein O, Weber C. Neutrophil extracellular traps in atherosclerosis and atherothrombosis. *Circ Res*. 2017;120:736–43.

54. Feinberg MW, Moore KJ. MicroRNA regulation of atherosclerosis. *Circ Res*. 2016;118:703–20.

55. Jaiswal S, Natarajan P, Silver AJ, Gibson CJ, Bick AG, Shvartz E, et al. Clonal hematopoiesis and risk of atherosclerotic cardiovascular disease. *N Engl J Med*. 2017;377:111–21.

56. Roy P, Orecchioni M, Ley K. How the immune system shapes atherosclerosis: Roles of innate and adaptive immunity. *Nat Rev Immunol*. 2022;22:251–65.

57. Wang Z, Klipfell E, Bennett BJ, Koeth R, Levison BS, Dugar B, et al. Gut flora metabolism of phosphatidylcholine promotes cardiovascular disease. *Nature*. 2011;472:57–63.

58. Glass CK, Witztum JL. Atherosclerosis. the road ahead. *Cell*. 2001;104:503–16.

59. Libby P, Ridker PM, Hansson GK. Progress and challenges in translating the biology of atherosclerosis. *Nature*. 2011;473:317–25.

60. Ference BA, Ginsberg HN, Graham I, Ray KK, Packard CJ, Bruckert E, et al. Low-density lipoproteins cause atherosclerotic cardiovascular disease. 1. Evidence from genetic, epidemiologic, and clinical studies. A consensus statement from the European Atherosclerosis Society Consensus Panel. *Eur Hear. J* 2017;38:2459–72.

61. Libby P. Inflammation in atherosclerosis. *Arter Thromb Vasc Biol*. 2012;32:2045–51.

62. Gimbrone Jr MA, Garcia-Cardena G. Vascular endothelium, hemodynamics, and the pathobiology of atherosclerosis. *Cardiovasc Pathol*. 2013;22:9–15.

63. Hedayatnia M, Asadi Z, Zare-Feyzabadi R, Yaghooti-Khorasani M, Ghazizadeh H, Ghaffarian-Zirak R, et al. Dyslipidemia and cardiovascular disease risk among the MASHAD study population. *Lipids Heal Dis*. 2020;19:42.

64. Gupta M, Blumenthal C, Chatterjee S, Bandyopadhyay D, Jain V, Lavie CJ, et al. Novel emerging therapies in atherosclerosis targeting lipid metabolism. *Expert Opin Investig Drugs*. 2020;29:611–22.

65. Hansson GK, Hermansson A. The immune system in atherosclerosis. *Nat Immunol*. 2011;12:204–12.

66. Bennett MR, Sinha S, Owens GK. Vascular smooth muscle cells in atherosclerosis. *Circ Res*. 2016;118:692–702.

67. Swirski FK, Nahrendorf M, Libby P. The ins and outs of inflammatory cells in atheromata. *Cell Metab*. 2012;15:135–6.

68. Libby P, Hansson GK. Inflammation and immunity in diseases of the arterial tree: Players and layers. *Circ Res*. 2015;116:307–11.

69. Gistera A, Robertson AK, Andersson J, Ketelhuth DF, Ovchinnikova O, Nilsson SK, et al. Transforming growth factor-beta signaling in T cells promotes stabilization of atherosclerotic plaques through an interleukin-17-dependent pathway. *Sci Transl Med*. 2013;5:196ra100.

70. Grabner R, Lotzer K, Dopping S, Hildner M, Radke D, Beer M, et al. Lymphotoxin beta receptor signaling promotes tertiary lymphoid organogenesis in the aorta adventitia of aged ApoE−/− mice. *J Exp Med*. 2009;206:233–48.

71. Clarke MC, Talib S, Figg NL, Bennett MR. Vascular smooth muscle cell apoptosis induces interleukin-1-directed inflammation: Effects of hyperlipidemia-mediated inhibition of phagocytosis. *Circ Res*. 2010;106:363–72.

72. Geng YJ, Libby P. Evidence for apoptosis in advanced human atheroma. Colocalization with interleukin-1 beta-converting enzyme. *Am J Pathol*. 1995;147:251–66.

73. Yurdagul Jr A, Doran AC, Cai B, Fredman G, Tabas IA. Mechanisms and consequences of defective efferocytosis in atherosclerosis. *Front Cardiovasc Med*. 2017;4:86.

74. Lavin B, Andia ME, Saha P, Botnar RM, Phinikaridou A. Quantitative MRI of endothelial permeability and (Dys)function in atherosclerosis. *J Vis Exp*. 2021.

75. Sriranjan RS, Tarkin JM, Evans NR, Le EP V, Chowdhury MM, Rudd JHF. Atherosclerosis imaging using PET: Insights and applications. *Br J Pharmacol*. 2021;178:2186–203.

76. Meng H, Ruan J, Yan Z, Chen Y, Liu J, Li X, et al. New progress in early diagnosis of athero-sclerosis. *Int J Mol Sci*. 2022;23.

77. Brown MS, Goldstein JL. Heart attacks: Gone with the century? *Science*. 1996;272:629.

78. Libby P. The forgotten majority: Unfinished business in cardiovascular risk reduction. *J Am Coll Cardiol*. 2005;46:1225–8.

79. Nissen SE, Nicholls SJ, Sipahi I, Libby P, Raichlen JS, Ballantyne CM, et al. Effect of very high-intensity statin therapy on regression of coronary atherosclerosis: The Asteroid trial. *JAMA*. 2006;295:1556–65.

80. Punch E, Klein J, Diaba-Nuhoho P, Morawietz H, Garelnabi M. Effects of PCSK9 targeting: Alleviating oxidation, inflammation, and atherosclerosis. *J Am Hear Assoc*. 2022;11:e023328.

14 Consideration of the Pathophysiology and Treatment of Type 1 and Type 2 Diabetes Mellitus and Other Diabetes Mellitus Subtypes

Paige DeBlieux, Monica Stevens, Richard Kang, and Charles Preuss

14.1 INTRODUCTION

"Diabetes" is a somewhat non-specific term that refers to several conditions of metabolic dysregulation. Diabetes mellitus, diabetes insipidus, gestational diabetes, and maturity-onset diabetes of the young are just a few categories that fall under this broader term of diabetes, with each encompassing further subsets. However, if you have heard someone use the term "diabetes" colloquially, they are most likely referring to *diabetes mellitus*, a condition in which a person's blood sugar concentrations are chronically elevated above normal physiologic levels. Diabetes mellitus classically falls under one of two categories: type 1 or type 2. In 2022, according to the Centers for Disease Control National Diabetes Statistics Report, 37.3 million adults in the United States, with or without a formal diagnosis, had diabetes (1), that is, 11.3% of the adult population, "adult" being defined as those of 18 years of age or older. Far surpassing that number are those who are considered "pre-diabetic", at 96 million, or 38% of the adult population. In the 65 and older age group, nearly 50% of adults have been diagnosed with pre-diabetes. These statistics elucidate just how pertinent this metabolic condition is among our population, especially older adults, and the need for education and awareness.

This disease is without doubt a life-altering diagnosis. At the very least, people are expected to change their lifestyle by avoiding processed sugars, to exercise regularly for weight management, and to undergo daily glucose checks. (2) More often, people are started on a medication regimen that can range from one pill (tablet or capsule) twice daily to complex routines involving multiple medications and close monitoring. These medications, as with all pharmacological therapies, have varying side effects that can include anything from gastrointestinal upset to lactic acidosis to serious hypoglycemia and death. (3, 4)

This chapter will discuss the pathology, treatment, and various disease processes involved in the broader term of *diabetes*. Other topics to be covered will include preventative measures, the physician's approach, and questions patients should know to ask. By the end of this chapter, the reader should have developed a more holistic understanding of the complexities of this disease and its management.

14.2 DIABETES: A Sweet History

The word "diabetes" comes from the Greek derivative *siphon*, or to pass through. "Mellitus" means *honeyed* or *sweet*. (5) This derivation makes sense as the initial clinical manifestations of the disease include side effects secondary to overly sweetened urine and blood. The Egyptians described symptoms similar to this as early as 3,000 years ago. The term "diabetes" was first recorded around AD 81–133 by Araetus of Cappadocia. Later, in 1675, Thomas Willis added the term "mellitus" after the discovery of sugar in the urine and blood of his patients. Although Willis's documentation of the sugar content in urine and blood was the first written documentation, other ancient civilizations had already acknowledged that people with this condition had sweet urine and blood. (6, 7) In 1857, nearly 200 years after the first recorded diagnosis, Claude Bernard of France discovered the process by which the liver stores and then utilizes glucose molecules for energy use. The storage is termed glycogenesis, while the utilization is termed glycolysis. With this discovery, he described the potential role that the liver and these processes play in diabetes. Finally, almost 30 years later, Mering and Minkowski isolated insulin and described the involvement of the pancreas in this pathology. (6, 7)

Generally, the metabolic condition of diabetes mellitus, either type 1 (DMT1) or type 2 (DMT2), refers to a relative insufficiency of the hormone insulin. Insulin regulates the uptake of glucose, a metabolite of the food products we consume and our main energy source. In addition, insulin plays an important role in lipid and protein metabolism. (8) The function of this hormone will be further discussed in the subsection "Therapies and Management". In DMT1, insulin deficiency develops because the body cannot adequately produce insulin. The most common reason for this is that the body's own immune system has been wired to damage those cells in the pancreas that produce it. In comparison, in DMT2, the body's insulin receptors have become desensitized and the body cannot produce enough insulin to elicit a response. (9) See Figure 14.1 for a comparison of

DOI: 10.1201/9781003384823-14

	Type 1	Type 2
Prevalence	1.9 million Americans	34 million Americans
Average Age of Onset	13 -14 years old	45 - 64 years old
Symptoms	Excessive thirst, increased urination, weight loss	Asymptomatic or increased thirst and urination. Numbness in hands or feet and vision loss
Pathogenesis	Inability to produce insulin	Reduced response to insulin
Treatment	Insulin replacement	Lifestyle changes and Blood glucose control

Figure 14.1   Type 1 and type 2 diabetes mellitus compared

type 1 and type 2 DM. When the body is unresponsive to a surge in insulin, or unable to create a surge in the first place, those glucose particles remain in the bloodstream rather than being transported to tissue for metabolism and storage. The next section contains a discussion of different types of diabetes, their pathophysiology, clinical manifestations, and, briefly, how management of them differs.

14.3 BACKGROUND AND BASICS

14.3.1 Diabetes Mellitus Type 1

DMT1 was traditionally thought of as childhood-onset, or juvenile, diabetes because of its early initial presentation. These patients often present with excessive thirst, increased urination, difficulty gaining weight, and, in more severe cases, a dangerous condition termed diabetic ketoacidosis. The early onset can be explained by its pathophysiology. Patients with DMT1 experience insulin-deficiency secondary to autoimmune destruction of their insulin-producing cells, as previously mentioned. (10) These specialized cells, known as *beta cells*, are found in the pancreas, an organ in the upper mid- to left abdomen. As the innate and adaptive immune systems develop, a genetic predisposition to the destruction of these specialized cells is triggered and the body's own protector cells begin damaging them. The exact mechanism by which this develops is characterized by much controversy and speculation. However, there are genotypic, environmental, and viral-associated mechanisms that are now better understood and accepted. Because these individuals cannot produce adequate endogenous insulin concentrations, they are started on exogenous insulin or insulin analogues. Therapeutic insulin delivery routes have undergone significant changes over the past decade as physician-scientists and researchers have worked to establish accessible routes for patients that will optimize adherence and patient comfort without compromising treatment efficacy. (11) Insulin therapies were initially administered via self-injections. This required patients to draw up the appropriate insulin dosage from one vial into a syringe, self-inject the insulin, and then properly dispose of the needle. In addition, patients had to keep those vials at appropriately cool temperatures to ensure the insulin's effectiveness. Thankfully, due to the efforts of experts in the field, great strides have been taken to allow patients improved delivery routes including oral, nasal, transdermal, and subcutaneous implantable insulin pumps, which lessen the burden of painful injections and the management of excessive equipment. (11) Continuous glucose monitoring (CGM), rather than intermittent finger sticks to check for capillary glucose concentrations, is more accurate in insulin administration and generally easier on the patient. CGMs also allow patients and physicians to more accurately observe daily fluctuations in blood glucose concentrations, which helps guide therapy adjustments. (12) Other considerations for the development of insulin-dependent diabetes mellitus include those circumstances in which damage to the pancreas is not incurred through a congenital etiology but rather through exogenous or iatrogenic factors, such as chronic pancreatitis, pancreatectomy (removal of a portion or the entire pancreas), acute-severe pancreatitis resulting in irreversible damage, endocrinopathies, infections, and even poorly managed type 2 diabetes. (13, 14) Regardless of the reason, patients with DMT1 remain at high risk of developing significant hyperglycemia and hypoglycemia, which can have substantial negative effects on these persons' health. These patients should be followed closely by their primary care physician and they should maintain a strict regimen of glucose checks and medical management.

14.3.2 Diabetes Mellitus Type 2

DMT2 is likely what comes to mind when the average person thinks of their middle-aged uncle who just got diagnosed with diabetes. These persons usually have an elevated body mass index (BMI) and present with symptoms of increased urination, increased thirst, and, in more prolonged cases, worsening vision, and a loss of sensation in the most distal extremities. BMI is measured by dividing a person's weight in kilograms by their height in meters squared (kg/m^2). This is currently the standard for determining if a person is underweight, of normal weight, overweight, obese, or severely obese. Any BMI between 18.5 and 24.9 is considered normal, while less than 18.5 is underweight. A BMI of 25 and over is considered elevated, with differing classes designated at certain increments. A BMI of 25–29.9 is denoted as overweight, 30–34.9 as obese, and 35 and higher as severely obese. (15)

DMT2 develops over time as the patient's insulin receptors become desensitized from overexposure, or when the beta cells of the pancreas become "worn out" from overuse. This typically takes years to develop and most commonly occurs because of chronically elevated glucose concentrations secondary to high rates of sugar consumption. (16) This is analogous to drowning out the background music at a restaurant. Constant inundation with stimuli, whether sound or insulin, causes us to become less responsive over time. The approach to this is not to introduce more insulin to the system, but rather to augment the responsiveness of those receptors to the insulin during a surge. See Figure 14.2 for step-up management of DMT2. It is important to note here that overlap can happen in the pathophysiology of those patients with chronic, uncontrolled type 2 diabetes and those with type 1 diabetes, as previously mentioned. Chronically elevated concentrations of glucose lead to glycosylated cell membranes and stepwise global organ dysfunction. As will be discussed later in the section on "Manifestations of Diabetes", one of the organs that can potentially become damaged is the pancreas. At this point, when the pancreas becomes damaged, type 1 and type 2 diabetics have essentially the same pathophysiology, in which neither can produce adequate amounts of insulin. Type 2 diabetics can then be referred to as insulin-dependent type 2 diabetes despite its previous distinction as insulin-independent, although such diabetes remains classified as DMT2 because of its etiology and insulin insensitivity.

14.3.3 Maturity-Onset Diabetes of the Young

Maturity-onset diabetes of the young, or MODY, is a rare form of inherited diabetes in which there is a defective enzyme that affects beta-cell functionality. (17) The discovery and description of this disease are fairly new, only having come to light in the past decade. The subtypes MODY I and MODY II can be managed with diet alone, whereas all other subtypes require other additional interventions, including insulin or sulfonylureas. (17)

14.3.4 Gestational Diabetes

Gestational diabetes, as the name implies, arises during pregnancy. In the first trimester, insulin sensitivity is increased to account for the additional need in glucose consumption as the fetus is developing rapidly. In the second and third trimesters, however, this need slows down leading to insulin insensitivity. (18, 19) Because of this change in regulation, childbearing women are at higher risk of hypoglycemia in the first trimester and are likely to present with gestational diabetes in the second and third trimesters. This occurs in 5–9% of all pregnancies and increases the risk of fetal and maternal morbidity and mortality. Patients are more likely to develop gestational diabetes if they have a history of gestational diabetes, an elevated BMI, have previously had an infant born with macrosomia, and/or have had recurrent pregnancy loss. (18, 19) Most patients

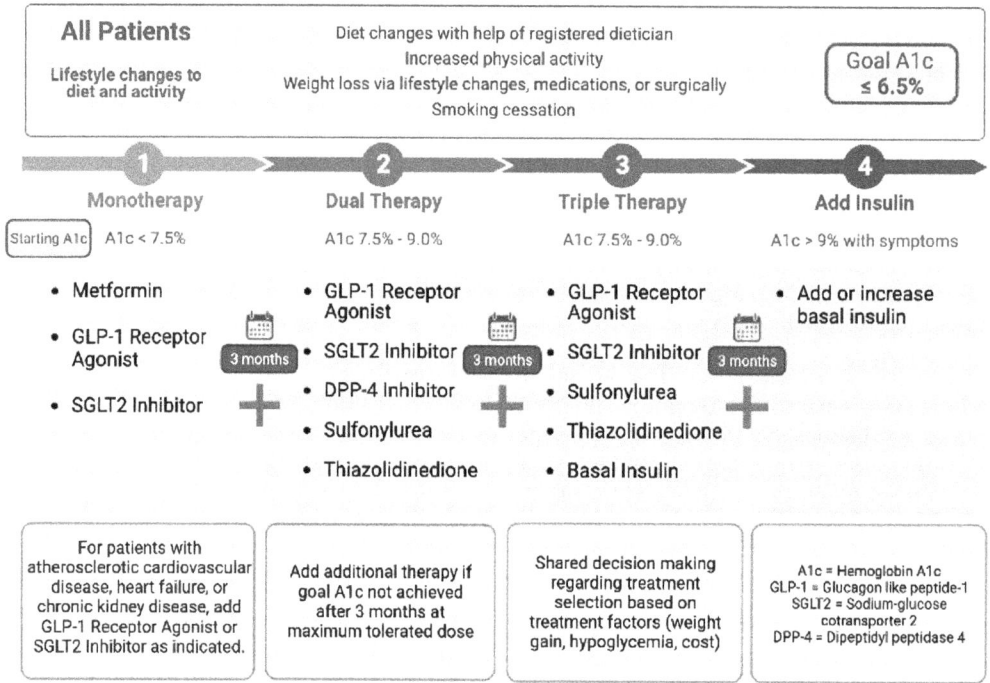

Figure 14.2 Type 2 diabetes mellitus step-up management plan

experience resolution of their diabetes after delivery; however, they are at increased risk of developing DMT2 after pregnancy. This is likely related to these people having an elevated BMI, higher glucose consumption, and already decreased insulin receptor sensitivity. These patients should be counseled on the importance of regular checkups during their pregnancy and continued follow-up with their primary care physicians after pregnancy.

14.3.5 Diabetes Insipidus

Diabetes insipidus (DI) is a metabolic condition in which there is no insulin insufficiency or dysregulation of glucose. Rather, these patients suffer from insufficiency of a hormone called anti-diuretic hormone, or ADH, and have dysregulation of free water retention. (20) This hormone is produced by a portion of the brain termed the hypothalamus. It functions to increase the uptake of free water in the renal system. Therefore, patients with DI experience excessive urination as free water loss is uninhibited. The development of DI is most commonly idiopathic. However, other secondary etiologies include brain tumors, iatrogenic injury from surgery, ischemia, infection, and traumatic brain injury. (20) These patients often present with dehydration and/or excessive thirst coupled with excessive urination, as well as elevated blood sodium concentrations. Sodium retention occurs as an effort to increase the osmotic gradient into the vasculature but results in hypernatremia as the free water loss is not appropriately compensated for. These losses can be catastrophic as the electrolyte imbalance can lead to organ dysfunction and eventually organ failure. These patients should be treated with ADH (which is also called vasopressin) as well as properly rehydrated.

14.4 DIAGNOSTICS

Patients suspected of having any of the aforementioned diseases require specific diagnostic studies to determine the condition. In addition, what the physician suspects and what he/she orders will differ depending on the patient's presentation. Before a discussion of the different diagnostic studies, it is important to consider which patients need to be screened.

Per the American Diabetes Association (ADA) 2021 guidelines, those patients who meet the following criteria should be screened for diabetes mellitus, type 2:

- 45 years of age or older.

- History of pre-diabetes or gestational diabetes.

- Patients 45 years of age or younger who are overweight or obese and have one or more risk factors for developing type 2 diabetes mellitus, including those which are modifiable (smoking, inactivity, excessive alcohol use) and non-modifiable (family history, age).

- Presence of risk-enhancing comorbidities including HIV, cystic fibrosis, and post-organ transplantation.

- And women planning to become pregnant or who have become pregnant and are overweight/obese or have a history of gestational diabetes.

As previously discussed, type 1 diabetes will typically present itself in younger individuals and in the setting of a more serious condition known as diabetic ketoacidosis, or DKA. This occurs when the patient has been chronically unable to utilize glucose they have consumed. Because glucose is not properly taken up and metabolized, the body believes it is in a state of starvation and therefore begins to form ketones to provide an energy source. The formation of ketones decreases the body's pH below normal physiologic levels and can cause significant organ damage. These patients often require critical care, which will be discussed in greater detail later in this chapter. Tests that should be ordered initially for the patient with type 1 diabetes include a hemoglobin A1c, glucose concentrations, creatinine kinase concentrations, and urinalysis, as a baseline. These studies will help guide which insulin regimen should be initiated, as well as determining the patient's renal function and any damage that has already occurred.

Type 2 diabetes mellitus is more typical in the older adult who has comorbid obesity. These patients will typically present with symptoms such as increased thirst (polydipsia) and increased urination (polyuria). In more chronic cases where a person has lived with undiagnosed type 2 diabetes for many years, the patient may present with numbness or tingling in their most distal extremities, and/or decreased visual acuity. This is secondary to prolonged hyperglycemia (elevated blood glucose concentrations), which leads to glycosylation and subsequent damage to the nerve endings and endothelial lining of the small blood vessels. Because the distal nerves and blood vessels of the eye are so small, manifestations of damage to these are the first to present clinically. Diagnostic tests for patients with suspected type 2 diabetes are similar to type 1 diabetics, including hemoglobin A1c, glucose concentrations, and urinalysis. In those patients whom the physician suspects have gone undiagnosed for a significant period, it may be appropriate to employ physical exam techniques such as the monofilament exam on the distal fingers and toes, temperature testing on those same sites, and a fundoscopic exam to see the retina and the posterior blood vessels of the eyes. These will give the physician a sense of the severity of the disease and the appropriate treatment plan that should be started.

In the patient that the physician suspects of new-onset diabetes mellitus, whether type 1 or type 2, it is important to approach the diagnostics systematically to ensure the most accurate results from testing. If the patient is asymptomatic, obtaining two or more abnormal blood glucose tests can be diagnostic. In those individuals who are symptomatic (i.e., hyperphagia, polydipsia, polyuria, unexplained weight loss), one abnormal glucose concentration is diagnostic. When testing for glucose concentrations, the physician can either order a fasting level, a post-prandial level, or a random level. While multiple random levels may show fluctuations throughout a patient's day, one random level will demonstrate very little in the way of diagnostics. On the other hand, a fasting glucose concentration, which needs to be 8 hours or more after the patient's last meal, will demonstrate the ability, or inability, of the body to either produce or react to an insulin surge and take up the glucose in the bloodstream. In contrast, an oral glucose tolerance test is most sensitive when determining the body's ability to utilize glucose. In this test, individuals are given 75 mg of glucose and, 2 hours later, their blood glucose is tested. Although this is a sensitive test, it is not as convenient or cost-effective as a random or fasting glucose concentration, and therefore not as likely to be utilized in the outpatient clinical setting.

Next, hemoglobin A1c, often abbreviated as HgbA1c, is a gold standard of diagnosis and prognosis in patients with diabetes. Hemoglobin A1c tells the percentage of hemoglobin molecules in the blood that are saturated with glucose molecules (i.e., *glycated*). This gives an average of the glucose concentrations over the past 8–12 weeks and can help steer management. A HgbA1c result is given in a percentage to demonstrate percentage saturation and should be 6.5% or less.

Lastly, in the patient with chronic diabetes mellitus, whether type 1 or 2, the clinician should consider several routine diagnostic tests that allow for following the disease process. A commonly used blood test that is cost-effective and offers a decent amount of information is the basic metabolic panel, or BMP. This test includes looking at metabolites in the blood, which indicate the health of a patient's kidneys, as well as electrolyte balance. These are important markers as prolonged, uncontrolled diabetes can cause kidney damage, as mentioned earlier. When there is damage to the smaller renal structures that regulate the elimination and retention of certain electrolytes, this can be revealed in a BMP. It is important to keep electrolytes adequately regulated as disturbance can have serious side effects on vital organs such as the brain and heart.

Other tests that should be routinely ordered are liver studies. This is because chronically elevated glucose concentrations can lead to issues such as non-alcoholic fatty liver disease/steatosis hepatitis (NASH). In addition, many of the common medications used in the management of diabetes, such as metformin, can lead to liver damage. Therefore, liver transaminases should be checked with some regularity.

On a broader scale, lipid concentrations should be monitored to maintain awareness of the patient's cardiovascular risk assessment. Elevated cholesterol concentrations, or hypercholesteremia, in conjunction with hyperglycemia, increase a patient's risk of developing arteriosclerosis and atherosclerosis, which directly increase risk of cardiovascular disease, e.g., myocardial infarction.

Finally, another routine test that should be performed in those diagnosed with diabetes mellitus is the spot urinary albumin-to-creatinine ratio. This test is another marker for kidney damage but can catch the damage in the very early stages. This test works by picking up traces of albumin in the urine, which should not be present in healthy kidneys.

While the diagnostic tests discussed up to this point can be more broadly applied to the initial diagnosis and routine follow-up of diabetes mellitus, both type 1 and 2, there are special tests that are not required but can be used to differentiate between the types of DM. In order to discuss these, a deeper dive into the physiology of insulin is required. The pancreas, as previously mentioned, produces and releases insulin in response to elevated glucose concentrations in the normal physiologic state to initiate glucose uptake. When endogenous insulin is produced, it comes from the starter protein known as "proinsulin". As proinsulin is metabolized, it leaves behind a metabolite known as protein C, along with the desired insulin molecule. This protein can be detected in high volumes in those patients with DMT2 who have released insulin but cannot respond to it. In comparison, those patients with DMT1 that cannot produce insulin in the first place will be found to have lower levels of protein C secondary to low levels of proinsulin being produced by the pancreas.

Maturity-onset diabetes of the young, or MODY, is a rarer condition in which there is a hereditary dysfunctional enzyme that impairs the functionality of beta cells in the pancreas. Current diagnostic criteria are largely clinical and include onset before age 25, two consecutive familial generations with diabetes, a lack of autoantibodies, and the presence of endogenous insulin production with C protein blood concentrations equal to or higher than 200 pmol/L. (21) Overall, there are 14 described subtypes of MODY, with 1–8 being the major types. As genetic testing remains cost-prohibitive and is significantly resource-dependent, clinical criteria remain the gold standard of diagnosis for this disease process – namely, diagnosis younger than age 30 with a family history of diabetes. That being said, as the field of molecular analysis progresses, appropriately diagnosing these patients and providing the proper treatment plan is becoming increasingly possible. (21)

In pregnancy, women are routinely monitored for the development of gestational diabetes, regardless of their history or risk factors. Although guidelines vary between societies, the American College of Obstetrics and Gynecologists (ACOG) continues to recommend the two-step approach. Women without significant risk factors or a history of gestational diabetes undergo a routine oral glucose test in the second trimester, around 24–28 weeks. (22) Those with increased risk factors should undergo testing prior to 24 weeks. The 50-gram oral glucose test is an initial screening test in which a woman receives 50 g oral glucose and, 1 hour later, her blood glucose concentrations are tested. Her glucose concentrations should be <135 mg/dL. If this is normal, there is no need for further testing. However, if her blood glucose concentrations are elevated, then a confirmation test with 100 g oral glucose is administered and her blood glucose is tested 3 hours later. If her blood glucose concentrations remain elevated, this time ≥140 mg/dL, then she can be officially diagnosed, and a management plan started. (22)

Diabetes insipidus is largely beyond the scope of this chapter and is a metabolic condition that is not a product of pancreatic damage. Instead, as previously mentioned, it is secondary to central nervous system dysregulation of ADH. Diagnostic criteria include the clinical features of polydipsia, polyuria, dehydration, and hypernatremia, as well as low ADH concentrations.

14.5 TREATMENT AND MANAGEMENT

This portion of the chapter will discuss various treatment and management options for diabetes mellitus, both pharmacologic and otherwise. This is by no means an exhaustive list and each potential avenue for a plan of care should be approached systematically but with the individual patient, their past medical history, needs, and resources in mind. In addition, risks and benefits should always be considered and compared against one another as none of these medications and interventions are completely benign. Just as hyperglycemia can lead to significant clinical problems, hypoglycemia can be a dangerous state depending on the severity. Figure 14.3 demonstrates drug classes in a consolidated manner and Table 14.1 lists the symptoms associated with hyper- and hypoglycemia depending on the severity of each.

14.5.1 Insulin and Its Analogues

Insulin, a naturally occurring endogenous hormone, is released by pancreatic beta cells in response to increasing serum glucose concentrations. Insulin facilitates cell glucose uptake and various anabolic processes in the human body, including glycogenesis and lipogenesis. Since its initial discovery in the 1920s, insulin supplementation has become an integral part of DM treatment, particularly for insulin-deficient type 1 diabetics. (23) Insulin is subdivided into several classes based on the onset of activity. (23) The rapidly acting insulins include aspart (Fiasp), glulisine (Apidra), and lispro (Humalog). They have a quick onset of action (approximately 10–15 minutes after administration) and have a relatively short duration of action (approximately 3–5 hours). (23) Long-acting insulins, such as glargine (Lantus), detemir (Levemir), and degludec (Tresiba) exist on the opposite end of the spectrum. These formulations take longer to take effect (1–3 hours) but exert effects for up to 48 hours. (23) Regular insulin (Humulin R) and intermediate-acting insulin/NPH (Humulin N) exist in the middle of the spectrum. Insulin is available for administration in several injectable forms, such as pens, syringes, or insulin pumps. As a polypeptide hormone that would be denatured and degraded by the digestive tract, it cannot be administered by mouth (PO). Given the wide variety of insulin formulations, clinicians often incorporate the various subtypes and tailor medication use for patients' specific needs. For example, a long-acting insulin such as glargine (Lantus) might be given to reign in blood sugar concentrations throughout the day and short-acting insulins such as aspart (Fiasp) might be given several minutes before mealtimes to blunt the transient spikes in blood sugar concentrations after eating. See Figure 14.4 for the timing of insulin and its analogues after administration.

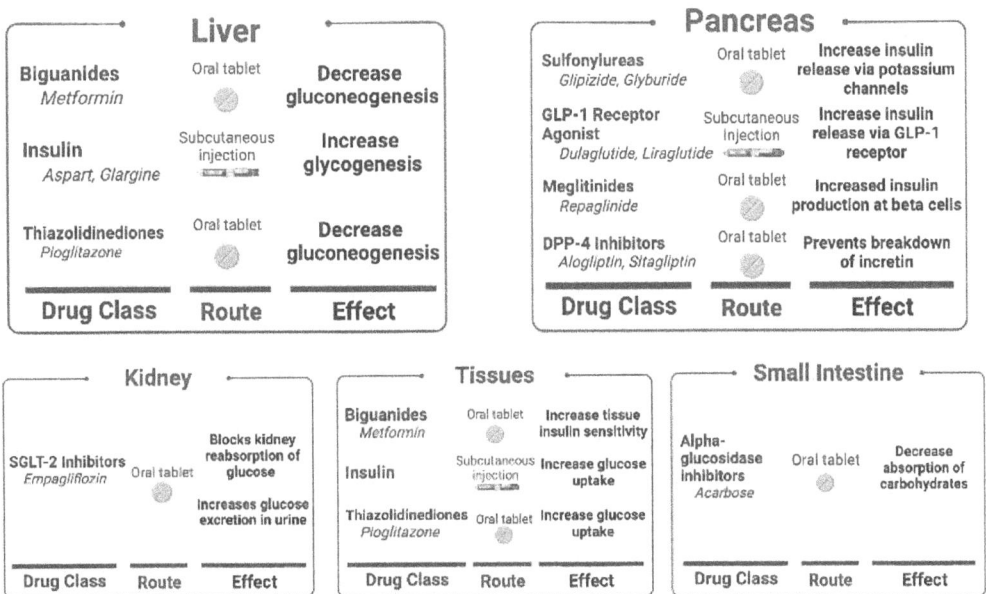

Figure 14.3 Drug classes: their routes and effects

Table 14.1 **Compared symptomology of hypo- and hyperglycemia based on severity**

	Mild	Moderate	Severe
Hyperglycemia	> 150 mg/dL Increased urination Increased thirst	> 200 mg/dL Dry mouth Blurred vision Abdominal pain Confusion	> 300 mg/dL Diabetic ketoacidosis Coma
Hypoglycemia	< 70 mg/dL Sweating Shaking Hunger Palpitations	< 55 mg/dL Irritability Sleepiness Confusion	< 40 mg/dL Loss of consciousness Seizures Coma

14.5.2 Sulfonylureas

Sulfonylureas interact with ATP-sensitive potassium channels in pancreatic beta cells, eventually leading to calcium influx into beta cells and subsequent insulin release. (24) In addition to directly stimulating insulin release, sulfonylureas increase insulin sensitivity in target organs and decrease glucagon secretion. (24) Sulfonylureas are subdivided into two classes of medications: first- and second-generation drugs. The first-generation sulfonylureas include tolazamide, tolbutamide, and chlorpropamide. The second-generation sulfonylureas include glyburide, glimepiride, and glipizide. Sulfonylureas are available only in oral formulations. As one of the oldest diabetic medications, sulfonylureas are still used in clinical medicine today, particularly due to their low cost. (24) They are often prescribed in conjunction with other diabetic medications such as metformin and are often used as an adjunct to lifestyle modifications, such as dieting and exercise. Hypoglycemia is a common adverse effect of sulfonylureas, which are known to have a narrow therapeutic index. (24) To mitigate this potential side effect, the American Diabetes Association recommends that patients on these medications routinely self-monitor blood glucose

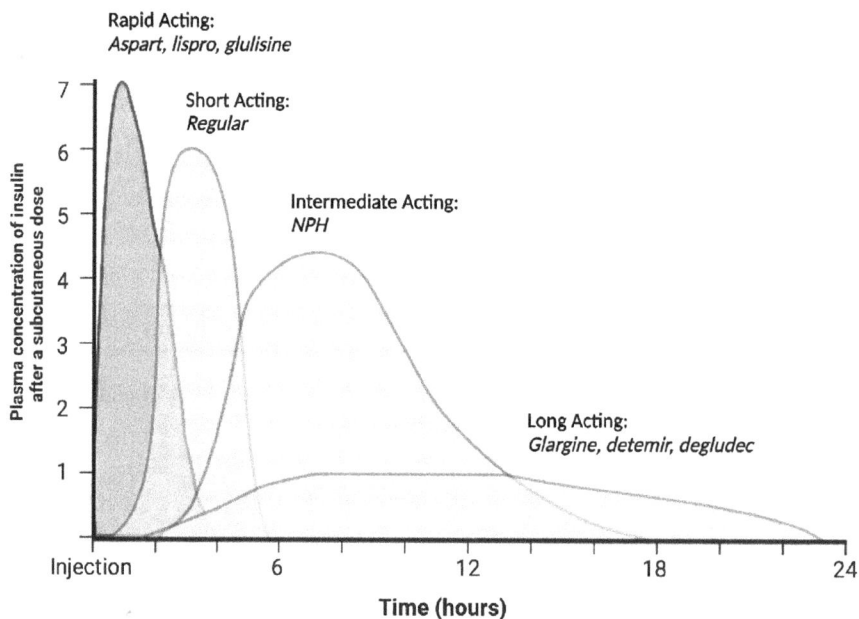

Figure 14.4 Timing of insulin and insulin analogues

concentrations. Furthermore, caution is to be used in prescribing these medications to patients with hepatic or renal insufficiency as these conditions may heighten the risk of hypoglycemia. (25) Hepatic injury is another potential adverse effect of sulfonylurea use. (26) These medications should also be avoided in patients with sulfa allergies.

14.5.3 Meglitinides

Meglitinides include the oral medications repaglinide and nateglinide. (27) By binding to ATP channels on pancreatic beta cells, these medications stimulate increased insulin production. (27) Concurrent use of meglitinides and sulfonylureas is contraindicated because of their similar mechanism of action. Some adverse side effects of meglitinides include weight gain, gastrointestinal symptoms such as diarrhea, and joint pain. (27) As with many diabetic medications, hypoglycemia is a common side effect of unintentional overdose or skipping meals. As repaglinide and nateglinide are both metabolized and excreted through the liver, they should be avoided in patients with liver disease but make good candidates for pharmacologic therapy in patients with comorbid kidney disease. (27)

14.5.4 Biguanides

Biguanides is a class of oral diabetic medications that most notably includes metformin. Metformin exerts its effects on the liver to decrease gluconeogenesis and glycogenolysis, as well as increasing tissue sensitivity to insulin, creating a three-pronged mechanism for decreasing blood glucose levels. Metformin is often used as a first-line medication to manage type 2 DM. (28) It has a relatively favorable side effect profile, including being weight neutral and unlikely to precipitate hypoglycemia. (29) However, some common adverse effects patients experience upon starting the medication include gastrointestinal symptoms, such as nausea and vomiting. (29) As metformin is renally excreted from the body, it is important to consider patient's renal status and to avoid use in patients with renal insufficiency or decreased glomerular filtration rate (GFR). (29) Some important off-label indications for starting metformin include gestational diabetes (well tolerated during pregnancy and nonteratogenic) or the treatment of oligomenorrhea in patients with polycystic ovary syndrome (PCOS). (29)

14.5.5 Thiazolidinediones

Thiazolidinediones consist of the drugs rosiglitazone and pioglitazone. (30) These oral medications work by promoting insulin sensitivity in various target organs and decreasing hepatic gluconeogenesis. (30) More specifically, they regulate gene expression in target organs through peroxisome proliferator-activated receptor-gamma (PPAR-gamma), which in turn promotes various anabolic processes, such cellular glucose uptake and lipid storage within adipocytes. Rosiglitazone and pioglitazone should be avoided in patients with cardiac comorbidities, such as congestive heart failure, because they promote edema and fluid retention in the body. (30) Unlike metformin, which is weight neutral, thiazolidinediones have also been associated with weight gain during use. (30) Additionally, thiazolidinediones have been associated with increased risk of bone fractures. (30) Due to this side effect profile, these drugs are considered second-line in diabetes compared to the better-tolerated biguanides.

14.5.6 Alpha-Glucosidase Inhibitors

Alpha-glucosidase inhibitors, such as acarbose, voglibose, and miglitolare, lower serum glucose concentrations by inhibiting carbohydrate absorption through the intestine. Some adverse side effects of alpha-glucosidase inhibitors include gastrointestinal symptoms, such as bloating, flatulence, and abdominal pain/discomfort. Because of these potential adverse effects, these medications should be avoided in patients with intestinal obstruction or inflammatory bowel disease, such as Crohn's disease or ulcerative colitis. One potentially rare complication of alpha-glucosidase inhibitors is acute liver injury. (31) Instances of liver injury are limited to case reports, however, and one cohort study in 2018 found no significant liver injury in patients treated with acarbose versus controls. (32)

14.5.7 DPP-4 Inhibitors

Dipeptidyl peptidase IV (DPP-4) inhibitors, otherwise known as "gliptins", because the different medications end with the suffix "gliptin", function to increase the endogenous incretin effect. Incretins are released from a portion of the stomach lining in response to nutrient intake to increase insulin secretion. Gliptins work to inhibit DPP-4, which would otherwise work to break down glucagon-like peptide-1 (GLP-1) and glucose-dependent insulinotropic peptide (GIP), thereby decreasing further the release of insulin and concomitantly increasing glucagon. (33) Here, it is pertinent to consider the role of the hormone glucagon in the disease of diabetes mellitus. Glucagon is a hormone that can be considered to work in the background, releasing stored glucose into the bloodstream when insulin is not actively working or when appropriate uptake is not occurring. So, if a patient consumes a meal and glucose is left in the blood because insulin either cannot be excreted or utilized, glucagon gets the go-ahead to continue increasing blood glucose concentrations, further worsening the problem. In light of this, there is a now a better understanding of the effect of DPP-4 inhibitors and their role in type 2 DM. They increase insulin to overcome the desensitized receptors, and decrease the work of glucagon, creating a double effort to decrease blood glucose. As with all medications, however, there are considerations for when this may be an appropriate or inappropriate pharmacotherapy. Patients with liver or renal failure, or those who are hypersensitive to the drug, should avoid use of DDP-4 inhibitors. Side effects include gastrointestinal effects such as constipation or diarrhea, arthralgias, worsening renal failure or pancreatitis, and increased feelings of satiety, among a few others. The satiety may be a favorable side effect as it will likely aid in weight loss and is secondary to delayed gastric emptying. It is important to note that these medications do not increase the risk of hypoglycemia unless taken with insulin or insulin-promoting medications.

14.5.8 SGLT-2 Inhibitors

Sodium-glucose co-transporter-2 (SGLT-2) inhibitors, or the "glifozins", work to reversibly inhibit the sodium-glucose linked transporter 2 in the kidneys to decrease glucose reabsorption. While this decreases glucose concentrations in the blood, it increases glucose in the urine, leading to glycosuria and polyuria. As a consequence of this, side effects of SGLT-2 inhibitors include urinary tract infections, genital yeast infections, especially in women, and dehydration. Another significant side effect is severe DKA. These medications are best used in young adults without renal failure or renal disease.

14.5.9 Glucagon-like Peptide Receptor Agonists

Glucagon-like peptide 1 (GLP-1) receptor agonists include liraglutide. These medications work like incretins by binding to the GLP-1 receptors to increase insulin release. GLP-1 receptor agonists are resistant to breakdown by DPP-4 enzymes, thereby prolonging the incretin effect. Side effects include gastrointestinal upset, like nausea and vomiting, as well as an increased risk of pancreatitis. Another side effect that may be viewed as beneficial rather than adverse is weight loss secondary to the incretin effect of delayed gastric emptying and subsequent early satiety.

14.5.10 Bile Acid Sequestrants

Bile acid sequestrants, although not first-line agents in the treatment of type 2 DM, have been shown to have some significance not only in lipid-lowering properties but also in glucose control. (34) While the exact mechanism behind their effects is still up for debate, a few potential leads have remained at the forefront of research. Bile acid sequestrants, or BASs, have some association with the farnesoid X receptors, TGR5 receptors, GLP-1 molecules, and glucose-dependent insulinotropic polypeptides, all of which are intertwined in the complex regulation of glucose, its uptake, and its metabolism on the molecular level. Currently, the only FDA-approved BAS in the United States for the treatment of type 2 DM is colesevelam.

14.5.11 Dopamine Agonists

Dopamine agonists (DAs), such as bromocriptine and cabergoline, were primarily designed for the management of neurological diseases such as restless leg syndrome, Parkinson's disease, and hyperprolactinemia. However, there has been promising evidence of DAs' positive effects on patients with DMT2, including glycemic control and weight loss. (35)

14.5.12 Surgical Intervention

The 2017 STAMPEDE Trial compared 5-year outcomes between three groups with DMT2: those who underwent intensive medical therapy alone, sleeve gastrectomy, and gastric bypass with or without medical therapy. (36) Five-year outcomes looked at glycated hemoglobin (HgbA1c), weight loss, reduction in medication, lower lipid concentrations, and quality of life. In all categories, surgical intervention was superior to medical therapy alone. (36)

Next, diabetes and its clinical manifestations will be explored.

14.6 DIABETES MELLITUS AND ITS MANIFESTATIONS

Diabetes mellitus can have profound systemic impacts on the human body, especially in the unmanaged state. Routine surveillance and maintenance treatments/lifestyle modifications are recommended to prevent deleterious effects to various organ systems (i.e., heart, kidneys, eyes, etc.). In the following subsection, the systemic ramifications of DM and appropriate treatment methods will be explored. See these global manifestations illustrated in Figure 14.5.

14.6.1 Cardiovascular

Inadequate glycemic control has been significantly associated with increased risk of cardiovascular disease, including coronary artery disease, myocardial infarction, and peripheral arterial disease. (37) Prior research has shown that patients with DM have approximately a 2.5 times higher risk of heart failure, independent of other comorbidities. As the number of Americans affected by DM is expected to increase by approximately 50% by 2030, the need for adequate blood sugar control to minimize cardiovascular risks becomes increasingly important. Current understanding of the interplay between DM and cardiovascular disease involves several biophysical pathways. Chronic hyperglycemic states promote a constant state of inflammation, which damages vessels and predisposes patients to thrombus formation and atherosclerotic changes. Excess glucose has been shown to activate nuclear factor kappa b (NF-kB), which promotes inflammatory cytokine release into the body. Additionally, hyperglycemia is directly related to elevated concentrations of cholesterol and fats in the body through lipogenic pathways. In patients with poorly managed DM,

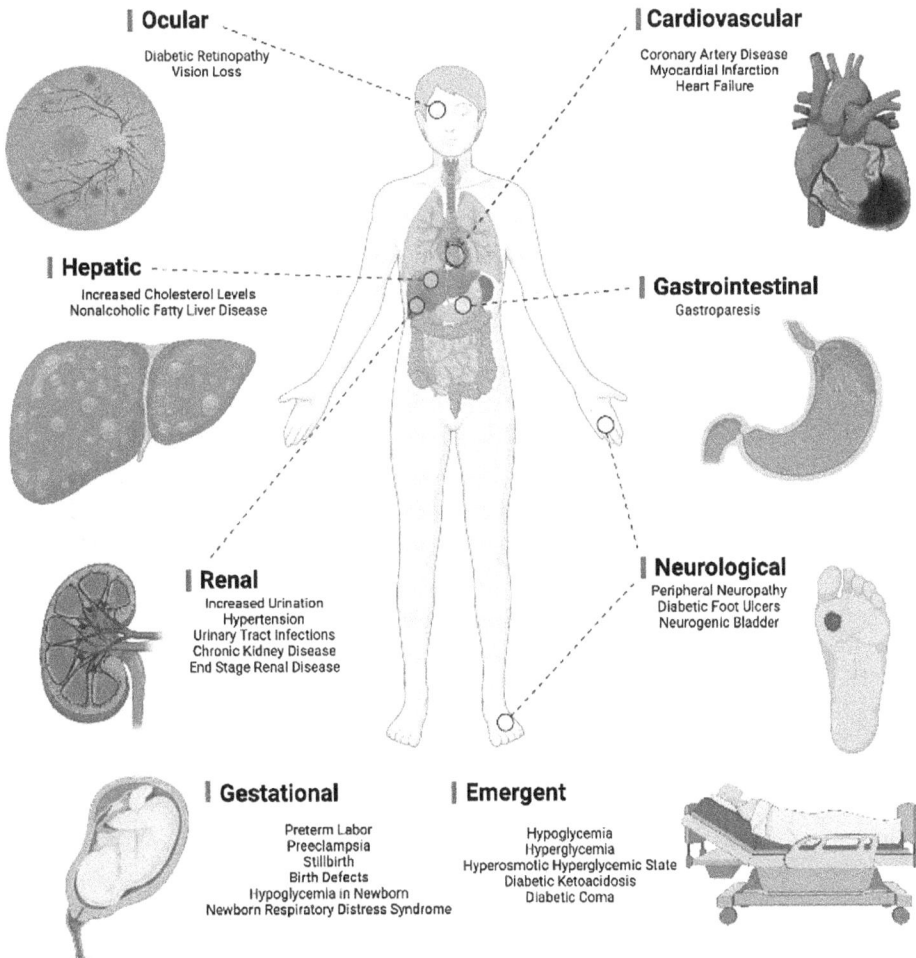

Ocular
Diabetic Retinopathy
Vision Loss

Cardiovascular
Coronary Artery Disease
Myocardial Infarction
Heart Failure

Hepatic
Increased Cholesterol Levels
Nonalcoholic Fatty Liver Disease

Gastrointestinal
Gastroparesis

Renal
Increased Urination
Hypertension
Urinary Tract Infections
Chronic Kidney Disease
End Stage Renal Disease

Neurological
Peripheral Neuropathy
Diabetic Foot Ulcers
Neurogenic Bladder

Gestational
Preterm Labor
Preeclampsia
Stillbirth
Birth Defects
Hypoglycemia in Newborn
Newborn Respiratory Distress Syndrome

Emergent
Hypoglycemia
Hyperglycemia
Hyperosmotic Hyperglycemic State
Diabetic Ketoacidosis
Diabetic Coma

Figure 14.5   Clinical manifestations of uncontrolled diabetes mellitus

the concentrations of low-density lipoproteins (LDLs), which have been correlated with atherosclerotic disease, are often found to be elevated. Due to these deleterious cardiovascular effects, many patients with chronic diabetes suffer from insufficient arterial perfusion to their distal extremities, one of the clinical manifestations being peripheral arterial disease (PAD). This often results in the formation of ulcers, particularly in the legs and feet, claudication, hair loss, delayed wound healing, and increased risk of infection.

For the clinical management of cardiovascular risk in patients with DM, the American College of Cardiologists outline several recommendations based on patients' atherosclerotic cardiovascular disease (ASCVD) risk stratification (2019). The ASCVD calculation incorporates several parameters, including age, gender, presence/absence of type 2 DM, smoking status, LDL, etc., to produce an easy-to-use numerical value for treatment cutoffs. For ASCVD >7.5%, patients are started on a high-intensity statin to lower lipid levels, and antihypertensives if necessary to maintain systolic blood pressures below 140 mm Hg and diastolic blood pressures below 90 mm Hg. Metformin, which is considered a first-line treatment for type 2 DM, is particularly useful in this context because of its low cardiovascular side effect profile. Other classes of diabetic medications such as SGLT-2 inhibitors, which have been shown to have some cardiorenal protective factors, can be added depending on patients' response to monotherapy, as well as other comorbid conditions. In the past, diabetic patients were often started prophylactically on a low dose of aspirin. However, recent studies have shown that this management may be harmful and is only justified in patients with other clinical indications for aspirin, such as a history of prior myocardial infarction.

14.6.2 Renal

In addition to significant adverse effects on the cardiovascular system, DM has been shown to play a role in progressive renal dysfunction. In fact, DM is the leading cause of chronic kidney disease (CKD) worldwide. Many patients will develop laboratory abnormalities, such as increased albumin concentration in urine, long before they develop any clinical or systemic symptoms of kidney damage. Over extended periods of time, however, DM induces changes in kidney structure that impair function. If left untreated, this kidney damage will progress to renal insufficiency and end-stage renal disease. Symptomatically, patients with DM will exhibit polyuria, or excessive urination, which is a hallmark of DM. Due to this fluid loss through urine, the body activates the renin–angiotensin–aldosterone system (RAAS) to elevate blood pressure. The elevation in blood pressure only exacerbates the cardiovascular complications of DM, which were discussed in the previous section. Additionally, DM induces a chronic state of inflammation, which weakens the immune response and predisposes diabetic patients to developing urinary tract infections (UTIs) and kidney infections (e.g., pyelonephritis). Another potential renal complication of DM is the formation of uric acid stones. It has been theorized that kidney damage leads to impaired production and secretion of ammonium in the urine, which decreases urinary pH and favors the formation of uric acid stones. Other than controlling the effects of DM through medications and lifestyle modifications, angiotensin-converting enzyme inhibitors (ACE-I) or angiotensin receptor blockers (ARB) are two mainstays in the prevention of kidney injury in diabetic patients. These two medications lower glomerular hypertension and delay the progression of kidney disease. Unfortunately, however, many patients eventually progress to end-stage renal disease, at which point lifelong dialysis will most likely be necessary.

14.6.3 Gastrointestinal

Another complication of uncontrolled diabetes is gastroenteropathy, which includes indigestion or dysmotility. Diabetes results in the loss of autonomic nerve function due to chronic ischemic changes. This nerve damage results in delayed gastrointestinal motility and delayed gastric emptying (gastroparesis), which commonly lead to symptoms such as abdominal pain, early satiety, and nausea. Common treatments include lifestyle modifications and medications. Commonly used medications include metoclopramide and erythromycin. However, metoclopramide cannot be used for more than 12 weeks because it increases the risk of developing tardive dyskinesia, a potentially irreversible condition in which the patient develops involuntary facial movements. For patients who do not see improvement with the combination of lifestyle modifications and medications, a gastric pacemaker may be considered to regulate intestinal motility.

14.6.4 Neurological

Chronic hyperglycemic conditions promote an environment of inflammation that gradually damages nerve fibers. It is estimated that 50–60% of all diabetic patients will eventually develop peripheral neurologic deficits. Distal extremities are commonly affected first, and patients will often develop sensory changes, including tingling, numbness, or burning sensations in "stocking-glove" distributions known as paresthesias. As nerve damage progresses, patients may develop concordant motor weakness, which can affect coordination and walking. Damage to the nerves that regulate autonomic functions can lead to a wide range of symptoms, such as diabetic gastroparesis, bladder control, or impotence. Furthermore, decreased sensation in distal extremities, particularly the feet, predisposes patients to being unaware of developing injuries or ulcerations. It is recommended that diabetic patients undergo routine foot examinations by a clinician and that they be taught how to perform foot examinations at home. For patients with chronic neural pain, medications such as pregabalin, gabapentin, or duloxetine can be prescribed.

14.6.5 Ocular

The Centers for Disease Control and Prevention (CDC) estimate that more than one-third of patients with diabetes developed diabetic retinopathy. Combined with direct optic nerve or retinal damage, diabetic patients are also predisposed to a lack of blood flow due to atherosclerotic occlusion. Without tight blood sugar control, patients can develop permanent visual deficits. As a preventative measure, the ADA recommends that patients see an eye doctor at least once a year. Early detection of eye changes, such as retinal neovascularization, has been shown to dramatically improve patient outcomes. In addition to preventative measures, such as lowering or maintaining healthy blood sugar concentrations and blood pressure, other treatment options exist. If early retinal changes are detected, laser photocoagulation has been shown to stop disease proliferation. Patients may also be started on vascular endothelial growth factor (VEGF) inhibitors, which work to reduce erratic formation of new blood vessels in the retina and can lead to vision loss.

14.6.6 Diabetic Ketoacidosis

Diabetic ketoacidosis is an emergent complication of diabetes occurring in the setting of insulin deficiency. The typical patient is one with undiagnosed type 1 diabetes on first presentation. Additionally, in a patient with type 1 or type 2 DM, insufficient insulin due to underdosing, or a physiologic stressor such as infection or ischemia, are common causes of DKA. DKA is diagnosed by the presence of serum ketones, an acidotic state with arterial pH less than 7.30, and an anion gap over 12. (38) It is often associated with blood glucose concentrations typically 300 mg/dL or higher, although patients can be euglycemic. (39) Due to a lack of insulin, the liver will begin to utilize triglycerides and amino acids for energy. (38) Insulin is an inhibitor of ketosis, so its absence coupled with increased fat breakdown leads to the elevation of ketones. The excess amount of glucose in the blood will be excreted by the kidneys, leading to osmotic diuresis and ultimately dehydration. Electrolyte imbalances also occur with DKA. The total body potassium is reduced due to excretion by the kidneys; however, the serum concentrations may be maintained as potassium moves extracellularly due to the acidosis. (40) It is important to be mindful of this during treatment, as insulin will drive the potassium back into the cells, which can result in life-threatening hypokalemia if potassium is not replaced.

The management of DKA focuses on the correction of the elevated anion gap acidosis, the replacement of volume with intravenous fluids, and the repletion of potassium. DKA must be treated in the intensive care setting due to frequent monitoring of electrolyte and glucose concentrations. Volume repletion is achieved through rapid infusion of normal saline at a rate of 1–1.5 liters in the first 1–4 hours, followed by a continuous infusion of 4–14 mL/kg/hr of a hypotonic 0.45% saline solution, ensuring the serum sodium is normal to high. (41) As the blood glucose concentrations decrease to 250 mg/dL, normal saline should be replaced entirely with dextrose 5% or with half normal saline and half dextrose 5% to allow for continued insulin infusion without causing hypoglycemia. (42) In severe acidosis (pH <6.9), the addition of bicarbonate is indicated. Potassium is often added during bicarbonate infusion if potassium is below 5.3 mmol/L, as the potassium will be driven intracellularly with the correction of the acidosis. Prior to giving insulin, it is imperative to ensure that potassium concentrations are over 3.3 mmol/L, with potassium being replaced intravenously until concentrations are above that threshold. (41) Patients should first be given a regular insulin bolus of 0.1 units/kg intravenously. Then, a continuous regular insulin infusion will be initiated. The continuous rate is 0.1 units of regular insulin per kilogram per hour. Blood glucose concentrations should be checked hourly, with the insulin infusion adjusted per hospital-specific protocols. Computerized software systems can be used to manage insulin infusion based on blood glucose readings of the patient. This is a new option for DKA management. By responding to blood glucose readings entered, the software adjusts the insulin protocol rate accordingly. Studies have shown that patients managed with computerized decision support systems have significantly reduced episodes of both hyperglycemia and serious hypoglycemia. (43–45) If the patient is in a DKA state with normal blood glucose concentrations, glucose will be administered in addition to insulin. (41, 46)

Resolution of DKA is achieved once the anion gap is decreased below 10–12, serum bicarbonate is over 15 mEq/L, and the venous blood pH is greater than 7.3. (41) The patient may be converted to subcutaneous insulin administration once the anion gap is closed, the bicarbonate is corrected, the patient is no longer acidotic, and the patient is able to eat without vomiting. Basal-bolus regimen should be implemented based on the insulin requirement over the 24 hours prior. It is important to continue the intravenous insulin for 2–4 hours after the first dose of basal insulin as discontinuation can cause hyperglycemia and recurrence of ketoacidosis. This is due to the onset of action being 2–4 hours after administration. (41) Typically, the basal dosage is 40–50% of the insulin needs over the last 24 hours. (46) For basal dosing, long-acting insulin glargine or detemir can be used, or intermediate-acting NPH. Additionally, short-acting insulin with meals should be administered three times per day.

14.6.7 Pregnancy

During pregnancy, diabetes management and glycemic control are imperative in minimizing the negative impact of the disease on the gestation. Pregnancy incurs increased insulin resistance. Patients can develop diabetes during the gestation or have pre-existing diabetes. Pre-gestational diabetes has been associated with preterm labor, an increased Cesarean section rate, and an increased rate of preeclampsia. (47, 48) For the baby, poorly controlled gestational diabetes can lead to low blood sugar at birth, respiratory distress syndrome, stillbirth, and an increased rate of birth trauma due to the increased size. (49–51) Patients with pre-gestational diabetes are more likely to give birth to a fetus with birth defects or a large fetal size. (52) It is standard to test all pregnant women for diabetes around week 24 of gestation. The regulation of blood glucose during pregnancy is critical as elevated blood glucose can lead to complications with the pregnancy, labor, and infant.

The first line of treatment for diabetes during pregnancy is modification of diet and exercise. Blood glucose concentrations should be monitored prior to insulin administration, as well as when fasting, 1 hour after eating, and 2 hours after eating. Blood glucose concentrations should be below 140 mg/dL 1 hour after eating, less than 120 mg/dL 2 hours after eating, and 70–95 mg/dL while fasting. If necessary to achieve glycemic control, insulin is the recommended pharmacologic treatment. (53–55) Insulin does not cross the placenta. Per the American College of Obstetrics and Gynecology, the recommended starting dose of is 0.7–1 unit/kg daily of an intermediate-acting basal insulin. The insulin dose or regimen can be categorized as long-acting or intermediate-acting insulin, as well as short-acting insulin. (53) Typically, treatment is individualized based on which blood glucose readings are abnormal. For long-acting insulin, NPH insulin, insulin glargine, and insulin detemir can be used. For short-acting insulin, insulin lispro and insulin aspart are preferred over regular insulin due to the rapid onset. (53) However, the administration and monitoring of insulin therapy can be cumbersome. Oral agents such as metformin are occasionally used for patients with gestational diabetes due to the convenience of oral administration, the cost, and administration frequency. Metformin in pregnancy is started at 500 mg nightly for 1 week and then increased to 500 mg two times per day. (53) Additionally, glyburide can be used at 2.5–20 mg in divided daily doses. (53) Both metformin and glyburide cross the placenta. Due to the intrauterine exposure of these medications, without superior outcomes compared to insulin, the American Diabetes Association (ADA) continues to recommend insulin only as first-line treatment. (53, 55) There are data to support the safety of metformin in pregnancy, although additional studies on long-term fetal outcomes are necessary. (53, 56, 57) With glyburide, there is an increased risk of low blood glucose in the newborn and increased size. (56, 58) These complications, in addition to inferior glycemic control compared to insulin, make glyburide a second-line treatment option. Additionally, patients with type 2 diabetes mellitus on oral agents are typically switched to insulin for glycemic control during pregnancy. Due to the increased risk of preeclampsia, patients with preexisting diabetes should initiate a daily low-dose aspirin between gestational weeks 12–28 until delivery. (54) Following pregnancy, insulin requirements often decrease over the first 48 hours postpartum to levels lower than pregestational. Due to this, insulin dosages should be about 30% lower than the requirements during pregnancy. Those with a diagnosis of gestational diabetes should be tested again with a glucose tolerance test 4–12 weeks postpartum. (55) The ADA additionally recommends that patients with gestational diabetes be tested every 1–3 years as the lifetime maternal risk for developing diabetes in this population is about 50%. (55) Insulin is safe for use during breastfeeding and mothers with gestational diabetes should be encouraged to breastfeed as this reduces the risk of developing type 2 diabetes. (55)

14.7 CONCLUSION

Diabetes mellitus is a common but complex and often misunderstood diagnosis. The term "diabetes mellitus" encompasses several categories of metabolic dysregulation, which involve significant life changes. From diabetes mellitus to MODY, each patient's diagnosis should be approached individually and with consideration of that patient's goals and resources. Given the considerable prevalence of diabetes mellitus and gestational diabetes in the population, education and awareness are of the utmost importance. Ensuring that patients know the potential clinical manifestations that can arise in the setting of poor glycemic control, and how comorbid conditions can beget new, devastating conditions, clinicians can open a line of communication with their patients on how to work together to not only improve management but also decrease the incidence of disease altogether. Early recognition and diagnosis are critical in tempering the clinical manifestations of patients encumbered with these conditions. By correctly identifying a patient's diagnosis, a proper management strategy can be initiated early on, improving outcomes and saving resources and time. In addition to early management, diligent follow-up and adjustment of the patient's regimen are vital to ensure the patient is being adequately treated, as both undertreatment and over-treatment can have equally catastrophic effects. As the scientific and clinical community continue to work together to improve the availability of educational resources, diagnostic tools, and treatment options, there is a collective movement toward a healthier population.

ABBREVIATIONS

ACOG:	American College of Obstetrics and Gynecologists
ADA:	American Diabetes Association
ADH:	Anti-diuretic hormone
BAS:	Bile acid sequestrants
BG:	Blood glucose
BMI:	Body mass index
BMP:	Basic metabolic panel
CGM:	Continuous glucose monitoring
CKD:	Chronic kidney disease
DA:	Dopamine agonists
DI:	Diabetes insipidus
DKA:	Diabetic ketoacidosis
DM:	Diabetes mellitus
DMT1:	Diabetes mellitus type 1
DMT2:	Diabetes mellitus type 2
GFR:	Glomerular filtration rate
HgbA1c:	Hemoglobin A1c
MODY:	Maturity-onset diabetes of the young
NASH:	Non-alcoholic steatosis hepatitis
PAD:	Peripheral arterial disease
PCOS:	Polycystic ovary syndrome

REFERENCES

1. National Diabetes Statistics Report [Internet]. *Centers for Disease Control and Prevention*. [cited 2023 Jan 25]. Available from: https://www.cdc.gov/diabetes/data/statistics-report/index.html.

2. Shrivastava SR, Shrivastava PS, Ramasamy J. Role of self-care in management of diabetes mellitus. *J Diabetes Metab Disord*. 2013 Dec 5;12(1):14. .

3. Niswender KD. Basal insulin: Physiology, pharmacology, and clinical implications. *Postgrad Med*. 2011 Jul 13;123(4):17–26.

4. Flory J, Lipska K. Metformin in 2019. *JAMA*. 2019 May 21;321(19):1926.

5. Shader RI. Some reflections on diabetes mellitus. *Clin. Ther.* 2022;38(6):1259–1261.

6. Ahmed AM. History of diabetes mellitus. *Saudi Med J*. 2002 Apr;23(4):373–8.

7. Eknoyan G. A history of diabetes mellitus – A disease of the kidneys that became a kidney disease. *J Nephrol.* 2006;19(Suppl 10):S71–4.

8. Norton L, Shannon C, Gastaldelli A, DeFronzo RA. Insulin: The master regulator of glucose metabolism. *Metabolism*. 2022 Apr;129:155142.

9. American Diabetes Association. Diagnosis and classification of diabetes mellitus. *Diabetes Care*. 2013 Jan 1;36(suppl_1):S67–74.

10. DiMeglio LA, Evans-Molina C, Oram RA. Type 1 diabetes. *The Lancet*. 2018 Jun;391(10138):2449–62.

11. Easa N, Alany RG, Carew M, Vangala A. A review of non-invasive insulin delivery systems for diabetes therapy in clinical trials over the past decade. *Drug Discov Today*. 2019 Feb;24(2):440–51.

12. Lee I, Probst D, Klonoff D, Sode K. Continuous glucose monitoring systems – Current status and future perspectives of the flagship technologies in biosensor research. *Biosens Bioelectron*. 2021 Jun;181:113054.

13. WHO. *Classification of Diabetes Mellitus*. WHO. 2019. p. 1–36.

14. American Diabetes Association. Classification and diagnosis of diabetes: Standards of medical care in diabetes—2020. *Diabetes Care*. 2020 Jan 1;43(Suppl_1):S14–31.

15. *Class III Obesity (Formerly Known as Morbid Obesity)* [Internet]. Cleveland Clinic. 2021 [cited 2023 Feb 15]. Available from: https://my.clevelandclinic.org/health/diseases/21989-class-iii-obesity-formerly-known-as-morbid-obesity.

16. Galicia-Garcia U, Benito-Vicente A, Jebari S, Larrea-Sebal A, Siddiqi H, Uribe KB, et al. Pathophysiology of type 2 diabetes mellitus. *Int J Mol Sci*. 2020 Aug 30;21(17):6275.

17. Anık A, Çatlı G, Abacı A, Böber E. Maturity-onset diabetes of the young (MODY): An update. *Journal of Pediatric Endocrinology and Metabolism*. 2015 Jan 1;28(3–4):251–263.

18. Allen SR. Gestational Diabetes. *Treat Endocrinol*. 2003;2(5):357–65.

19. Pillay J, Donovan L, Guitard S, Zakher B, Gates M, Gates A, et al. Screening for Gestational Diabetes. *JAMA*. 2021 Aug 10;326(6):539.

20. Christ-Crain M, Bichet DG, Fenske WK, Goldman MB, Rittig S, Verbalis JG, et al. Diabetes insipidus. *Nat Rev Dis Primers*. 2019 Aug 8;5(1):54.

21. Urakami T.. Maturity-onset diabetes of the young (MODY): current perspectives on diagnosis and treatment. *Diabetes Metab Syndr Obes*. 2019 Jul;12:1047–56.

22. Sweeting A, Wong J, Murphy HR, Ross GP. A clinical update on gestational diabetes mellitus. *Endocr Rev*. 2022 Sep 26;43(5):763–93.

23. Lee SH, Yoon KH. A century of progress in diabetes care with insulin: A history of innovations and foundation for the future. *Diabetes Metab J*. 2021 Sep 30;45(5):629–40.

24. Lv W, Wang X, Xu Q, Lu W. Mechanisms and characteristics of sulfonylureas and glinides. *Curr Top Med Chem*. 2020 Jan 22;20(1):37–56.

25. Costello R, Nicolas S, Shivkumar A. *Sulfonylureas*. In [cited 2023 Feb 24]. Available from: https://www.ncbi.nlm.nih.gov/books/NBK513225/.

26. LiverTox: Clinical and research information on drug-induced liver injury [Internet]. 2012 [cited 2023 Feb 24]. Available from: https://www.ncbi.nlm.nih.gov/books/NBK548361/.

27. Milner Z, Akhondi H. *Repaglinide*. Treasure Island (FL): StatPearls Publishing; 2022 [cited 2023 Feb 24]. Available from: https://www.ncbi.nlm.nih.gov/books/NBK559305/.

28. Flory J, Lipska K. Metformin in 2019. *JAMA*. 2019 May 21;321(19):1926.

29. Corcoran C, Jacobs TF. Metformin. In: *StatPearls* [Internet]. Treasure Island (FL): StatPearls Publishing; 2022.

30. Eggleton JS, Jialal I. Thiazolidinediones. In: *StatPearls* [Internet]. Treasure Island (FL): StatPearls Publishing; 2022.

31. Zhang, L, Chen, Q, Li, L, Kwong, JS, Jia, P, Zhao, P, ... Sun, X. Alpha-glucosidase inhibitors and hepatotoxicity in type 2 diabetes: a systematic review and meta-analysis. *Scientific Reports*. 2016;6(1):32649.

32. Chao CT, Wang J, Huang JW, Chien KL. Acarbose use and liver injury in diabetic patients with severe renal insufficiency and hepatic diseases: A propensity score-matched cohort study. *Front Pharmacol*. 2018 Aug 7;9:860.

33. Deacon CF. Dipeptidyl peptidase 4 inhibitors in the treatment of type 2 diabetes mellitus. *Nat Rev Endocrinol*. 2020;16(11):642–53.

34. Handelsman Y. Role of bile acid sequestrants in the treatment of type 2 diabetes. *Diabetes Care*. 2011 May 1;34(Suppl_2):S244–50.

35. Kabir MdT, Ferdous Mitu J, Akter R, Akhtar MF, Saleem A, Al-Harrasi A, et al. Therapeutic potential of dopamine agonists in the treatment of type 2 diabetes mellitus. *Environmental Science and Pollution Research*. 2022 Jul 29;29(31):46385–404.

36. Schauer PR, Bhatt DL, Kirwan JP, Wolski K, Aminian A, Brethauer SA, et al. Bariatric Surgery versus Intensive Medical Therapy for Diabetes — 5-Year Outcomes. *New England Journal of Medicine*. 2017 Feb 16;376(7):641–51.

37. Sartore G, Ragazzi E, Caprino R, Lapolla A. Long-term HbA1c variability and macro-/microvascular complications in type 2 diabetes mellitus: A meta-analysis update. *Acta Diabetol*. 2023 Jan 30;60:721–738.

38. Kitabchi AE, Umpierrez GE, Miles JM, Fisher JN. Hyperglycemic crises in adult patients with diabetes. *Diabetes Care* [Internet]. 2009 Jul [cited 2023 Jan 29];32(7):1335. Available from: https://www.ncbi.nlm.nih.gov/pmc/articles/PMC2699725/.

39. Peters AL, Buschur EO, Buse JB, Cohan P, Diner JC, Hirsch IB. Euglycemic diabetic ketoacidosis: A potential complication of treatment with sodium–glucose cotransporter 2 inhibition. *Diabetes Care* [Internet]. 2015 Sep 1 [cited 2023 Jan 29];38(9):1687. Available from: https://www.ncbi.nlm.nih.gov/pmc/articles/PMC4542270/.

40. Adrogué HJ, Wilson H, Boyd AE, Suki WN, Eknoyan G. Plasma acid-base patterns in diabetic ketoacidosis. *N Engl J Med* [Internet]. 1982 Dec 23 [cited 2023 Jan 29];307(26):1603–10. Available from: https://pubmed.ncbi.nlm.nih.gov/6815530/.

41. Gosmanov AR, Gosmanova E, Dillard-Cannon E. Management of adult diabetic ketoacidosis. *Diabetes Metab Syndr Obes*. 2014 Jun;255.

42. Kitabchi AE, Umpierrez GE, Murphy MB, Barrett EJ, Kreisberg RA, Malone JI, et al. Management of hyperglycemic crises in patients with diabetes. *Diabetes Care*. 2001 Jan 1;24(1):131–53.

43. Fogel SL, Baker CC. Effects of computerized decision support systems on blood glucose regulation in critically ill surgical patients. *J Am Coll Surg*. 2013 Apr;216(4):828–33.

44. John SM, Waters KL, Jivani K. Evaluating the implementation of the EndoTool glycemic control software system. *Diabetes Spectrum*. 2018 Feb 1;31(1):26–30.

45. Juneja R, Roudebush CP, Nasraway SA, Golas AA, Jacobi J, Carroll J, et al. Computerized intensive insulin dosing can mitigate hypoglycemia and achieve tight glycemic control when glucose measurement is performed frequently and on time. *Crit Care*. 2009;13(5):R163.

46. Pasquel, FJ, Tsegka, K, Wang, H, Cardona, S, Galindo, RJ, Fayfman, M, ... Umpierrez, GE. Clinical outcomes in patients with isolated or combined diabetic ketoacidosis and hyperosmolar hyperglycemic state: a retrospective, hospital-based cohort study. *Diabetes Care*. 2020; 43(2): 349–357.

47. Sibai BM, Caritis SN, Hauth JC, MacPherson C, VanDorsten JP, Klebanoff M, et al. Preterm delivery in women with pregestational diabetes mellitus or chronic hypertension relative to women with uncomplicated pregnancies. *Am J Obstet Gynecol*. 2000 Dec;183(6):1520–4.

48. Holmes VA, Young IS, Patterson CC, Pearson DWM, Walker JD, Maresh MJA, et al. Optimal glycemic control, pre-eclampsia, and gestational hypertension in women with type 1 diabetes in the diabetes and pre-eclampsia intervention trial. *Diabetes Care* [Internet]. 2011 Aug [cited 2023 Jan 29];34(8):1683–8. Available from: https://pubmed.ncbi.nlm.nih.gov/21636798/.

49. Langer O, Berkus MD, Huff RW, Samueloff A. Shoulder dystocia: Should the fetus weighing greater than or equal to 4000 grams be delivered by cesarean section? *Am J Obstet Gynecol* [Internet]. 1991 [cited 2023 Jan 29];165(4 Pt 1):831–7. Available from: https://pubmed.ncbi.nlm.nih.gov/1951539/.

50. Piper JM, Xenakis EMJ, Langer O. Delayed appearance of pulmonary maturation markers is associated with poor glucose control in diabetic pregnancies. *J Matern Fetal Med*. 1998 May;7(3):148–53.

51. Starikov R, Dudley D, Reddy UM. Stillbirth in the pregnancy complicated by diabetes. *Curr Diab Rep* [Internet]. 2015 Mar 1 [cited 2023 Jan 29];15(3). Available from: https://pubmed.ncbi.nlm.nih.gov/25667005/.

52. Macintosh MCM, Fleming KM, Bailey JA, Doyle P, Modder J, Acolet D, et al. Perinatal mortality and congenital anomalies in babies of women with type 1 or type 2 diabetes in England, Wales, and Northern Ireland: Population based study. *BMJ* [Internet]. 2006 Jul 22 [cited 2023 Jan 30];333(7560):177–80. Available from: https://pubmed.ncbi.nlm.nih.gov/16782722/.

53. Holt, RIG, Lambert, KD. The use of oral hypoglycaemic agents in pregnancy. *Diabetic Medicine*. 2014;31(3): 282–291.

54. American College of Obstetricians and Gynecologists. ACOG practice bulletin no. 201: Pregestational diabetes mellitus. *Obstetrics and Gynecology*. 2018;132(6):e228–48.

55. ElSayed NA, Aleppo G, Aroda VR, Bannuru RR, Brown FM, Bruemmer D, et al. 15Management of diabetes in pregnancy: Standards of care in diabetes—2023. *Diabetes Care*. 2023 Jan 1;46(Suppl_1):S254–66.

56. Rowan JA, Hague WM, Gao W, Battin MR, Moore MP. Metformin versus insulin for the treatment of gestational diabetes. *N Engl J Med* [Internet]. 2008 May 8 [cited 2023 Jan 30];358(19):2003–15. Available from: https://pubmed.ncbi.nlm.nih.gov/18463376/.

57. Wouldes TA, Battin M, Coat S, Rush EC, Hague WM, Rowan JA. Neurodevelopmental outcome at 2 years in offspring of women randomised to metformin or insulin treatment for gestational diabetes. *Arch Dis Child Fetal Neonatal Ed* [Internet]. 2016 Nov 1 [cited 2023 Jan 30];101(6):F488–93. Available from: https://fn.bmj.com/content/101/6/F488.

58. Spaulonci CP, Bernardes LS, Trindade TC, Zugaib M, Francisco RPV. Randomized trial of metformin vs insulin in the management of gestational diabetes. *Am J Obstet Gynecol*. 2013 Jul;209(1):34.e1–34.e7.

15 Clinical Management of Cardiovascular Diseases

Jenifer L. Ferreir, Santhana Kumar, Arun Soni, Niyati Acharya, and Sanjeev Acharya

15.1 INTRODUCTION

Cardiovascular illnesses are the leading cause of death globally, accounting for 17.9 million deaths annually and over 32% of all deaths worldwide (1). In 2019, 38% of almost 17 million fatalities in people under the age of 70 were related to CVDs (2). Cardiovascular diseases are a group of conditions that impact the heart and blood vessels. These illnesses may have an influence on one or more parts of the heart and/or blood vessels. Any individual exhibiting symptoms of CVD is referred to as symptomatic and those not exhibiting any symptoms are referred to as asymptomatic (3). Coronary heart disease, cerebrovascular illness, peripheral arterial disease, rheumatic heart disease, congenital heart disease, deep vein thrombosis, and pulmonary embolism are six main categories of disorders included under this umbrella term (4).

Numerous variables, such as hypertension, diabetes, obesity, and age-related factors, contribute to the development of CVD. The differences in CVD risk factors and outcomes between men and women due to sex are primarily caused by sex hormones and the associated receptors. The greatest risk factors for coronary artery disease are being male and above 50 years of age (5, 6). The behavioural risk factors include unhealthy eating habits, drug and cigarette use, and excessive physical activity. Stress, loss and melancholy, rage and aggression, and inappropriate behaviour by a partner are among the psychological risk factors (7). People with CVD might exhibit an array of characteristics and symptoms, depending on where the condition originated. These patients frequently complain of chest stiffness or pain, difficulty breathing regularly, exhaustion, and strange feelings and numbness in their arms and/or legs (8).

Despite the variables in the factors contributing to CVD, it can be treated when diagnosed in time and by maintaining a sustainable lifestyle. The disease can thus be prevented or treated through a healthy lifestyle, regular exercise, quitting smoking and other abuses, and close observation of medications.

15.2 THE CARDIOVASCULAR SYSTEM

The circulatory system is a closed-loop system that moves oxygenated blood from the heart to the body's tissues and organs while returning the blood that has lost oxygen to the heart to be sent to the lungs for purification. The circulatory system's important function in maintaining homeostasis depends on the continuous and steady flow of blood through the millions of capillaries entering every tissue and reaching every cell in the body. The diverse actions and component parts of the circulatory system must be coordinated, regulated, and integrated in order to deliver blood to specific body areas as needed (9). The cardiovascular system is mainly comprised of three major components: the heart, the systemic and pulmonary circulation, and the microvasculature (10).

15.2.1 The Heart

Every day, the hollow, muscular heart beats more than one million times to pump blood through the body's veins. The right side of the heart receives blood and transfers it to the lungs for oxygenation and purification, whereas the left side of the heart distributes oxygenated blood from the lungs to the body's tissues. The three layers that compose the heart wall are the endocardium, which is the inner layer, the epicardium, which is the outer protective layer, and the myocardium, which is the middle layer. The pericardium, the protective membrane, is a thick-walled fibrous sac covering the heart that shields it from any external damage (11).

The human heart is divided into four chambers: the lower heart's right and left ventricles and the upper heart's right and left atria. A regular heartbeat involves the contraction of the ventricles first while the atria relax, and then the atria contract and the ventricles relax. In order to prevent the backward flow of blood during the intervals between ventricular contractions, there are valves that allow blood to travel between the chambers of the heart in one direction only (12).

15.2.2 Systemic and Pulmonary Circulation

The circulatory system is made up of the heart, as well as the arteries and veins that aid in the transport of blood throughout the whole body. Blood must constantly flow to sustain life. It moves oxygen from the air we breathe to every cell in the body. This blood is moved by the heart's

DOI: 10.1201/9781003384823-15

pumping motion through the arteries, capillaries, and veins. In order to exchange gases, blood is pushed into the lungs by one network of blood vessels: arteries. The other blood vessels, veins, support the rest of the body (13, 14).

Systemic circulation transports blood throughout the body. By supplying the cells with oxygenated blood, it returns blood that has lost oxygen to the heart. Pulmonary circulation carries blood from the heart to the lungs. It transports deoxygenated blood to the lungs, where an exchange of oxygen and carbon dioxide takes place. The oxygenated blood then flows back to the heart (15, 16).

The respiratory and circulatory systems work in tandem to rid the body of carbon dioxide and provide it with oxygen. Pulmonary circulation facilitates external breathing, whereas systemic circulation facilitates interior respiration (17).

By way of the pulmonary loop, deoxygenated blood exits the right ventricle of the heart, travels via the pulmonary trunk, divides into the right and left pulmonary arteries, and eventually arrives at the pulmonary arterioles and capillary beds. Following that, venules carry the oxygenated blood from the capillary beds into the pulmonary veins. The pulmonary veins carry it to the left atrium of the heart. The pulmonary arteries are the only vessels that carry deoxygenated blood, while the pulmonary veins carry oxygenated blood (18).

The aorta, systemic arteries, arterioles, and capillary beds are all parts of the systemic loop, which carries oxygenated blood from the left ventricle of the heart to the body's tissues. Following that, venules carry the deoxygenated blood from the capillary beds into the systemic veins. The systemic veins penetrate the inferior and superior venae cavae, which subsequently provide deoxygenated blood to the right atrium of the heart (19, 20).

15.2.3 The Microvasculature

The microcirculation, which consists of microvessels of less than 20 μm, is the ultimate vascular network of the systemic circulation. These microvessels are made up of arteries, post-capillary venules, capillaries, and their (sub)cellular constituents. The oxygen is transported to the parenchymal cells by RBC in the capillaries, where it is used to meet the energy requirements of the tissue cells for their functional activity. The cardiovascular system's eventual endpoint is the microcirculation (21).

The microvasculature serves to transport nutrients and oxygen to tissues, as well as eliminating metabolic waste products like CO_2 from tissues. The microvasculature is made up of arteries and veins, which have a great capacity and are in charge of quickly moving blood towards or away from organs. The network of the microvasculature controls regional blood perfusion and carries out blood–tissue exchange (22, 23).

15.3 DISEASES ASSOCIATED WITH THE CARDIOVASCULAR SYSTEM

Serious health problems might arise from anomalies or any injury to the cardiovascular system. There Is a chance that such problems could be fatal and severe. By being aware of problems that can affect the cardiovascular system, people may be better equipped to receive adequate and immediate medical guidance.

There are many circulatory system diseases that can occur when the complex process of the normal working of the heart, as well as the circulatory system, gets interrupted. The diseases that can affect the cardiovascular system include the following.

15.3.1 Atherosclerosis

Atherosclerosis is a condition that develops as a result of plaque build-up on interior artery walls. Plaque, a gooey substance made of fat, cholesterol, calcium, and other components, accumulates on the blood vessel walls, which then gives rise to various problems, thus disrupting the blood flow through the arteries. Arteries harden and narrow as plaque builds up (24).

It is possible for a piece of plaque to break away, get stuck in the blood vessels, and affect the body. Moreover, a blood clot might form in a small artery. It might eventually get dislodged and pass through the artery. This can cause the artery to constrict and get blocked, restricting the flow of blood, oxygen, and other nutrients, and causing narrowing of the arteries. In time, obstructions may cause tissue death or infection in the affected part of the body (25).

15.3.2 Heart Attack

When the blood flow that supplies oxygen to the heart muscle is significantly reduced or entirely stopped, a heart attack happens. In medical terms, this is also referred as myocardial infarction. This occurs when plaque accumulates in the atrial blood vessels, which provide blood to the heart muscle. A blood clot develops around plaque that ruptures in a cardiac artery, thus preventing the blood, which carries the oxygen, from reaching the heart through the arteries. If blood flow is not restored quickly, then such an event may lead to permanent heart damage, eventually leading to death.

An intermittent spasm or temporary contraction of a coronary artery causes the artery to constrict, which reduces or ceases blood flow to a region of the heart muscle. This can also be a cause of heart attacks. Both blood vessels that appear normal and vessels that have atherosclerosis partially blocking them can experience spasms. The resultant severe spasms might contribute to the occurrence of heart attack (26, 27).

3.3 Angina Pectoris

Angina pectoris refers to chest pain brought on by metabolite build-up as a result of myocardial ischaemia. Atheromatous blockage of the major coronary vessel is by far the most typical cause of angina. An imbalance between the amount of oxygen the heart needs and the amount of oxygen delivered to it by the coronary veins is the main factor causing angina pectoris (28).

Effort angina, sometimes referred to as classic angina, is the outcome of inadequate blood flow when coronary artery disease is present (29). Vasospastic or variant angina refers to the pain caused by the brief spasm of specific, localized parts of these arteries, which is frequently linked to underlying atheroma and can significantly worsen myocardial ischaemia (30). Small platelet clots or periods of elevated epicardial coronary artery resistance that happen close to an atherosclerotic plaque are the two main causes of unstable angina (31).

15.3.4 Cardiac Ischaemia

Cardiac ischaemia is a condition where there is insufficient oxygen-rich blood flowing to the heart muscle as a result of decreased heart blood flow. This might be caused by the coronary arteries, which are the blood vessels that provide blood to the heart muscle, being partially or totally blocked. Cardiac ischaemia is primarily caused by atherosclerosis; however, it can also be caused by other factors, like blood clots or coronary artery spasms (32).

15.3.5 Heart Failure

Congestion, fatigue, and shortness of breath are all typical signs of heart failure. These signs are related to fluid retention and insufficient blood supply to the tissues during physical activity. The inefficiency of the heart's ability to appropriately fill or empty the left ventricle and its inadequacy in supplying sufficient blood to maintain body functions are the major factors responsible for heart failure. This may give rise to frequent pooling of blood, which causes accumulation in the limbs and lungs. The accumulated fluid may cause difficulty in breathing and oedema in the limbs and feet. (33).

15.3.6 Hypertension

When measuring blood pressure, consideration is given to how much blood is flowing through blood arteries and how much resistance the blood encounters as the heart pumps. When the amount of blood that flows through the vessels is continually too high, this results in elevated blood pressure, also known as hypertension. The flow of blood via arteries and other small blood vessels is more difficult. As the arteries narrow because of increased resistance, blood pressure will rise. Over time, the increased pressure may cause health issues like heart disease (34).

15.3.7 Stroke

When blood circulation to the brain is blocked, a stroke, often termed a "brain attack", happens, resulting in the death of the affected brain portion. While a heart attack affects the heart, a stroke affects the blood arteries circulating in the brain. When a blood clot prevents the brain's blood supply from reaching the brain, an ischaemic stroke ensues (35). Another type of stroke known as a transient ischaemic attack, sometimes also referred as a "mini stroke", is brought on by a transitory clot. When a blood artery in the brain rupture and bleeds, it results in a haemorrhagic stroke that damages the brain by starving an area of blood (36).

15.3.8 High Cholesterol

Fatty deposition in the arteries occurs when the level of cholesterol is excessive. Once large enough, these deposits prevent enough blood from flowing through the blood capillaries, preventing the organs and tissues from receiving adequate blood. When the cholesterol level in the body rises above 200mg/dl, and the body produces bad cholesterol in the form of LDL, this condition is called as hyperlipidaemia (37).

15.3.9 Congenital Heart Disease

Structural abnormalities of the heart give rise to congenital heart disease (CHD). "Congenital" refers to a condition that develops from birth. When a baby's heart does not develop normally during pregnancy, several problems arise. The way the heart pumps blood can be altered by congenital cardiac abnormalities. These may cause blood to flow too slowly or in the wrong direction, or they may entirely stop blood flow (38).

CHD is a structural flaw or issue with the heart that exists from birth. Examples include problems with the heart valves or problems with the blood arteries. Nearly one-third of all significant congenital malformations are caused by CHD. It is believed that the prevalence of CHD births varies globally and across time (39).

15.3.10 Arrhythmia and Dysrhythmia

Simply put, a cardiac arrhythmia is a deviation from the regular heartbeat's rhythm or rate that is not supported by the body's physiological needs. The two main groups of cardiac arrhythmia-causing processes are as follows: intensified or aberrant impulse production, and disturbances in conduction (40).

Arrhythmia generally means "without rhythm", while dysrhythmia roughly means "poor rhythm". A research overview states that a person's dysrhythmia and arrhythmia type might differ because of several factors, for instance, the site of origin, the frequency of disturbances, the appearance of electrocardiogram, and the mechanism of disturbance (41).

15.3.11 Mitral Stenosis

A medical disorder known as mitral stenosis causes the mitral valve of the heart to narrow, which impairs blood flow from the left atrium to the left ventricle. The left atrium and left ventricle of the heart are divided by the mitral valve, which also controls blood flow between them. The mitral valve orifice or aperture narrows when left undiagnosed. Mitral stenosis restricts blood flow from the left atrium to the left ventricle. As a result, there is a reduction in the amount of blood carrying oxygen from the lungs. The rise in the blood volume remaining in the atrium, as well as blood pressure, causes the left atrial to enlarge and fluid to accumulate in the lungs (42).

15.3.12 Mitral Valve Prolapse (MVP)

The mitral valve leaflets (MVL) expand and move superiorly during systole, which is what causes mitral valve prolapse. The hallmark characteristic of MVP is the myxomatous degeneration of the mitral valve leaflets, which ultimately leads to constructional impotence and superior displacement of either or any mitral leaflets into the left atrium during systole (43). Mid-systolic clicks, late systolic murmurs, and catastrophic side effects like bacterial endocarditis, severe mitral regurgitation, and unexpected mortality have all been linked to this valve anomaly (44).

15.3.13 Mitral Valve Regurgitation

The valves present in between of the left chambers of the heart not closing entirely, thus allowing blood to leak backward through the valve, gives rise to an ailment referred as mitral valve (MV) regurgitation. Complications and ailments of the MV leaflets, anomalies of the MV apparatus, or dysfunction of the left ventricles can all cause mitral regurgitation (45).

There are two types of mitral regurgitation mechanisms: primary and secondary. Primary mitral regurgitation, also termed organic/degenerative, is brought on by an innate lesion of the MV mechanism. Secondary mitral regurgitation, also referred as functional/ischaemic, affects the left ventricle. Dilated cardiomyopathy or ischaemic cardiomyopathy can cause the papillary muscles to move laterally and apically, which tethers and misaligns the MV leaflets and results in secondary mitral regurgitation (46).

15.3.14 Aortic Aneurysms

Aortic aneurysms are a medical condition that results in the permanent enlargement of the aorta or the formation of a bulge-like aorta. They are most frequently found in the infrarenal and proximal thoracic areas. Progressive aneurysmal dilatation, albeit typically asymptomatic, is linked to the disastrous effects of aortic rupture (47). How much dilatation has occurred is arguable, but one standard is an increase in diameter of at least 50% over what would be anticipated for the same aorta section in normal people of a similar age and gender. Aneurysms of the aorta are classified according to their size, location, morphology, and cause. Blood that is pumped at great speed can thus rupture the aorta, which would lead to leakage (48).

15.3.15 Peripheral Artery Disease

Atherosclerotic narrowing and/or blockage associated with all arterial disorders, with the exception of coronary arteries and the aorta, is referred to as peripheral artery disease (PAD). Plaque accumulation in arteries in the legs causes PAD, which makes it more difficult for blood to supply oxygen and nutrients to the tissues there (49). PAD can cause limb-related consequences such as intermittent claudication, ischaemic rest discomfort, ischaemic ulcer, gangrene, and functional impairment (50).

15.3.16 Venous Thromboembolisms

Deep vein thrombosis (DVT) is an obstructive disease that hinders venous reflux. The venous system of the legs is frequently affected by DVT, with the production of clots originating in the veins of the calf and progressing proximally (51).

The term "venous thromboembolism" (VTE) refers to the generation of blood clumps (thrombus) in veins that may move away from their place of origin and travel through the blood, a condition known as an embolism. DVT most frequently affects the legs, when a thrombus forms there (52).

15.3.17 Cardiomyopathy

Cardiomyopathies are a diverse set of diseases marked by changes to the heart's structure and function. Heart failure can result from this congenital or acquired cardiac muscle condition, which makes it challenging for the heart to transport blood throughout the body (53). Numerous changes in myocardial function are grouped together under the umbrella term "cardiomyopathies". Cardiomyopathies that are dilated and ischaemic are the most prevalent types. While the latter has a clearly characterized aetiology – ischaemia and infarction, followed by a loss of contractility and remodelling – the former does not (54).

15.3.18 Rheumatic Heart Disease

Chronic heart valve illness, called rheumatic heart disease, is brought on by bacterial pathogens referred as Group A Streptococcus (Strep A), which has the ability to produce an immunological reaction in the body that manifests as acute rheumatic fever. The only cardiovascular illness with significant morbidity and death is RHD.

At least one of the four heart valves may suffer lasting harm as a result of ARF-associated carditis (55). Rheumatic heart disease is a severe type of congenital heart disorder that equally impacts adolescents and adults globally. Rheumatic fever bouts, whether they are singular or recurrent, can cause the valve cusps to become rigid or deformed, the fusion of the commissures, or the shortening and fusion of the chordae tendineae (56).

15.3.19 Raynaud's Disease

The body adapts to decreases in temperature by reducing blood circulation to the skin. This acts as a thermoregulatory mechanism, maintaining the body's internal temperature and prohibiting additional heat loss (57). Vasoconstriction of the digital arteries and cutaneous arterioles occurs in Raynaud's phenomenon and is characterized by increased cold-induced vasoconstriction. The sympathetic nervous system's reflex response to cooling and the local activation of 2C adrenoceptors (2C-AR) are both responsible for this increased vasoconstriction (58). Typically, the fingers change colour from white to blue to red to depict vasospasm, deoxygenation, and reperfusion hyperaemia respectively (59).

15.3.20 Buerger's Disease

Buerger's disease, frequently termed thromboangiitis obliterans (TAO), is a non-atherosclerotic segmental occlusive vascular disease brought on by inflammation of the peripheral blood vessels, which causes coagulation, critical limb ischaemia, and reduced blood flow. Blood vessels throughout the body are affected, most frequently in the arms and legs. Blood clots can form as a result of blood vessel swelling, which can restrict blood flow. Pain, tissue damage, and even the perishing of body tissues may result from this (60).

15.4 RISK FACTORS FOR DEVELOPING CARDIOVASCULAR DISEASE

Specific habits, actions, situations, or conditions are responsible for development of the cardiovascular disease.

Factors that majorly contribute to the development of CVD are as follows.

15.4.1 Hyperlipidaemia

Hyperlipidaemia involves the deposition of fatty substances on the walls of the blood vessels due to a rise in cholesterol levels. This makes it more difficult for the blood to flow through these arteries. When these deposited fats come loose, clots form and these can result in a heart attack or heart stroke. It has been demonstrated that lowering levels of low-density lipoprotein cholesterol, also termed "bad cholesterol", reduces the incidence of heart attacks and morbidity due to CAD (61).

15.4.2 Hypertension

When the elasticity of the arteries lessens, the flow of blood passing through these arteries is affected. When the continuous flow of blood is disrupted due to fluctuations in blood pressure, this gives rise to many ailments of the heart. Unchecked hypertension can result in the arteries hardening and thickening (62). The circulation of blood is disrupted by these alterations.

15.4.3 Smoking

Nicotine and carbon monoxide are the two substances produced by smoking that have significant impact on the cardiovascular system. People may have an elevated heart rate and decreased tolerance to exercise when high doses of carbon monoxide enter the bloodstream at a concentration above 1%. Cigarettes and other tobacco products contain nicotine, which is dangerous and addictive. This can make arteries harder and result in increased blood pressure and heart rate.

Smoking also causes the accumulation of plaque on the walls of arteries. Plaque is a waxy substance consisting of cholesterol, scar tissue, calcium, fat, and other substances found in the body. It becomes significantly more challenging for blood to flow through the vessels as plaque accumulates on the walls of the arteries. Atherosclerosis is a disorder caused by plaque accumulation. Heart attacks and strokes are substantially more likely to occur in people with this illness (63).

15.4.4 Lack of Physical Activity

Inactivity can also cause the accumulation of plaque on the walls of the artery. When plaque builds up, it can cause clogging of the arteries and disruptions to the flow of blood, which can result in a heart attack (64).

Even in the absence of comorbidities, excessive adiposity disrupts heart appearance and function, in addition to causing metabolic inefficiency. Therefore, being overweight or obese can have an impact on the heart through factors like dyslipidaemia, hypertension, glucose intolerance, and inflammatory markers, as well as other as yet unidentified pathways (65).

15.4.5 Unhealthy Diet

Unhealthy eating habits act as a major trigger for acquiring CVD, for example, consuming too much sodium and processed food and not enough veggies, fruits, fibrous foods, seafood, whole grains, and nuts. Diet is a significant contributor to the growth in major ailments such as high blood pressure, glucose intolerance, obesity, and other illnesses of CVD, according to the Global Burden of Disease research (66).

15.4.6 Obesity

The pathophysiology of obesity is influenced by the state of balance between calories consumed and energy expended, accompanied by increased body weight (67).

Obesity increases the risk of disorders such dyslipidaemia, insulin resistance, high blood pressure, and atherosclerosis, irrespective of the age group, and it is an independent risk factor for various CVDs. An increase in the level of adipose tissue and a lower level of adinopectin, which restricts the ability of protein to suppress inflammation procedures and perpetuate the inflammation conditions, are factors that make obesity a state of inflammation. These adipocyte dysregulations contribute to the body's homeostasis being out of balance, together with the pro- and anti-inflammatory mechanisms, which causes metabolic difficulties associated with being obese and results in cardiometabolic changes (68).

The atherosclerotic inflammatory process, which is linked to obesity, leads to coronary calcification. Diabetes and obesity are usually associated with vitamin D or vitamin K2 insufficiency, which may be a factor in the high prevalence of vascular calcification. High levels of leptin and elevated blood pressure are linked to obesity. Leptin stimulates the sympathetic nervous system and impacts the synthesis of nitric oxide, which results in salt retention, systemic vasoconstriction, and raised blood pressure (69, 70).

15.4.7 Age as a Factor
There is a gradual accumulation of CVD risk factors as people age. Age still functions as an independent risk factor even if these risk factors are included in a multivariable regression model. With ageing, there is a significant increase in CHD risk (71). The majority of the population experiences an increase in blood total cholesterol with ageing. Similar to serum cholesterol, blood pressure also tends to rise with age, which weakens the heart and results in older people being more likely to develop cardiovascular disease than younger people (72).

15.4.8 Genetics
Studies on twins and familial aggregation imply that genetic factors are involved in the progression of CVD and hypertension. Younger individuals with coronary heart disease are more likely to have genetic predispositions to the condition. The heritable hyperlipidaemias have received the majority of genetic attention, but family clustering of coronary heart disease that is unrelated to lipid variables shows that nonlipid-related genes may also play a role in the interaction of the environment and genes. Due to one of the various LDL receptor abnormalities, familial hypercholesterolemia can result in premature coronary heart disease (73).

15.4.9 Socioeconomic Status
Socioeconomic status (SES) and the likelihood of CVD mortality are inversely related, according to research on the socioeconomic determinants of CVD, particularly in developing nations. Although cardiovascular risk factors and diseases first appeared in upper SES categories, over the past 50 years, the risk factors for the disease have gradually migrated to the lower SES groups. Numerous studies have demonstrated that, in comparison to the lower SES groups, cardiac patients with better SES receive care at hospitals with a greater level of specialization and better-prescribed medications. For those with lower SES, access to rehabilitation services is likewise more limited. Additionally, socioeconomic factors, such as job and money, have an impact on risk factors linked to previous and subsequent lifestyle choices, which in turn affects the death rate (74).

15.4.10 Diabetes
The upregulation of numerous cytokines by adipose tissue, including tumour necrosis factor, interleukin (IL)-1, IL-6, leptin, resistin MCP-1, PAI-1, fibrinogen, and angiotensin, is linked to diabetes mellitus and insulin resistance. These cytokines are overexpressed, which results in increased inflammation and fat accumulation, which negatively affects blood vessels and can cause various heart diseases. (75).

C-reactive protein (CRP) levels are also high in diabetic patients, which could be a factor in the dysfunctioning of the endothelium. Surveys demonstrate that CRP can reduce the production of endothelial prostacyclin and nitric oxide (NO); both are equally indispensable for vascular assent. The uptake of oxidized low-density lipoprotein (LDL) in the walls of coronary vasculature is also increased by CRP, which has been shown to lead to the dysfunctioning of the endothelium and atherosclerotic plaque formation (76).

In patients with diabetes mellitus, insulin resistance is also associated with an increase in plasma free fatty acids, which causes an increase in muscle triglyceride storage, hepatic glucose synthesis, and insulin production (77, 78).

15.4.11 Chronic Inflammatory Conditions
Atherothrombosis, the primary root cause of over 80% of all coronary heart deaths, involves inflammation. However, ongoing, mild inflammation irritates blood vessels. Inflammation may encourage plaque growth, loosen plaque in arteries, and cause blood clots, all of which are key contributors to irregular blood circulation in the entire body and are responsible for the development of CVD (79).

15.4.12 Chronic Kidney Conditions

Heart attacks and strokes are significantly more likely to occur in CKD patients. One of the biggest risk factors for CVD is CKD. A detectable diversification is caused when there is any injury to the kidney or when there is inadequacy in the kidney; in such cases, the kidney releases enzymes, hormones, or cytokines into the vasculature. Haemodynamic changes and CKD-associated mediators also contribute to heart injury. When the heart becomes tired, this results in difficulty pumping blood, causing high blood pressure, thus further damaging the blood vessels. When such occurs, the kidney faces difficulty filtering the blood as effectively as the high blood pressure harms the veins in the kidney (80).

15.4.13 Excessive Alcohol Consumption

Numerous studies have been done on alcohol consumption as a modifiable risk factor for cardio-vascular illnesses (81). It is widely established that excessive alcohol use >60 ml/day for males and >40 ml/day for women increases mortality and the burden of CVDs. One of several potential reasons for alcohol's effects is cell dysfunction that results in plaque accumulation in the arteries and disturbs the functioning of atrio-vascular blood vessels, as well as an imbalance of the hormones that regulate the blood volume and pressure (82).

15.4.14 Stress

Stress can raise the body's need for oxygen, cause coronary blood vessels to spasm, and disrupt the electrical conduction of the heart. Persistent stress has been demonstrated to raise heart rate and blood pressure, putting more strain on the heart as it pumps blood to the body's various organs. One important risk factor for cardiovascular disease is psychological stress. Stress can raise inflammation in the body, which is connected to heart-harming variables like increased blood pressure and a decreased level of "good" high-density lipoprotein (HDL) cholesterol (83).

15.5 DIAGNOSIS

Cardiovascular problems are diagnosed using a wide variety of laboratory testing and imaging techniques. A substantial component of the diagnosis is based on the patient's medical and familial background, contributing factors, physical assessment, and coordination of these research results with the findings of tests and procedures.

15.5.1 Blood Tests

Laboratories run tests to find the risk factors for heart diseases. These consist of lipid blood component measurements. Blood sugar and glycosylated haemoglobin levels are measured to diagnose diabetes. To identify inflammation that could result in cardiac disorders, C-reactive protein and diverse protein-markers, including apo-lipoprotein A1 and B, are employed. Proteins are released in the bloodstream when heart muscle dies as a result of a heart attack; thus, such proteins play a vital role in indicating a heart attack (84).

15.5.2 Electrocardiogram (EKG/ECG)

This quick and painless examination captures the electrical activity of the heart. A patient is strapped to the device, multiple patches or leads are affixed to the patient's wrists, ankles, and chest, and the instrument graphically records the heart's action on paper.

The heart's rhythm and rate of beat is examined in the test. Moreover, the timing and strength of the heart's electrical signals are visible. An EKG/ECG can aid in the early detection of heart attacks, angina attacks, arrhythmias, etc. (85).

15.5.3 Echocardiography

This examination creates an visual representation of the movement of the heart using sound-waves. A probe is rolled along a region of chest during this painless test, and the device projects a picture of the heart onto the monitor. This gives details about the structure, dimensions, function, valves, and chambers of the heart.

Doppler echocardiography can be used to reveal the parts of the heart with inadequate blood flow. It displays previously damaged cardiac muscle, as well as heart muscle regions that are not pumping regularly (86).

15.5.4 Cardiac Catheterization

A heart artery occlusion may be discovered by this examination. A lengthy, slender, flexible tube (catheter) is inserted into a blood vessel, commonly in the wrist or groin, to deliver medication to the heart. Dye travels through the catheter and into the arteries of the heart. The dye used during the examination increases the visibility of the arteries on X-rays. (87).

15.5.5 Electro-Beam Computed Tomography (EBCT)

The coronary artery walls' calcifications or calcium deposits can be determined using EBCT. These are early indicators of coronary heart disease and atherosclerosis (88).

15.5.6 Cardiac Magnetic Resonance Imaging (MRI)

A kind of magnetic resonance imaging called cardiac MRI employs radio frequencies, magnets, and a computer to create images of the heart. In addition to static pictures, this offers a three-dimensional representation of the beating heart (89).

15.5.7 Chest X-Ray

The structural representation of the heart, lungs, and major blood vessels are shown by this examination. Due to the fact that it offers little additional information not offered by echocardiography and other imaging procedures, chest X-rays are rarely used to diagnose cardiac problems (90).

15.5.8 Stress Testing

These tests often involve walking on a treadmill or cycling at a constant speed while the heart rate is monitored. These tests can help evaluate whether exercising triggers heart disease symptoms and how the heart reacts to exercise. If one is unable to exercise, medication may be prescribed (91).

15.5.9 Cardiac Computed Tomography Scan

An imaging technique called computed tomography (CT) scans the heart using X-rays to produce detailed images of the heart and its blood vessels. The X-ray tube and the photon detectors are arranged so that they are facing each other and are constructed so that they may rotate around the patient in a single direction for the full 360 degrees(92).

15.5.10 Cardiac Angiography

An invasive diagnostic procedure called cardiac catheterization gives vital details regarding the composition and operation of the heart. Via the catheter, a specialized dye known as contrast medium is injected, and X-ray photographs (angiograms) are obtained (93).

15.6 MANAGEMENT OF CARDIOVASCULAR DISEASE

Management of CVD involves a combination of lifestyles changes, medications, and other interventions to prevent or treat the underlying conditions (Figure 15.1). The epidemiology and monitoring of CVDs have established the groundwork for public healthcare initiatives that could lessen the burden of diseases.

15.6.1 Managing blood pressure

Because high blood pressure damages blood arteries and raises the risk of heart attacks, strokes, and other consequences, controlling blood pressure is crucial for those with CVD. The following can be adopted for maintaining and/or lowering blood pressure (94).

■ Following a heart-healthy diet: A diet that is heart-healthy, including plenty of fruits, vegetables, whole grains, and lean proteins, should be adopted. It is crucial to keep sodium, cholesterol, and saturated and trans fats to a minimum (95).

■ Regular medications should be taken as prescribed: Common medications used to treat high blood pressure include ACE inhibitors, calcium channel blockers, diuretics, and beta blockers (96).

■ Exercise regularly: Consistent exercise can enhance cardiovascular health and reduce blood pressure (97).

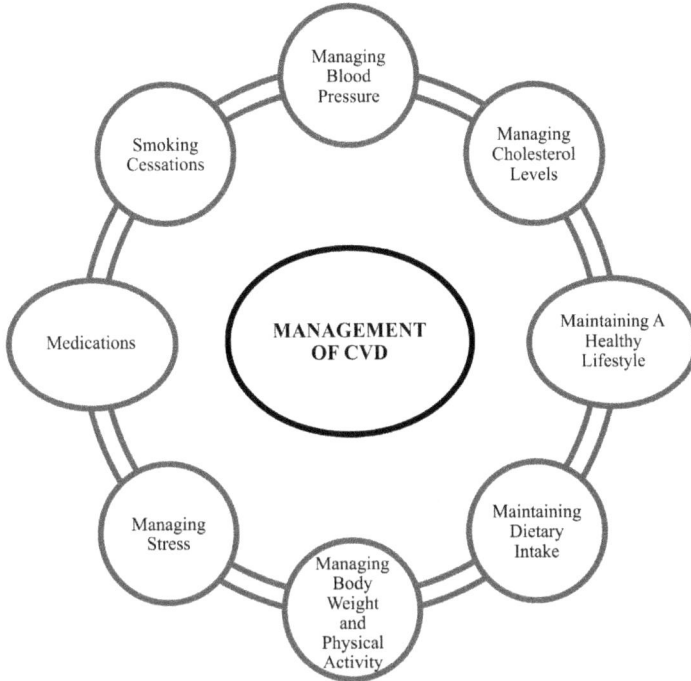

Figure 15.1 Management options for cardiovascular diseases

■ Maintain a healthy weight: High blood pressure and cardiovascular disease risk can both be increased by being overweight or obese. Blood pressure can be lowered and general health can be improved by losing weight (98).

15.6.2 Managing Cholesterol Level

Managing cholesterol is an important part of managing CVD as increased levels of cholesterol are a major risk factor for stroke and heart diseases (99). In order to prevent cardiovascular disease, regulate cholesterol via following measures.

■ Adopt a healthy diet: Plenty of fruits, vegetables, whole grains, and lean proteins are part of a heart-healthy diet. It is also crucial to keep sodium, cholesterol, and saturated and trans fats to a minimum. Constructing a tailored food plan with the assistance of the physician or a qualified dietitian is advised (100).

■ Exercise regularly: Moderate exercise can help decrease cholesterol levels and strengthen the heart. To maintain a sustainable lifestyle, at least 150 minutes of moderate-intensity activity or 75 minutes of intense exercise is recommended (101).

■ Maintain a healthy weight: Obesity and excess weight can raise cholesterol levels and CVD risk. Losing weight can help lower cholesterol and improve overall health (102)

■ Manage stress: Chronic stress can increase cholesterol levels and worsen CVD. Finding stress management techniques, such as practising relaxation methods, can help lower cholesterol and improve overall health (103).

■ Take medications as prescribed: Some medications that are prescribed for the treatment of high cholesterol are statins, bile acid sequestrants, and PCSK9 inhibitors (104).

15.6.3 Maintaining a Healthy Lifestyle

Maintaining a healthy lifestyle is crucial to managing CVD. Premature deaths, which are defined as fatalities that occur before people's expected death dates, account for about half of all recorded premature deaths. The following changes can be made to maintain a healthy lifestyle

■ Quit smoking, due to the fact that smoking can elevate the probability of CVD and other health issues. One of the most crucial actions a person can take is to stop smoking (105).

■ Keep body weight in check, as CVD risk can be raised by being overweight or obese. Weight loss can help decrease blood pressure, raise cholesterol levels, and minimize the risk of heart disease (106).

■ Reduce stress as the risk of CVD can grow with ongoing stress. Discovering ways of dealing with stress, including using relaxation methods or doing fun things, might be a helpful way to enhance overall health (107).

■ Get enough sleep as sleeping and resting for the adequate amount of time is vital for overall health, and a lack of sleep can increase the chance of CVD. Aim for 7–9 hours of sleep per night (108).

■ Consume alcohol in moderation: Drinking too much alcohol can elevate blood pressure and the chance of developing cardiovascular disease. Limit alcohol intake to not much more than one drink per day for women and two drinks per day for men (109).

15.6.4 Managing Dietary Intake

Diet is a major area of concern in coronary heart disease. Heart disease risk can be considerably reduced by eating a diet rich in fibre, plant-based foods, and less saturated fat. Even if there is no one single cause of heart disease, an unhealthy diet could be among the risk factors. Paying heed to what you eat and ingesting a variety of nutritious meals is one of the most important preventative measures you can take (110).

■ Consume a variety of fruits and vegetables as they are rich in vitamins, minerals, and fibre, and essential for a balanced diet. At least five servings of fruits and vegetables should be consumed each day.

■ Choose whole grains: Whole grains, such as brown rice, quinoa, and whole wheat bread, are high in fibre and can help lower cholesterol and improve blood sugar control.

■ Reduce intake of food containing saturated and trans fats because they can raise cholesterol and increase your chance of developing cardiovascular disease. Reduce intake of processed meals, full-fat dairy products, and fatty meats as these are sources of these fats (111).

■ Opt for lean proteins. Instead of high-fat meats, opt for lean proteins like skinless chicken, fish, and legumes. A diet that is heart-healthy can also include lean poultry and eggs in moderation. Make sure to buy lean red meat, and limit weekly consumption to one to three servings.

■ Reduce intake of sodium because it elevates the blood pressure and increases the chances of CVD. Reduce daily salt consumption to 2.300 grams per day. Reduce intake of processed foods, avoid fast food, and use herbs and spices for flavour as a quick and easy strategy to lower salt intake.

■ Choose healthy fats: Monounsaturated and polyunsaturated fats, which can help decrease cholesterol and enhance cardiovascular health, are examples of healthy fats. Nuts, seeds, avocado, and fatty fish are examples of excellent sources of healthy fats. The risk of getting heart disease can be decreased by swapping out saturated and trans dietary fats for unsaturated fats ("good fats").

■ Limit added sugars. Added sugars, such as those found in soda, candy, and processed foods, can increase your risk of developing CVD. Limit added sugar intake to less than 10% of daily calories (112, 113, 114, 115).

15.6.5 Managing Body Weight and Physical Activity

To minimize the chance of developing any heart complications, and to improve blood pressure and lipid levels in obese people suffering from coronary heart disease, weight loss is strongly advised.

■ Consume a nutritious diet: Eating a healthy diet will help you manage weight and enhance cardiovascular health. A healthy diet should be high in fruits, whole grains, lean meats, vegetables, and healthy fats.

■ Control portion sizes: Controlling portion sizes can help manage calorie intake and control weight. Use smaller plates and bowls and be mindful of serving sizes.

■ Monitor food intake: Maintaining a food journal will help you keep track of intake and find areas where your diet needs work (116, 117).

15.6.6 Managing Stress

Individuals who are in good mental health also tend to have physical characteristics that minimize their risk of heart complications. It is beneficial to health and wellbeing to manage stress.

■ Determine the sources of stress in life and take action to control the factors resulting in the stress (118).

■ Exercise relaxation strategies: Stress reduction and blood pressure-lowering strategies include deep breathing, meditation, yoga, and tai chi.

■ Sleep well: Sleep is crucial for general health and can help you feel less stressed. Sleep for 7–9 hours every night (119).

■ Connect with others: Social support can aid in stress reduction and general health improvement.

■ Time management is important since it can reduce stress. Create a timetable and establish priorities for better time management.

■ Get professional assistance from a mental health professional or counsellor if required (120).

15.6.7 Medications

There are several types of medications that are used to treat cardiovascular disease, depending on the specific condition and individual needs. Here are a few drugs commonly used to treat cardiovascular disease.

■ Antiplatelet agents that include aspirin and clopidogrel. Antiplatelet medications help prevent blood clots from developing on the walls and clogging the arteries by making platelets less sticky. As a result, they aid in the prevention of blood spots and are used to treat diseases including heart attack and stroke (121).

■ Medicines known as anticoagulants lengthen the time it takes for blood to clot. They are often referred to as blood thinners. In addition to treating disorders like atrial fibrillation and deep vein thrombosis, anticoagulants like warfarin and dabigatran can prevent blood clots (122).

■ Blood pressure medications: These medications, such as ACE inhibitors, beta blockers, and calcium channel blockers, help lower blood pressure and are used to treat conditions such as hypertension and heart failure (123).

■ Cholesterol-lowering medication: The quantity of cholesterol the body produces is decreased by cholesterol-lowering drugs. Certain drugs, including ezetimibe and statins, reduce cholesterol levels and are used to treat atherosclerosis and hyperlipidaemia, among other disorders (124).

■ Diuretics lower intravascular volume, which lowers the blood filling pressures of all the chambers of heart including pulmonary arteries as well as central venous pressure. As venous capacitance rises, intrapulmonary fluid enters the bloodstream once more. Certain drugs, such furosemide and hydrochlorothiazide, assist the body in getting rid of extra fluid and are used to treat diseases like heart failure and hypertension (125).

■ Antiarrhythmic agents, commonly known as heart rhythm drugs, are used for the prevention and treatment of irregular beats, as well as abnormal beating of the heart. Certain drugs, such as amiodarone and sotalol, help control cardiac rhythm and are used to treat diseases like ventricular tachycardia and atrial fibrillation. Several of these medications blocks the erratic and excessive electrical impulses while the others help in preventing accelerated impulses passing through the tissues of the heart (126).

15.6.8 Smoking Cessation

Smoking is a major contributing factor in the development of CVD. Ceasing smoking can majorly reducing the risk of heart ailments and other related conditions. The following can be done in order to prevent smoking.

- Employ nicotine replacement treatment to ease the withdrawal symptoms you might experience by replacing some of the nicotine you used to get from smoking. Patches, gum, or lozenges that contain nicotine can help control cravings and withdrawal symptoms (127).

- Consider prescription medicines. Certain drugs, including bupropion or varenicline, can help control nicotine cravings and withdrawal symptoms.

- Avoid triggers: Identify triggers that make you want to smoke, such as stress or social situations, and develop strategies to avoid or manage them (128).

- Join a programme to stop smoking: Participating in a programme to stop smoking, whether in person or online, can offer additional support and resources. Make a plan to stop smoking and discuss it with family, close friends, or a healthcare professional. They could provide assistance and inspiration.

- Get moving: Frequent exercise might help cope with stress and curb appetite (129–131).

15.7 INTERVENTIONS

Depending on the nature and severity of the illnesses, there are a number of additional therapies that can be used in the treatment of cardiovascular diseases. In these situations, medical procedures are a crucial component of the CVD therapy plan. These interventions need to be personalized for each person and should be managed by trained medical specialists.

The following are some of the interventions that could be used.

15.7.1 Angioplasty and Stents

An angioplasty procedure is used to relieve obstructed or constrained arteries. It involves pushing back the plaque and restoring blood flow inside the blocked artery using a tiny balloon that is inflated by a catheter with a balloon tip. A stent may be implanted to help keep the artery open after it has been expanded. During angioplasty, a small mesh tube made of metal called a stent is inserted into the artery to give it structural support and stop it from contracting or narrowing again. The stent keeps the blocked portion of the artery open permanently and permits blood to flow through it. Stents are available in a variety of shapes and sizes and are made of high-quality alloy to prevent corrosion. To help prevent re-blockage, they can also be coated with medications that are gradually released into the artery. Coronary artery disease is frequently treated through angioplasty and stent implantation. These therapies reduce the chance of a heart attack and aid in re-establishing blood flow to the heart. They are not, however, suitable for everyone and come with hazards, like bleeding, infection, and blood clots. (132,133)

15.7.2 Pacemakers

A pacemaker is a tiny, battery-powered device used to control the rhythm of the heart that is implanted beneath the skin, typically in the chest region. It helps to regularize the heartbeat by sending electrical impulses to the organ. Bradycardia, a disorder in which the heart beats too slowly or irregularly, is frequently treated using pacemakers. The generator and the leads are the two major components of pacemakers. The battery and the electronic circuitry that generate the electrical signals are within the generator. The generator is connected to the leads, which are little cables that travel through a vein into the heart. The leads track the electrical signals from the heart and transmit them to the generator, which generates electrical impulses to promote the heartbeat. Pacemakers come in a variety of designs, including single-, dual-, and biventricular pacemakers. The atrium or ventricle's heartbeat can be controlled using single-chamber pacemakers, which have one lead. Dual-chamber pacemakers control the heartbeat in both the atrium and the ventricle and contain two leads. Three-lead biventricular pacemakers are used in treatment of heart failure by controlling the electrical activity of both the ventricles of the heart.

Pacemakers are typically inserted via a small surgical operation, and the battery can last for several years. After the treatment, some people may feel a little discomfort or soreness, but the majority can return to their regular activities within a few days.

Although pacemakers are generally safe, problems like infection, bleeding, or lead displacement can occur (134, 135).

15.7.3 Implantable Cardioverter-Defibrillator

A small, battery-operated device called an implantable cardioverter-defibrillator (ICD), inserted under the skin of the chest region, can monitor and treat irregular cardiac beats, or arrhythmias.

In those who are at greater risk of developing fatal arrhythmias, it is used to prevent sudden cardiac death.

The generator and the leads are the two primary components of an ICD. The battery and electronic circuitry that track the heart's rhythm and, if necessary, shock the patient are housed inside the generator. The generator is connected to the leads, which are little cables that travel through a vein into the heart. The leads pick up electrical impulses from the heart and relay them to the generator, which tracks the heartbeat and administers shocks as necessary. ICDs have two electrical shock-delivery options: defibrillation shocks and pacing shocks. When the heart is beating too quickly or irregularly, defibrillation shocks are given to the heart to bring it back to normal rhythm. Low-energy shocks known as pacing shocks are given to the heart to pace the heartbeat when it beats too slowly.

ICD implantation is often performed as a minor surgical operation, and the majority of patients can return to their regular activities in a few days. Following the operation, some people may feel a little discomfort or soreness. Although ICDs are generally safe, problems like infection, haemorrhage, or lead displacement can occur (136, 137).

15.7.4 Heart Bypass Surgery

Cardiovascular bypass surgery, also referred to as coronary artery bypass graft (CABG) surgery, is a procedure carried out by surgeons to treat blockages or constriction of the coronary arteries, which supply blood to the heart muscle. In the course of the procedure, a surgeon makes a fresh passageway (bypass) for blood to travel through to get around the blocked or constricted area of the artery. In the most common type of bypass surgery, a healthy blood vessel from a different part of the body, like the leg or chest, is utilized to create a new conduit around the obstructed or constrained segment of the artery. Blood can circulate freely around the blockage thanks to the new vessel's attachment to the coronary artery above and below the obstruction.

A heart-lung bypass machine is required for bypass surgery, which is normally carried out while the patient is under general anaesthesia and during which the heart and lungs are artificially replaced. Most patients remain in the hospital for several days following the surgery, which typically lasts several hours.

Bypass surgery reduces the chance of heart attack, enhances the circulation of blood to the heart, and eases angina symptoms. However, as it involves a significant procedure, there is a chance of bleeding, infection, stroke, and heart attack (138, 139).

15.7.5 Valve Disease Treatment

When the heart's valves are unhealthy, blood flow into and out of the heart is impeded, which is referred to as valve disease. Depending on the type and severity of the condition, valve disease may be treated surgically or medically. The initial line of treatment for valve disease is typically medication, which aims to manage symptoms and avoid consequences. For valve disease, surgical procedures include the following:

■ Surgically repairing the damaged valve so it can operate again. This can entail bending the valve, patching it up, or reattaching damaged valve flaps.

■ Replacement of the valve may be necessary if it is significantly damaged or cannot be repaired. Mechanical and biological valve replacement are the two basic varieties. Metal or plastic mechanical valves are strong and long-lasting, but they necessitate lifelong anticoagulation medication to prevent blood clots. The lifespan of biological valves may be less than that of mechanical valves; however, they are manufactured from animal or human tissue and do not necessitate anticoagulant medication.

■ Transcatheter aortic valve replacement (TAVR): This invasive surgery uses a catheter introduced through a tiny incision in the leg or chest to replace the aortic valve.

■ To enlarge the valve and improve blood flow, a balloon catheter is inserted through the valve and inflated. This operation is known as balloon valvuloplasty (140, 141).

15.7.6 Heart Transplants

The irregular or damaged heart of a patient is substituted by a healthy heart obtained from a suitable donor during a heart transplant procedure. End-stage heart failure, in which the heart is unable to pump enough blood to meet needs of the body, is the most common ailment for which this is used as a treatment. Usually carried out under anaesthesia, the transplant procedure can last for many hours. As the healthy heart is attached to the patient's remaining blood vessels and the arteries and veins are connected, the surgeon removes the diseased or damaged heart and replaces it. The patient will need to adjust their lifestyle significantly to preserve their health after the transplant and is prescribed medications so the body does not reject the replaced heart. For those with end-stage heart failure, a heart transplant may be a life-saving procedure. Nevertheless, it is a major surgery with risks, including infection, haemorrhage, organ rejection, and the necessity of lifelong immunosuppressive drugs (142).

15.7.7 Left Ventricular Assist Device (LVAD)

A LVAD is a mechanical pump, placed in the chest, that helps the heart to pump blood. LVADs are frequently used to treat advanced heart failure, a disease in which the heart can no longer circulate enough blood to sustain the needs of the body.

The left ventricle, which regulates the pumping of oxygen-rich blood throughout the body, is attached to the LVAD during open-heart surgery. The aorta, which is the major artery that circulates blood from the heart to the body, is then filled with blood by the device as it pumps blood from the left ventricle into it.

While a patient waits for a suitable donor heart, LVADs can be utilized as a temporary measure, preserving life and enhancing health. For those who are not candidates for a heart transplant or who are not anticipated to recover from their heart failure, LVADs can also be utilized as a long-term treatment (143).

15.7.8 Enhanced External Counterpulsation Therapy

Angina, which is typically pain in the chest brought on by decreased flow of blood to the heart, can be treated non-invasively with enhanced external counterpulsation (EECP) therapy. This entails putting on leg cuffs that inflate and deflate in accordance with the wearer's heartbeat to help the heart receive greater blood flow. The subject lies on a table during an EECP session with cuffs around their hips, thighs, and calves. A "squeezing" effect that enhances blood circulation to heart is produced by timing the inflation and deflation of the cuffs. The normal course of treatment comprises of 35 one-hour sessions spread out over a few weeks.

According to the theory, EECP therapy works by producing a "counterpulsation" effect that lessens the burden on the heart and enhances its capacity to pump blood. Moreover, it might encourage the development of new blood vessels and enhance circulation of blood throughout the body. EECP therapy is not a substitute for other angina treatments; rather, it can be used in conjunction with them or as a stand-alone therapy for those who are not candidates for other interventions (144).

15.7.9 Cardioversions

For patients with specific types of irregular heartbeats, such as atrial fibrillation or atrial flutter, cardioversion is a medical procedure that is performed to restore a normal heart rhythm. An electric shock or medicine are frequently used to perform cardioversion. Delivering a regulated electric shock to the heart in order to return it to its normal rhythm is known as electrical cardioversion. To reduce pain during the treatment, the patient is typically given an anaesthetic, as well as being sedated. The entire operation usually takes less than 30 minutes, and the shock is administered through patches or paddles applied to the back or chest. Electrical cardioversion may occasionally be combined with or substituted by medicines. Pharmacological cardioversion uses medications to assist in controlling the heart's rhythm (145).

Even though all these interventions are frequently carried out, it is crucial to carefully follow all pre- and post-procedure instructions and to have a discussion with a skilled healthcare practitioner about the dangers and advantages of such therapies.

15.8 COPING AND SUPPORT

It can be challenging to deal with a diagnosis of a cardiovascular disease, so it is critical to look for assistance and resources to help with the condition's practical, emotional, and physical elements. The following coping and support techniques may be useful.

15.8.1 Cardiac Rehabilitation

A regimen of exercise, education, and counselling known as cardiac rehabilitation is intended to aid in the recovery from a CVD or a surgical procedure, as well as to improve general CVD. Those who have had a heart attack or heart surgery, or who have certain other CVDs are frequently advised to undergo cardiac rehabilitation. It is frequently carried out under supervision in a facility like a hospital or outpatient clinic and is customized to the patient's specific requirements and objectives.

Cardiac rehabilitation has been demonstrated to be successful in improving CVD and lowering the risk of problems, including subsequent heart attacks.

15.8.2 Plant-Based Diets

Many health advantages of plant-based diets have been demonstrated, including a lower risk of CVD. Whole grains, vegetables, nuts, fruits, seeds, and legumes are consumed in abundance in a plant-based diet, which eliminates or restricts the use of animal products.

These diets have been recognized as a very beneficial approach. Studies have shown that adopting these diets reduces cholesterol levels, blood pressure, and the chance of many fatal cardiac ailments.

It is crucial to acknowledge that not all plant-based diets are beneficial. Although they can still be consumed as part of a plant-based diet, processed foods that are high in sugar and refined carbs raise the risk of cardiovascular disease. To ensure that all nutrient demands are met, it is crucial to eat a balanced, diversified, plant-based diet that includes a variety of whole foods.

15.8.3 A Safe Exercise Plan after Cardiac Complications

Exercise is crucial for healing and lowering the risk of future incidents, but it must be done cautiously. To begin engaging in safe exercise, one should consult a healthcare professional, specifically a cardiologist, to ensure that one is ready, given the severity of the heart complications.

Low-impact exercises are less stressful and easier on the heart. It is important to regularly monitor the heart rate to remain in the safe range and to listen to the body if experiencing any symptoms. When such events occur, it is of the utmost importance to include a cool-down period and provide enough resting time during the entire exercise routine.

15.8.4 Educating and Counselling

Patients should be educated regarding their illness, how to treat it, and minimizing the chances of developing cardiac ailments. They should receive advice on healthy lifestyle choices, such as food, exercise, and quitting smoking. Moreover, counselling is offered to assist the patient in navigating the difficulties of rehabilitation, as well as the emotional and psychological repercussions of the ailment (146–148).

15.9 CONCLUSION

Keeping the heart in good shape is crucial for overall health and wellbeing. A nutritious diet, consistent exercise, stress management, and minimizing substance abuse are examples of lifestyle changes that can lower the possibility of cardiovascular disease. CVD can be treated early to reduce the risk of complications and improve results. It is critical to consult a healthcare professional in relation to major concerns associated with CVD. People can take charge of their CVD and enhance their quality of life by adopting healthy lifestyle choices and collaborating with healthcare professionals.

ABBREVIATIONS

BP: Blood pressure
CAD: Coronary artery disease
CKD: Chronic kidney disease
CHD: Congenital heart disease
CVS: Cardiovascular system
DM: Diabetes mellitus
DVT: Deep vein thrombosis
HDL: High-density lipoprotein
ICD: Implantable cardioverter defibrillator
LDL: Low-density lipoprotein
LVAD: Left ventricular assist device
MVL: Mitral valve leaflet
PAD: Peripheral artery disease
VTE: Venous thromboembolism

REFERENCES

1. Yang, M., Ta, N., Bai, X., Wei, C., Sun, C., Han, C., 2023. The effectiveness of personalized nursing on quality of life in cardiovascular disease patients: A systematic review and meta-analysis. *Evidence-Based Complementary & Alternative Medicine: eCAM, 2023,* 4689732.

2. World Health Organization, 2022. Cardiovascular diseases (CVDs). https://www.who.Int/ News-Room/Fact-Sheets/Detail/Cardiovascular-Diseases-(cvds).

3. https://my.clevelandclinic.org/health/diseases/21493-cardiovascular-disease.

4. World Health Organization (WHO). Cardiovascular diseases (CVDs). https://www.who.int/ newsroom/fact-sheets/detail/cardiovascular-diseases-(cvds), 2021a.

5. Rodgers, J.L., Jones, J., Bolleddu, S.I., et al., 2019. Cardiovascular risks associated with gender and aging. *Journal of Cardiovascular Development & Disease, 6*(2), p. 19. https://doi.org/10.3390/ jcdd6020019.

6. Garcia, M., Mulvagh, S.L., Merz, C.N., Buring, J.E., Manson, J.E., 2016. Cardiovascular disease in women: Clinical perspectives. *Circulation Research, 118*(8), pp. 1273–1293.

7. Komasi, S., Saeidi, M., 2016. Presentation of new classification of perceived risk factors and etiologies of cardiovascular diseases. *ARYA Atherosclerosis, 12*(6), pp. 295–296.

8. Jurgens, C.Y., Lee, C.S., Aycock, D.M., et al., 2022. State of the science: The relevance of symptoms in cardiovascular disease and research: A scientific statement from the American Heart Association. *Circulation, 146*(12), pp. e173-e184.

9. Training, NIH SEER. *Classification & Structure of Blood Vessels.* https://training.seer.cancer.gov /anatomy/cardiovascular/blood/classification.html.

10. Quarteroni, A., Manzoni, A., Vergara, C., 2019. *Mathematical Modelling of the Human Cardiovascular System: Data, Numerical Approximation, Clinical Applications,* (Vol. 33). Cambridge University Press.

11. Farrell, A.P., Jones, D.R., Hoar, W.S., Randall, D.J., 1992. The heart. *Cardiovascular System, 12,* pp. 1–88.

12. Katz, A.M., 2010. *Physiology of the Heart.* Lippincott Williams & Wilkins.

13. Noordergraaf, A., 2012. *Circulatory System Dynamics,* (Vol. 1). Elsevier.

14. Kroeker, C.G., 2018. Cardiovascular system: Anatomy and physiology. *Cardiovascular Mechanics, 2*(5), p. 1.

15. Peate, I., 2020. The circulatory system. *British Journal of Healthcare Assistants, 14*(11), pp. 548–553.

16. Hislop, A., 2005. Developmental biology of the pulmonary circulation. *Paediatric Respiratory Reviews, 6*(1), pp. 35–43.

17. Magder, S., 2016. Mechanical interactions between the respiratory and circulatory systems. *Sleep Apnea,* pp. 60–80.

18. Saikia, D., Mahanta, B., 2019. Cardiovascular and respiratory physiology in children. *Indian Journal of Anaesthesia, 63*(9), pp. 690–697

19. Miller, T.A., 2013. Structure and physiology of the circulatory system. *Comprehensive Insect Physiology. Biochemistry & Pharmacology, 3*, pp. 289–353.

20. Pugsley, M.K., Tabrizchi, R., 2000. The vascular system: An overview of structure and function. *Journal of Pharmacological & Toxicological Methods, 44*(2), pp. 333–340.

21. Guven, G., Hilty, M.P., Ince, C., 2020. Microcirculation: Physiology, pathophysiology, and clinical application. *Blood Purification, 49*(1–2), pp. 143–150.

22. Levick, J.R., 2013. *An Introduction to Cardiovascular Physiology.* Butterworth-Heinemann.

23. Yuan, S.Y., Rigor, R.R., 2011. Regulation of endothelial barrier function. *Colloquium Series on Integrated Systems Physiology, 3*(1), 1–146.

24. Davies, M.J., Woolf, N., 1993. Atherosclerosis: What is it and why does it occur? *British Heart Journal, 69*(1), pp. S3–11. doi: 10.1136/hrt.69.1_suppl.s3; PMID: 8427761; PMCID: PMC1025252.

25. Ross, R., 1986. The pathogenesis of atherosclerosis—an update. *New England Journal of Medicine, 314*(8), pp. 488–500.

26. Reddy, L. and Thangam, S., 2022. Predicting relapse of the myocardial infarction in hospitalized patients. In 2022 3rd International Conference for Emerging Technology (INCET) (pp. 1–7). Belgaum: IEEE.

27. Lu, L., Liu, M., Sun, R., Zheng, Y., Zhang, P., 2015. Myocardial infarction: Symptoms and treatments. *Cell Biochemistry & Biophysics, 72*(3), pp. 865–867.

28. Katzung, B.G., Chatterjee, K., 1989. 12 vasodilators & the treatment of angina pectoris. *Basic & Clinical Pharmacology, 4*, p. 140.

29. Pepine, C.J., Abrams, J., Marks, R.G., Morris, J.J., Scheidt, S.S., Handberg, E. and TIDES investigators, 1994. Characteristics of a contemporary population with angina pectoris. *American Journal of Cardiology, 74*(3), pp. 226–231.

30. Picard, F., Sayah, N., Spagnoli, V., Adjedj, J., Varenne, O., 2019. Vasospastic angina: A literature review of current evidence. *Archives of Cardiovascular Diseases, 112*(1), pp. 44–55.

31. Yeghiazarians, Y., Braunstein, J.B., Askari, A., Stone, P.H., 2000. Unstable angina pectoris. *New England Journal of Medicine, 342*(2), pp. 101–114.

32. https://www.mayoclinic.org/diseases-conditions/myocardial-ischemia/symptoms-causes/syc-20375417#:~:text=Myocardial%20ischemia%2C%20also%20called%20cardiac,cause%20serious%20abnormal%20heart%20rhythms.

33. Cohn, J.N., 1996. The management of chronic heart failure. *New England Journal of Medicine, 335*(7), pp. 490–498.

34. Hypertension. https://www.healthline.com/health/high-blood-pressure-hypertension.

35. Sirsat, M.S., Fermé, E., Câmara, J., 2020. Machine learning for brain stroke: A review. *Journal of Stroke & Cerebrovascular Diseases, 29*(10), p. 105162.

36. Chen, Z., Venkat, P., Seyfried, D., Chopp, M., Yan, T., Chen, J., 2017. Brain–heart interaction: Cardiac complications after stroke. *Circulation Research, 121*(4), pp. 451–468.

37. Subczynski, W.K., Pasenkiewicz-Gierula, M., Widomska, J., Mainali, L., Raguz, M., 2017. High cholesterol/low cholesterol: Effects in biological membranes: A review. *Cell Biochemistry & Biophysics, 75*(3–4), pp. 369–385.

38. Liu, Y., Chen, S., Zühlke, L., et al., 2020. Global prevalence of congenital heart disease in school-age children: A meta-analysis and systematic review. *BMC Cardiovascular Disorders*, *20*(1), pp. 488.

39. Van Der Linde, D., Konings, E.E., Slager, M.A., et al., 2011. Birth prevalence of congenital heart disease worldwide: A systematic review and meta-analysis. *Journal of the American College of Cardiology*, *58*(21), pp. 2241–2247.

40. Antzelevitch, C., Burashnikov, A., 2011. Overview of basic mechanisms of cardiac arrhythmia. *Cardiac Electrophysiology Clinics*, *3*(1), pp. 23–45. https://doi.org/10.1016/j.ccep.2010.10.012.

41. Kronhaus, K.D., 1979. Dysrhythmia vs arrhythmia. *JAMA*, *241*(1), pp. 28–28.

42. Chandrashekhar, Y., Westaby, S., Narula, J., 2009. Mitral stenosis. *The Lancet*, *374*(9697), pp. 1271–1283.

43. Morningstar, J.E., Nieman, A., Wang, C., Beck, T., Harvey, A., Norris, R.A., 2021 Mitral Valve Prolapse and Its Motley Crew-Syndromic Prevalence, Pathophysiology, and Progression of a Common Heart Condition. *Journal of the American Heart Association*, *10*(13), p. e020919.

44. Devereux, R.B., Kramer-Fox, R., Kligfield, P., 1989. Mitral valve prolapse: Causes, clinical manifestations, and management. *Annals of Internal Medicine*, *111*(4), pp. 305–317.

45. Apostolidou, E., Maslow, A.D., Poppas, A., 2017. Primary mitral valve regurgitation: Update and review. *Global Cardiology Science & Practice*, *2017*(1), e201703.

46. Nishimura, R.A., Otto, C.M., Bonow, R.O., et al., 2014. Heart Association task force on practice guidelines. 2014 AHA/ACC guideline for the management of patients with valvular heart disease: A report of the American College of Cardiology/American Heart Association Task Force on Practice Guidelines. *Journal of the American College of Cardiology*. American College of Cardiology/American, *63*(22), pp. 2438–2488.

47. Davis, F.M., Daugherty, A., Lu, H.S., 2019. Updates of recent aortic aneurysm research. *Arteriosclerosis, Thrombosis, & Vascular Biology*, *39*(3), pp. e83–90.

48. Wanjari, M.B., Mendhe, D., Wankhede, P., 2021. Abdominal aortic aneurysm-a case report. *Journal of Pharmaceutical Research International*, *33*(43A), pp. 265–269.

49. Tran, B., 2021. Assessment and management of peripheral arterial disease: What every cardiologist should know. *Heart*, *107*(22), pp. 1835–1843.

50. Bevan, G.H., White Solaru, K.T., 2020. Evidence-based medical management of peripheral artery disease. *Arteriosclerosis, Thrombosis, & Vascular Biology*, *40*(3), pp. 541–553.

51. Iverson, R. E., Gomez, J. L., 2013. Deep venous thrombosis: prevention and management. *Clinics in Plastic Surgery*, *40*(3), pp. 389–398.

52. Centre–Acute, N.C.G. and UK, C.C., 2010. *Venous Thromboembolism: Reducing the Risk of Venous Thromboembolism (deep vein thrombosis and pulmonary embolism) in patients admitted to hospital.*

53. Ciarambino, T., Menna, G., Sansone, G., Giordano, M., 2021. Cardiomyopathies: An overview. *International Journal of Molecular Sciences*, *22*(14), p. 7722.

54. Lüscher, T.F., 2016. Cardiomyopathies: Definition, diagnosis, causes, and genetics. *European Heart Journal*, *37*(23), pp. 1779–1782.

55. Peters, F., Karthikeyan, G., Abrams, J., Muhwava, L., Zühlke, L., 2020. Rheumatic heart disease: Current status of diagnosis and therapy. *Cardiovascular Diagnosis & Therapy, 10*(2), pp. 305–315.

56. Dass, C., Kanmanthareddy, A., 2019. *Rheumatic Heart Disease.*

57. Butendieck, R. R., Murray, P. M., 2014. Raynaud disease. *Journal of Hand Surgery, 39*(1), pp. 121–124.

58. Fardoun, M.M., Nassif, J., Issa, K., Baydoun, E., Eid, A.H., 2016. Raynaud's phenomenon: A brief review of the underlying mechanisms. *Frontiers in Pharmacology, 7*, p. 438.

59. Wigley, F. M., Flavahan, N. A., 2016. Raynaud's phenomenon. *New England Journal of Medicine, 375*(6): 556–565.

60. Dash, C., Peyvandi, H., Duan, K., et al., 2020. Stem cell therapy for thromboangiitis obliterans (Buerger's disease). *Processes, 8*(11), p. 1408.

61. Stewart, J., McCallin, T., Martinez, J., Chacko, S., Yusuf, S., 2020. Hyperlipidemia. *Pediatrics in Review, 41*(8), pp. 393–402.

62. Poznyak, A.V., Sadykhov, N.K., Kartuesov, A.G., et al., 2022. Hypertension as a risk factor for atherosclerosis: Cardiovascular risk assessment. *Frontiers in Cardiovascular Medicine, 9*, 959285.

63. https://www.modernheartandvascular.com/how-smoking-affects-the-heart/.

64. Zhang, X., Cash, R.E., Bower, J.K., Focht, B.C., Paskett, E.D., 2020. Physical activity and risk of cardiovascular disease by weight status among US adults. *PLoS One, 15*(5), p. e0232893.

65. Poirier, P., Giles, T.D., Bray, G.A., et al., 2006. Obesity and cardiovascular disease: Pathophysiology, evaluation, and effect of weight loss: An update of the 1997 American Heart Association Scientific Statement on Obesity and Heart Disease from the Obesity Committee of the Council on Nutrition, Physical Activity, and Metabolism. *Circulation, 113*(6), pp. 898–918.

66. Anand, S.S., Hawkes, C., De Souza, R.J., et al., 2015. Food consumption and its impact on cardiovascular disease: Importance of solutions focused on the globalized food system: A report from the workshop convened by the World Heart Federation. *Journal of the American College of Cardiology, 66*(14), pp. 1590–1614.

67. Schwartz, M.W., Seeley, R.J., Zeltser, L.M., et al., 2017. Obesity pathogenesis: An endocrine society scientific statement. *Endocrine Reviews, 38*(4), pp. 267–296.

68. Gomes, F., Telo, D.F., Souza, H.P., Nicolau, J.C., Halpern, A., Serrano Jr, C.V., 2010. Obesity and coronary artery disease: Role of vascular inflammation. *Arquivos Brasileiros de Cardiologia, 94*(2), pp. 273–279.

69. Bravo, P.E., Morse, S., Borne, D.M., Aguilar, E.A., Reisin, E., 2006. Leptin and hypertension in obesity. *Vascular Health & Risk Management, 2*(2), pp. 163–169.

70. Cercato, C., Fonseca, F.A., 2019. Cardiovascular risk and obesity. *Diabetology & Metabolic Syndrome, 11*(1), pp. 74.

71. Dhingra, R., Vasan, R.S., 2012. Age as a risk factor. *Medical Clinics of North America*. Medical Clinics, 96(1), pp. 87–91.

72. Jousilahti, P., Vartiainen, E., Tuomilehto, J., Puska, P., 1999. Sex, age, cardiovascular risk factors, and coronary heart disease: A prospective follow-up study of 14 786 middle-aged men and women in Finland. *Circulation*, *99*(9), pp. 1165–1172.

73. Motulsky, A.G. The role of genetics as a risk factor in cardiovascular disease. In *Multiple Risk Factors in Cardiovascular Disease*, 1992, 27–29.

74. Davari, M., Maracy, M.R., Khorasani, E., 2019. Socioeconomic status, cardiac risk factors, and cardiovascular disease: A novel approach to determination of this association. *ARYA Atherosclerosis*, *15*(6), pp. 260–266.

75. Matheus, A.S.D.M., Tannus, L.R.M., Cobas, R.A., Palma, C.C.S., Negrato, C.A., Gomes, M.B., 2013. Impact of diabetes on cardiovascular disease: An update. *International Journal of Hypertension*, *2013*, 653789.

76. Chait, A., Han, C.Y., Oram, J.F., Heinecke, J.W., 2005. Lipoprotein-associated inflammatory proteins: Markers or mediators of cardiovascular disease. *Journal of Lipid Research*, *46*(3), pp. 389–403.

77. Belke, D.D., Betuing, S., Tuttle, M.J., et al., 2002. Insulin signaling coordinately regulates cardiac size, metabolism, and contractile protein isoform expression. *Journal of Clinical Investigation*, *109*(5), pp. 629–639.

78. Leon, B.M., Maddox, T.M., 2015. Diabetes and cardiovascular disease: Epidemiology, biological mechanisms, treatment recommendations and future research. *World Journal of Diabetes*, *6*(13), pp. 1246–1258.

79. Willerson, J.T., Ridker, P.M., 2004. Inflammation as a cardiovascular risk factor. *Circulation*, *109*(21_suppl_1), p. II-2.

81. Hoek, A.G., van Oort, S., Mukamal, K.J., Beulens, J.W.J., 2022. Alcohol consumption and cardiovascular disease risk: Placing new data in context. *Current Atherosclerosis Reports*, *24*(1), pp. 51–59.

82. Piano, M.R., 2017. Alcohol's effects on the cardiovascular system. *Alcohol Research: Current Reviews*, *38*(2), pp. 219–241.

83. Torpy JM, Lynm C, Glass RM, 2007. Chronic stress and the heart. *JAMA*, *298*(14), pp. 1722–1722.

84. Adams, J., Apple, F., 2004. Cardiology patient page. New blood tests for detecting heart disease. *Circulation*, *109*(3), pp. E12-E14.

85. Stern, S., 2006. Electrocardiogram: still the cardiologist's best friend. *Circulation*, 113(19), pp. 753–756.

86. Steeds, R.P., 2011. Echocardiography: Frontier imaging in cardiology. *British Journal of Radiology*, *84*(special_issue_3), pp. S237-S245.

87. Kosova, E., Ricciardi, M., 2017. Cardiac catheterization. *JAMA*, *317*(22), pp. 2344–2344.

88. Nallamothu, B.K., Saint, S., Bielak, L.F., et al., 2001. Electron-beam computed tomography in the diagnosis of coronary artery disease: A meta-analysis. *Archives of Internal Medicine*, *161*(6), pp. 833–838.

89. Busse, A., Rajagopal, R., Yücel, S., et al., 2020. Cardiac MRI—update 2020. *Radiologe*, *60*(suppl. 1), 33–40.

90. Singh, R., Kalra, M.K., Nitiwarangkul, C., et al., 2018. Deep learning in chest radiography: Detection of findings and presence of change. *PLoS One*, 13(10), p. e0204155.

91. Kharabsheh, S.M., Al-Sugair, A., Al-Buraiki, J., Al-Farhan, J., 2006. Overview of exercise stress testing. *Annals of Saudi Medicine*, 26(1), pp. 1–6.

92. Sun, Z., 2012. Cardiac CT imaging in coronary artery disease: Current status and future directions. *Quantitative Imaging in Medicine & Surgery*, 2(2), pp. 98–105.

93. Kumamaru, K.K., Hoppel, B.E., Mather, R.T., Rybicki, F.J., 2010. CT angiography: Current technology and clinical use. *Radiologic Clinics*, 48(2), pp. 213–235.

94. Fuchs, F.D., Whelton, P.K., 2020. High blood pressure and cardiovascular disease. *Hypertension*, 75(2), pp. 285–292.

95. Antonakoudis, G., Poulimenos, L., Kifnidis, K., Zouras, C., Antonakoudis, H., 2007. Blood pressure control and cardiovascular risk reduction. *Hippokratia*, 11(3), pp. 114–119.

96. *Types of Heart Medications*. https://www.heart.org/en/health-topics/heart-attack/treatment-of-a-heart-attack/cardiac-medications.

97. Nystoriak, M.A., Bhatnagar, A., 2018. Cardiovascular effects and benefits of exercise. *Frontiers in Cardiovascular Medicine*, 5, p. 135.

98. Katsoulis, M., Stavola, B.D., Diaz-Ordaz, K., et al., 2021. Weight change and the onset of cardiovascular diseases: Emulating trials using electronic health records. *Epidemiology (Cambridge, Mass)*, 32(5), pp. 744–755.

99. Soliman, G.A., 2018. Dietary cholesterol and the lack of evidence in cardiovascular disease. *Nutrients*, 10(6), p. 780.

100. Lichtenstein, A.H., Appel, L.J., Vadiveloo, M., et al., 2021. American Heart Association Council on Lifestyle and Cardiometabolic Health; Council on Arteriosclerosis, Thrombosis and Vascular Biology; Council on Cardiovascular Radiology and Intervention; Council on Clinical Cardiology; and Stroke Council. 2021 dietary guidance to improve cardiovascular health: A scientific statement from the American Heart Association. *Circulation*. 144(23), pp. e472–e487.

101. Zhao, S., Zhong, J., Sun, C., Zhang, J., 2021. Effects of aerobic exercise on TC, HDL-C, LDL-C and TG in patients with hyperlipidemia: A protocol of systematic review and meta-analysis. *Medicine*, 100(10).

102. Verschuren, W.M.M., Boer, J.M.A., Temme, E.H.M., 2022. Optimal diet for cardiovascular and planetary health. *Heart*, 108(15), pp. 1234–1239.

103. Cortes, V. A., Busso, D., Maiz, A., Arteaga, A., Nervi, F., Rigotti, A., 2014. Physiological and pathological implications of cholesterol. *Frontiers in Bioscience-Landmark*, 19(3, pp. 416–428.

104. Zodda, D., Giammona, R., Schifilliti, S., 2018. Treatment strategy for dyslipidemia in cardiovascular disease prevention: Focus on old and new drugs. *Pharmacy*, 6(1), p. 10.

105. Faseru, B., Fagan, P., Okuyemi, K.S., 2022. Additional benefits of maintaining a healthy lifestyle after quitting smoking. *JAMA Network Open*, 5(9), p. e2232784–2232784.

106. Rippe, J. M., 2019. Lifestyle strategies for risk factor reduction, prevention, and treatment of cardiovascular disease. *American Journal of Lifestyle Medicine*, 13(2), pp. 204-212.

107. Kris-Etherton, P.M., Sapp, P.A., Riley, T.M., Davis, K.M., Hart, T., Lawler, O., 2022. The dynamic interplay of healthy lifestyle behaviors for cardiovascular health. *Current Atherosclerosis Reports*, 24(12), 969–980.

108. Grandner, M.A., Alfonso-Miller, P., Fernandez-Mendoza, J., Shetty, S., Shenoy, S., Combs, D., 2016. Sleep: Important considerations for the prevention of cardiovascular disease. *Current Opinion in Cardiology*, 31(5), pp. 551–565.

109. Biddinger, K.J., Emdin, C.A., Haas, M.E., et al., 2022. Association of habitual alcohol intake with risk of cardiovascular disease. *JAMA Network Open*, 5(3), p. e223849–223849.

110. Jakše, B., Jakše, B., Pinter, S., et al., 2019. Dietary intakes and cardiovascular health of healthy adults in short-, medium-, and long-term whole-food plant-based lifestyle program. *Nutrients*, 12(1), p. 55.

111. Brandhorst, S., Longo, V.D., 2019. Dietary restrictions and nutrition in the prevention and treatment of cardiovascular disease. *Circulation Research*, 124(6), pp. 952–965.

112. Dietary management of cardiovascular diseases. http://www.myhealth.gov.my/en/diet-management-for-cardiovascular-disease-cvd/.

113. *Nutritional Manament of Cardiovascular Diseases.* https://peerlesshospital.com/blog/?p=308.

114. *Diet and Heart Diseases Risk.* https://www.betterhealth.vic.gov.au/health/conditionsandtreatments/heart-disease-and-food.

115. Pallazola, V.A., Davis, D.M., Whelton, S.P., et al., 2019. A clinician's guide to healthy eating for cardiovascular disease prevention. *Mayo Clinic Proceedings. Innovations, Quality & Outcomes*, 3(3), pp. 251–267.

116. Buttar, H.S., Li, T., Ravi, N., 2005. Prevention of cardiovascular diseases: Role of exercise, dietary interventions, obesity and smoking cessation. *Experimental & Clinical Cardiology*, 10(4), pp. 229–249.

117. Ravera, A., Carubelli, V., Sciatti, E., et al., 2016. Nutrition and cardiovascular disease: Finding the perfect recipe for cardiovascular health. *Nutrients*, 8(6), p. 363.

118. Dimsdale, J.E., 2008. Psychological stress and cardiovascular disease. *Journal of the American College of Cardiology*, 51(13), pp. 1237–1246.

119. Levine, G.N., Lange, R.A., Bairey-Merz, C.N., et al., 2017. Meditation and cardiovascular risk reduction: A scientific statement from the American Heart Association. *Journal of the American Heart Association*, 6(10), p. e002218.

120. Stress and heart health. https://www.heart.org/en/healthy-living/healthy-lifestyle/stress-management/stress-and-heart-health.

121. Gremmel, T., Michelson, A.D., Frelinger III, A.L., Bhatt, D.L., 2018. Novel aspects of antiplatelet therapy in cardiovascular disease. *Research & Practice in Thrombosis & Haemostasis*, 2(3), pp. 439–449.

122. Gradolí, J., Vidal, V., Brady, A.J., Facila, L., 2018. Anticoagulation in patients with ischaemic heart disease and peripheral arterial disease: Clinical implications of COMPASS study. *European Cardiology*, 13(2), pp. 115–118.

123. Patel, P., Ordunez, P., DiPette, D., et al., 2016. Improved blood pressure control to reduce cardiovascular disease morbidity and mortality: The standardized hypertension treatment and prevention project. *Journal of Clinical Hypertension*, 18(12), pp. 1284–1294.

124. Hadjiphilippou, S., Ray, K.K., 2019. Cholesterol-lowering agents? *Circulation Research*, 124(3), pp. 354–363.

125. Roger, V. L., 2013. Epidemiology of heart failure. *Circulation Research*, 113(6), pp. 646–659.

126. Dan, G.A., Martinez-Rubio, A., Agewall, S., et al., 2018 May 1 Corrigendum. *Europace*, 20(5), pp. 738–738.

127. Rigotti, N.A., Tesar, G.E., 1985. Smoking cessation in the prevention of cardiovascular disease. *Cardiology Clinics*, 3(2), pp. 245–257.

128. Pisinger, C., Wennike, P., Tønnesen, P., 1999. Nicotine replacement therapy in patients with coronary heart disease: Recommendations for effective use. *CNS Drugs*, 12(2), pp. 99–110.

129. Reid, R.D., Mullen, K.A., Pipe, A.L., 2018. Tackling smoking cessation systematically among inpatients with heart disease. *CMAJ*, 190(12), pp. E345-E346.

130. Whats the best ways to quit smoking. https://www.health.harvard.edu/blog/whats-best-way-quit-smoking-201607089935.

131. *Five Ways to Quit Smoking by Hannah Nichols.* https://www.medicalnewstoday.com/articles/319460.

132. Malik, I., Berger, A., 2002. Coronary angioplasty and stenting. *BMJ*, 325(7363), p. 519.

133. Al Suwaidi, J., Berger, P.B., Holmes Jr, D.R., 2000. Coronary artery stents. *JAMA*, 284(14), pp. 1828–1836.

134. Cingolani, E., Goldhaber, J.I., Marbán, E., 2018. Next-generation pacemakers: From small devices to biological pacemakers. *Nature Reviews. Cardiology*, 15(3), pp. 139–150.

135. DiFrancesco, D., 2019. A brief history of pacemaking. *Frontiers in Physiology*, 10, p. 1599.

136. Higgins, S.L., 2002. Automatic implantable cardiac defibrillators. *Current Treatment Options in Cardiovascular Medicine*, 4(4), pp. 287–293.

137. Ammannaya, G.K.K., 2020. Implantable cardioverter defibrillators–the past, present and future. *Archives of Medical Science – Atherosclerotic Diseases*, 5(1), pp. 163–170.

138. Diodato, M., Chedrawy, E.G., 2014. Coronary artery bypass graft surgery: The past, present, and future of myocardial revascularisation. *Surgery Research & Practice*, 2014, 726158.

139. Ziv-Baran, T., Mohr, R., Yazdchi, F., Loberman, D., 2019. The epidemiology of coronary artery bypass surgery in a community hospital: A comparison between 2 periods. *Medicine*, 98(13), e15059.

140. Bhandari, S., Subramanyam, K., Trehan, N., 2007. Valvular heart disease: diagnosis and management. Japi, 55, pp. 575–584.

141. Hinton, R.B., 2014. Advances in the treatment of aortic valve disease: Is it time for companion diagnostics? *Current Opinion in Pediatrics*, 26(5), pp. 546–552.

142. Kim, I.C., Youn, J.C., Kobashigawa, J.A., 2018. The past, present and future of heart transplantation. *Korean Circulation Journal*, 48(7), pp. 565–590.

143. Eisen, H.J., 2019. Left ventricular assist devices (LVADS): History, clinical application and complications. *Korean Circulation Journal*, 49(7), pp. 568–585.

144. Sharma, U., Ramsey, H.K., Tak, T., 2013. The role of enhanced external counter pulsation therapy in clinical practice. *Clinical Medicine & Research, 11*(4), pp. 226–232.

145. Brandes, A., Crijns, H.J.G.M., Rienstra, M., et al., 2020. Cardioversion of atrial fibrillation and atrial flutter revisited: Current evidence and practical guidance for a common procedure. *Europace, 22*(8), pp. 1149–1161.

146. Blikman, M.J., Jacobsen, H.R., Eide, G.E., Meland, E., 2014. How important are social support, expectations and coping patterns during cardiac rehabilitation. *Rehabilitation Research & Practice, 2014*, 973549.

147. Svensson, T., Inoue, M., Sawada, N., et al., 2016. Coping strategies and risk of cardiovascular disease incidence and mortality: The Japan Public Health Center-based prospective Study. *European Heart Journal, 37*(11), pp. 890–899.

148. Albus, C., Waller, C., Fritzsche, K., et al., 2019. Significance of psychosocial factors in cardiology: Update 2018: Position paper of the German Cardiac Society. *Clinical Research in Cardiology, 108*(11), pp. 1175–1196.

16 The Biochemical Basis of Neurological Disorders

Ngurzampuii Sailo, Dhritiman Roy, Rajashri Bezbaruah, and Bibhuti Bhusan Kakoti

16.1 INTRODUCTION

The term "neurological disorders" (ND) refers to diseases that occur as a result of the functional loss of neuronal cells and synapses in the central nervous system (CNS). This functional loss impairs cognition and memory, movement and locomotor functions, thinking abilities, and decision-making (1). NDs account for 9 million deaths annually, making them the second leading cause of death in the world after disability-adjusted life years (DALYs) (2). Neurodegeneration, a multifactorial process that involves the deposition of misfolded proteins as a result of genetic, environmental, and endogenous stress and stimuli, is the term used to describe the death and degeneration of neurons in the spinal cord and the brain (3). Older people are very much susceptible to neurodegenerative diseases. From 55–65 years old to 90 years old, the frequency of NDs rises (4). One important aspect of neurological disorders is their biochemical basis, which refers to the complex network of biochemical reactions and signaling pathways involved in normal brain function (5, 6). The biochemical reactions necessary for normal nerve function are often disrupted by many factors, including excitotoxicity and neurotransmitter abnormalities, neuroinflammation, oxidative stress, calcium intake, abnormalities, altered ion homeostasis, impaired axonal transport, impaired synaptic plasticity, mitochondrial dysfunction, stressed endoplasmic reticulum (ER), impaired bioenergetics such as the loss of adenosine triphosphate (ATP), and impaired protein synthesis and weakness. In this chapter, we will delve into the biochemical aspects of neurological disorders, exploring some of the key mechanisms involved.

16.2 CLASSIFICATION OF NEUROLOGICAL DISORDERS

Different and distinct types of ND have been reported in the human population. NDs can be classified into three main categories: traumatic, neurodegenerative, and neuropsychiatric disorders (Figure 16.1). Neurotraumatic diseases are associated with neurological dysfunction caused by trauma to the head or spine, including stroke, traumatic brain injury (TBI), spinal cord injury (SCI), and traumatic encephalopathy chronic injury (CTE). Alzheimer's disease (AD), Parkinson's disease (PD), and Huntington's disease (HD) are the main prevalent neurodegenerative diseases. Multiple sclerosis (MS) is a chronic autoimmune disease of the central nervous system characterized by inflammation, demyelination, gliosis, and neurodegeneration. Amyotrophic lateral sclerosis (ALS) is a neurodegenerative disease characterized by progressive muscle paralysis that reflects degeneration of the primary motor cortex, cortical regions, brain stem, and spinal cord. Anxiety, major depressive disorder, autism, seizures, epilepsy, post-traumatic stress, attention-deficit/hyperactivity, and schizophrenia are some common neuropsychiatric disorders. The aberrant release of neurotransmitters, such as gamma-aminobutyric acid (GABA), dopamine, serotonin, and glutamate, and the disruption of their release, associated with neuroinflammation and mild oxidative stress, have been implicated in neuropsychiatric disorders.

16.3 BIOCHEMICAL BASIS OF THE NEUROLOGICAL DISEASES

16.3.1 Neurotraumatic Diseases

In neurotraumatic diseases, ATP levels drop quickly, ion homeostasis fails, neuroinflammation and oxidative stress develop rapidly, and interaction of aberrant neuron-glia occurs. Acute neurodegeneration that occurs within minutes to hours is a common complication of neurotraumatic diseases (40). A schematic diagram of traumatic brain injury and its consequences in the brain is illustrated in Figure 16.2.

16.3.1.1 Stroke

Stroke is a complex metabolic injury in the brain caused by a substantial decrease in or blockage of blood flow within the brain, which results in a decrease in the transport of glucose and oxygen to the brain tissue, the accumulation of possibly toxic substances in the brain, and the breakdown of the blood–brain barrier (BBB). Ischemic and hemorrhagic strokes are the two types of strokes. Ischemic strokes occur due to a severe reduction in blood supply to different parts of the brain, which leads to neurodegeneration. It is sub-classified as embolic and thrombotic strokes, where embolic stroke results from a clot that first develops anywhere in the body and then travels via

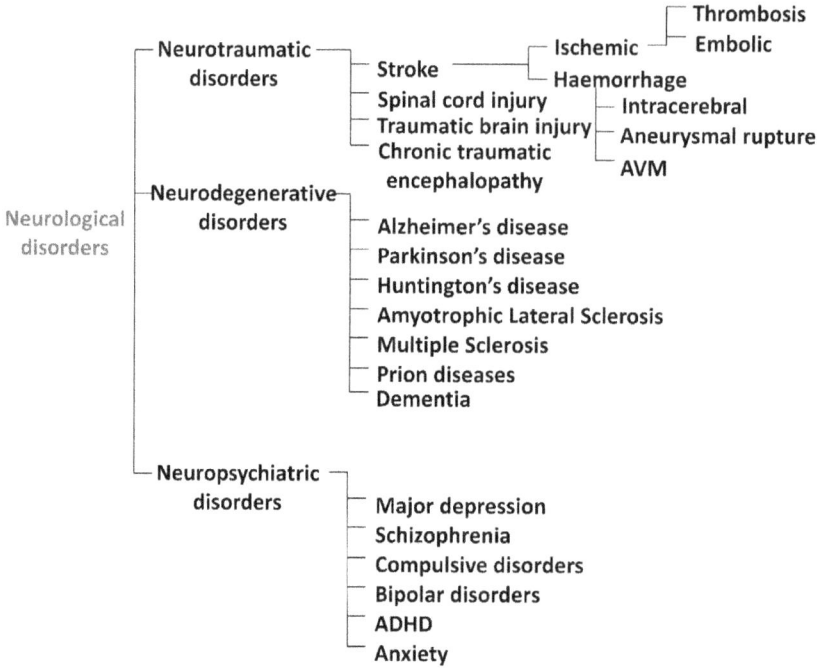

Figure 16.1 Neurological disorders and their classification

the bloodstream to the brain; and thrombotic stroke or infarction happens when a clot forms within the artery that travels to the brain. Hemorrhagic strokes occur due to a rupture in the artery wall, causing blood to flow throughout the brain (41). The major risk factor of stroke is age.

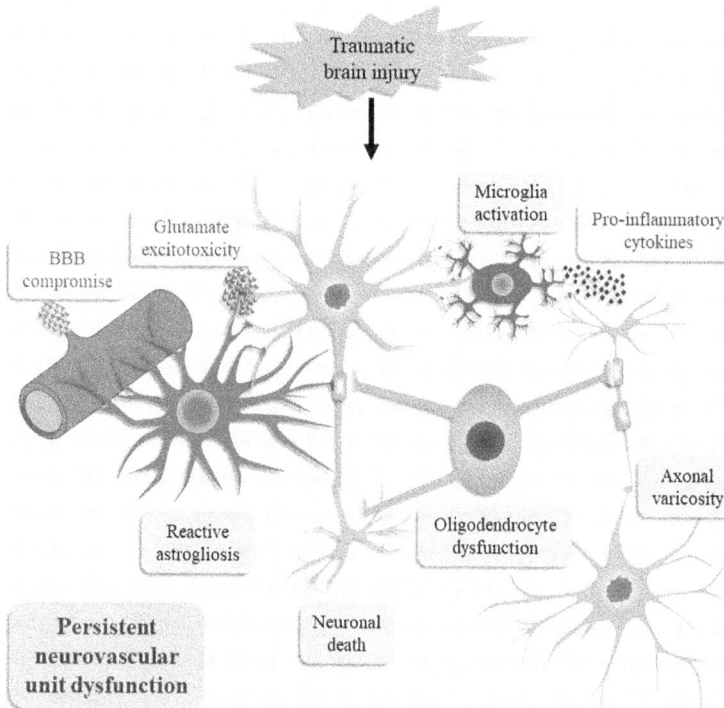

Figure 16.2 Traumatic brain injury causing persistent neurovascular unit dysfunction

The synaptic spine loss appears to be an initial indication of cerebral ischemia and usually plays a role in subsequent brain injury. The extracellular glutamate overstimulates glutamate receptors at the beginning of a stroke, causing rapid Ca2+ influx, stimulating phospholipases A_2, C, and D, calmodulin-dependent kinases, nitric oxide synthases, mitogen-activated protein kinases such as extracellular signal-regulated kinase, c-Jun N-terminal kinase, and p38, calcineurin, calpains, and endonucleases that cause hydrolysis of phospholipids, proteolysis, and defective phosphorylation leading to the interruption of the docking of glutamate-containing vesicles; these are all mechanisms by which stroke causes neural excitotoxicity. Many of these enzymes cause neuronal injury by boosting reactive oxygen species (ROS) generation through the oxidation of cell membrane-bound nicotinamide adenine dinucleotide phosphate (NADPH), mitochondrial malfunction, and unregulated arachidonic acid cascade (through the activation of PLA2, cyclooxygenase, and lipoxygenase). Stroke also sets off a strong inflammatory response that includes endogenous microglia activation and peripheral leukocyte infiltration into cerebral parenchyma (41). Through the necrotic and apoptotic cell death, there is an elevated number of oxidants, calcium influx, and mitochondrial dysfunction, all of which lead to neurodegeneration. These conditions result in a lack of energy (ATP) supply. Nitric oxide production may also increase as a result of excessive glutamate receptor stimulation, which can be dangerous to neural cells since nitric oxide reacts with superoxides, generating the toxic substance peroxynitrite. The high level of peroxynitrite and other oxidants induces the death of neurons. Dysphagia, sensory impairment, dysarthria aphasia, visual impairment, cognitive impairment, and poststroke depression are all stroke-related injuries (40).

16.3.1.2 Traumatic Brain Injury (TBI)

Traumatic brain injuries occur due to an external force impacting the head during motor accidents, as well as resulting from sports like football, boxing, hockey, skiing, wrestling, etc., among young adults (15–24 years). Military veterans (20–30 years) are exposed to repeated concussions as well as mild traumatic brain injuries, and the leading cause of TBI among seniors (75 years and above) is injuries from falls. The primary injury in TBI happens immediately and the symptoms are seen in the rise in intracranial pressure, neural cell death, diffuse axonal shearing, the rupture of blood–brain barrier permeability, and microvessel and microglial rupture. Contrarily, secondary TBI happens at a later point in time, when Ca^{2+} influx, microglial cell and astrocyte activation, the development of cellular stress and neuroinflammation, as well as the death of apoptotic cells, occurs as an outcome of secondary damage. This secondary injury takes time to show its clinical symptoms; this may be days, weeks, or months. Primary injury happens in a matter of moments, and its biological effects remain for a lifetime, inducing excitotoxicity, a rise in Ca^{2+} influx, the activation of Ca^{2+}-dependent enzymes, viz. cPLA2, COX-2, NOS, MMPs, and calpains, oxidative stress, a reduction in ATP, the destruction of the blood–brain barrier, an increase in the production of proinflammatory chemokines and cytokines, as well as changes in cellular redox. Cerebral ischemia is also another factor of the secondary TBI that results in the reduction of cerebral blood flow after TBI, causing mitochondrial damage, changes in ion homeostasis, the formation of edema, in addition to affecting the interactions of neurons and glial cells, leading to neuroinflammation (40).

16.3.1.3 Spinal Cord Injury (SCI)

SCI is a fatal neurological condition that can cause loss of sensory and motor function, paralysis, and death, depending on the severity of the injuries (41). It can be classified into primary and secondary events. The primary event is mainly caused by the mechanical trauma during which the spinal cord tissue is acutely stretched, which ruptures the neural cell membranes and changes the BBB's permeability, causing the intracellular contents to be released (40). This primary event is instantaneous and results in damage to neuronal fiber and neuronal cell death (41). In the secondary event, pathophysiological alterations and systemic and local neurochemical alterations, like an increase in excitatory amino acids, edema, ischemia, and reactive oxygen species, occur in the tissue of spinal cord after the primary traumatic injury. In addition to the growth of glial cells like astrocytes, microglia, and oligodendrocytes, these neurochemical changes also cause leukocyte infiltration, macrophage activation, and the activation of vascular endothelial cells, which leads to neurodegeneration. Spinal cord injury also develops a systemic, syndrome of neurogenic immune depression, which is indicated by a sharp decline in CD14+ monocytes, CD19+ B-lymphocytes, CD3+ T-lymphocytes, and MHC class II (HLA-DR)+ cells that starts within 24 hours and reaches a minimum level during the first week (40). Autoantibodies that attach to nuclear antigens like DNA and RNA are also produced due to spinal cord injury. There is also a release of glutamate, the production of reactive oxygen species (ROS) and reactive nitrogen species (RNS), the induction of NF-κB, an increase in the production and expression of IL-1β, IL-6, and TNF-α, along with the activation of the proteases at the site of injury. Therefore, changes in the cellular redox, ion homeostasis, and enzymatic activity, mitochondrial issues, the stimulation of neurodestructive and neuroprotective genes, and an increase in the production of proinflammatory cytokines and chemokines occur after these neurochemical events (40).

16.3.1.4 Chronic Traumatic Encephalopathy (CTE)

Repetitive moderate brain trauma (RMBT) is a risk factor for the neurodegenerative tauopathy known as chronic traumatic encephalopathy (CTE). CTE is a significant public health concern since RMBTs, subconcussive insults, and traumatic brain injury are all common among numerous athletes and military personnel. An uncertainty surrounds the link between CTE and concussion. The frequency of concussions, however, is said to not be considerably correlated with the pathology of CTE. Sudden changes in mood, behavior, and cognition are frequently brought on by CTE. Movement and speech problems are brought on by the stimulation of astrocytes and microglia, cytokine production, the development of neuroinflammation, and other late-stage symptoms of CTE. The tau neurofibrillary tangles (NFTs) have a specific topographic position and cellular architecture that can be used to distinguish CTE from other neurodegenerative disorders. CTE is identified utilizing antibodies against the phosphorylated tau (p-tau) protein; it is also characterized by changes in the BBB and postmortem tissues (40).

16.3.2 NEURODEGENERATIVE DISEASES

Neurodegeneration is associated with the dysfunction of synapses and the neural network, and the deposition of physico-chemically altered variants of proteins in the brain (Figure 16.3). Neurodegenerative diseases mainly refer to illnesses that have neurodegeneration as their defining characteristic (7). Although age is the single most important risk factor for the onset of all neurodegenerative diseases, recent research has shown that genetic make-up and environmental factors may significantly increase the risk of neurodegenerative disorders. The onset of neurodegenerative diseases occurs when neurons fail to respond adaptively to an age- and lifestyle-related

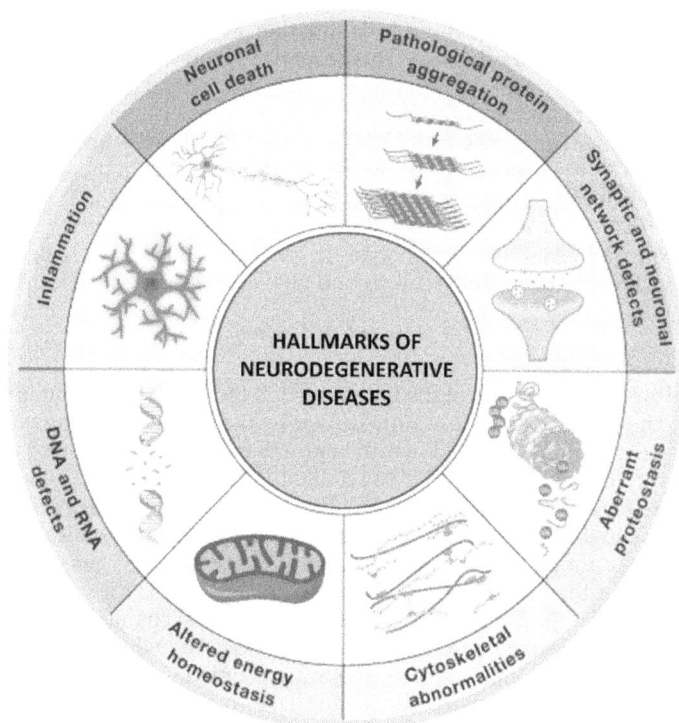

Figure 16.3 Hallmarks of neurodegenerative diseases

increase in oxidative stress and neuro-inflammation. Glutathione, glutathione peroxidase, gluta-thione-S-transferase, and superoxide dismutase levels often fall significantly when oxidative stress and neuro-inflammation persists.

16.3.2.1 Alzheimer's Disease

AD is a progressive neurodegenerative disorder that causes cognitive decline, memory loss, behavioral and personality changes, difficulties reasoning, disorientation, and language difficul-ties in the geriatric population. AD is identified within the brain by the aggregation of amyloid-beta (Aβ) plaques and tau protein-based neurofibrillary tangles (NFTs) (8). Initially, the breakdown of amyloid precursor protein (APP) by β-secretase 1 (BACE-1) enzyme leads to the release of a soluble N-terminus exodomain (APPβ) into the lumen and a membrane-bound β-C-terminus frag-ment (β-CTF). This membrane-bound β-CTF then undergoes cleavage by gamma secretase, which produces Aβ peptides, including Aβ38, Aβ40, and Aβ42 (9). The production of Aβ plaques is mainly accompanied by activated microglial cells and astrocytes, along with overexpressed proinflamma-tory markers such as TNF-α, IL-1β, and IL-6 (10). Meanwhile, the tau protein is obtained from an alternative splicing of the microtubule-associated protein tau (MAPT) gene, resulting in differ-ent soluble protein isoforms. The imbalance in the Aβ aggregation and its clearance lead to the formation of soluble Aβ oligomers, Aβ plaques, and intraneuronal Aβ, causing synaptic damage, neurodegeneration, and ultimately dementia (11). Interestingly, Aβ toxicity appears to depend on the presence of hyperphosphorylated forms of tau, which are deposited as NFTs in the brains of those with AD. Synaptic loss is a reliable predictor of clinical symptoms, even though there is no link between the load of Aβ plaque and tau hyperphosphorylation, on the one hand, and memory problems in AD patients on the other.

AD is biochemically associated with oxidative stress, mitochondrial dysfunction, neuroinflam-mation, and various enzyme changes that can lead to the depletion of neurotransmitter systems in the hippocampus and cerebral cortex, such as cholesterol hydroxylases (CYP46), phospholipases A2 (PLA2), and sphingomyelinases (SMase) (12, 13). The levels of neurotransmitters such as sero-tonin (5-HT), acetylcholine (Ach), norepinephrine, glutamate, and somatostatin are often reduced due to Aβ plaque formation. Low levels of Ach in the brain lead to the impairment of learning and memory in AD patients (14). The hyperphosphorylation of tau protein and NFT in AD brains leads to the impairment of misfolded protein degradation machinery called the ubiquitin-proteasome system (UPS) and ATP supply, along with disruption of antioxidant defense mechanisms, which leads to an abrupt increase in reactive oxygen species (ROS) (15). The Aβ plaques not only induce abnormal calcium influx and impair calcium homeostasis; they also promote the release of proin-flammatory cytokines by modulating COX-2 and NOS activities (16–18).

16.3.2.2 Parkinson's Disease

PD is a chronic and progressive movement disorder that affects 15 out of 100,000 old-age individu-als globally (19). It is primarily characterized by the degeneration of dopaminergic neurons in the substantia nigra pars compacta of the brain and the accumulation of misfolded α-synuclein proteins, leading to the depletion of the neurotransmitter dopamine (DA) (20). The degeneration of dopaminergic neurons causes irregular neurotransmission in the basal ganglia motor circuit that results in movement and locomotor dysfunction. Clinical features consist of motor and non-motor symptoms, such as akinesia, tremors, bradykinesia, rigidity, depression, apathy, cognitive dysfunction, and sleep disorders (21, 22). PD can be both familial and sporadic. The mutation of several genes has been identified as a cause of PD, including α-synuclein, PINK1, LRRK2, DJ-1, Parkin, and UCHL1 (23). An over-accumulation of α-synuclein due to mutation and other stimuli, such as stress and environmental factors, results in the formation of Lewy bodies that disrupt neurotransmission in the brain (24). The aggregated α-synuclein is known to induce mitochondrial dysfunction and cause apoptosis of dopaminergic neurons. The activity of PINK1, which initiates autophagy and helps to remove toxic aggregates of α-synuclein, is disrupted by its mutation in PD (25). The dysfunction of DJ-1 can induce mitochondrial dysfunction and oxidative stress, which are also implicated in the onset of PD (26). Cases of sporadic PD may be caused by a variety of genetic and environmental risk factors, which can result in mitochondrial dysfunction, oxidative stress, neuroinflammation, excitotoxicity, the misfolding and aggregation of α-synuclein, deficiencies in proteasomal function, the autophagy-lysosomal degradation of damaged proteins, and cell-auton-omous mechanisms (27).

Protein misfolding and accumulation in intracellular regions have become the hypoth-esized reasons for PD. The phosphorylation, nitration, and truncation of α-synuclein lead to the production of its oligomeric species with abnormal solubility, which can aggregate into fibrils and be ubiquitinated (28). Extracellular α-synuclein is known to modulate the activities of astrocytes and microglial cells, which results in the secretion of proinflammatory cytokines. Studies have shown that a proportion of α-synuclein resides within the mitochondria and over-accumulation can lead to downregulation of mitochondrial complex I activity, disrupting the energy metabolism of ATP production. This leads to the generation of ROS that can trigger the transcription of inflammation cascades, such as nuclear factor-kappa B (NF-KB) (29). The UPS remains disrupted by the toxicity induced and abnormal molecular signaling caused by the formation of Lewy bodies (30). Disrupted cystatin expression and cathepsin activity are also reported in patients and animal models of PD (31–32). The high levels of α-synuclein within the blood can contribute to CNS pathology, as levels of plasma in α-synuclein are significantly higher than the level of CSF (33). Besides DA, other neurotransmitters are often altered in PD; this includes decreased levels of GABA and serotonin and increased levels of Ach, glutamate, and histamine (34).

16.3.2.3 Huntington's Disease

Huntington disease (HD) is an autosomal dominant disorder that occurs due to the elongation of CAG repeats on the short arm of chromosome 4p16.3 in the HTT gene (35). This gene codes for the huntingtin protein. The mutation responsible for producing the disease is characterised by the amplification of a CAG repeat sequence within exon 1 of the HD gene. The wild type contains a CAG repetition that codes for a polyglutamine stretch in the protein at that site in the range 6 to 26. HD is associated with 36 repeats or more. The clinical manifestation happens when the number of repeats exceeds 40. The range 36–39 leads to an incomplete penetrance of the disease or very late onset. The range between 29 and 35, the so-called intermediate alleles, is unstable, which means that these alleles are prone to changes during reproduction. Copying the gene may lead to mistakes and very often leads to elongation and seldom to shortening. This phenomenon is seen mainly in the reproduction of males (36).

HD is an inherited neurodegenerative disorder that causes the loss of neurons that are medium spiny projection neurons within the brain, primarily in the cortex and striatum, as well as the hippocampus regions. The disease usually develops between the ages of 30 and 50 and progresses for an average of 17–20 years, causing physical, cognitive, and emotional deterioration, involuntary movements, dementia, and personality changes. It ultimately leads to premature death, most commonly from pneumonia or suicide. The HTT protein is expressed in all glial cells and neurons, but in HD, proteolytic fragments of huntingtin accumulate in both the cytoplasm and nucleus, leading to various cellular dysfunctions, such as altered signaling pathways, synaptic transmission impairments, protein trafficking defects, proteasome dysfunction, and mitochondrial alterations. Mutant huntingtin produces toxicity through protein aggregation, defective energy metabolism, transcriptional dysregulation, excitotoxicity, oxidative stress, inflammation, and the loss of beneficial functions of wild-type huntingtin (37). Mounting evidence shows that the mutant huntingtin disrupts mitochondrial functions, leading to energetic defects, reactive oxygen species overload, and the release of proapoptotic molecules. Impairment of mitochondrial complex II/III activity has been observed in HD patients, and downregulation of peroxisome proliferator-activated receptor gamma coactivator-1-alpha (PGC-1α), a key transcriptional coactivator that controls mitochondrial biogenesis and energy metabolism, has been shown to occur in HD due to interference with the CREB/TAF4-dependent transcriptional pathway (38). Recent studies have linked fragmented mitochondria to HD due to the increased activity of dynamin-related protein 1, highlighting the role of mitochondrial damage in the development of HD (39).

16.3.3 NEUROPSYCHIATRIC DISEASES

Mild chronic oxidation and neuroinflammation are associated with neuropsychiatric disorders. Neuronal network-mediated anomalies, unbalanced neurotransmission, and over- or under-expression of genes that regulate behavioral symptoms may all contribute to abnormalities in neuropsychiatric illnesses at the nuclear level (Figure 16.4). Hormonal dysfunctions and environmental variables, such as heavy metals or other poison exposure, can also play a role in the etiology of neuropsychiatric illnesses. The reduction in neuronal and glial size, the rise in density of the cellular pack, the disruption of neuronal connection, mainly in the dorsolateral prefrontal cortex, and the distortion of neuronal direction are further factors that contribute to grey-matter atrophy in neuropsychiatric illnesses (40).

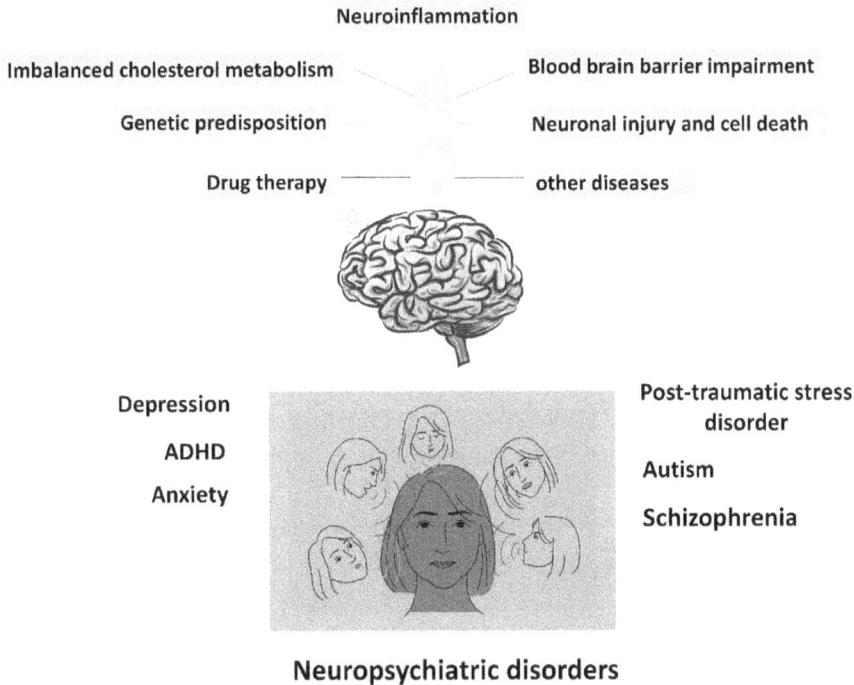

Figure 16.4 Causes of neuropsychiatric disorders

16.3.3.1 Anxiety

Anxiety neurosis is characterized by feelings of tension and apprehension, shortness of breath, palpitations, nervousness, irritability, chest pain and discomfort, easy fatigue, dizziness, numbness and tingling of the skin, trembling, and faintness, as well as acute anxiety attacks. An excessive increase in lactate, a typical metabolic product, is observed in patients with anxiety neurosis. A study has demonstrated that lactate infusions can cause anxiety symptoms and attacks (42). It is thought that anxiety disorders are extremely complicated and polygenic. Although it is well recognized that genetics may impact how anxiety symptoms manifest, more anxiety disorders are caused by the interplay of genetics and stressful environmental factors than by genetics alone. The increased risk of developing anxiety disorders may be influenced by several genes that have been discovered. A serotonin transporter gene, also known as SERT, has been a promising discovery. The serotonin transporter plays a critical role in controlling serotonin levels in synapses. In the neuronal circuitry that regulates mood and temperament, serotonin synapses are important. Numerous psychiatric diseases are known to be influenced by issues in the serotonin system. Mutations in the SERT gene have been linked to increased anxiety-related personality characteristics and decreased serotonin activity. The increased anxiety reactions frequently observed in anxiety disorders may be caused by several brain structures and pathways. The prefrontal cortex, hippocampus, and amygdala in particular have been associated with anxiety disorders (43).

16.3.3.2 Depression

A multisystem and multifactorial mental condition, depression is characterized by sad mood, anhedonia (limited capacity to enjoy natural pleasures), irritability, concentration problems, irregular eating, and abnormal sleep patterns (neurovegetative symptoms). Several studies on depression have found that depressed people have altered cerebral structures, glial density and decreased grey-matter volume in the hippocampal regions and the prefrontal cortex, elevated blood levels of TNF-α and IL-6, low levels of magnesium, and an overactive hypothalamic pituitary adrenal axis. Uncertainty remains regarding the chemical basis of depression (40). Major depression is distinguished from the other types by a persistently depressed mood that lasts longer than 2 weeks, as well as other symptoms like difficulty concentrating, a loss of interest in activities, changes in appetite and sleeping, feelings of unworthiness, and suicide attempts (44).

The pathophysiology of depression, however, is thought to entail changes in the neurotransmitters, including dopamine, norepinephrine, and serotonin, as well as a rise in inflammation, faults in neurogenesis, a decline in synaptic plasticity, mitochondrial malfunction, and redox imbalance. Additionally, modifications to vasopressin, cytokines, and interactions between genes within the external environment may contribute to the pathophysiology of depression (40). The cause of depression is unclear and may involve both hereditary and the environment risk factors (44).

16.3.3.3 Attention-Deficit Hyperactivity Disorder (ADHD)

The attention-deficit hyperactivity disorder (ADHD) affects about 5% of children and adults and affects men more often than women. Its symptoms include inattention, hyperactivity and impulsivity, and executive functioning issues, all of which go beyond which is typical for the development stage. A variant of ADHD called attention-deficit disorder (ADD) is sometimes identified in people who do not exhibit the hyperactive component of symptoms. Many patients who have ADHD also exhibit comorbidity, or the occurrence of secondary conditions on top of ADHD (45).

Although there is no known cause of ADHD, research suggests that there may be delays and dysfunctions in the prefrontal cortex's development, along with complications in neurotransmission. Research conducted on twins revealed a substantial hereditary component. Although no clear relations have been identified, there are several possible genes that may cause ADHD. An external factor, like exposure to various pesticides, may potentially play a role in the emergence of ADHD. Behavioral therapy and the administration of stimulant drugs are frequently used in the treatment of ADHD, having a calming effect on patients (45).

16.3.3.4 Post-traumatic Stress Disorder

Witnessing an incident that is life-threatening or that has the potential to harm the person or others can cause psychological distress. These events, which are frequently accompanied by extreme terror, horror, and helplessness, might contribute to the onset of post-traumatic stress disorder (PTSD). PTSD is an extreme case, with the severity of the response relating to the degree of the trauma or stressor. When thinking about the interactions between stressful situations, stress responses, and disease, a variety of factors need to be considered. The principal controller of the human neuroendocrine stress response systems, the hypothalamic-pituitary-adrenal (HPA) axis, has been the focus of much attention in studies on PTSD patients. Numerous studies have investigated the neurobiological alterations found in PTSD patients that are indicators of neural susceptibility to the disorder upon exposure to extreme stress, as opposed to abnormalities acquired through traumatic exposure. For instance, low cortisol levels immediately following a trauma indicate the later development of PTSD. Therefore, low levels of cortisol may be one risk factor in the development of PTSD. Low levels of cortisol may disinhibit corticotropin-releasing hormone circuits and thus stimulate unopposed autonomic and neuroendocrine responses to stress (46).

16.3.3.5 Autism Spectrum Disorder

An autism spectrum disorder (ASD) is distinguished by limitations in social interaction, communication, as well as confined and repetitive interests and behaviors. Patients with ASD have a wide range of symptoms, and several animal models of the disorder have been created with mutations that closely resemble those discovered in the ASD patients. The origins of ASD are generally unclear, except for a few well-known, hereditary types of autism like Rett's syndrome and Fragile X. ASD is correlated with variations in several genes, although for any patient, the illness may need several mutations in various genes. ASD is often considered to be a disorder of "incorrect" wiring. As a result, some ASD patients do not exhibit the same degree of synaptic pruning as healthy individuals. There is uncertainty regarding the molecular processes involved in the pathophysiology of ASD. However, it is hypothesized that an aberrant immune response, autoimmunity, and persistent neuroinflammation may have a detrimental effect on neurodevelopment, thereby contributing to the etiology of autism. The cerebellum, amygdala, hippocampus, and insular cortex of autistic individuals have all been linked to structural abnormalities. Studies using animal models show that stress decreases brain-derived neurotrophic factor (BDNF) expression or activity in the hippocampus, and that this decrease may be stopped by taking antidepressants. Recent data supports the idea that chronic neuroinflammation and significant environmental influences may also play a role in the pathophysiology of autism, in addition to hereditary factors. Some evidence also frames autism as a neuropsychiatric illness with an unknown pathophysiology. Neuroinflammation, abnormalities in the peripheral immune system, and environmental factors are characteristics of ASD. These variables may interact to cause the symptoms of ASD (40, 47).

16.3.3.6 Schizophrenia

Schizophrenia is a severe and frequently disabling mental disorder. An inability to distinguish between fantasy and reality, uncontrolled and inappropriate emotional reactions, difficulty thinking, and social interaction issues are all signs of the illness. People who have schizophrenia may experience delusions and hallucinations and they may hear voices. Additionally, patients also experience "negative" symptoms, such as a loss of pleasure, a flattened emotional state, and a loss of fundamental drives (44, 45). Dopaminergic neurons that are not performing normally are considered to have a role in the onset of schizophrenia, and glutamate signaling issues might also play a role. Antipsychotic drugs are typically needed to treat the disorder because they block dopamine receptors and reduce dopamine neurotransmission within the brain. Some people may experience symptoms like Parkinson's disease as a result of dopamine reduction. The majority of patients must use antipsychotic medications for the rest of their lives, despite the fact that few classes of these medications can be highly effective in the treatment of the condition (44).

16.3.4 OTHERS

There are several other neurological disorders, such as dystonia, amyotrophic lateral sclerosis, neuromuscular disease, multiple sclerosis, epilepsy, dementia, motor neuron disease, neurological infections, etc. Dystonia is characterized by excessive muscular contractions that result in abnormal and involuntary movements. Its clinical signs vary depending on the muscles involved and the intensity of their contractions, but the underlying biological issue is excessive muscular contraction (48).

Motor neurons, which are specialized nerve cells in the brain and spinal cord, gradually deteriorate in motor neuron disease. The reason is still unclear. Amyotrophic lateral sclerosis (ALS) is the most prevalent kind of motor neuron disease. Motor neurons, specialized nerve cells in the brain and spinal cord, malfunction and die too soon in motor neuron disease. Muscle movements such as grasping, walking, speaking, eating, and breathing are all controlled by motor neurons.

An adult-onset neurodegenerative disease called amyotrophic lateral sclerosis (ALS) selectively kills motor neurons, resulting in paralysis and death. A portion of ALS cases are brought on by mutations in the Cu, Zn superoxide dismutase (SOD1) gene, which give this antioxidant enzyme a harmful increase in function. It is generally accepted that this neurotoxic feature results from either a tendency to lose stabilizing post-translational modifications or a greater propensity to misfold and aggregation caused by a loss in the stability of the original homodimer. A complex network of interconnected pathological processes, including glutamate excitotoxicity, dysregulation of neurotrophic factors and axon guidance proteins, defects in axonal transport, mitochondrial dysfunction, inadequate protein quality control, and abnormal RNA processing, have been identified through the study of the molecular mechanisms of SOD1-related ALS. Misfolded and aggregated SOD1 and/or cytosolic calcium excess directly worsen many of these diseases, indicating the importance of these occurrences in disease etiology and their potential as therapeutic targets (49).

Multiple sclerosis (MS) is a persistent inflammatory demyelination disorder affecting the central nervous system (CNS) in humans. Over the course of several years, it can progress into a neurodegenerative state characterised by significant clinical deficits.. It is most likely to develop as the consequence of a complicated interaction of genetic variables, environmental triggers, and viral events. The reason for this is the autoimmune condition in which the immune system mistakenly targets certain substances. As a result, the CNS myelin is formed and recognized as foreign, after which it is triggered to be destroyed. Axonal injury and neurodegeneration eventually results from the development of demyelinated plaques due to multiple sclerosis (50).

Epilepsy mainly occurs after stroke. When there is excessive firing in the cortical neurons, hypersynchronously, or in both, this temporarily disrupts the normal brain function and manifests as recurring, unprovoked seizures. According to predictions, up to 3% of Americans experience epilepsy at some point in their lives. Even though epilepsy comes in many forms, all of them have recurring seizures as a characteristic. Epilepsy may be a sign of brain disorder, disease, or another sickness. For instance, persons with intellectual disabilities or autism spectrum disorder (ASD) may suffer from seizures, possibly due to the same issues that led to their problems. For many patients, the underlying cause of their epilepsy has not been found , and is believed to be a combination of genetic and environmental factors. The use of anticonvulsant drugs can frequently control seizures; removing the part of the brain that causes seizures, however, may be necessary for patients in severe cases (45). The acute symptomatic seizures might not reoccur once the root cause has been treated or after the acute phase has passed.

Dementia is a chronic illness that results from a brain disorder that impairs many of higher cortical functions, including memory, reasoning, direction, understanding, calculations, learning ability, language, and judgment (47, 51). These are just a few of the higher cortical skills that are disrupted in dementia, which can be either chronic or progressive. There is no obscuration of consciousness and 2% of dementia cases begin before the age of 65. It primarily affects older people. With every 5-year increase in age, the prevalence doubles. The main cause of impairment in later life is dementia. When strokes or other blood vessel disorders frequently interrupt the brain's flow of oxygenated blood, causing significant cumulative damage to brain tissue and function, vascular dementia (VaD) is identified. A few uncommon dementia-causing conditions, such as hypercalcemia, subdural hemorrhages, hydrocephalus with normal pressure, and deficiencies in thyroid hormone, vitamin B12, and folic acid, may be successfully treated with prompt medical or surgical intervention (51).

When viruses, bacteria, parasites, or fungi enter the brain system through the circulation or peripheral neurons, neurological infection develops. When some viral diseases, like the rabies virus, enter the brain, they can result in uncertainty and seizures. Some neurological infections, including syphilis, tuberculosis, and brain abscesses, are caused by bacteria. Neuroinfections or brain inflammation like encephalitis and meningitis are caused by viral or bacterial inflammation. Viral neuroinfections can either be chronically sluggish or acutely fast. Encephalitis, aseptic meningitis, and encephalomyelitis are examples of acute viral infections. Panencephalitis and retrovirus diseases are examples of chronic viral infections (47).

16.4 CONCLUSION

The biochemical basis of neurological disorders is a multifaceted and complex area of research that has significantly advanced our understanding of these conditions. By unraveling the intricate biochemical mechanisms underlying disorders such as Parkinson's disease, Alzheimer's disease, Huntington's disease, multiple sclerosis, and amyotrophic lateral sclerosis, researchers have made strides in developing targeted therapies and interventions. The identification of specific biochemical abnormalities, such as protein misfolding, neurotransmitter imbalances, oxidative stress, mitochondrial dysfunction, and inflammation, has paved the way for the development of novel treatment approaches. From acetylcholinesterase inhibitors and dopamine replacement therapy to amyloid-beta and tau-targeting therapies, researchers are actively exploring various strategies to alleviate symptoms and modify the progression of neurological disorders.

Looking to the future, continued research in the field of the biochemical basis of neurological disorders holds great promise. Advances in technology, including genomics, proteomics, and imaging techniques, offer opportunities to gain deeper insights into the intricate molecular processes involved. This knowledge may contribute information that could lead to the discovery of new therapeutic targets and the development of personalized medicine approaches that consider individual variations in biochemistry and genetics. Furthermore, emerging fields, such as neuropharmacology, gene therapy, and neurodegeneration, hold exciting potential for the treatment and prevention of neurological disorders. By leveraging our understanding of the biochemical basis of these conditions, researchers can design interventions that directly target the underlying molecular abnormalities, potentially providing more effective and tailored treatments.

In summary, the exploration of the biochemical basis of neurological disorders has already yielded significant advancements in our understanding and treatment of these complex conditions. Continued research efforts, along with interdisciplinary collaborations and technological innovations, will likely propel us toward more precise diagnostics, targeted therapies, and ultimately improved outcomes for individuals affected by neurological disorders in the future.

REFERENCES

1. Farooqui AA. Neurodegeneration in Neural Trauma, neurodegenerative diseases, and neuropsychiatric disorders. In: AA Farooqui (Ed.) *Neurochemical Aspects of Neurotraumatic and Neurodegenerative Diseases*. 2010. p. 1–25.

2. Feigin VL, Nichols E, Alam T, Bannick MS, Beghi E, Blake N, et al. Global, regional, and national burden of neurological disorders, 1990–2016: A systematic analysis for the Global Burden of Disease Study 2016. *Lancet Neurol*. 2019;18(5):459–80.

3. Deleidi M, Jäggle M, Rubino G. Immune ageing, dysmetabolism and inflammation in neurological diseases. *Front Neurosci.* 2015;9(APR):172 (1–14).

4. Callixte KT, Clet TB, Jacques D, Faustin Y, François DJ, Maturin TT. The pattern of neurological diseases in elderly people in outpatient consultations in Sub-Saharan Africa. *BMC Res Notes.* 2015;8(1):159 (1–6).

5. Sahu S, Nag DS, Swain A, Samaddar DP, Sanjay Nag D. Biochemical changes in the injured brain. *World J Biol Chem.* 2017;26(81):21–31.

6. Barman KP. Biochemical changes in the brain and metabolism as risk factors of neurological disorders. *World J Neurosci.* 2022;12(02):45–56.

7. Li M. The role of P53 up-regulated modulator of apoptosis (PUMA) in ovarian development, cardiovascular and neurodegenerative diseases. *Apoptosis.* 2021;26(5–6):235–47.

8. Calderon-Garcidueñas, A. L., Duyckaerts, C.. Alzheimer disease. *Handbook of Clinical Neurology.* 2018;145:325–337.

9. Roda A, Serra-Mir G, Montoliu-Gaya L, Tiessler L, Villegas S. Amyloid-beta peptide and tau protein crosstalk in Alzheimer's disease. *Neural Regener Res.* 2022;17:1666–74.

10. Heppner FL, Ransohoff RM, Becher B. Immune attack: The role of inflammation in Alzheimer disease. *Nat Rev Neurosci.* 2015;16:358–72.

11. Jalbert JJ, Daiello LA, Lapane KL. Dementia of the Alzheimer type. *Epidemiol Rev.* 2008;30:15–34.

12. Schaeffer EL, da Silva ER, de A Novaes B, Skaf HD, Gattaz WF. Differential roles of phospholipases A2 in neuronal death and neurogenesis: Implications for Alzheimer disease. *Prog Neuro-Psychopharmacol Biol Psychiatry.* 2010;34:1381–9.

13. Heii A, Yosuke I, Kenji K, Takashi M, Reiji I. Neurotransmitter changes in early- and late-onset alzheimer-type dementia. *Prog Neuropsychopharmacol Biol Psychiatry.* 1992;16(6):883–90.

14. Levey AI. Muscarinic acetylcholine receptor expression in memory circuits: Implications for treatment of Alzheimer disease. *Proc Natl Acad Sci USA.* 1996;93(24):13541–6.

15. Ihara Y, Morishima-Kawashima M, Nixon R. The ubiquitin-proteasome system and the autophagic-lysosomal system in Alzheimer disease. *Cold Spring Harb Perspect Med.* 2012;2(8).

16. Supnet C, Bezprozvanny I. The dysregulation of intracellular calcium in Alzheimer disease. *Cell Calcium.* 2010;47:183–9.

17. Minghetti L. Cyclooxygenase-2 (COX-2) in inflammatory and degenerative brain diseases. *J Neuropathol Exp Neurol.* 2004;63:901–10.

18. Dorheim MA, Tracey WR, Pollock JS, Grammas P. Nitric oxide synthase activity is elevated in brain microvessels in alzheimer's disease. *Biochem Biophys Res Commun.* 1994;205(1):659–65.

19. Tysnes O-B, Storstein A. Epidemiology of {Parkinson}'s disease. *J Neural Transm.* 2017;124(8):901–5.

20. Lebouvier T, Chaumette T, Paillusson S, Duyckaerts C, Bruley Des Varannes S, Neunlist M, et al. The second brain and Parkinson's disease. *Eur J Neurosci.* 2009;30(5):735–41.

21. Moustafa AA, Chakravarthy S, Phillips JR, Gupta A, Keri S, Polner B, et al. Motor symptoms in Parkinson's disease: A unified framework. *Neurosci Biobehav Rev.* 2016;68:727–40.

22. Poewe W. Non-motor symptoms in Parkinson's disease. *Eur J Neurol*. 2008;15(s1):14–20.

23. Klein C, Westenberger A. Genetics of Parkinson's disease. *Cold Spring Harb Perspect Med*. 2012;

24. Poewe W, Seppi K, Tanner CM, Halliday GM, Brundin P, Volkmann J, et al. Parkinson disease. *Nat Rev Dis Prim*. 2017;3(1):1–21.

25. Song S, Jang S, Park J, Bang S, Choi S, Kwon KY, et al. Characterization of PINK1 (PTEN-induced putative kinase 1) mutations associated with parkinson disease in mammalian cells and drosophila. *J Biol Chem*. 2013;288(8):5660–72.

26. Pankratz N, Pauciulo MW, Elsaesser VE, Marek DK, Halter CA, Wojcieszek J, et al. Mutations in DJ-1 are rare in familial Parkinson disease. *Neurosci Lett*. 2006;408(3):209–13.

27. Dextera DT, Jenner P. Parkinson disease: From pathology to molecular disease mechanisms. *Free Radicals Biol Med*. 2013;62:132–44.

28. Fields CR, Bengoa-Vergniory N, Wade-Martins R. Targeting alpha-synuclein as a therapy for Parkinson's disease. *Front Mol Neurosci*. 2019;42:299 (1–14).

29. Bellucci A, Bubacco L, Longhena F, Parrella E, Faustini G, Porrini V, et al. Nuclear factor-κB dysregulation and α-Synuclein pathology: Critical interplay in the pathogenesis of Parkinson's disease. *Front Aging Neurosci*. 2020;12:68 (1–13).

30. Behl T, Kumar S, Althafar ZM, Sehgal A, Singh S, Sharma N, et al. Exploring the role of Ubiquitin–Proteasome system in Parkinson's disease. *Mol Neurobiol*. 2022;59:4257–73.

31. Xu J, Chen J, Mao C, Yang Y, Liu C. Preliminary relationship between serum cystatin C level and Parkinson's disease. *Natl Med J China*. 2014;94(11):804–7.

32. McGlinchey RP, Lacy SM, Huffer KE, Tayebi N, Sidransky E, Lee JC. C-terminal α-synuclein truncations are linked to cysteine cathepsin activity in Parkinson's disease. *J Biol Chem*. 2019;294(25):9973–84.

33. Chang CW, Yang SY, Yang CC, Chang CW, Wu YR. Plasma and serum alpha-synuclein as a biomarker of diagnosis in patients with Parkinson's disease. *Front Neurol*. 2020;10:1388 (1–7).

34. Di Michele F, Luchetti S, Bernardi G, Romeo E, Longone P. Neurosteroid and neurotransmitter alterations in Parkinson's disease. *Front Neuroendocrinol*. 2013;34:132–42.

35. MacDonald ME, Ambrose CM, Duyao MP, Myers RH, Lin C, Srinidhi L, et al. A novel gene containing a trinucleotide repeat that is expanded and unstable on Huntington's disease chromosomes. *Cell*. 1993;72(6):971–83.

36. Trottier Y, Biancalana V, Mandel JL. Instability of CAG repeats in Huntington's disease: Relation to parental transmission and age of onset. *J Med Genet*. 1994;31(5):377–82.

37. Rüb U, Vonsattel JPG, Heinsen H, Korf HW. The neuropathology of huntington's disease: Classical findings, recent developments and correlation to functional neuroanatomy. *Adv Anat Embryol Cell Biol*. 2015;217:1–146.

38. La Spada AR. PPARGC1A/PGC-1α, TFEB and enhanced proteostasis in Huntington disease. *Autophagy*. 2012;8(12):1845–7.

39. Vantaggiato C, Castelli M, Giovarelli M, Orso G, Bassi MT, Clementi E, et al. The fine tuning of drp1-dependent mitochondrial remodeling and autophagy controls neuronal differentiation. *Front Cell Neurosci*. 2019;13.

40. Farooqui AA. Neurochemical aspects of neurological disorders. *Curcumin Neurol Psychiatr Disord Neurochem Pharmacol Prop*. 2019;1–22.

41. Farooqui AA. Neurochemical aspects of neurological disorders. *Trace Amin Neurol Disord Potential Mech Risk Factors*. 2016;237–56.

42. Pitts FN. The biochemistry of anxiety. 2016;220(2):1–23.

43. Brawman-Mintzer, O., Lydiard, R. B.. Biological basis of generalized anxiety disorder. *Journal of Clinical Psychiatry*. 1997;58(3): 16–26.

44. Westin J. *Biological Bases of Nervous System Disorders*. pp. 1–8. https://jackwestin.com/resources/mcat-content/psychological-disorders/biological-bases-of-nervous-system-disorders.

45. Lange, K. W., Reichl, S., Lange, K. M., Tucha, L., Tucha, O.. The history of attention deficit hyperactivity disorder. *ADHD Attention Deficit and Hyperactivity Disorders*. 2010;2:241–255.

46. Sherin JE, Nemeroff CB. Post-traumatic stress disorder: The neurobiological impact of psychological trauma. *Dialogues Clin Neurosci*. 2011;13(3):263–78.

47. Fouad GI, Aly HH. Neurological disorders: Causes and treatments strategies. *Int J Public Ment Heal Neurosci*. 2018;5(1):32–3.

48. Jinnah HA, Sun Y V. Dystonia genes and their biological pathways. *Neurobiol Dis*. 2019;129(September):159–68.

49. Redler RL, Dokholyan N V. The complex molecular biology of Amyotrophic Lateral Sclerosis (ALS). *Prog Mol Biol Transl Sci*. 2012;107:215–262.

50. Lassmann, H.. Axonal injury in multiple sclerosis. *Journal of Neurology, Neurosurgery & Psychiatry*. 2003;74(6):695–697.

51. Moritz DJ, Fox PJ, Luscombe PA, Kraemer HC. Neurological and psychiatric predictors of mortality in patients with Alzheimer disease in California. *Arch Neurol*. 1997;54(7):878–85.

17 Clinical Management of Neurological Disorders

Mohit Agrawal, Manmohan Singhal, Yash Jasoria, Hema Chaudhary, and Bhupendra Prajapati

17.1 INTRODUCTION

The most prevalent neurological disorders (NDs) include Alzheimer's disease (AD), Parkinson's disease (PD), amyotrophic lateral sclerosis (ALS), and Huntington's disease (HD). These conditions are characterized by atrophy of the central nervous system (CNS) components (Figure 17.1). Despite substantial studies in the sector, the frequency of NDs is rising quickly. The disorders affect the patient's personality, intelligence, social skills, and vocational function since they are sporadic and familial, impacting specific areas of the brain , and cause motor and/or cognitive issues, such as aphasia, apraxia, and agnosia. The identification of genetic patterns and symptoms that disclose the kind of illness while the patient is still alive poses a major difficulty since the neuropathological symptoms of common NDs overlap. These ambiguities frequently cause incorrect diagnoses, which are followed by incorrect treatment. To enable better diagnostic approaches and to promote information sharing between scientists and medical practitioners, it is necessary to provide details on the fast-expanding insights into the genetic and molecular processes that cause NDs. Identification of genetic markers that may be connected to NDs is made easier by evaluating frequently occurring genetic alterations. Studies on diverse animal models and epidemiological research on humans provided conclusive proof that genetic and environmental variables may raise the risk of dementia [1]. The term "health-related quality of life" (HRQOL) refers to how neurological disorders and their treatments can impact a variety of aspects of social, psychological, and physical functioning. Treatment strategies frequently center on symptom control, lowering the severity of impairment, and stopping disease progression because many neurologic disorders are chronic and irreversible. Although certain medications can alter the course of many disorders, rehabilitation is the main goal of care. In essence, by lessening the effects of the condition, therapy often tries to enhance the social, physical, and mental elements of the individual's life. The entire impact of these illnesses and their therapies is not captured by conventional clinical and functional markers of disease state. In this context, multifaceted patient-reported outcome measures, such as HRQOL tools that evaluate social, physical, and mental health, might be more valuable, especially in clinical trials where variations in clinical assessments may or may not be relevant [2]. Whether the conceptual framework of the instrument adequately represents the HRQL experience of the population of interest is a critical factor in the creation and implementation of an HRQL instrument. This study presents the results of formative research that was concerned with identifying the subject matter for a neurology-specific HRQL measuring system [3]. Many chronic disorders with extremely complex etiologies are included in the category of neurological conditions. Several acute, as well as ongoing, neurological illnesses that cause persistent impairment have neuroaxonal loss and destruction as their pathological basis. In determining disease activity, tracking treatment outcomes, and predicting prognosis, the capacity to quickly identify and track such damage would be extremely helpful. Consequently, a biomarker that truly depicts neuroaxonal damage would be crucial for making individual treatment decisions and assessing the impact of medications in clinical management. Cerebrospinal fluid (CSF) proteins, magnetic resonance imaging (MRI), magnetic resonance spectroscopy, and metabolic imaging have all been investigated in the search for such a biomarker, and each method has offered a unique perspective with its own set of drawbacks [4].

17.2 GENERAL UNDERLYING MECHANISMS CONTRIBUTING TO NEUROLOGICAL DISORDERS

17.2.1 Network Dysfunction

The neurobiological underpinnings of functional decline in normal aging are less clear than those in neurodegenerative illnesses, which are characterized by significant neuron loss and impaired functioning. While ubiquitous neuron death in the neocortex and hippocampus has long been thought to be an inherent consequence of brain aging, recent statistical studies indicate that neuron death is restricted in healthy aging and is unlikely to be the cause of age-related impairment of neocortical and hippocampal functions [5]. The majority of medical professionals and family members who care for persons with neurological illnesses are fully aware of the significant changes in functional status that these patients experience, sometimes within the same day and

DOI: 10.1201/9781003384823-17

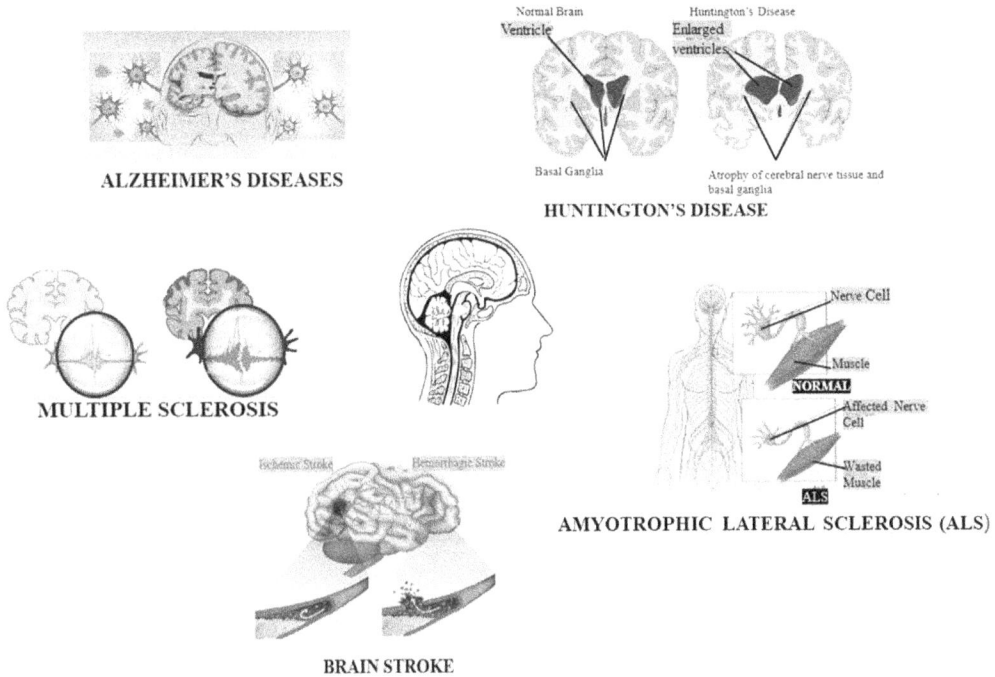

Figure 17.1 Some common neurological disorders

spanning a startling range of functional (dis)abilities. It is impossible for the abrupt loss or growth of nerve cells to be the source of these oscillations. Instead, they most likely represent changes in the activity of neuronal networks and perhaps prolonged poisoning by aberrant proteins that the brain is only momentarily able to overcome. The therapeutic implications of these concepts are extensive [6]. Eliminating aberrant proteins may help transgenic mice recover from their neurological abnormalities without altering their number of neurons [7]. So, instead of being the result of neuronal death, neurological impairments linked to NDs might be brought on by neuronal malfunction. Effective neural plasticity enables the brain to adapt to even severe neuronal losses, which lends credence to this idea [8].

17.2.2 Synaptic Dysfunction Leading to Network Failure

Protein structural changes that cause misfolding, aggregation, and the deposition of amyloid fibrils inside or outside of neurons are the hallmarks of many neurodegenerative diseases. Among the most effective inhibitors of neurodegeneration found in animal models of human illness, molecular chaperones serve as a first line of defense against misfolded, aggregation-prone proteins [9]. Excitotoxicity, inflammation, stress, and other processes are only a few of the many mechanisms that might be at play. In AD, synaptic loss outweighs neuronal loss, and a decrease in synapses and synaptic proteins is more closely associated with cognitive impairment than an increase in Aβ plaques or neurofibrillary tangles (NFTs) [10]. In relation to gene–environment interactions and experience-dependent plasticity in the healthy and sick brain, namely the cerebral cortex, the consequences of different environmental interventions are examined [11]. Apolipoprotein E4 (apoE4) is significantly more than just a cause of neurodegeneration. Repairing damaged neurons, maintaining synapto-dendritic connections, scavenging toxins, and redistributing lipids across CNS cells are all important roles played by apoE. ApoE4-associated neuropathology is caused by certain structural characteristics of this protein. Although in dynamic equilibrium, the structures of apoE2, apoE3, and apoE4 are more likely to adopt a disordered conformation in apoE4, which is harmful in a number of neurological illnesses [12].

17.2.3 Survival of Neurons

During various phases of NDs, a wide range of events may have an impact on the survival of neurons. These include co-morbid conditions like vascular disease, hereditary variables like apoE isoforms, the functionality of neurons in afflicted regions, and people's capacity to apply certain learning mechanisms to overcome impairments. Aside from that, different brain networks might make up for the missing neurons [13]. The comparatively minor deficiencies in fibroblast growth factor 2 (FGF2) knockout in mice are not the result of fibroblast growth factor 1 (FGF1) compensating for them, which suggests that both proteins have very limited functions throughout normal physiological and developmental processes [14]. A big myth is that for a neural network to operate effectively, certain cellular and synaptic parameters must be controlled to certain values. There may be significant animal-to-animal variation in many of the parameters that control network activity, and a variety of combinations of synaptic strengths and intrinsic membrane properties can be consistent with effective network performance. Virtually indistinguishable network activity can arise from widely divergent sets of underlying mechanisms, indicating that different animals may differ in many of the parameters that control network activity [15].

17.3 CLINICAL MANAGEMENT IN NEUROLOGICAL DISORDER
17.3.1 Alzheimer's Diseases Overview
17.3.1.1 Alzheimer's Disease

Alzheimer's disease (AD), the most prevalent type of irreversible dementia, is putting a significant and growing burden on patients, carers, and society as more humans live long enough to be afflicted. Clinically, Alzheimer's disease (AD) is defined by development from recurrent memory issues to a gradual deterioration in cognitive ability, which renders individuals with end-stage AD immobile and dependent on others to meet their care needs. [16]. The population with younger-onset AD is made up of around 200,000 persons under the age of 65 who have the disease. . By 2050, it is predicted that there will be about a million new cases of Alzheimer's disease (AD) worldwide, with a prevalence of 13.8 million. A new case is predicted to arise every 33 seconds [17]. It is commonly acknowledged that Alois Alzheimer, a German neuroscientist and physician, was responsible for the discovery of the disease that bears his name. He did so following a histopathological examination of Auguste D., a 51-year-old woman who had symptoms of dementia syndrome. Neurofibrillary tangles and senile plaques were discovered during the pathological examination of her brain [18]. Genetic factors operate as predisposing agents in the majority of sporadic AD cases, raising the risk of illness above that of the general population but without the power to actually cause the disease. To exert their harmful impact, they presumably interact with physiologic or pathologic states, environmental variables, or both (Figure 17.2). To further increase the likelihood of causing the disease, they may potentially interact with one another. A multidisciplinary strategy combining clinical and neurophysiological characterization of AD subtypes, in vivo functional brain imaging studies, and molecular examinations of genetic components may be successful in identifying the complex etiology that underlies AD [19].

17.3.1.2 Clinical Management in Alzheimer's Disease

The current emphasis in treating AD includes endogenous molecules linked to the generation and clearance of Aβ, such as the β- and γ-secretases, insulin-degrading enzymes, such as neprilysin, and immunotherapeutic-based methods. Recent research using preclinical transgenic mouse models has suggested that specific endogenous inflammatory mechanisms might be modulated to eliminate accumulated Aβ [20]. Treatment for AD frequently involves the use of acetylcholinesterase inhibitors (AChEI). The preliminary experiment showed that rivastigmine was safe and efficient in terms of cognitive, general functioning, and daily living activities. High-dose rivastigmine treatment was safe and well tolerated for a total of 5 years in this open-label extension. In the first high-dose rivastigmine group during the double-blind phase, two-thirds of the people in the group were still participating at week 234, indicating that early treatment may have some advantage in slowing the course of symptoms over time. There were no discontinuations owing to side effects after the initial titration phase, indicating that rivastigmine's long-term cholinesterase inhibition treatment was well tolerated. Early treatment start-up with titration to high-dose medication may be advantageous in preventing sickness progression [21]. Galantamine usage in AD patients in the United States may decrease the need for expensive resources like nursing homes and formal home care, eventually resulting in cost savings [22].

The symptoms of AD are reduced by modulating N-methyl-D-aspartate (NMDA) receptors to lessen glutamate-induced excitotoxicity. This brand-new neurochemical strategy differs from the cholinomimetic process used by all presently authorized Alzheimer's disease therapies. NMDA

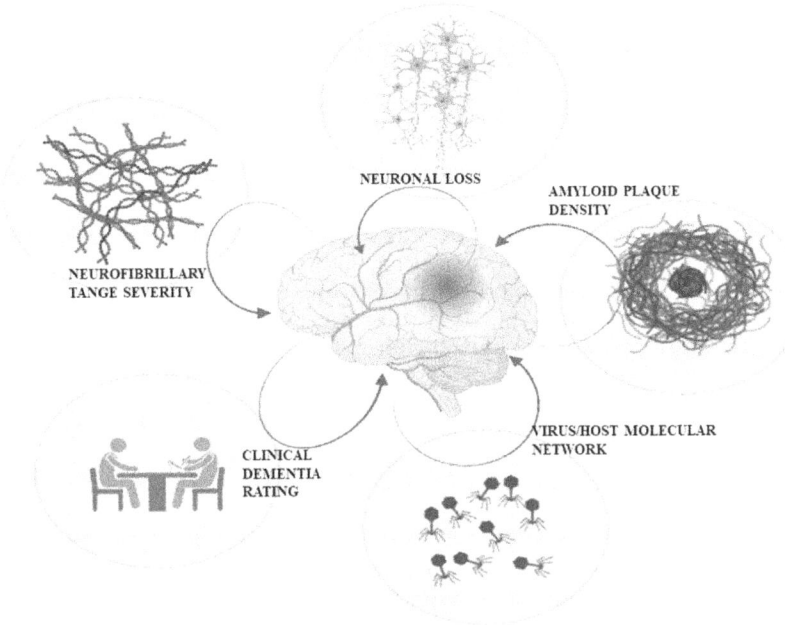

Figure 17.2 Neuropathophysiological state of Alzheimer's disease

receptor antagonists are a class of drugs that includes memantine. In particular, senile dementia is treated with memantine in the management of AD [23].

There is growing proof that CNS inflammatory processes in AD act as a mediator of neurotoxicity. These mechanisms entail the production of pro-inflammatory cytokines such as IL-1β, IL-6, and TNF-α as a result of amyloid-β activating microglia. Inhibition of hippocampus neurogenesis, promotion of apoptosis, diminished synaptic function as shown by suppression of long-term potentiation, and direct neuronal death are all examples of neurotoxic processes that may be mediated by these cytokines. CNS inflammation may be a more accurate indicator of prodromal AD since it may appear before the onset of senile plaques and neurofibrillary tangles in AD. Novel nonsteroidal anti-inflammatory agents and opioid antagonists may be new anti-inflammatory medications used to treat or prevent AD. With regard to anti-amyloid treatments for AD, these advances provide an alternative or possible complement [24].

Dale Schenk and colleagues found in 1999 that vaccination of Aβ protein transgenic mice with senile plaques and the prevention of new beta-amyloid deposits lower senile plaques. Antibodies against Aβ also have a comparable impact, according to their research. As mice that had been inoculated showed improved cognitive abilities, a human test of an active vaccination technique was conducted. This is a potential strategy to treat and prevent AD since Th1 immune responses are inhibited in the gut immune system [25]. The development of Aβ-plaque formation, neuritic dystrophy, and astrogliosis was substantially inhibited in young mice by immunization. The degree and development of these AD-like neuropathologies were significantly slowed down in older animals who had received treatment, hence the potential for Aβ to be used as a vaccine for AD prevention and treatment [26].

17.3.2 Parkinson's Disease Overview

17.3.2.1 *Parkinson's Disease*

Parkinson's disease is a degenerative neurological disorder characterized by the malfunction or death of dopamine-producing neurons in the brain. Lewy bodies, which are cytoplasmic aggregations of the protein α-synuclein in brain neurons, and the degeneration of dopaminergic neurons in the substantia nigra pars compacta of the midbrain are the pathologic characteristics of the illness. These characteristics are linked to the clinical symptoms of the illness. Parkinson's disease is characterized by decreasing levels of dopamine (DA), resulting in problems with both voluntary and involuntary movements. Dopamine is a neurotransmitter that helps the body carry out coordinated movement. Parkinson's disease also causes non-motor signs and symptoms, including sadness, restlessness, and orthostatic hypotension [27]. In 1817, James Parkinson reported "shaking palsy", a disease that would later be given his name. Since then, Parkinson's disease has remained widespread on a global scale. Clinicians will increasingly frequently notice the disease's symptoms as it affects the elderly, who make up a growing portion of the population. Much remains unclear about this degenerative neurologic condition despite several advances in knowledge and care, including the creation of medications that can enhance the quality of life of people affected. About 150 people worldwide have Parkinson's disease (PD), and that number is rising quickly in people over 70. Population characteristics including age, sex, ethnicity, and geography are risk factors. In Europe, for example, PD occurs more frequently than in North America. Older White males in industrialized areas are at greater risk of acquiring PD compared to their counterparts in less industrialized areas. A significant risk is also posed by past exposure to viral encephalitis lethargica and exposure to low dosages of methylphenyl-tetrahydropyridine (MPTP). Amazing research suggests that PD is less common among smokers than it is in those who have never smoked. Genetics, external toxins, endogenous toxins, and viral infection have been the main areas of focus so far. The main characteristics of PD are tremor, muscle stiffness, bradykinesia, postural instability, and micrographia [28]. Parkinson's disease is a slowly progressive neurological condition that impairs motor function and results in sluggish movements, tremors, and abnormalities of gait and balance. Parkinson's disease is frequently accompanied by a number of non-motor symptoms. Constipation and urine disturbances, a range of sleep abnormalities, and a spectrum of neuropsychiatric symptoms are some of them. These symptoms also include disrupted autonomic function with orthostatic hypotension [29].

17.3.2.2 Clinical Management in Parkinson's Disease

Decreased DA concentrations in the basal ganglia are the neurochemical result. The pathology caused by α-synuclein in the autonomic nerves and ganglia is one of the clinical indicators of Parkinson's disease (PD), which also involves mass loss and gastrointestinal symptoms including indigestion and constipation. Due to the lack of effective laboratory-based diagnostic techniques, the diagnosis of PD now relies on observing clinical trends. As conventional imaging is useless, positron emission tomography (PET) is the sole method employed [30]. While such testing can rule out other illnesses, medical science lacks an effective blood or imaging diagnostic test for Parkinson's disease. It is recommended that PD medical experts evaluate symptoms in order to get a diagnosis. The rate at which PD progresses varies; therefore, therapy is tailored to the patient's specific needs and concentrates on reducing adverse effects of medication while resolving symptoms of the disability. While there is no known cure for Parkinson's disease, medicines can reduce symptoms and improve function and quality of life for persons who have the condition. Levodopa (L-dopa) and other DA agonists are used in an effort to restore DA activity, despite the fact that PD is incurable and that medications cannot change the underlying cause of the illness. If given systemically, DA has no therapeutic benefit since it cannot penetrate the BBB [31]. L-dopa therapy for PD is frequently accompanied by dyskinesias and variations in motor responsiveness. Thus, directly acting dopamine receptor agonists have been developed in order to combat the negative consequences of long-term L-dopa usage. Nonetheless, L-dopa continues to be the most efficient treatment for the tremor, increased muscular tone, and slowness of movement that characterize PD. Compared to dopamine receptor agonists, L-dopa-derived dopamine has a wider range of effects. Dopamine may also activate adrenoceptors, new dopamine sites, the dopamine transporter, and trace amine receptors, in addition to D1- and D2-like dopamine receptors. These additional mechanisms may all play a role in the superior impact of L-dopa in PD [32].

For treating Parkinson's symptoms, levodopa is the most effective drug. Swedish research revealed that levodopa usage was increasing despite the availability of dopamine agonists and catechol-O-methyltransferase (COMT) inhibitors on the market. In treating fragile elderly individuals, levodopa is typically first used by professionals. Patients frequently require extra levodopa for symptom management after a few years of medication, even when they initially get dopamine agonist treatment [33]. In order to reduce the frequency and severity of motor fluctuations in PD patients, transdermal administration of dopamine agonists (DA) is a viable treatment option [34]. To balance the variations in response to L-dopa, a powerful D1 and D2 agonist called apomorphine is infused subcutaneously using a metered dosage infusion. A second-generation monoamine-oxidase type B (MAO-B) inhibitor, rasagiline has been studied as a potential therapy for PD. It is a powerful, irreversible, and specific inhibitor of MAO-B. In addition to its ability to inhibit MAO, rasagiline also has neuroprotective qualities. In the treatment of early PD, rasagiline shows demonstrably positive results when used alone [35].

The idea behind using cells as treatment modalities for PD and other neurodegenerative illnesses is that by replacing the injured cell population, patient functionality will be enhanced. These cells are predicted to live, develop neurites, create functional synapses, integrate most effectively and durably with the host tissue, particularly in the striatum, repair the damaged wiring, and result in significant clinical improvement. In animal models of PD, non-neuronal cells have previously been implanted to boost the production of dopamine, either naturally or after the insertion of genes like tyrosine hydroxylase. These cells did not grow under control, did not integrate well into the brain parenchyma, and had low survival rates since they were not of neuronal origin. The majority of these studies made use of fetal dopaminergic cells derived from fetuses' ventral mesencephalic region. While it has been demonstrated that the transplanted cells survived and some patients have benefitted from this therapy, other patients have experienced severe dyskinesia, which is most likely due to the graft's excessive and uncontrolled synthesis and release of dopamine. The ability of the transplanted cells to synthesize dopamine, regulate release and reuptake, and metabolize dopamine, as well as other functions, must be comparable to the abilities of the original dopaminergic neurons for the cell replacement technique to be effective in PD [36].

17.3.3 Huntington's Disease Overview

17.3.3.1 *Huntington's Disease*

Huntington's disease (HD) is an autosomal dominant neurological disorder characterized by a slew of symptoms and indications, including mobility dysfunction, cognitive impairment, and psychiatric abnormalities. Any one of these disorders may prevail in a person and they can all occur separately or in combination. There are 4–7 cases of Huntington's disease per 100,000 people globally. Before developing a movement issue, up to half of all people exhibit just psychological symptoms [37]. Trinucleotide (cytosine-adenine-guanine [CAG]) repeats that code because glutamine are abnormally expanded at the N-terminal of a protein known as "huntingtin" (IT15 at 4p16.3), which is the etiology of HD [38]. A highly sensitive and specific marker for the inheritance of the illness mutation, CAG trinucleotide expansion is the molecular cause of HD globally [39]. HD is marked by behavioral instability, cognitive deterioration, and mobility abnormalities. The main modification is a decrease in striatal medium spiny γ-aminobutyric acid (GABA) neurons, which is most pronounced in the caudate but also in the globus pallidus. Reduced D1- and D2-receptor binding in the striatum has been seen in HD patients, and this has been linked to the severity of the disease according to receptor studies (Figure 17.3) [40].

17.3.3.2 *Clinical Management in Huntington's Disease*

The several hyperkinetic and hypokinetic movement problems, as well as the behavioral and psychological symptoms, that accompany HD, which is a progressive heredodegenerative illness, cause a significant amount of impairment and cognitive deterioration, all of which degrade the patient's functional status and make them dependent on others. While the immediate family normally bears the majority of the load in caring for a HD patient, a multidisciplinary approach is necessary. So far, no medications have been identified to halt or stop the course of the illness, and neuroprotective therapy for HD remains elusive. The degeneration of medium spiny neurons in the caudate nucleus in HD may be directly correlated with aberrant Ca^{2+} signaling, according to recent findings; as a result, calcium channel blockers may be effective in treating HD. Clinical studies for gene treatments or the delivery of trophic factor genes through viral vectors, such as brain-derived neurotrophic factor, ciliary neurotrophic factor, neurotrophin, or neurturin, are currently thought to be imminent. While employing symptomatic remedies, it is crucial to individually adjust the treatment to each patient's demands and keep a close eye out for the onset of any negative side effects [41]. Antiglutamatergic medicines, antidepressants, DA antagonists, GABA agonists, antiepileptics, acetylcholinesterase inhibitors, and botulinum toxin are only a few of the medication types that have been utilized to treat the varied symptoms of HD. The antipsychotic medicine olanzapine has a considerable short-term impact on behavioral changes and may be particularly helpful for people who first have severe mental symptoms. It could be taken into account as a potential therapeutic option for HD therapy [42].

In order to lower the dosage of antipsychotic medicine and thereby help avoid side effects that may result in medication rejection, the combination of valproate, administered as a mood stabilizer, and olanzapine was chosen. We come to the conclusion that the lowest effective dosages of

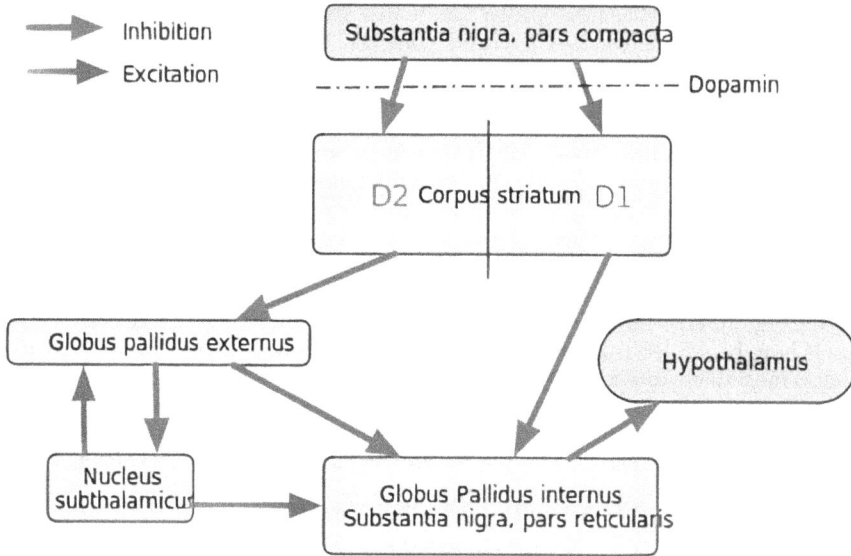

Figure 17.3 Huntington's disease basal ganglia

valproate and olanzapine may be beneficial for treating agitation and aggressiveness in individuals with HD or a related condition, as well as for treating movement disorders and psychosis [43].

17.3.4 Amyotrophic Lateral Sclerosis Review

17.3.4.1 Amyotrophic Lateral Sclerosis

Amyotrophic lateral sclerosis (ALS) is a heterogeneous neurodegenerative illness that causes both motor and extra-motor symptoms due to the degeneration of both upper motor neurons and lower motor neurons, which are the neurons that project from the cortex to the brainstem and spinal cord, respectively. When ALS first manifests, individuals might appear in one of two ways: either with spinal-onset illness, which causes the development of muscular weakness in the limbs, or with bulbar-onset disease, which causes speech and swallowing difficulties. Whilst some people have familial ALS, which is linked to abnormalities in genes with a variety of activities, , the majority of patients have ALS for which there is no known cause [44]. Epidemiological studies on ALS have been made more challenging by a number of factors, including the difficulty in pinpointing the exact time at which the disease first manifested itself and the potentially protracted interval between the onset of pathological changes and the appearance of clinical symptoms. It is possible that the common delay between the commencement of the disease and the onset of symptoms reflects neuronal populations' redundancy. In order to support various disease-causing processes, a variety of epidemiological studies with rigorous designs and the use of impartial patient cohorts have produced diverse degrees of evidence. According to population-based research, there are 216 cases of ALS for every 100 000 people aged over 1 year in Europe. The actual prevalence of ALS is unknown, despite the fact that it affects individuals everywhere [45]. Several neuro-inflammation-related genes, including TNF- α, IL-RA, CD86, CD200R, and Groα, are regulated differently [46]. The neurodegenerative effects of defective microglial function on G93A SOD1 are accompanied by glutamate neurotoxicity, oxidative stress, improper metal ion regulation, apoptosis, and inflammatory neuropathology [47]. The proapoptotic activity of mutant SOD-1 in cultured brain cell lines and the neuroprotective effect of overexpressing Bcl-2 in mutant SOD-1-transgenic mice point toward a role for apoptosis in familial ALS. Moreover, ALS patients' spinal cords and the spinal cords of mutant SOD-1-transgenic mice can both show signs of activated caspase-1 and caspase-3. Significantly, the suppression of caspase-1 activity prevents the development of illness in SOD-1-transgenic animals. By boosting interleukin-1 synthesis, which is a pro-inflammatory cytokine, and by directly activating caspase-3, caspase-1 may result in a predisposition to neuronal cell death (Figure 17.4). According to all available information, activation may be a key factor in the pathogenesis of ALS, and early therapy with inhibitors that target certain caspases may be able to stop the death of motor neurons [48].

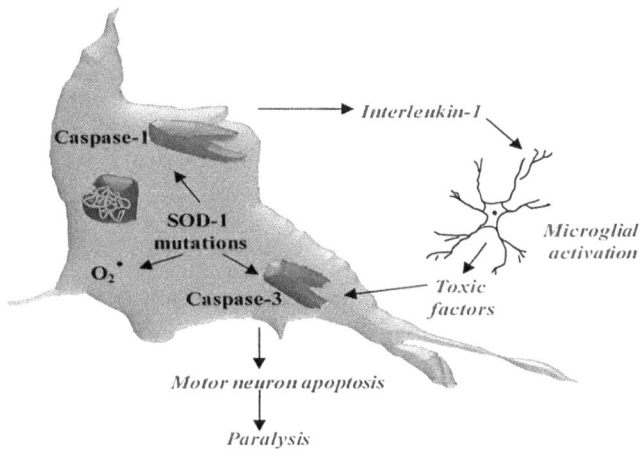

Figure 17.4   Activation of cell death pathways by SOD-1 mutations in familial amyotrophic lateral sclerosis

17.3.4.2 *Clinical Management in Amyotrophic Lateral Sclerosis*

Even though there is currently no therapy for ALS, recent advancements in clinical staging systems, genetic research, novel medicines, and the 2019 coronavirus pandemic have all had an influence on how clinical care of ALS is currently conducted. The recent coronavirus pandemic has provided opportunities to develop telemedicine and remote monitoring of disease, increasing accessibility to care and lowering the burden of traveling to centers for those living with the disease and their carers. An enhanced understanding of genetics has helped provide insights into pathophysiology. Staging systems and clinical measures have helped provide tools for monitoring disease clinically [49]. For the assessment and treatment of dysphagia and dysarthria in patients with bulbar amyotrophic lateral sclerosis (ALS), speech therapists and otolaryngologists/head and neck surgeons are frequently consulted. Due to the progressive and multi-system nature of their condition, these individuals make up an uncommon group. Many symptoms linked to eating, speaking, and breathing are brought on by the neuromuscular impairments caused by bulbar ALS. To help the doctor create an organized plan of management for this progressive condition, the development of symptoms is associated with particular therapy suggestions [50].

In individuals with ALS, the daily dose of riluzole, 100 mg, is probably safe and increases median life by two to three months. Bulbar and limb function both showed a slight improvement, but muscular strength did not. More patients using riluzole than controls saw a threefold rise in serum alanine transferase [51].

17.3.5. Other Related Atypical Neurological Disorders

Hepatic encephalopathies come in a variety of unusual forms, including acquired hepatocerebral degeneration (AHD). Similar to Wilson's disease (hepatolenticular degeneration), it is characterized by neuropsychiatric and extrapyramidal symptomatology. AHD is an uncommon illness, and because of its many clinical presentations, it can be challenging to identify. Yet, in our opinion, an accurate diagnosis benefits from a comprehensive examination and comprehension of the ailment.. In Pick body disease (PBD) brains, the immunolocalization of 14-3-3 protein isoforms in connection to Pick bodies was studied. In the neurons of normal participants' and brains affected by Pick body disease, weakly granular immunoreactivity of 14-3-3 proteins was discovered. Pick bodies showed immunostaining patterns similar to those seen with anti-14-3-3 proteins when they were probed with isoform-specific antibodies and found to be positive for the isoforms beta, gamma, epsilon, eta, tau, and zeta (common) [52]. Furthermore, it was surprisingly discovered that Pick bodies, healthy hippocampus neurons, and brain homogenate from age-matched controls had immunoreactivity of the sigma isoform, which was previously thought to be exclusively extraneuronal. While 14-3-3 proteins are found in Pick bodies, which implies their participation in Pick body formation, their role may vary depending on the isoforms that are differentially expressed in various brain regions [53].

Axonal degeneration induced by persistent demyelination in the absence of active inflammation may also contribute to increasing impairment in the later stages of the disease. Both investigations employing magnetic resonance imaging and magnetic resonance spectroscopy have shown brain shrinkage in the early stages of multiple sclerosis, which is consistent with the hypothesis that axonal loss starts at the time of the ER initiation. Without accompanying disability progression, brain shrinkage increases throughout the relapsing-remitting illness stage [54].

17.4 FUTURE PERSPECTIVE

From a neurotherapeutic standpoint, it is critical to distinguish the progression of the initial neuropathogenic process from the appearance of co-pathogens and the age-related failure of compensatory mechanisms, as well as to identify whether the early increases in neural activity are compensatory or neuropathogenic mechanisms [55]. Certain requirements must be met for stem cell (SC) treatment for neurological illnesses to be successful. The transplanted cell must first undergo in vitro and in vivo cell type differentiation. The transplanted cells must then integrate into the neighborhood neural network. Lastly, the grafted cell's half-life needs to be increased. Fourthly, and most significantly, there should be no tumor growth. Moreover, the safety and effectiveness of SC treatment may be impacted by the diseased microenvironment of an animal model [56]. On the basis of existing clinical criteria, it is inadequate to make a clinical diagnosis of significant neurological illnesses, such as AD and PD. Emerging metabolomics is a potent method for locating novel biomarkers and biochemical pathways to enhance diagnosis, as well as for figuring out prognosis and treatment. With recent developments in metabolomics, which are more accurate than standard clinical practice, the identification of several new biomarkers for neurological illnesses has been considerably improved [57]. Current strategies primarily focus on building a precise viral vector, plasmid transfection, nanotechnology, microRNA, and in vivo CRISPR-based treatment for enhanced gene delivery. Treatment of common neurological and neurodevelopmental disorders, such as Parkinson's disease, Alzheimer's disease, and autism spectrum disorder, as well as uncommon illnesses, has greatly benefitted from the use of these most recent approaches. Many of these delivery strategies do, however, have certain drawbacks, such as immunogenic responses, off-target effects, and a lack of useful biomarkers to assess the efficacy of the therapy [58]. For the development of therapeutic and diagnostic techniques for the treatment of neurodegenerative illnesses, systemic distribution of oligonucleotides (ODN) to the central nervous system is required [59].

17.5 CONCLUSION

These sophisticated neurodegenerative diseases include AD, PD, ALS, and HD. Most of the time, their cause is unclear. Based on prior research, the fundamental mechanisms of action that contribute to the emergence of neurological diseases are still being studied. Different pathophysiological factors will be connected with the treatment of various neurological diseases; as a result, transplantation therapy must be carried out safely and under ideal circumstances. Basic research is still necessary prior to conducting transplants on humans. This serves as a good example of how combining fundamental neurology, pharmacology, and cutting-edge drug delivery techniques may justify tackling a variety of approaches to the clinical management of neurological disorders. For a wider group of researchers, conceptualizing the molecular foundation and pathophysiology of neurological disorders will provide valuable and illuminating knowledge of the neurological disease. Moreover, shorter clinical trial durations and the evaluation of a wider variety of neuroactive drugs may be made possible by future research that may validate the neuropathogenic importance of reversible network disruption in NDs. This might quicken the process of medication validation and result in clear financial savings. Even though these regimens are challenging to evaluate in clinical studies, they have shown potential for the treatment of other multifaceted conditions, including epilepsy, hypertension, and cancer. They are also likely necessary for the successful management of neurological diseases. Additionally, this challenge includes a sizeable portion of the most recent discoveries in novel therapeutic targets and therapies, which expose innovative drug delivery pathways.

REFERENCES

1. Choonara YE, Pillay V, Du Toit LC, Modi G, Naidoo D, Ndesendo VM, Sibambo SR. Trends in the molecular pathogenesis and clinical therapeutics of common neurodegenerative disorders. *International Journal of Molecular Sciences*. 2009 Jun 3;10(6):2510–57.

2. Cella D, Nowinski C, Peterman A, Victorson D, Miller D, Lai JS, Moy C. The neurology quality-of-life measurement initiative. *Archives of Physical Medicine and Rehabilitation*. 2011 Oct 1;92(10):S28–36.

3. Perez L, Huang J, Jansky L, Nowinski C, Victorson D, Peterman A, Cella D. Using focus groups to inform the Neuro-QOL measurement tool: Exploring patient-centered, health-related quality of life concepts across neurological conditions. *Journal of Neuroscience Nursing*. 2007 Dec 1;39(6):342–53.

4. Khalil M, Teunissen CE, Otto M, Piehl F, Sormani MP, Gattringer T, Barro C, Kappos L, Comabella M, Fazekas F, Petzold A. Neurofilaments as biomarkers in neurological disorders. *Nature Reviews Neurology*. 2018 Oct;14(10):577–89.

5. Morrison JH, Hof PR. Life and death of neurons in the aging brain. *Science*. 1997 Oct 17;278(5337):412–9.

6. Palop JJ, Chin J, Mucke L. A network dysfunction perspective on neurodegenerative diseases. *Nature*. 2006 Oct 19;443(7113):768–73.

7. Lewin R. Is your brain really necessary? John Lorber, a British neurologist, claims that some patients are more normal than would be inferred from their brain scans. *Science*. 1980 Dec 12;210(4475):1232–4.

8. Chen R, Cohen LG, Hallett M. Nervous system reorganization following injury. *Neuroscience*. 2002 Jun 6;111(4):761–73.

9. Muchowski PJ, Wacker JL. Modulation of neurodegeneration by molecular chaperones. *Nature Reviews Neuroscience*. 2005 Jan 1;6(1):11–22.

10. Lazarov O, Robinson J, Tang YP, Hairston IS, Korade-Mirnics Z, Lee VM, Hersh LB, Sapolsky RM, Mirnics K, Sisodia SS. Environmental enrichment reduces Aβ levels and amyloid deposition in transgenic mice. *Cell*. 2005 Mar 11;120(5):701–13.

11. Van Dellen A, Grote HE, Hannan AJ. Gene–environment interactions, neuronal dysfunction and pathological plasticity in Huntington's disease. *Clinical and Experimental Pharmacology and Physiology*. 2005 Dec;32(12):1007–19.

12. Mahley RW, Weisgraber KH, Huang Y. Apolipoprotein E4: A causative factor and therapeutic target in neuropathology, including Alzheimer's disease. *Proceedings of the National Academy of Sciences*. 2006 Apr 11;103(15):5644–51.

13. Stern Y. What is cognitive reserve? Theory and research application of the reserve concept. *Journal of the International Neuropsychological Society*. 2002 Mar;8(3):448–60.

14. Miller DL, Ortega S, Bashayan O, Basch R, Basilico C. Compensation by fibroblast growth factor 1 (FGF1) does not account for the mild phenotypic defects observed in FGF2 null mice. *Molecular and Cellular Biology*. 2000 Mar 15;20(6):2260–8.

15. Prinz AA, Bucher D, Marder E. Similar network activity from disparate circuit parameters. *Nature Neuroscience*. 2004 Dec 1;7(12):1345–52.

16. Citron M. Alzheimer's disease: Strategies for disease modification. *Nature Reviews Drug Discovery*. 2010 May;9(5):387–98.

17. Kumar A, Singh A. A review on Alzheimer's disease pathophysiology and its management: An update. *Pharmacological Reports*. 2015 Apr 1;67(2):195–203.

18. Ramirez-Bermudez J. Alzheimer's disease: Critical notes on the history of a medical concept. *Archives of Medical Research*. 2012 Nov 1;43(8):595–9.

19. Rocchi A, Pellegrini S, Siciliano G, Murri L. Causative and susceptibility genes for Alzheimer's disease: A review. *Brain Research Bulletin*. 2003 Jun 30;61(1):1–24.

20. Chang WP, Koelsch G, Wong S, Downs D, Da H, Weerasena V, Gordon B, Devasamudram T, Bilcer G, Ghosh AK, Tang J. In vivo inhibition of Aβ production by memapsin 2 (β -secretase) inhibitors. *Journal of Neurochemistry*. 2004 Jun;89(6):1409–16.

21. Farlow MR, Lilly ML. Rivastigmine: An open-label, observational study of safety and effectiveness in treating patients with Alzheimer's disease for up to 5 years. *BMC Geriatrics*. 2005 Dec;5(1):1–7.

22. Migliaccio-Walle K, Getsios D, Caro JJ, Ishak KJ, O'Brien JA, Papadopoulos G, AHEAD Study Group. Economic evaluation of galantamine in the treatment of mild to moderate Alzheimer's disease in the United States. *Clinical Therapeutics*. 2003 Jun 1;25(6):1806–25.

23. Reisberg B, Doody R, Stöffler A, Schmitt F, Ferris S, Möbius HJ. Memantine in moderate-to-severe Alzheimer's disease. *New England Journal of Medicine*. 2003 Apr 3;348(14):1333–41.

24. Rosenberg PB. Clinical aspects of inflammation in Alzheimer's disease. *International Review of Psychiatry*. 2005 Jan 1;17(6):503–14.

25. Tabira T. Vaccination therapy for Alzheimer's disease. *Brain Nerve*. 2007 Apr 1;59(4):375–82.

26. Schenk D, Barbour R, Dunn W, Gordon G, Grajeda H, Guido T, Hu K, Huang J, Johnson-Wood K, Khan K, Kholodenko D. Immunization with amyloid-β attenuates Alzheimer-disease-like pathology in the PDAPP mouse. *Nature*. 1999 Jul 8;400(6740):173–7.

27. Lew M. Overview of Parkinson's disease. *Pharmacotherapy: The Journal of Human Pharmacology and Drug Therapy*. 2007 Dec;27(12P2):155S–60S.

28. Conley SC, Kirchner JT. Parkinson's disease—The shaking palsy: Underlying factors, diagnostic considerations, and clinical course. *Postgraduate Medicine*. 1999 Jan 1;106(1):39–52.

29. Sveinbjornsdottir S. The clinical symptoms of Parkinson's disease. *Journal of Neurochemistry*. 2016 Oct;139(Suppl 1):318–24.

30. Seibyl J, Jennings D, Tabamo R, Marek K. Neuroimaging trials of Parkinson's disease progression. *Journal of Neurology*. 2004 Oct 1;251(Suppl 7):vii9.

31. Albin RL, Frey KA. Initial agonist treatment of Parkinson disease: A critique. *Neurology*. 2003 Feb 11;60(3):390–4.

32. Mercuri NB, Bernardi G. The 'magic'of L-dopa: Why is it the gold standard Parkinson's disease therapy?. *Trends in Pharmacological Sciences*. 2005 Jul 1;26(7):341–4.

33. Thanvi BR, Lo TC. Long term motor complications of levodopa: Clinical features, mechanisms, and management strategies. *Postgraduate Medical Journal*. 2004 Aug 1;80(946):452–8.

34. Woitalla D, Müller T, Benz S, Horowski R, Przuntek H. *Transdermal Lisuride Delivery in the Treatment of Parkinson's Disease*. Vienna: Springer; 2004.

35. Siddiqui MA, Plosker GL. Rasagiline. *Drugs Aging*. 2005 Jan;22:83–91.

36. Levy YS, Stroomza M, Melamed E, Offen D. Embryonic and adult stem cells as a source for cell therapy in Parkinson's disease. *Journal of Molecular Neuroscience*. 2004 Nov;24:353–85.

37. Harper PS. The epidemiology of Huntington's disease. *Human Genetics*. 1992 Jun;89:365–76.

38. MacDonald ME, Ambrose CM, Duyao MP, Myers RH, Lin C, Srinidhi L, Barnes G, Taylor SA, James M, Groot N, MacFarlane H. A novel gene containing a trinucleotide repeat that is expanded and unstable on Huntington's disease chromosomes. *Cell*. 1993 Mar 26;72(6):971–83.

39. Kremer B, Goldberg P, Andrew SE, Theilmann J, Telenius H, Zeisler J, Squitieri F, Lin B, Bassett A, Almqvist E, Bird TD. A worldwide study of the Huntington's disease mutation: The sensitivity and specificity of measuring CAG repeats. *New England Journal of Medicine*. 1994 May 19;330(20):1401–6.

40. Hersch SM, Ferrante RJ. Neuropathology and pathophysiology of Huntington's disease. Movement disorders. *Neurologic Principles and Practice*. New York: McGraw-Hill. 1997:503–18.

41. Adam OR, Jankovic J. Symptomatic treatment of Huntington disease. *Neurotherapeutics*. 2008 Apr 1;5(2):181–97.

42. Squitieri F, Cannella M, Porcellini A, Brusa L, Simonelli M, Ruggieri S. Short-term effects of olanzapine in Huntington disease. *Cognitive and Behavioral Neurology*. 2001 Jan 1;14(1):69–72.

43. Grove Jr VE, Quintanilla J, DeVaney GT. Improvement of Huntington's disease with olanzapine and valproate. *New England Journal of Medicine*. 2000 Sep 28;343(13):973–4.

44. Hardiman O, Al-Chalabi A, Chio A, Corr EM, Logroscino G, Robberecht W, Shaw PJ, Simmons Z, Van Den Berg LH. Amyotrophic lateral sclerosis. *Nature Reviews Disease Primers*. 2017 Oct 5;3(1):1–9.

45. Kiernan MC, Vucic S, Cheah BC, Turner MR, Eisen A, Hardiman O, Burrell JR, Zoing MC. Amyotrophic lateral sclerosis. *The Lancet*. 2011 Mar 12;377(9769):942–55.

46. Chen LC, Smith AP, Ben Y, Zukic B, Ignacio S, Moore D, Lee NM. Temporal gene expression patterns in G93A/SOD1 mouse. *Amyotrophic Lateral Sclerosis and Other Motor Neuron Disorders*. 2004 Sep 1;5(3):164–71.

47. Andersen PM, Sims KB, Xin WW, Kiely R, O'Neill G, Ravits J, Pioro E, Harati Y, Brower RD, Levine JS, Heinicke HU. Sixteen novel mutations in the Cu/Zn superoxide dismutase gene in amyotrophic lateral sclerosis: A decade of discoveries, defects and disputes. *Amyotrophic Lateral Sclerosis and Other Motor Neuron Disorders*. 2003 Jun 1;4(2):62–73.

48. Yuan J, Yankner BA. Apoptosis in the nervous system. *Nature*. 2000 Oct 12;407(6805):802–9.

49. Norris SP, Likanje MF, Andrews JA. Amyotrophic lateral sclerosis: Update on clinical management. *Current Opinion in Neurology*. 2020 Oct 1;33(5):641–8.

50. Hillel AD, Miller R. Bulbar amyotrophic lateral sclerosis: Patterns of progression and clinical management. *Head & Neck*. 1989 Jan;11(1):51–9.

51. Miller RG, Mitchell JD, Moore DH. Riluzole for amyotrophic lateral sclerosis (ALS)/motor neuron disease (MND). *Cochrane Database of Systematic Reviews*. 2012(3):1–36.

52. Feany MB, Dickson DW. Neurodegenerative disorders with extensive tau pathology: A comparative study and review. *Annals of Neurology*. 1996 Aug;40(2):139–48.

53. Umahara T, Uchihara T, Tsuchiya K, Nakamura A, Ikeda K, Iwamoto T, Takasaki M. Immunolocalization of 14–3-3 isoforms in brains with Pick body disease. *Neuroscience Letters*. 2004 Nov 23;371(2–3):215–9.

54. Trapp BD, Ransohoff R, Rudick R. Axonal pathology in multiple sclerosis: Relationship to neurologic disability. *Current Opinion in Neurology*. 1999 Jun 1;12(3):295–302.

55. Oldstone MB. Molecular mimicry, microbial infection, and autoimmune disease: Evolution of the concept. *Molecular Mimicry: Infection-Inducing Autoimmune Disease*. 2005:1–7.

56. Rahman MM, Islam MR, Islam MT, Harun-Or-Rashid M, Islam M, Abdullah S, Uddin MB, Das S, Rahaman MS, Ahmed M, Alhumaydhi FA. Stem cell transplantation therapy and neurological disorders: Current status and future perspectives. *Biology*. 2022 Jan 7;11(1):147.

57. Zhang AH, Sun H, Wang XJ. Recent advances in metabolomics in neurological disease, and future perspectives. *Analytical and Bioanalytical Chemistry*. 2013 Oct;405:8143–50.

58. Mani S, Jindal D, Singh M. Gene therapy, A potential therapeutic tool for neurological and neuropsychiatric disorders: Applications, challenges and future perspective. *Current Gene Therapy*. 2023 Feb 1;23(1):20–40.

59. Vinogradov SV, Batrakova EV, Kabanov AV. Nanogels for oligonucleotide delivery to the brain. *Bioconjugate Chemistry*. 2004 Jan 21;15(1):50–60.

18 Endothelial Dysfunction and Its Related Disorders

Jigar Vyas, Nensi Raytthatha, and Bhupendra Prajapati

18.1 INTRODUCTION TO ENDOTHELIAL CELLS

Endothelial cells (ECs) comprise a singular cell membrane that covers all capillary vessels and regulates blood-to-tissue exchange. Endothelial cell signals coordinate the development and establishment of the connective tissue cells, which form the outermost layer of the blood vessel walls. ECs have an exceptional ability to alter their amount and configuration to meet regional needs. They build an adaptive life network that extends all through the body via cellular proliferation.

18.1.1 Structure and Function of Endothelial Cells

The blood vessels are composed of three layers: the outermost layer, known as the adventitia, which consists of connective components (like collagen, as well as fibroblasts and fibres), neuronal endings, as well as perivascular adipose tissues; the middle layer is composed of smooth musculature, which also moderates arterial contraction or dilatation produced by inducer or mechanical forces such as tensile strain; and the innermost and most complicated layer is known as the endothelium.

The endothelium is a one-cell-thick layer comprised of endothelial cells (ECs) that lines the innermost wall of blood arteries, establishing a selective porous wall in between blood in the vessels and the adjacent tissue. It is an extremely centred structure that is found throughout the body. Blood vessels are made up of an inner endothelium layer, which is an endothelial cell monolayer that covers functioning cells, such as pericytes and vascular smooth muscle cells. The endothelial cells include a variety of membrane-bound protein receptors, including growth factors, coagulant and anticoagulant molecules, fat-transporting molecules, metabolites, and hormones. [1] Furthermore, the angiotensin-converting enzyme (ACE) in ECs is mechanosensory and is accountable for ECs detecting physical stresses and translating them into chemical signals that control cell–cell and cell–matrix interconnections in the vasculature. Mural cells are closely connected to one other, partially via integrins, and this helps to preserve vascular integrity. The endothelium is made up of $1 - 6 \times 10^{13}$ endothelial cells that cover the body, with a total surface area of more than 1,000 m^2 throughout the body.

The intimal layer not only serves as a mechanical wall between the arterial wall and the circulatory blood, but it also secretes a variety of mediators that operate in an autocrine and paracrine approach to maintain the cardiovascular (CV) system's homeostasis. ECs perform a variety of tasks, including the interchange of fluids and chemicals among blood and tissues, the formation of new vascular beds, and the control of immunological, fibrinolytic, and coagulating responses. [2] Furthermore, ECs play a significant part in controlling vasculature tone, and vasoreactivity studies are a well-known approach to detecting modifications in ECs and the capillary network in many clinical situations, as well as the modification of vasculature resistance in physiologic reactions such as physical exercise.

Endothelial cells both produce and release vasodilators and vasoconstrictors, which must be balanced in order to sustain vascular homeostasis. Endothelin-1 and angiotensin II are the primary mediators of vascular constriction, following by thromboxane A2, prostaglandin (PGH2), and reactive oxygen species (ROS). Factors such as nitric oxide (NO), endothelium-derived prostacyclins, and hyperpolarizing factor influence the vasodilation impact of ECs.

Although all of these mediators play critical roles in the circulatory system, NO is considered the most significant of the endothelium-derived factors.

18.1.2 Role of Endothelial Cells in Healthy Humans

Figure 18.1 demonstrates the activities of endothelial cells.

18.1.2.1 *Maintenance of Blood Flow*

ECs play an important part in the regulation of blood flow. They also play a role in vasodilation and vasoconstriction.

DOI: 10.1201/9781003384823-18

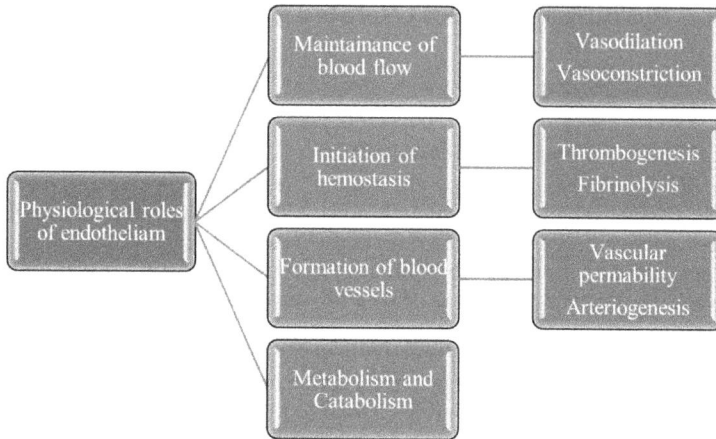

Figure 18.1   Activities of endothelial cells

18.1.2.1.1 Vasodilation and Vasoconstriction

The endothelium normally modulates vasculature homeostasis by coordinating with blood circulation, distributing nutrition, hormones, and other macronutrients, as well as regulating vascular smooth muscle cell (VSMC) migration and proliferation; it also controls coagulation and fibrinolysis actions, decreases vascular tone, modulates cellular and vascular adhesions, impedes leukocyte adhesions, and helps regulate inflammation actions and angiogenesis. [3] ECs serve an essential role in blood flow regulation, specifically through their capability to mediate anti-thrombotic and prothrombotic properties. The antithrombotic properties of the vascular endothelium inhibit the formation of thrombi, as well as the impairment of antithrombotic properties, which is generally the result of the prolonged effect of physiological stresses, such as inflammatory conditions, shear stress, radiation, and low-flow situations.

Antithrombotic compounds that change and control connective tissue components are produced and secreted by ECs. These compounds have a range of actions, including vasodilation and vasoconstriction, as well as having procoagulant and anti-coagulant properties. All antithrombotic medications help to prevent the formation of non-physiological thrombi. [4]

PGI2, i.e., prostaglandin, is a strong vasodilator produced by ECs in response to biochemical and mechanical impulses. PGI2 has properties that include the prevention of platelet agglomeration via the cyclic adenosine monophosphate (cAMP) pathways [5], which directly contravene the actions of thromboxane via cell receptor interaction. [6] NO, another strong vasodilator produced by ECs, promotes smooth muscle relaxation by elevating the intracellular level of cyclic guanosine monophosphate (cGMP). [7]

18.1.2.2 Inhibition of Haemostasis

The two processes constantly engage in haemostasis include: primary, which uses platelets, and secondary, which involves fibrin formation or blood coagulation. Circulating blood in the heart, arteries, capillaries, and veins usually comes into contact with the normal endothelium and remains liquid. The luminal membrane of dormant ECs works as an anti-coagulant and it is not thrombogenic; platelets and leukocytes do not react to it and the clotting mechanism remains dormant. The basal lamina's macromolecules are highly thrombogenic, so stimulated endothelial cells promote thrombus formation. Endothelial cells therefore regulate haemostasis, thrombo-resistance, and thrombosis.

18.1.2.2.1 Thrombogenesis

The endothelium's prothrombotic action, known as thrombogenesis, works in opposition to its anticoagulant effect. This is a complicated set of processes that result in the formation of a matrix of platelets, erythrocytes, and insoluble fibrin; this material deposition provides a mechanical obstacle to blood circulation. [8] The cell makeup of thrombi differs between the artery and vein routes; artery thrombi are more firmly packed with platelets, whereas venous thrombi are loosely loaded with erythrocytes, leukocytes, and fibrin. In the circulatory systems, thrombogenesis and thrombolysis are constantly occurring, and their control is almost entirely dependent on the endothelium.

18.1.2.3 Formation of Blood Vessels

The endothelium is essential for blood vessel synthesis, and two distinct processes, vasculogenesis and angiogenesis, which are closely involved in the progeny of new vessels. Angiogenesis is the formation of blood vessels from existent vessels by the proliferation and migration of mature ECs; vasculogenesis involves the differentiation of mesodermal precursors into ECs. [9]

18.1.2.3.1 Angiogenesis

Angiogenesis is a physiological or pathologic process that results in the formation of new capillary channels from pre-existing ones. Angiogenesis is crucial in development and growth, tissue repair, ischaemic heart disease, cardiovascular complications in diabetic patients, and malignant cancers. Angiogenesis includes the branching, splitting, sprouting, and differential development of blood vessels from the main plexus or a former vessel into the circulatory system. An optimal equilibrium of antiangiogenic and proangiogenic aspects is required for angiogenesis control, including tumour angiogenesis. [10] Angiogenic factors, both pro-angiogenic and anti-angiogenic factors, are important in the control of angiogenesis. In human iliac and femoral artery ECs, vascular endothelial cell growth factor (VEGF) has been found to enhance Notch1 and DLL4 appearance via a PI3kinase/Akt signalling route rather than a MAPK/Erk pathway, indicating the contribution of Akt signalling in angiogenesis and arteriogenesis. [5]

18.1.3 The Relation between Endothelial Dysfunction and the Occurrence of Diseases

Endothelial dysfunction (ED) should be diagnosed promptly in order to prevent and possibly identify a reversible stage in the progression of such cardiometabolic ailments.

Diabetes: When ECs are exposed to hyperglycaemia, a chain of unfavourable intracellular events begins, resulting in ED. In diabetics, the coronary circulation constricts rather than dilating in response to increased levels of Ach. [6] When endothelium stability is impaired, the M3 subtype of muscarinic receptor in the vascular system regulates contractions rather than vasodilation. This reaction shows that endothelium cells subjected to hyperglycaemia undergo apoptosis, resulting in intimal denudation. Mechanical strain causes cell death through a complicated sequence of actions following integrin stimulation. Mechanical stretch increases p38 mitogen-activated protein kinase and c-Jun N-terminal protein kinase initiation, culminating in the induction of apoptosis. Down-regulation of vascular endothelial cadherin triggers the caspase protein family, causing endothelial cell death mostly in atherosclerotic arterial sites. The apoptotic process results in the detachment of endothelial cells, which are transferred into the circulation and may be identified and monitored as circulatory ECs. The apoptotic process causes arterial denudation, which causes crucial proatherosclerotic activities, such as smooth muscle cell growth, migration, and matrix secretion. As a result, endothelial repair processes are critical in restoring vessel integrity. [11] Previous research on insulin resistance found that endothelial vasodilator-stimulated phosphoprotein (VASP)/NO mediated inflammatory suppression in fat tissues and liver. It is worth noting that VASP/NO signalling activation promotes a phenotypic shift into an M2 macrophage's state. A high-fat diet increases M1 activation and polarization of M2 in Kupffer cells, leading to insulin resistance in the liver. All these data imply that a therapeutic strategy targeting the VASP/NO signalling pathway would enhance anti-inflammatory activities and, as a result, could be utilized in therapy for the treatment of metabolic ailments such as obesity and diabetes.

Obesity: Obesity is linked to endothelial dysfunction, which is produced by a range of processes, including low-grade inflammation induced by the perivascular adipose tissue or the vasculature itself. Because a dysfunctioning endothelium is now well recognized as a predictive measure of cardiovascular events in high-risk individuals, this change might be one of the processes through which fat increases cardiovascular risk. Obesity-related endothelial dysfunction involves a vascular ET-1/NO imbalance in favour of aberrant endogenous ET-1 activation. [12]

Nephrological disorders: The endothelium of the kidney possesses a distinctive structural composition characterised by the presence of oval or round transcytoplasmic pores that serve as conduits for the filtration of substances across the renal capillary membrane. The presence of glycocalyx and holes in the filtration barrier plays a crucial role in restricting the passage of proteins from the bloodstream to the urine, therefore contributing to the occurrence of proteinuria. Because the regulation of openings is challenging to examine, it has not been well described. Pre-eclampsia is the most prevalent cause of endothelial dysfunction in the context of abnormal fenestrations.

Interestingly, this disease is linked with decreased glomerular filtration rate and proteinuria, suggesting the degradation of the glycocalyx during the fenestrations, enabling proteins to enter the urine. [13] Inflammation, oxidative stress, chronic renal disease, mineral and bone condition including lack of vitamin D, hyperphosphatemia, and excessive fibroblast growth factor are the key risk factors underpinning this systemic disorder in CKD patients. Systemic levels of IL-6, CRP, and TNF-K-beta are elevated in the majority of CKD patients.

Atherosclerosis: Endothelial cells are activated after being exposed to atherogenic stimuli, such as oxidized low-density lipoprotein (oxLDL), its atherogenic elements, cholesterol crystals, inflammatory stimulation, and interrupted blood flow. A decrease in endothelial-derived NO and increased OS are the main sources of endothelial phenotypic changes that manifest as decreased endothelium-dependent vasodilation. Endothelial cells that have been activated release many molecules of adhesion, such as intercellular monocyte chemoattractant protein-1, adhesion molecule-1, vascular adhesion molecule-1, P-selectin, and E-selectin, which engage neutrophils and monocytes that bind to the activated ECs and enter the artery wall. [14] ECs' exposure to distinctive stimuli causes oxidative stress, which exacerbates the continuous cycle of inflammatory processes and atherosclerosis. Increased endothelial dysfunction, as demonstrated by enlarged endothelium–platelet–endothelium contacts, will condense unstable plaques, as well as plaques vulnerable to rupture in advanced stages of atherosclerosis due to the excessive generation of pro-thrombotic substances (such as plasminogen activator inhibitor-1 and thrombins), as well as inefficient fibrinolytic, antithrombotic, and antiaggregatory functional areas and inflammatory resolution. Alterations to the endothelium glycocalyx microstructure aid the generation and propagation of plaques by controlling vascular tone, stability, and mechanotransduction.

Polycystic ovary syndrome (PCOS): This is an ordinary endocrine ailment that affects up to 19.9% of reproductive-age women. The combination of elevated androgens and insulin resistance in PCOS increases the risk of developing cardiometabolic syndrome. According to research, ED is often linked to PCOS. Endothelial failure in PCOS has been linked to insulin resistance (IR), hyperandrogenism, and obesity/adipocyte malfunction. [15] Endothelial dysfunction has previously been linked to IR, however, individuals with IR can exhibit normal endothelial function. [16] Research has determined that hyperandrogenaemia is the primary risk factor for ED and CVD in women with PCOS. The lectin-like oxidized low-density lipoprotein receptor-1 (LOX1) was discovered to be a key receptor for oxLDL identified in ECs. Increased levels of soluble LOX-1 (sLOX-1) and reduced NO levels may be an early indicator of ED. Continuously high oxLDL concentrations can also excite vascular endothelial cells, resulting in vascular endothelial apoptosis.

Hypothyroidism: Hypothyroidism is linked to an elevated risk of coronary artery disease (CAD) and NO that extends beyond what can be clarified by its relationship with traditional cardiovasular system (CVS) risk aspects. ED in the coronary arteries that precedes atherosclerosis is associated with unfavourable CVS events, and it may explain the elevated risk of CV events for hypothyroid individuals. The exact processes by which hypothyroidism impairs endothelial function are unknown. Receptors for the thyroid hormone and its isoforms have been found in aortic vascular smooth muscle cells in humans, indicating that thyroid hormones might act directly on the vascular bed and regulate vasomotion. Other research has linked hypothyroidism to the existence of anti-endothelial cell antibodies, which may be connected to the autoimmune aetiology in many cases. [17]

Spondylitis: Inflammation in spondylitis is related to arterial endothelial dysfunction, which accelerates atherosclerosis (AS). In spondylitis, increased atherosclerosis contributes to early cardiovascular disease and higher cardiovascular mortality. In AS, inflammatory cytokines released into the systemic circulation from enthesis and synovium modify the function of distant tissues, such as fatty tissue, skeletal muscle, liver, and the vascular endothelium, resulting in a spectrum of proatherogenic alterations. TNF-blockade improves endothelial dysfunction in spondylitis, which is an important sign and a strong predictor of atherosclerosis. [18]

Dengue haemorrhagic fever (DHF): Dengue viral infection can cause a wide range of clinical symptoms, from a vague febrile state to DHF, which is characterized by increased vascular permeability and haemorrhage, including shock. Researchers studying capillary leakage due to an increase in free VEGF factor in dengue disease are particularly interested in the endothelial barrier. ECs, smooth muscle cells, an extracellular matrix, basement membranes, a cytoskeleton, and cell–cell junctions are all components of the barrier that alter normal physiology [19] Endothelial cell activation can cause coagulation alterations in dengue, such as procoagulation, fibrinolysis, and, in rare cases, disseminated intravascular coagulation.

Erectile dysfunction: Erectile dysfunction is almost a vascular disorder. It is well known that it rises rapidly in males with diabetes, hypercholesterolemia, and CVS ailments. It has a significant occurrence and primarily affects men between the ages of 40 and 70. The loss of endothelial functional integrity and subsequent endothelial dysfunction is critical in the development of erectile dysfunction. Long-term hyperglycaemia is thought to promote the formation of advanced glycation end products and ROS, which may hasten endothelial dysfunction by impairing endothelial NO synthase (eNOS) activities and NO synthesis. As a result, there is a discrepancy between vasocontractors and vasomediators, which changes vascular permeability and disrupts endothelial integrity. Endothelial walls decrease their sensitivity to vasodilator mediators and increase their reactions to vasoconstrictor stimuli in this environment, resulting in reduced vasculature and smooth muscle relaxation and causes clinical ED. [20]

Cardiovascular disease: ED occurs if there is an overall imbalance in NO generation and intake, favouring usage and decreasing synthesis. This pathological condition facilitates the initiation and adhesion of platelets and leukocytes, along with the activation of cytokines that boost the permeability of blood vessel walls to oxidised low-density lipoprotein (oxLDL) and inflammatory mediators, ultimately causing mechanical impairment of the walls of arteries, smooth muscle cell proliferation, and atherosclerotic plaque development. ED is common, since people with recognized atherosclerosis have ED in the periphery of circulatory beds that are not impacted by frank atherosclerosis. It is also observed in populations with a family history of initial CVD with no additional risk factors, hypertriglyceridaemia, lowered high-density lipoprotein (HDL) and increased LDL, tobacco use, overweight patients insulin-resistant patients with first-degree family with diabetes mellitus, cardiac syndrome X, and elderly patients, regardless of other comorbidities and physiological stress. High oxidative stress and inflammation are linked to abnormal endothelial function; both processes result in unusual NO metabolic activities that can be aggravated by other ailments (cold, psychological stress, frustration) that are known to cause global vasoconstriction. Increased oxidative stress is defined by a quantifiable increase in ROS, which may be caused by impaired NO synthesis, decreased L-arg absorption, increased oxidized cholesterol level (Ox-LDL), or reduced superoxide dismutase (an enzyme essential for ROS clearance). [21]

18.2 ASSESSMENT OF ENDOTHELIAL DYSFUNCTION

Ludmer et al. demonstrated ED in arteries using intracoronary acetylcholine infusion and quantitative coronary angiography in 1986. Less invasive procedures were also developed, primarily using the forearm circulation as a proxy for coronary arteries. All techniques have benefits and drawbacks; most importantly, various vascular beds are investigated. The fundamental premise, though, is the same: healthy arteries, such as the brachial or coronary artery, dilate as a result of reactive hyperaemia (flow-mediated vasodilation) or in response to pharmacological stimuli, such as intra-arterial infusion of endothelium-dependent vasodilators such as Ach, serotonin, or bradykinin, via NO or other endothelial-derived vasoactive agents. Endothelial-dependent dilatation is decreased or absent in disease conditions.

18.2.1 Invasive Approach for Diagnosis of Endothelial Dysfunction

Intra-arterial infusion of vasoactive drugs is used in the invasive procedure. High-resolution ultrasound (HRU) or strain-gauge pletismography (SGP) are used to assess response. Through intravascular administration of vasoactive stimuli, intra-arterial assessment can be integrated into intravascular examination. The response is then assessed using intravascular ultrasonography.

18.2.1.1 Intracoronary Infusion

Intracoronary infusion in combination with quantitative angiography is the preferred strategy for direct measurement of endothelium activity in the vessels and arteries, because it permits the examination of dose-response correlations of endothelium antagonists and protagonists allowing for the measurement of baseline endothelium functioning through the transfusion of NOS (nitric oxide synthase) antagonists. [22] It is widely established that intracoronary cholinergic infusion does cause dilatation of healthy arteries with the presence of intact endothelial cells via receptor-mediated activation of nitric oxide formation. Acetylcholine, on the other hand, causes vasoconstriction in the context of endothelial dysfunction (ED) due to its direct influence on smooth muscles. It is the most commonly used vasodilator and also activates endothelial cells and increases nitric oxide production. In patients with a typical endothelial response, acetylcholine causes limited access to vasodilators, resulting in blood vessel dilatation and hyperaemia.

This mechanism is disrupted in individuals with endothelial dysfunction, resulting in reduced vasodilation.

In brief, a Doppler-tipped guidewire is installed through a 6 French Judkins catheter in the proximal segment of a blood vessel (adjacent portion of the left anterior descending coronary artery), and the Doppler flow velocity is constantly monitored. Ach is administered at rising rates into the blood vessel via the Judkins catheter (such as 1 mg/min, 3 mg/min) and saline (medium) is co-administered; the overall administration flow is maintained using an arterial infusion pump. Each dosage is administered for 1–2 minutes. Coronary blood flow velocity is recorded by an online spectrum analyzer and stored. Volumetric coronary flow of blood, a method established by Doucette et al., is computed. [23]

In addition to Ach, intracoronary infusions of vasoactive drugs like substance P, serotonin, and bradykinin have been employed as nitric oxide stimuli. The vasodilatory impact of cholinergic or other dilators is typically contrasted with the reaction to glyceryl trinitrate that causes endothelial-independent vessel dilatation. [24] The main advantage of this technique is that it allows the examination of the coronary arteries' vasculature via dosage response curves to EC antagonists and agonists and the analysis of baseline endothelial function by endothelial NO synthase antagonist infusion. Although intracoronary investigations are regarded as the gold standard for detecting ED in the blood vessels, they are costly and invasive, with the risk of cardiac catheterization, and in the population, they are not suitable as a diagnostic test. [25]

18.2.1.2 Venous Occlusion Plethysmography (VOP)

Venous occlusion plethysmography has been used to assess blood flow for a decade. This approach is appropriate for studying endothelial function, vasodilation responsiveness to different stimuli both in healthy and pathologic conditions, and regulation of autonomic nerbous system's (ANS) blood flow. Under local anaesthetic (2% lidocaine), a polyethylene cannula (typically 21 gauge) is placed into the brachial arteries and attached to a pressure transducer through stopcocks for the continuous measurement of systemic mean heart rates and blood pressures (BPs). Gauge-strain plethysmography is used to assess forearm blood flow (FBF), which can simultaneously be used for both experimental and contralateral forearms. The circulation of the arm is restricted for less than 1 minute before and throughout each FBF assessment by inflating a paediatric clamp over the wrist at suprasystolic BP. [26]

This stimulation might be mechanical, inducing responsive hyperaemia, or chemical and invasive, including intra-arterial administration of vasoactive substances. The infusion of NO precursors, such as sodium nitroprusside, is used to assess endothelium-independent vasodilation. This approach assesses blood flow rather than artery diameter and is dependent on baseline circumstances, but lacks consistency between laboratories. Considering the drawbacks, VOP with intra-arterial administration of vasoactive chemicals is regarded as the gold standard for evaluating vascular function. The brachial arteries are relatively accessible and simpler to cannulate using this procedure. Despite the requirement for artery cannulation, it provides meaningful and reliable surrogate measurements in a less invasive way than 3D quantitative coronary angiography, allowing dosage response curves to EC antagonists and agonists and the study of baseline endothelial function with eNOS antagonist infusion. [27]

18.2.2 Non-invasive Approach for Diagnosis of Endothelial Dysfunction

A wide range of non-invasive techniques for assessing endothelium function in humans have recently been developed. These approaches are simple to use in individuals and can be used as screening tests to detect ED. It is often the forearm or arm that is used to assess endothelium functioning in the brachial arteries or upper arm resistance arteries.

18.2.2.1 Ultrasound Flow-Mediated Dilatation (FMD)

FMD is a typical method for assessing brachial arterial vascular functioning that uses imaging, most commonly ultrasonography, to quantify artery dilatation during post-occlusive reactive hyperaemia (PORH).

It should be connected with 2D imaging, colour, an internal electrocardiogram (ECG) monitor, and a spectral doppler as well as a high-frequency vascular linear array transducer with a minimum frequency of 7 MHz. The timing of every picture frame in relation to the heart cycle is accomplished by simultaneous ECG recording on the ultrasound (US) video display. PORH is accomplished by compressing an air cuff across the arm, reaching suprasystolic pressures for 5 minutes. Reactive hyperaemia would then be produced by promptly lowering the pressure; this phenomenon is caused by NO-mediated ED in the brachial artery. Because NO is the primary medium of FMD in the brachial artery, this offers a much more precise substitute for assessment ofendothelial NO production. [28] Poor dilation suggests impaired endogenous vasodilation release in response to ischaemia, and subsequently endothelial dysfunction. Ultrasound for FMD is limited to a clearly visible artery and necessitates a high-frequency transducer and a skilled ultrasonologist for precise results. Otherwise, substantial errors in flow estimates may arise. [29] To ensure repeatability, a defined procedure for subject preparation and FMD evaluation is also essential. [30] Magnetic resonance imaging (MRI) has been verified as another approach for measuring FMD. [31]

To overcome some of the constraints described above, new approaches such as enclosed zone FMD (ezFMD) have been developed. Oscillometry is used in ezFMD to assess alterations in the magnitude of intra-arterial pressure fluctuations and hence variation in vascular volume. [32]

18.2.2.2 *Pulse Wave Analysis (PWA)*

For measuring FMD, blood vessel imaging using ultrasound or magnetic resonance allows for the determination of arterial compliance using sonographic rigidity indices such as the augmentation index. Pulse wave velocity may also be used to calculate arterial stiffness, with carotid-femoral pulse wave velocities becoming the gold standard for determining large arterial stiffness. [33] To conveniently evaluate arterial compliance, one-point pulse wave velocity, and oscillometric approaches have been developed. [34] Although arterial stiffness is higher in those with CVD risk factors and heart failure, it is not consistent throughout all arteries. Pulse wave velocity monitoring is not yet suggested for normal clinical use as it is not practical. The administration of ACE antagonists and angiotensin receptor blockers can improve pulse wave velocity, but the therapeutic implications of this enhancement have not been thoroughly shown.

18.2.2.3 *Pulse Contour Analysis (PCA)*

In 1904, Erlanger and Hooker developed the concept of pulse contour analysis. They proposed a relationship between cardiac output and arterial pulse pressure. Today's pulse contour devices are based on the same idea. The contour of artery blood pressure waveforms is related to stroke volume and system arterial stiffness. To calculate heart function and provide a consistent readout, an algorithm is used. Each device displays a variety of functional parameters, like heart rate, cardiac index, and cardiac output. All of these sensors also provide information on stroke volume variation (SVV) and breathing as a measurement of liquid sensitivity. There are many devices in clinical use that use the pulse waveform to calculate continuous cardiac output. The three main devices are the PiCCO device, a blood flow sensor, and the LiDCO monitor, which are used to calculate cardiac output in distinct ways. The PiCCO device measures the aortic trace waveform morphology using a thermistor-tipped artery line in a proximal artery. [35]

A blood flow sensor linked to a normal arterial catheter is also used in the FloTrac/Vigileo systems. [36] A recently updated method calculates cardiac output every 20 seconds. The LiDCO monitor employs pulse power assessment rather than PCA. For continuous cardiac monitoring, it employs an algorithm based on the law of conservation of mass for continuous cardiac output calculation.

18.2.2.4 *Pulse Amplitude Tonometry (PAT)*

Emerging research suggests that digital PAT can be employed to assess endothelial function. PAT is used to evaluate vascular functioning by monitoring pulse amplitude within the fingertip at rest and after inducing reactive hyperaemia. The EndoPAT device (Itamar Medical, Caesarea, Israel) is a commercially accessible, FDA-approved apparatus that consists of a fingertip plethysmograph that can monitor volume changes in the digit with each arterial pulse.

The constant applied pressure field throughout the finger minimizes venous pooling and relieves some of the stress on the artery wall. Volume variations in the fingertip are digitally captured as pulse amplitude, which may be followed over time. The three steps of a comprehensive digital PAT endothelial function test are baseline, occlusion, and hyperaemia. A PAT probe is placed on one finger of each hand and set by the computer system to inflate to 10 mm Hg lower diastolic pressure or 70 mm Hg higher diastolic pressure (the lower value is selected). Throughout the investigation, recordings are made from both fingers at the same time. To compensate for systemic effects, the reaction in the control finger that is not experiencing hyperaemia might be employed. Following the collection of baseline data, a blood pressure cuff is raised to suprasystolic pressure on one arm for 5 minutes.

The pulse amplitude in the hyperaemic finger rises once the cuff is released. An automated, proprietary programmer automates and analyzes the pulse amplitude records. For up to 5 minutes following cuff occlusion, the average pulse amplitude is determined at 30-second intervals. The amplitude of the baseline pulse is likewise measured and given in standardized, arbitrary units. [37]

18.2.2.5 Strain-Gauge plethysmography

Strain-gauge plethysmography is another measure currently being employed for endothelial function in the brachial artery to assess changes in forearm blood flow in reactive hyperaemia. The approach measures the percentage difference in flow from zero, i.e., base to maximum flow in responsive hyperaemia after 5 minutes of distal forearm ischaemia. Furthermore, assessing the maximal hyperaemic flow and the overall time-flow curve during reactive hyperaemia may provide useful data in assessing endothelium functioning. [38]

A mercury-filled silastic strain-gauge plethysmograph is used to measure FBF. The strain gauge is fastened to the upper forearm at its widest point; it is held just above the threshold of the right atrium and therefore is linked to a plethysmography system. The upper arm is puffed up to 40 mm Hg for 7 seconds in each 15-second cycle using a rapid cuff inflator to encase vascular flow through the arm. The FBF is calculated using the slope of the line of the curves during the initial cardiac phase and is represented in millilitres per hundred millilitres of forearm tissue volume per minute. The final forearm blood flow is derived by taking the mean of ten successive measurements, which are performed by two independent viewers. The intra-viewer variance coefficient should be less than 4%. To create ischaemia, a second cuff (on the wrist) is kept in the distal part of the strain gauge and inflated at 50 mm Hg above the systolic BP for 5 minutes. The FBF is recorded every 15 seconds after the ischaemia cuff is released, and a time-flow curve is displayed. By measuring the maximum blood flow in reactive hyperaemia and the percentage of flow change between rest and maximum hyperaemic flow, and by analyzing the time-flow curves during reactive hyperaemia, endothelium functioning can be measured. [39]

18.2.2.6 Markers

Several endothelial function biomarkers with clinical implications have been found. For example, studies have linked measures of angiopoietins, selectins, and growth factors with the degree of sepsis. The vast majority of biomarkers can be evaluated using enzyme-linked immunosorbent assays (ELISAs) or liquid chromatography mass spectrometry (LC/MS).

Asymmetric dimethylarginine (ADMA) has recently surfaced as a mediator, an independent risk factor, and possibly a viable ED marker. ADMA is endogenously produced by arginine methylation and effectively suppresses eNOS, resulting in reduced NO generation and perhaps eNOS uncoupling. [40] Because elevated ADMA levels have been seen in individuals with dyslipidaemia, hypertension, and atherosclerotic cardiovascular disease, they may be a valuable indicator of endothelial health, as well as a possible marker for cardiovascular risk in clinical practice. [41]

Chronic inflammation causes ED and promotes reactions between altered monocyte-derived macrophages, T cells, lipoproteins, and normal cellular components of the arterial wall, promoting both late and early atherosclerotic processes. This model has stimulated research assessing inflammation indicators of atherosclerosis, with high-sensitivity C-reactive protein (CRP) becoming one of the most significant indicators. As a result, CRP is a strong independent predictor of myocardial infarction, strokes, and vascular fatality in a variety of contexts, and it appears to be a stronger predictor of cardiovascular events than LDL cholesterol. CRP should be viewed as an indirect, yet crucial, marker of endothelial function. The main benefits of biochemical measurements of endothelial function are their low cost and high repeatability. However, it is not yet obvious what the link is between these indicators, which are measures of endothelial-dependent vasodilation, and cardiovascular outcomes. This is an area that is being researched. Preliminary research indicates that individuals with increased CRP levels have impaired endothelium-dependent vasodilation, implying that CRP might be a valuable therapeutic tool for endothelial vasomotion. [42]

18.3 TREATMENT FOR ENDOTHELIAL DYSFUNCTION

In this context, identifying the mechanism of drugs that prevent ED is critical. Medical therapies can have either short- or long-term outcomes, and some have both. These may have an immediate effect on EC and minimize cardiovascular risk. Because the therapy for ED is dependent on the symptoms, the disease's treatment is discussed in the context of various symptoms/conditions in the following sections.

18.3.1 Diabetes

Several treatment strategies have been investigated in clinical trials with the goal of enhancing endothelium functioning in diabetic patients. There are a number of medications with many mechanisms of action that are used to treat patients with high blood sugar and other metabolic abnormalities of diabetes that influence endothelium functioning. [43]

Postprandial hyperglycaemia, which is more common in Asian patients who consume a carb-rich diet, has been associated with arterial endothelial dysfunction, which can lead to various cardiovascular issues. [44] As a result, medications intended to decrease blood glucose peaks, such as α-glucosidase inhibitors like voglibose, dipeptidyl peptidase-4 inhibitors like sitagliptin, and sodium-linked glucose transporter-2 (SGLT2) inhibitors like glifozins may enhance vascular function in diabetes patients.

Insulin sensitivity has been identified as a common factor in type 2 diabetes and cardiovascular complications. It involves fundamentally shifting insulin receptors downstream, signalling from PI3K-Akt to the MAPK/ERK cascade. Metformin, a popular medication among diabetes patients, works largely by enhancing hepatic insulin sensitivity and total systemic glucose status. Metformin has been proven in clinical investigations to improve impaired endothelial functioning in type 2 diabetic individuals. It has been found in experimental models to activate the AMPK/eNOS pathway, contributing to better vascular function in metabolic syndrome. [45] Metformin has also been found to protect from hyperglycaemia-induced ED in db/db mouse thoracic aortas via processes involving enhanced phosphorylation of the eNOS and Akt signalling pathway. [46] Thiazolidinediones, often known as glitazones, are another family of insulin-sensitizing oral hypoglycaemic medicines that can be used alone or in conjunction with biguanides like metformin. These medications activate the gamma subtype of the peroxisome proliferator-activated receptor. Though this family of drugs is traditionally known to operate on adipocytes by boosting non-esterified fatty acid absorption from the circulatory system, they exhibit pleiotropic activity with tissue-specific activities, endothelial being one of them. Pioglitazone is a clinically authorized member of this class.

18.3.2 Obesity

Some obese people might not react to lifestyle modifications. In certain cases, pharmacological and/or surgical procedures may be beneficial in the management of obesity. Bariatric surgery is a successful technique for weight loss in obese people. The American Heart Association (AHA)/American College of Cardiology (ACC)/The Obesity Society (TOS)'s guidelines suggest bariatric surgical procedures in persons with BMIs of 40 kg/m2 or 35 kg/m2 who have obesity-linked ailments. [47] A meta-analysis performed on the long-term results of bariatric surgery found that weight reduction peaks at 2 years and is reasonably steady from 2 to 20 years, with a mean weight loss of 24.8 kg. [48] Several studies have found that bariatric surgery lowers cardiovascular risk factors and the occurrence of CVS events.

Individuals with a BMI of 30 kg/m2 or a BMI of 27 kg/m2 who have obesity-related comorbidities may consider medication in addition to lifestyle changes as a treatment option. [49] There are five USFDA-permitted medications for the treatment of obesity: pancreatic lipase inhibitors (orlistat), phentermine-topiramate combinations (phentermine-topiramate), bupropion-naltrexone combinations (bupropion-naltrexone), and glucagon-like peptide 1 (GLP-1) receptors agonists (semaglutide and liraglutide). According to a recent meta-analysis, phentermine-topiramate has a median weight reduction of 8.07 kg and GLP-1 receptor agonists have a median weight loss of 4.96 kg for decreasing weight. [50] Figure 18.2 shows the correlation between ED and various ailments.

18.3.3 Nephrological Disorders

Statins are the first approved pharmaceutical treatments used to treat hypercholesterolemia & CVD. They have lipid-lowering properties, as well as extra cholesterol-independent or pleiotropic properties. [51] Statins have been shown to increase endothelial function and stabilize susceptible lesions, and also have antioxidant, anti-inflammatory, and antithrombotic properties. Mechanistic studies revealed that statin-mediated benefits were caused by the following mechanisms: lowering the effect of low-density lipoprotein, enhancing nitric oxide bioavailability, having a protective effect against oxLDL aiding eNOS phosphorylation at Ser1177 via the PI3K/Akt signalling pathway, aiding the agonist-stimulated eNOS-HSP90 interaction, as well as recoupling eNOS by increasing the vascular BH4 level and reducing vascular NOX-dependent O2 generation. Statins also increase eNOS mRNA stability, which increases eNOS expression. Additionally, the Ca

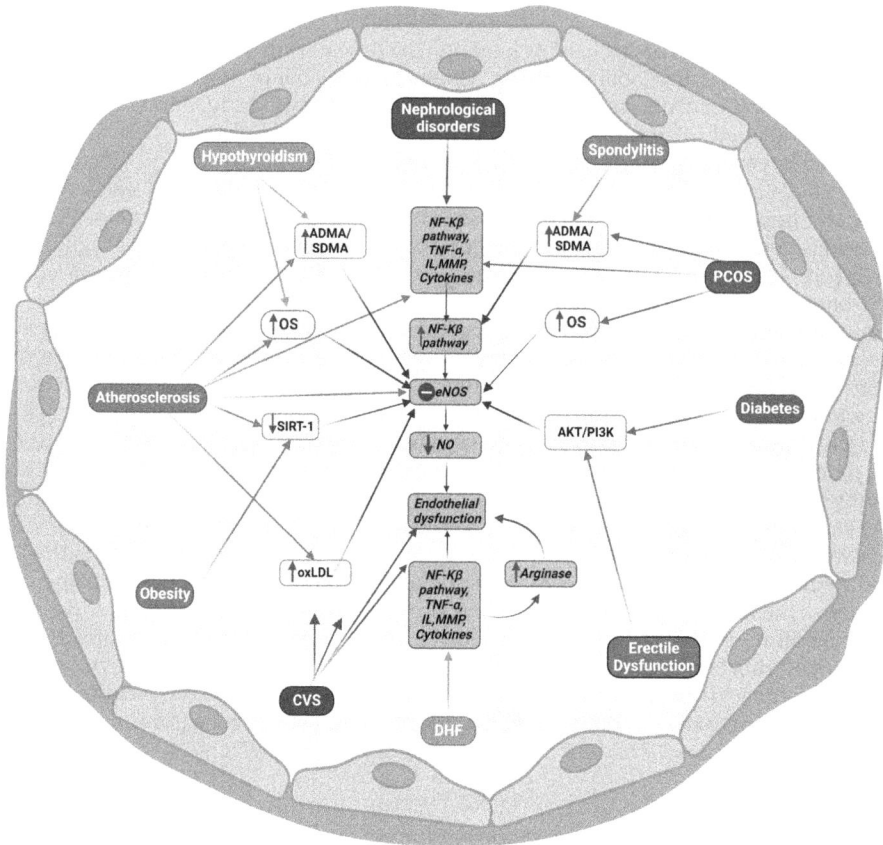

Figure 18.2 Correlation of ED with various ailments

channel inhibitor nifedipine can be used to treat nephrological disorders due to both its systemic and specific activities in terms of its involvement in preventing or improving glomerular endothelial function. [52]

18.3.4 Atherosclerosis

The glucocorticoids have pleiotropic activities relevant to CV health and endothelial functioning. Anti-inflammatory glucocorticoids have a number of effects on endothelium functioning and CV health. Selective and non-selective COX-2 inhibitors have been shown to boost endothelium functioning in those with existing atherosclerosis and high CVS risk factors. Because of their inhibitory impact on the trafficking of blood-borne lymphocytes and leukocytes, glucocorticoids have been shown to have anti-inflammatory effects on chemokine-cytokine synthesis and endothelium activation. Aside from nonsteroidal anti-inflammatory drugs, medicines targeting the NLRP3 inflammasome, including such colchicine as traditional Chinese medicine, have entered clinical trials for the treatment of CVD and ED. So, although it seems that the NLRP3 inflammasome plays a key role in atherosclerosis, it is unclear whether new NLRP3 inflammasome agents (such as MCC950) may be used as innovative therapeutics for related CVD and ED. [53]

18.3.5 PCOS

Impaired glucose tolerance, type 2 diabetes mellitus, obesity, dyslipidaemia metabolic syndrome, and non-alcoholic fatty liver disorder have all been linked to PCOS. [54] PCOS has now been linked to subclinical atherosclerosis indicators, such as coronary and aortic calcification, higher carotid intima-media thickness, and endothelial dysfunction, as compared to healthy controls. Metformin administration improves ovulatory frequency as well as insulin sensitivity and hyperandrogenism. Metformin therapy has been linked to obesity treatment and an enhanced blood lipid profile in women with PCOS; however, this is not consistently observed in all PCOS patients.

[55] There is also conflicting evidence about metformin's influence on endothelial function. Metformin slows ageing by boosting adenosine monophosphate-activated protein kinase, which leads to augmented nitric oxide synthesis in the endothelium and, as a result, greater vascular relaxation. Metformin reduces mammalian targeting of rapamycin, which can lead to a rise in nitric oxide. It reduces oxidative stress and inflammation, which may lead to improved endothelium functioning and vascular dilatation. It has anti-inflammatory properties and can prevent endothelial cell damage and apoptosis induced by mitochondrial membrane damage. [56]

Another therapy, hormone replacement therapy, has garnered a lot of interest as a primary and secondary preventative method in relation to cardiovascular disease. This interest was sparked by population-based research that linked hormone replacement treatment to a lower incidence of cardiovascular disease. [57] There is significant evidence that continuous oestrogen therapy enhances endothelial function in women. There have been reports of oestrogen improving endothelium functioning through antioxidant characteristics that boost nitric oxide expression and enhance superoxide anion radical degradation. [58] Oestrogen has the ability to enhance peripheral and coronary endothelial function, which is independent of the favourable effects on profiles of lipid and control vasculature via a nitric oxide-dependent pathway.

18.3.6 Hypothyroidism

Several investigations have found that thyroxine improves non-invasively assessed flow-mediated dilatation in hypothyroid individuals. The sample size in two of these trials was quite small, i.e., 8 and 14, and the found difference in flow-mediated dilatation of 1.7% in the third study may not be clinically meaningful. In another trial, FMD did not recover in hypothyroid individuals until they had been on thyroid replacement therapy for at least 6 months; thus, the length of thyroid replacement therapy treatment may be significant. While thyroid replacement therapy has been found to result in beneficial improvements in CV risk factors in hypothyroidism, its specific involvement in altering ED deserves additional investigation. [59] As a result, the latest research highlights the necessity for innovative therapies for endothelial dysfunction that can be target-specific. Oestrogen is thought to enhance thyroid-binding globulin concentrations; globulin binds thyroxine and decreases free thyroxine levels, reducing their effects on tissues. In comparison, androgens (testosterone) inhibit the formation of thyroid-binding globulin, leading to transiently elevated amounts of free thyroxine. Androgen administration has been demonstrated to induce clinical signs of hyperthyroidism in hypothyroid women. [60]

18.3.7 Spondylitis

Spironolactone, an aldosterone blocker, has been demonstrated to suppress the generation of proinflammatory cytokines such as TNF-alpha and IFN-gamma, and hence has potential as a form of arthritis therapy. Spironolactone reduces endothelial dysfunction and inflammatory disorder activities in rheumatoid arthritis, and it improves endothelial dysfunction and survival in congestive heart failure. TNF-alpha inhibition is responsible for spironolactone's therapeutic impact on heart failure. [61]

18.3.8 Dengue Haemorrhagic Fever (DHF)

There is currently no particular therapy for dengue. To ensure efficient intravascular volume and tissue perfusion, the primary therapy is cautious fluid replacement. The transfusion of blood components, corticosteroids or IV immunoglobulin, carbazochrome sodium sulfonate, and recombinant-activated factor VII have all been suggested as possible beneficial techniques. There is very little data to justify full implementation of these techniques. Because high viral load is frequently linked to severe dengue, reducing the viral burden with antiviral medicines is essential. Corticosteroids' anti-inflammatory and vasoactive actions provide a rationale for their usage in dengue. Potential treatment medicines include mediators that improve vascular integrity via diverse pathways, such as angiopoietin-1 phosphate and sphingosine-1-phosphatase. In vitro, vaculotide, an experimental chemical and an angiopoietin-1 receptor agonist, inhibited endothelial cell VE-cadherin loss and cytoskeleton rearrangement. Additionally, peptide beta15-42 decreased vascular leak and death in rats with DHF and in models of animals treated with lipopolysaccharide. [62]

18.3.9 Erectile Dysfunction

PDE5 inhibitors (PDE5Is) keep the level of cGMP high by inhibiting its breakdown, facilitating sexual excitement and erection. Since 1998, three PDE5Is have been on the market: sildenafil, tadalafil, and vardenafil. All three molecules have been shown to be effective in the treatment of erectile dysfunction. [63] As a result, taking a PDE5 inhibitor like sildenafil every night may improve Another potential benefit of erectile rehabilitation is the potential improvement in erectile dysfunction (ED) patients with severe illness or those with low scores in the international indicator of erectile function domain (IIEF) ranging from 1 to -10. These individuals may not respond well to short-term phosphodiesterase (PDE) inhibition, but they might experience better results with on-demand oral therapy if they undergo a sufficient period of erectile rehabilitation.

18.3.10 Cardiovascular Disease

Nifedipine has antioxidant properties, as well as having an impact on the expression and activity of endothelial nitric oxide synthase. Ranolazine is a Na channel inhibitor that may be used to treat angina. It is also proven to relieve indications of microvascular angina discomfort, but no substantial improvement in microvascular function was seen. Furthermore, endothelial function improved in smaller randomized control clinical studies involving patients with diabetes and individuals with chronic stable angina.

Combining ACE inhibitors and statins has also been found to promote endothelium-dependent relaxing of the coronary vascular system via nitric oxide-dependent pathways.

Fibrate treatment, like omega-3 fatty acid supplementation, improves fasting and postprandial endothelial function in type 2 diabetic patients. This might be due to an increase in HDL and a reduction in postprandial lipemia and oxidative stress. Metformin is widely considered to increase peripheral endothelium functioning, as indicated by smaller randomized control trials in metabolic and diabetic patients. According to these findings, metformin and rosiglitazone are promising candidates for enhancing endothelium functioning.

18.4 CONCLUSION

The endothelium is essential for regulating blood vessel activity and maintaining vascular homeostasis. The endothelium and inflammation play a critical role in all disease conditions. It is now known that inflammatory processes play an important role in the onset and development of many disease states. ED can be detected via various techniques that allow an early diagnosis and may make it possible to prevent ED. Angiotensin-converting enzyme (ACE) inhibitors, statins, insulin sensitizers, and L-arginine, as well as medicines that target endothelial nitric oxide synthase (eNOS) coupling, have been shown to enhance endothelial function.

REFERENCES

1. Aird WC. Phenotypic heterogeneity of the endothelium: I. Structure, function, and mechanisms. *Circ Res*. 2007;100:158–173.

2. Donato, A. J., Morgan, R. G., Walker, A. E., & Lesniewski, L. A.. Cellular and molecular biology of aging endothelial cells. *J Mol Cell Cardiol*. 2015;89(Pt B):122–135.

3. Sena, C.M., Carrilho, F., Seiça, R.M. *Endothelial Dysfunction in Type 2 Diabetes: Targeting Inflammation. Endothelial Dysfunction—Old Concepts and New Challenges, Helena Lenasi.* IntechOpen. 2018.

4. Verhamme, P, and M F Hoylaerts. The pivotal role of the endothelium in haemostasis and thrombosis. *Acta Clin Belg* 2006;61(5):213–9.

5. Ren B, Deng Y, Mukhopadhyay A, et al. ERK1/2–Akt1 crosstalk regulates arteriogenesis in mice and zebrafish. J Clin Invest. 2010;120(4):1217–1228.

6. Nitenberg A, Valensi P, Sachs R, Dali M, Aptecar E, Attali JR. Impairment of coronary vascular reserve and ACh-induced coronary vasodilation in diabetic patients with angiographically normal coronary arteries and normal left ventricular systolic function. *Diabetes*. 1993;42:1017–1025.

7. Furchgott RF, Zawadzki JV. The obligatory role of endothelial cells in the relaxation of arterial smooth muscle by acetylcholine. *Nature*. 1980;288:373–376.

8. Fernández-Ortiz A, Badimon JJ, Falk E, Fuster V, Meyer B, et al. Characterization of the relative thrombogenicity of atherosclerotic plaque components: Implications for consequences of plaque rupture. *J Am Coll Cardiol*. 1994;23:1562–1569.

9. Marcelo KL, Goldie LC, Hirschi KK. Regulation of endothelial cell differentiation and specification. *Circ Res*. 2013;112:1272–1287.

10. Ren B, Yee KO, Lawler J, et al. Regulation of tumor angiogenesis by thrombospondin-1. Biochim Biophys Acta. 2006;1765(2):178–188.

11. Civelek M, Manduchi E, Riley RJ, Stoeckert CJ Jr, Davies PF. Chronic endoplasmic reticulum stress activates unfolded protein response in arterial endothelium in regions of susceptibility to atherosclerosis. *Circ Res*. 2009;105:453–461.

12. Tesauro M, Schinzari F, Rovella V, Di Daniele N, Lauro D, Mores N, et al. Ghrelin restores the endothelin 1/nitric oxide balance in patients with obesity-related metabolic syndrome. *Hypertension*. 2009;54(5):995–1000.

13. Chistiakov DA, Melnichenko AA, Grechko AV, Myasoedova VA, and Orekhov AN. Potential of anti-inflammatory agents for treatment of atherosclerosis. *Exp Mol Pathol*. 2018;104:114–124.

14. Rajendran P, Rengarajan T, Thangavel J, Nishigaki Y, Sakthisekaran D, Sethi G, et al. The vascular endothelium and human diseases. *Int J Biol Sci*. 2013;9:1057–1069.

15. Dube R. Does endothelial dysfunction correlate with endocrinal abnormalities in patients with polycystic ovary syndrome? *Avicenna J Med*. 2016;6(4):91–102.

16. Wiweko B, Maidarti M, Priangga MD, Shafira N, Fernando D, Sumapraja K, et al. Anti-mullerian hormone as a diagnostic and prognostic tool for PCOS patients. *J Assist Reprod Genet*. 2014;31:1311–6.

17. Sara JD, Zhang M, Gharib H, Lerman LO, Lerman A. Hypothyroidism Is Associated With Coronary Endothelial Dysfunction in Women. *J Am Heart Assoc*. 2015;4(8):e002225. doi: 10.1161/JAHA.115.002225. PMID: 26224049; PMCID: PMC4599474.

18. Syngle A, Vohra K, Sharma A, Kaur L. Endothelial dysfunction in ankylosing spondylitis improves after tumor necrosis factor-α blockade. *Clin Rheumatol*. 2010;29:763–770.

19. Djamiatun K, van der Ven AJ, de Groot PG, Faradz SM, Hapsari D, Dolmans WM, Sebastian S, Fijnheer R, de Mast Q. Severe dengue is associated with consumption of von Willebrand factor and its cleaving enzyme ADAMTS-13. *PLoS Negl Trop Dis*. 2012;6:e1628.

20. Castela, Â., Costa, C. Molecular mechanisms associated with diabetic endothelial-erectile dysfunction. *Nat Rev Urol*. 2016;13: 266–274.

21. Widmer RJ, Lerman A. Endothelial dysfunction and cardiovascular disease. *Glob Cardiol Sci Pract*. 2014;2014(3):291–308. doi: 10.5339/gcsp.2014.43. PMID: 25780786; PMCID: PMC4352682.

22. Widlansky ME, Gokce N, Keaney JF, et al. The clinical implications of endothelial dysfunction. *J Am Coll Cardiol*. 2003;42:1149–60.

23. Doucette JW, Corl PD, Payne HM, et al. Validation of Doppler guide wire for intravascular measurement of coronary artery flow velocity. *Circulation*. 1992;85:1899–911.

24. Widlansky ME, Gokce N, Keaney JF, et al. The clinical implications of endothelial dysfunction. *J Am Coll Cardiol*. 2003;42:1149–60.

25. Porto I, Biasucci LM, De Maria GL, Leone AM, Niccoli G, Burzotta F, Trani C, Tritarelli A, Vergallo R, Liuzzo G, Crea F. Intracoronary microparticles and microvascular obstruction in patients with ST elevation myocardial infarction undergoing primary percutaneous intervention. *Eur Heart J*. 2012;33:2928–38.

26. Kraemer-Aguiar LG, de Miranda ML, Bottino DA, Lima Rde A, de Souza Md, Balarini Mde M, Villela NR, Bouskela E. Increment of body mass index is positively correlated with worsening of endothelium-dependent and independent changes in forearm blood flow. *Front Physiol*. 2015;6:223.

27. Libby P, Buring JE, Badimon L, Hansson GK, Deanfield J, Bittencourt MS, Tokgözoğlu L, Lewis EF. Atherosclerosis *Nat Rev Dis Primers*. 2019;5:56.

28. Gutterman DD, Chabowski DS, Kadlec AO, Durand MJ, Freed JK, Ait-Aissa K, et al. The human microcirculation: Regulation of flow and beyond. *Circ Res*. 2016;118:157–72.

29. Hoskins PR, Fish PJ, Mcdicken WN, Moran C. Developments in cardiovascular ultrasound. part 2: arterial applications. *Med Biol Eng Comput*. 1998;36:259–69.

30. Pyke KE, Tschakovsky ME. The relationship between shear stress and flow-mediated dilation: Implications for the assessment of endothelial function. *J Physiol*. 2005;568:357–69. doi: 10.1113/jphysiol.2005.089755.

31. Leeson CP, Robinson M, Francis JM, Robson MD, Channon KM, Neubauer S, et al. Cardiovascular magnetic resonance imaging for non-invasive assessment of vascular function: Validation against ultrasound. *J Cardiovasc Magn Reson*. 2006;8:381–7. doi: 10.1080/10976640500526993.

32. Hirano H, Takama R, Matsumoto R, Tanaka H, Hirano H, Soh Z, et al. Assessment of lower-limb vascular endothelial function based on enclosed zone flow-mediated dilation. *Sci Rep*. 2018;8:9263. doi: 10.1038/s41598-018-27392-3.

33. Van Bortel LM, Laurent S, Boutouyrie P, Chowienczyk P, Cruickshank JK, De Backer T, et al. Expert consensus document on the measurement of aortic stiffness in daily practice using carotid-femoral pulse wave velocity. *J Hypertens*. 2012;30:445–8. doi: 10.1097/HJH.0b013e32834fa8b0.

34. Vriz O, Driussi C, La Carrubba S, Di Bello V, Zito C, Carerj S, et al. Comparison of sequentially measured Aloka echo-tracking one-point pulse wave velocity with SphygmoCor carotid-femoral pulse wave velocity. *SAGE Open Med*. 2013;1:2050312113507563. doi: 10.1177/2050312113507563.

35. Funk DJ, Moretti EW, Gan TJ. Minimally invasive cardiac output, *Anesth Analg* 2009;108:887–97.

36. De Waal EEC, Wappler F, Buhre WF. Cardiac output monitoring, *Curr Opin Anaesthesiol*. 2009;22:71–7.

37. Hamburg NM, Keyes MJ, Larson MG, et al. Cross-sectional relations of digital vascular function to cardiovascular risk factors in the Framingham Heart Study. *Circulation*. 2008;117:2467–2474.

38. Higashi Y, Sasaki S, Keigo N, et al. Effect of angiotensin-converting enzyme inhibitor imidapril on reactive hyperemia in patients with essential hypertension: Relationship between treatment periods and resistance artery endothelial function. *J Am Coll Cardiol*. 2001;37:863–70.

39. Tousoulis D, Antoniades C, Tentolouris. et al Antioxidant vitamins C and E administration in smokers: Effects on endothelial function and adhesion molecules. *Atherosclerosis*. 2003;170:263–9.

40. Böger RH, Vallance P, Cooke JP. Asymmetric dimethylarginine (ADMA): A key regulator of nitric oxide synthase. *Atheroscler Suppl*. 2003;4:1–3.

41. Lekakis J, Abraham P, Balbarini A, Blann A, Boulanger CM, Cockcroft J, Cosentino F, Deanfield J, Gallino A, Ikonomidis I, et al. Methods for evaluating endothelial function: A position statement from the European Society of Cardiology Working Group on Peripheral Circulation. *Eur J Cardiovasc Prev Rehabil*. 2011;18:775–89.

42. Fichtlscherer S, Rosenberger G, Walter DH, et al. Elevated C-reactive protein levels and impaired endothelial vasoreactivity in patients with coronary artery disease. *Circulation*. 2000;102:1000–1006.

43. Triggle CR, Ding H, Marei I, Anderson TJ, Hollenberg MDc. Why the endothelium? The endothelium as a target to reduce diabetes-associated vascular disease. *Can J Physiol Pharmacol*. 2020;98:415–430.

44. Kitasato L, Tojo T, Hatakeyama Y et al. Postprandial hyperglycemia and endothelial function in type 2 diabetes: Focus on mitiglinide. *Cardiovasc Diabetol*. 2012;11(1):1.

45. Yu JW, Deng YP, Han X et al. Metformin improves the angiogenic functions of endothelial progenitor cells via activating AMPK/eNOS pathway in diabetic mice. *Cardiovasc Diabetol*. 2016;15(1):88.

46. Ghosh S, Lakshmanan AP, Hwang MJ et al. Metformin improves endothelial function in aortic tissue and microvascular endothelial cells subjected to diabetic hyperglycaemic conditions. *Biochem Pharmacol*. 2015;98(3):412–421.

47. Jensen, M.D., Ryan, D.H., Apovian, C.M., Ard, J.D., Comuzzie, A.G., Donato, K.A., Hu, F.B., Hubbard, V.S., Jakicic, J.M., Kushner, R.F., et al. 2013 AHA/ACC/TOS guideline for the management of overweight and obesity in adults: A report of the American College of Cardiology/American Heart Association task force on practice guidelines and the obesity society. *Circulation*. 2014;129(Suppl 2):S102–S138.

48. O'Brien, P.E., Hindle, A., Brennan, L., Skinner, S., Burton, P., Smith, A., Crosthwaite, G., Brown, W. Long-term outcomes after bariatric surgery: A systematic review and meta-analysis of weight loss at 10 or more years for all bariatric procedures and a single-centre review of 20-year outcomes after adjustable gastric banding. *Obes Surg*. 2019;29:3–14.

49. Shi, Q., Wang, Y., Hao, Q., Vandvik, P.O., Guyatt, G., Li, J., Chen, Z., Xu, S., Shen, Y., Ge, L., et al. Pharmacotherapy for adults with overweight and obesity: A systematic review and network meta-analysis of randomised controlled trials. *Lancet*. 2021;399:259–269.

50. Oesterle A, Laufs U, Liao JK. Pleiotropic effects of statins on the cardiovascular system. *Circ Res*. 2017;120:229–243

51. Ishizawa K, Yamaguchi K, Horinouchi Y, Fukuhara Y, Tajima S, Hamano S, et al. Drug discovery for overcoming chronic kidney disease (CKD): Development of drugs on endothelial cell protection for overcoming CKD. *J Pharmacol Sci*. 2009;109:14–19.

52. Vander Heijden T, Kritikou E, Venema W, van Duijn J, van Santbrink PJ, Slütter B, Foks AC, et al. NLRP3 inflammasome inhibition by MCC950 reduces atherosclerotic lesion development in apolipoprotein E-deficient mice-brief report. *Arterioscler Thromb Vasc Biol*. 2017;37:1457–1461.

53. Macut D, Božić-Antić I, Bjekić-Macut J, Tziomalos K. Management of endocrine disease: Polycystic ovary syndrome and nonalcoholic fatty liver disease. *Eur J Endocrinol.* 2017;177(3):R145–R158.

54. Conway G, Dewailly D, Diamanti-Kandarakis E, et al.; ESE PCOS Special Interest Group. The polycystic ovary syndrome: A position statement from the European Society of Endocrinology. *Eur J Endocrinol.* 2014;171(4):P1–P29.

55. Kulkarni AS, Brutsaert EF, Anghel V, et al. Metformin regulates metabolic and nonmetabolic pathways in skeletal muscle and subcutaneous adipose tissues of older adults. *Aging Cell.* 2018;17(2):e12723.

56. Scherer T, Wolf P, Winhofer Y, Duan H, Einwallner E, Gessl A, Luger A, Trattnig S, Hoffmann M, Niessner A, Baumgartner-Parzer S, Krssak M, Krebs M. Levothyroxine replacement in hypothyroid humans reduces myocardial lipid load and improves cardiac function. *J Clin Endocrinol Metab.* 2014;99:E2341–E2346.

57. Barrett-Connor E, Bush TL. Estrogen and coronary heart disease in women. *JAMA.* 1991;265:1861–1867.

58. Collins P, Shay J, Jiang C, Moss J. Nitric oxide accounts for dose-dependent estrogen-mediated coronary relaxation after acute estrogen withdrawal. *Circulation.* 1994;90:1964–8.

59. Sara JD, Zhang M, Gharib H, Lerman LO, Lerman A. Hypothyroidism is associated with coronary endothelial dysfunction in women. *J Am Heart Assoc.* 2015;4(8):1–11.

60. Syngle A, Vohra K, Kaur L, Sharma S. Effect of spironolactone on endothelial dysfunction in rheumatoid arthritis. *Scand J Rheumatol.* 2009;38:15–22.

61. Srikiatkhachorn A, Kelley JF. Endothelial cells in dengue hemorrhagic fever. *Antiviral Res.* 2014;109:160–70. doi: 10.1016/j.antiviral.2014.07.005; Epub 2014 Jul 12. Erratum in: *Antiviral Res.* 2015;114:47.

62. Cirino G, Fusco F, Imbimbo C, et al. Pharmacology of erectile dysfunction in man. *Pharmacol Ther.* 2006;111:400–23.

63. Villano A, Di Franco A, Nerla R, Sestito A, Tarzia P, Lamendola P, Di Monaco A, Sarullo FM, Lanza GA, Crea F. Effects of ivabradine and ranolazine in patients with microvascular angina pectoris. *Am J Cardiol.* 2013;112(1):8–13.

19 Alcoholic and Non-alcoholic Liver Diseases
Biochemical Aspects

Kamaruz Zaman, Pompy Patowary, Arpita Paul, Nilayan Guha, and Madhusmita Gogoi

19.1 INTRODUCTION TO LIVER DISEASES

Alcoholic liver disease (ALD) is directly linked to excessive alcohol intake (Rehm et al., 2009). Diseases related to alcohol consumption have plagued humanity since the practice of distilling alcohol became common in the fifteenth century (Schwartz and Reinus, 2012). According to a recent review, alcohol is responsible for 4.6% of disability-adjusted life years and 3.8% of all fatalities worldwide (Rehm et al., 2009). In addition, alcohol has a negative impact on economic operations; in high-income nations, the cost of excessive social drinking is 1% or more of GDP (Mohapatra et al., 2010). Overeating is a contributing factor to excess body fat. Body mass index (BMI) of 25 kg/m2 or greater was seen in an estimated 1.46 billion persons worldwide in 2008 (Finucane et al., 2011). Non-alcoholic fatty liver disease (NAFLD) is the hepatic manifestation of metabolic syndrome, which is commonly seen in obese people (Marchesini et al., 2003). American researchers showed that people with metabolic syndrome had annual healthcare costs that were 1.6% greater than those of people without metabolic syndrome (Boudreau et al., 2009). ALD and NAFLD are both associated with substantial health and economic costs around the world. Although the pathological spectra of ALD and NAFLD are similar, ranging from simple hepatic steatosis through steatohepatitis and liver cirrhosis (Tannapfel et al., 2011), there are significant distinctions between these disorders. Understanding and treating both ALD and NAFLD could benefit from a comparison of the two conditions (Toshikuni, Tsutsumi, and Arisawa, 2014; Idalsoaga et al., 2020; Ikejima, Kon, and Yamashina, 2020). To fully describe ALD, we compared its biochemical aspects, therapies, and outcomes to those of NAFLD in this chapter.

19.1.1 Epidemiology

There are reports of geographical distinctions between how much people drink. For instance, the yearly per capita consumption is highest in Eastern Europe (15.7 L) and lowest in North Africa and the Middle East (1.0 L) (Rehm, Samokhvalov, and Shield, 2013). Studies in Europe, the United States, and Asia that evaluated hepatic steatosis with ultrasonography or magnetic resonance imaging revealed a prevalence of NAFLD between 12.9% and 46.0% (Hamaguchi et al., 2005; Adams and Lindor, 2007; Williams et al., 2011; Eguchi et al., 2012), although this may vary depending on patterns of alcohol consumption. According to one study, the percentage of NAFLD prevalence in Japan rose from 12.6% in 1989 to 28.4% in 2000 (Kojima et al., 2003). In addition, a recent study from China indicated that the prevalence rates of ALD and NAFLD were 4.5% and 15.0%, respectively, and both rates are predicted to increase in the future (Fan, 2013) as the average yearly alcohol consumption in China is 4–6 L per person (Rehm, Samokhvalov, and Shield, 2013).

According to a study conducted in the United States, the peak age range for alcohol-related hospitalizations was between 45 and 69 years old (Adams et al., 1993). In contrast, a large Japanese study indicated that the prevalence of NAFLD peaked between the ages of 40 and 49 in men and 60 and 69 in women (Eguchi et al., 2012). However, a large Chinese study found that the prevalence of NAFLD in both sexes rose between the ages of 60 and 69 (Fan et al., 2005). Also, a recent autopsy research conducted in the United States found that NAFLD was present in approximately 10% of children (Schwimmer et al., 2006).

It seems to be predominantly males who develop ALD. Patients with alcoholic liver cirrhosis, for instance, tended to be male (9:1), according to a cross-sectional study (Bellentani et al., 1997). There were 4.5 cases of acute alcoholic hepatitis for every 100,000 people in the United States, with a male to female ratio of 1.83:1, and 13.7 cases of chronic alcoholic hepatitis with cirrhosis for every 100,000 people, with a male to female ratio of 2.64:1 (Yang et al., 2008). NAFLD is also more common in men than in women, according to research. One US study indicated that 58.9% of NAFLD patients were male (Williams et al., 2011); another, larger study in Japan found that the prevalence of NAFLD was 41.0% in men and 17.7% in women. Males had a higher incidence of NAFLD across all age groups, while the prevalence in females rose progressively with age (3.3% in the second decade to 31.3% beyond the sixth decade) (Eguchi et al., 2012). In China, we see the same tendencies (Shen et al., 2003).

DOI: 10.1201/9781003384823-19

The prevalence rates of ALD and NAFLD have been shown to vary according to ethnicity. For instance, South Asian males had a 32.8% higher incidence rate of alcoholic liver cirrhosis than Afro-Caribbean males (1.9%) in the United Kingdom (Douds et al., 2003). Hispanics (24.2%) have a greater prevalence of NAFLD than non-Hispanic whites (17.8%) or non-Hispanic blacks (13.5%), according to a recent large study of individuals with NAFLD (Lazo et al., 2013; Toshikuni, Tsutsumi, and Arisawa, 2014; Idalsoaga et al., 2020; Ikejima, Kon, and Yamashina, 2020).

19.1.2 Risk Factors

Most people who consume excessive amounts of alcohol (Schwartz and Reinus, 2012) or food (Sullivan, 2010) develop simple hepatic steatosis. However, only a minority of those affected will progress to cirrhosis or advanced liver fibrosis. Patients with ALD who underwent repeated liver biopsies at 4-year intervals showed that 11% of those with simple hepatic steatosis and 39% of those with alcoholic hepatitis developed liver cirrhosis (Mathurin et al., 2007). Patients with simple hepatic steatosis had a 5-year risk of cirrhosis estimated at 6.9%, whereas those with steatohepatitis had a risk of 16.0%, according to a recent cohort analysis of patients with ALD (Deleuran et al., 2012). Liver cirrhosis developed in 0–8% of patients without hepatic fibrosis and 11.3–17.6% of patients with hepatic fibrosis, according to studies investigating the histological course of NAFLD over a mean follow-up time of 3.2–13.8 years (Adams et al., 2005; Ekstedt et al., 2006). In a long-term study of individuals with simple hepatic steatosis (about 20 years), 22% of those with ALD and 1.2% of those with NAFLD progressed to liver cirrhosis (Dam-Larsen et al., 2009). According to a recent autopsy investigation, the ratio of patients with simple hepatic steatosis to those with steatohepatitis or liver cirrhosis was 2.33:1 (Dunn et al., 2012). Environment–host interactions may be to blame for the divergent disease progression. Recent genetic research has shed light on risk factors that can influence disease development.

19.1.3 Environmental Factors

Increased alcohol consumption is associated with an elevated risk of developing and progressing ALD (Becker et al., 1996; Bellentani et al., 1997; Naveau et al., 1997). ALD development could be affected by the types of drinks consumed. Deaths from cirrhosis were linked to the consumption of spirits, but not beer or wine. This was evident in a pooled cross-sectional time-series analysis (Kerr, Fillmore, and Marvy, 2000). Habitual alcohol consumption is also a risk factor for ALD. Heavy drinking on a daily or near-daily basis, as opposed to occasional or binge drinking, has been shown to have a strong correlation with the onset of ALD (Bellentani et al., 1997; Hatton et al., 2009). Drinking outside of mealtimes and consuming a variety of alcoholic beverages have also been shown to enhance the chance of getting ALD (Bellentani et al., 1997). Similarly, NAFLD development is promoted by a high total energy intake (Sullivan, 2010), and the pathophysiology of this disease is influenced by certain dietary components. An increased incidence of NAFLD was found in a cross-sectional study when participants ate more processed meats and consumed more soft drinks (Zelber-Sagi et al., 2007). n-3 polyunsaturated fatty acids may contribute to decrease intrahepatic fat deposition (Spadaro et al., 2008); fructose plays a role in disease progression (Abdelmalek et al., 2010) and contributes to disease development (Ouyang et al., 2008).

19.1.4 Host factors

19.1.4.1 Age

Aging reduces liver size and blood supply to the liver, which in turn reduces the activity of enzymes involved in alcohol metabolism, like alcohol dehydrogenase, acetaldehyde dehydrogenase, and cytochrome P-4502E1 (Seitz and Stickel, 2007; Meier and Seitz, 2008). Therefore, as people age, their livers become more susceptible to alcohol toxicity. Indeed, studies in patients with ALD showed that advanced fibrosis or liver cirrhosis was positively correlated with age (Naveau et al., 1997; Raynard et al., 2002). Aging was also found to be strongly linked to increasing fibrosis in a systematic analysis of NASH patients (Argo et al., 2009). The prevalence of ALD and NAFLD will certainly change as the world's population ages.

19.1.4.2 Gender

Researchers have shown that women are more vulnerable to the liver damage caused by drinking than men. The amount of alcohol consumed weekly at which the relative risk of ALD is greater than 1 was also found to be lower in women (7–13 drinks in a week) than in men (14–27 drinks in a week) in a large prospective study (Becker et al., 1996), and multivariate analyses showed that the female gender was more significantly associated with increased fibrosis in patients with ALD than the male gender (Naveau et al., 1997; Raynard et al., 2002). Females have been observed to have a higher risk of cirrhosis than males in studies of patients with uncomplicated alcoholic steatosis (Dam-Larsen et al., 2009; Deleuran et al., 2012). Although a gender gap in NAFLD prevalence was found, no such gender gap was found in the risk of increased fibrosis among patients with NASH (Argo et al., 2009).

19.1.4.3 Metabolic Syndrome

The risk of developing both ALD (Naveau et al., 1997) and NAFLD (Lazo et al., 2013) is increased in people who are overweight. Fibrosis was substantially related with higher body mass index in patients with ALD (Naveau et al., 1997; Raynard et al., 2002), although this was not the case in those with NAFLD (Argo et al., 2009). Type 2 diabetes and metabolic syndrome both have insulin resistance (IR) as a major contributing factor (Cornier et al., 2008). Recent research has shown a connection between ALD and IR (Longato et al., 2012), and links have been proposed between ALD and metabolic syndrome and type 2 diabetes (Kotronen et al., 2010). While IR/metabolic syndrome and type 2 diabetes were found to be strongly associated with NAFLD onset (Dixon, Bhathal, and O'Brien, 2001; Kotronen et al., 2010; Lazo et al., 2013), they were not found to be associated with NAFLD progression (Argo et al., 2009).

19.1.4.4 Ethnicity

The pathogenesis of ALD and NAFLD may vary according to ethnic background. The activity of the liver enzymes alanine aminotransferase (AST) and gamma-glutamyl transpeptidase (GGT) is twice as high in black non-Hispanic and Mexican Americans than in white non-Hispanic Americans, according to a large cross-sectional study (Stewart, 2002). Another study found that, compared to whites, African Americans were more likely to experience alcohol-induced hepatotoxicity (Stranges et al., 2004). Ethnicity may modulate the effects of IR on the risk of NASH, as the homeostasis model assessment of insulin resistance (HOMA-IR) was not a significant risk factor for NASH among Latinos (OR = 0.93; 95%CI: 0.85–1.02), but it was significant among non-Latino whites (OR = 1.06; 95%CI: 1.01–1.11) (Bambha et al., 2012).

19.1.4.5 Genetic Factors

Many researchers have put in a lot of time and energy into trying to figure out what genes play a role in the development of ALD and NAFLD (Daly et al., 2011; Stickel and Hampe, 2012). DNA variations called single nucleotide polymorphisms (SNPs) have been linked to illness risk and severity in a wide range of conditions. Adiponutrin, encoded by the PNPLA3 gene, is considered to play a significant role in lipid metabolism by hydrolyzing triacylglycerols (Wilson et al., 2006) and other lipids (Sookoian and Pirola, 2012). Increased hepatic fat content and hepatic inflammation have both been linked to the PNPLA3 SNP I148M (rs738409 C/G), according to a recent genome-wide association study (GWAS) of NAFLD (Romeo et al., 2008). Patients with the GG genotype had 73% more hepatic fat than those with the CC genotype, and the pooled ORs of the GG vs the CC genotype were 3.25 for having higher necroinflammatory scores and 3.26 for developing fibrosis, confirming the strong correlation between this SNP and hepatic fat content and disease progression. Notably, these results were true for people of all different ethnicities. Patients with ALD had similar outcomes (Tian et al., 2010; Stickel et al., 2011; Trépo et al., 2011). For instance, a multivariate analysis demonstrated that the PNPLA3 SNP was the greatest independent predictor of the advancement of alcoholic liver cirrhosis (OR = 2.08) and was more common in ALD patients than controls (OR = 1.54). These results regarding the PNPLA3 SNP may account, at least in part, for the disparities in the risk for and prevalence of ALD and NAFLD seen across different ethnic groups. The highest frequency of the PNPLA3 SNP is observed in the Hispanic population (Romeo et al., 2008), which is consistent with reports that Hispanics are more prone to ALD (Stewart, 2002) and have the highest prevalence rate of NAFLD [11]. Additional PNPLA3 SNPs have been found to be associated with NAFLD in recent studies (Kawaguchi et al., 2012; Kitamoto et al., 2013). Researchers have found two SNPs, rs2896019 and rs381062, in a recent genome-wide association study (GWAS) of Japanese people with NAFLD. This GWAS also identified SAMM50 and PARVB SNPs, which were thought to be important in the transition from basic steatosis to NASH after a second bout of NAFLD. However, SNPs in FDFT1 and COL13A1 were found in a GWAS of people of European ancestry with NAFLD (Chalasani et al., 2010). One further GWAS of Caucasian NAFLD patients found SNPs that link with hepatic steatosis in NCAN, PPP1R3B, and PNPLA3 (rs738409). Histological lobular inflammation/fibrosis was also observed to be linked with single nucleotide polymorphisms (SNPs) in the NCAN, GCKR, LYPLAL1, and PNPLA3 genes (Speliotes et al., 2011). Additional evidence suggests that some SNPs beyond the PNPLA3 SNP may be involved in the pathogenesis of ALD. One TNFA SNP (rs361525) was found to have a significant association with ALD in a meta-analysis (Marcos et al., 2009). Furthermore, the CD14 -159 C/T SNP has been found to be more common in patients with alcoholic cirrhosis compared to the general population in several studies (Daly et al., 2011). The PNPLA3 rs738409 G genotype is one of the few confirmed genetic variables contributing to a patient's vulnerability to both ALD and NAFLD and to the advancement of both diseases, despite significant genome-wide searching. More research is needed to determine whether or not this SNP can be used to effectively screen and manage high-risk patients and whether or not it can serve as a therapeutic target (Toshikuni, Tsutsumi, and Arisawa, 2014; Idalsoaga et al., 2020; Ikejima, Kon, and Yamashina, 2020).

19.2 MOLECULAR MECHANISMS

The pathogenesis of NAFLD involves a multitude of molecular mechanisms that are regulated by various factors such as lipid metabolic dysfunction, oxidative stress, insulin resistance (IR), and inflammation. This is supported by studies conducted by Friedman et al. in 2018, Hardy and Mann in 2016, and Eslam et al. in 2018.

The Nrf2/FXR/LXRα/RXR/SREBP-1c signaling pathway maintains intracellular redox balance and regulates lipid metabolism. Nrf2 is an upstream transcription factor that regulates oxidative stress and redox homeostasis (Dodson et al., 2019). Nrf2 recruits p300 to promote the deacetylation of farnesoid X receptor (FXR), which induces small heterodimer partner (SHP) to inhibit liver X receptor α (LXRα)-dependent gene transcription, thus negatively regulating LXRα and sterol regulatory element binding protein-1c (SREBP-1c). LXRα and retinoid X receptor (RXR) form a heterodimer, which activates SREBP-1c, the main transcription factor regulating fatty acid synthesis. Tissue-restricted FXR agonists improve insulin sensitivity and reduce hepatic steatosis (Fan et al., 2021). The PI3K/AKT/SREBP-1c pathway can reduce mitochondrial oxidative stress, inhibit adipogenesis, delay lipid deposition, and alleviate hepatic steatosis (Pan et al., 2018). Poly ADP-ribose polymerase 1 (PARP-1) inhibition can activate PI3K/AKT signaling, which down-regulates SREBP-1c to reduce lipid biosynthesis and improve fatty liver disease (Cantó and Auwerx, 2012). PARP-1 also affects energy metabolism by affecting nicotinamide adenine dinucleotide (NAD^+) consumption and sirtuin 1 (SIRT1) activity. The inhibition of PARP-1 increases NAD^+ content and SIRT1 activity, enhances lipid metabolism, and improves hepatic steatosis (Kraus and Hottiger, 2013).

On the other hand, in AFLD, excessive alcohol consumption leads to the accumulation of acetaldehyde, which is caused by the relative deficiency of acetaldehyde dehydrogenase (ALDH). This excess acetaldehyde produces reactive oxygen species (ROS), leading to oxidative stress and damage to hepatocytes (Xu et al., 2017).

The development of AFLD involves several signaling pathways in the liver, including SIRT1/AMPK/Lipin-1, PI3K/AKT/Nrf2/PPARγ, p62/Nrf2/KEAP1, and STING-IRF3-Bax. The SIRT1/AMPK/Lipin-1 pathway plays a crucial role in regulating lipid metabolism and inflammation in AFLD. The excessive consumption of alcohol impairs the function of this pathway and disrupts the balance between Lipin-1 and PGC-1α/PPARα signaling, leading to the development of AFLD (You et al., 2017). The PI3K/AKT/Nrf2/PPARγ pathway regulates oxidative stress and inflammation in AFLD. The p62/Nrf2/KEAP1 pathway regulates the activation of Nrf2, which plays a critical role in the antioxidant response to resist internal and external stimuli. The STING-IRF3-Bax pathway induces inflammation, ER stress, and apoptosis, leading to hepatocyte injury and dysfunction. Inhibition of this pathway could improve AFLD (Petrasek et al., 2013). Additionally, acetaldehyde can form various proteins and DNA complexes that act as antigens to activate adaptive immunity and increase inflammation (Anty and Gual, 2019). Furthermore, ethanol can cause dyslipidemia and lipid accumulation, resulting in the formation of lipid droplets (LDs). Excessive LDs are susceptible to attack by ROS produced during ethanol metabolism, thereby further exacerbating oxidative stress and liver damage. The SIRT1/AMPK/SREBP-1c pathway is shared by both NAFLD and AFLD for regulating lipid metabolism (Chen et al., 2012).

19.3 HOW TO DISTINGUISH ALCOHOLIC AND NON-ALCOHOLIC FATTY LIVER DISEASES?

It can be challenging to distinguish between ALD and NAFLD as both diseases exhibit similar pathological characteristics, ranging from mild fat accumulation to liver cirrhosis. However, certain histological findings can aid in the differential diagnosis. NAFLD typically displays a greater degree of fatty degeneration of liver cells, while ALD is characterized by more prominent inflammatory cell infiltration. Additionally, venous or perivenular fibrosis, phlebosclerosis, and lymphocytic phlebitis are more frequently observed in ALD than in NAFLD.

ALD and NAFLD are commonly differentiated based on a patient's alcohol intake history, as well as laboratory and imaging examinations. However, these methods may not always be reliable. As a result, discriminant indices based on clinical parameters have been developed, such as the ALD/NAFLD index (ANI). The ANI considers a patient's gender, BMI, aspartate aminotransferase (AST)/alanine aminotransferase (ALT) ratio, and mean corpuscular volume (MCV) to determine the likelihood of ALD or NAFLD. This index has demonstrated a high level of diagnostic accuracy. However, the diagnostic accuracy of the ANI may be reduced in patients with end-stage liver disease, as these patients often have elevated MCV and an elevated AST/ALT ratio.

19.4 BIOCHEMICAL PROFILE

19.4.1 Alcoholic

Careful examination of the biochemical profile of the patient may help in differentiating both. High blood gamma-glutamyl transferase (GGT) and serum alkaline phosphatase (ALP) levels may indicate alcohol-induced enzyme induction followed by severe liver damage, whereas normal to mild GGT elevation implies non-alcoholic hepatic injury (Torkadi et al., 2014).

19.4.2 Non-alcoholic Fatty Liver Diseases

It has been well established that many biochemical abnormalities occur in chronic liver diseases. An elevated serum transaminases level remains the most common or sometimes the only abnormal laboratory finding. Although the prime abnormality, liver enzymes may be normal in greater than 70% of patients with NAFLD (Pardhe et al., 2018). Several studies have shown that NAFLD patients have a significant increase in triglycerides (TG), total cholesterol, very low-density lipoprotein (VLDL), and low-density lipoprotein (LDL) cholesterol, whereas decreased high-density lipoprotein (HDL) was noticed. Similarly, deranged aspartate transaminase (AST) and alanine transaminase (ALT), γ-glutamyl transferase (GGT), and ALP were observed in greater percentages in patients with NAFLD than those without NAFLD (Maharjan et al., 2016). Diagnosis of NAFLD is based on abnormal serum AST and ALT in most of the studies. Some studies have shown a non-linear correlation between the level of ALT elevation and the histopathologic severity or grade of NAFLD, as well as showing that higher ALT levels carried a higher risk of NASH (Swain et al., 2017). However, there is ongoing debate regarding the cut-off for serum aminotransferases, at which a patient must be referred for liver biopsy to exclude NASH. An increase in TG, total cholesterol (TC), VLDL-C, and LDL-C and a decrease in HDL-C levels indicate possible atherogenic dyslipidemia. Moreover, the influx of high fatty acids in the liver causes liver toxicity and, additionally, inflammatory cytokines; TNF-6 also plays a major role in the development of hepatocellular injury mediated NAFLD and fatty liver with a mild to moderate increase in liver enzymes (Pardhe et al., 2018).

Where the liver function test results are mildly or moderately raised (transaminases 50–150 U/L [1 to 3 times the upper limit of normal] with AST levels less than those of ALT) and the information regarding body weight, lipids, HbA1c or glucose, family history of type 2 diabetes, and alcohol intake suggests NAFLD, patients should also be asked to return for repeat liver function tests in 2–3 months. The patients must be advised to reduce any alcohol intake or preferably discontinue it and to pursue lifestyle improvements to sustainably reduce weight. Noticeable increases in transaminases (>150 U/L [>3 times the upper limit of normal] with AST levels less than those of ALT) or the additional increase of alkaline phosphatase (ALP) should signal the possibility of other causes and the potential for progressive liver disease, whether due to NAFLD or another cause. These patients should be seen again within a few weeks for repeat testing and consideration for referral to a specialist (Sattar et al., 2014).

A novel technique called elastography has been explored in a variety of liver diseases, including NAFLD. The technique works through a vibration produced by the probe which induces an elastic shear wave. Propagation of this wave through the liver, measured by an ultrasonic transducer, is correlated to liver stiffness. Measurement of hepatic vein transit time (HVTT) of levovist from the antecubital fossa to the hepatic vein can predict functional hemodynamic changes correlated to disruption of the hepatic architecture. In cirrhosis, intrahepatic shunting will have an obvious effect on the HVTT but there is the possibility that more subtle changes in sinusoidal hemodynamics occurring in early fibrosis may also be detected using this technique.

The platform technologies of genomics, proteomics, and metabonomics may reveal new biomarkers in addition to giving insights into the mechanisms of liver fibrosis. Moreover, combinations of simple blood parameters, novel biomarkers, and functional imaging will increase diagnostic accuracy and allow greater separation of stages of fibrosis.

19.5 DIAGNOSIS OF ALCOHOLIC AND NON-ALCOHOLIC FATTY LIVER DISEASES

Diagnosis of alcoholic fatty liver disease (AFLD) and non-alcoholic fatty liver disease (NAFLD) typically involves a combination of clinical features, blood tests, imaging studies, and liver biopsy (Table 19.1).

19.5.1 Clinical Features

Clinical features are important for diagnosing FLD, as patients with these conditions may exhibit a variety of symptoms. Patients with AFLD may have a history of heavy alcohol consumption and may present with abdominal pain, nausea, and jaundice. In contrast, patients with NAFLD may be asymptomatic or may complain of fatigue, abdominal discomfort, and weight loss (Louvet and Mathurin, 2015; Jennison et al., 2019).

19.5.2 Blood Tests

Blood tests can also be useful in diagnosing FLD. In both AFLD and NAFLD, liver enzymes such as alanine transaminase (ALT) and aspartate transaminase (AST) may be elevated. Additionally, other markers of liver function such as bilirubin and albumin may be abnormal. However, these tests are not specific for FLD and may be elevated in other liver diseases as well (Papatheodoridi and Cholongitas, 2019; Chalasani et al., 2012; Louvet and Mathurin, 2015).

19.5.3 Imaging

Imaging studies such as ultrasound, computed tomography (CT), and magnetic resonance imaging (MRI) can be used to assess the extent of liver fat accumulation and to rule out other liver diseases. Ultrasound is often the first imaging modality used as it is non-invasive, widely available, and relatively inexpensive. CT and MRI can provide more detailed images of the liver and may be useful in identifying complications such as cirrhosis (Jennison et al., 2019).

19.5.4 Liver Biopsy

Liver biopsy is the gold standard for diagnosing FLD and can provide a definitive diagnosis. During a biopsy, a small piece of liver tissue is removed and examined under a microscope. This can help determine the extent of liver damage and the presence of inflammation or scarring. However, liver biopsy is an invasive procedure and carries a small risk of complications, such as bleeding and infection (Jennison et al., 2019). In conclusion, the diagnosis of FLD requires a multi-faceted approach, including a careful history and physical examination, blood tests, imaging studies, and liver biopsy. While each of these tests has its own advantages and limitations, a combination of these modalities can provide a more accurate diagnosis and guide treatment decisions. Early diagnosis and management of FLD can prevent or delay the progression to more severe liver disease (Chalasani et al., 2012; Louvet and Mathurin, 2015; Marchesini et al., 2016; Younossi et al., 2016)

Table 19.1   Diagnostic criteria for AFLD and NAFLD, based on current guidelines

Diagnostic Criteria	AFLD	NAFLD
Alcohol consumption history	Heavy alcohol consumption (>40 g/day in men)	Minimal or no alcohol consumption (<20 g/day in men)
Laboratory tests	Elevated liver enzymes (AST, ALT)	Elevated liver enzymes (AST, ALT)
Imaging studies	Ultrasound, CT, MRI	Ultrasound, CT, MRI
Liver biopsy	Histological evidence of fatty liver	Histological evidence of fatty liver
Other diagnostic criteria	Exclusion of other liver diseases	Exclusion of other liver diseases, metabolic risk factors (e.g., obesity, insulin resistance)

19.6 CURRENT THERAPIES FOR ALCOHOLIC AND NON-ALCOHOLIC FATTY LIVER DISEASES

19.6.1 Pharmacological Therapy

There are various pharmacological therapies available for ALD that aim to manage its symptoms and slow down the progression of the disease. Some of the current pharmacological therapies for ALD include the following.

Corticosteroids: Corticosteroids, such as prednisolone and pentoxifylline, are commonly used to treat severe alcoholic hepatitis, a complication of ALD. These drugs help reduce inflammation and improve liver function. However, they may have some side effects, including increased susceptibility to infection and osteoporosis.

Ursodeoxycholic acid (UDCA): UDCA is a naturally occurring bile acid that is used to treat cholestasis, a condition in which bile flow from the liver is obstructed. Studies have shown that UDCA may also have a protective effect on liver cells and reduce the risk of developing liver cirrhosis.

Naltrexone: It is an opioid antagonist that is used to reduce alcohol cravings and relapse in people with alcohol dependence. It works by blocking the effects of endogenous opioids, which are released when alcohol is consumed. Naltrexone is typically used in combination with other therapies, such as counseling and support groups.

Acamprosate: Acamprosate is another drug used to reduce alcohol cravings and help maintain abstinence in people with alcohol dependence. It works by stabilizing the balance of neurotransmitters in the brain that are disrupted by long-term alcohol use.

Nalemfene: Nalemfene is an opioid antagonist that is used to reduce alcohol cravings and relapse in some people with alcohol dependence. It results in fewer heavy drinking days per month.

Topiramate: Topiramate facilitates GABA transmission and reduces the alcohol-associated dopamine release in the limbic system. It results in fewer heavy drinking days per month.

Baclofen: Baclofen is a GABA agonist. It reduces alcohol withdrawal syndrome and safe for those with liver impairments. It is thus used to manage alcohol use disorder (AUD).

Disulfiram: Disulfiram inhibits aldehyde dehydreogenase, with the result that the accumulation of toxic acetaldehyde occurs at the time of alcohol consumption.

Vitamin supplements: ALD is often associated with malnutrition and vitamin deficiencies. Therefore, vitamin supplements, such as thiamine and folic acid, are frequently prescribed to people with ALD to help improve their nutritional status and prevent complications (Siddiqi, Sajja, and Latt, 2020; Ayares et al., 2022; Nielsen, Askgaard, and Thiele, 2022).

19.6.2 Non-pharmacological Therapy

Non-pharmacological therapies can play an important role in the management of alcoholic liver disease (ALD). These therapies aim to address the underlying lifestyle factors that contribute to the development and progression of the disease. Some of the current non-pharmacological therapies for ALD include the following.

Alcohol cessation: The most effective non-pharmacological therapy for ALD is the cessation of alcohol consumption. It is important for individuals with ALD to completely stop drinking alcohol to prevent further liver damage and improve liver function.

Nutritional therapy: Nutritional therapy involves working with a registered dietitian to develop a healthy eating plan that is tailored to the individual's needs. Nutritional therapy can help manage the malnutrition and vitamin deficiencies that are often associated with ALD and improve overall liver function.

Exercise: Regular exercise can help reduce inflammation, improve liver function, and manage other health conditions that may contribute to ALD, such as obesity and diabetes. It is recommended that individuals with ALD engage in moderate physical activity for at least 30 minutes per day, 5 days per week.

Psychosocial interventions: Psychosocial interventions, such as cognitive-behavioral therapy and motivational interviewing, can help individuals with ALD overcome addiction, manage stress, and improve mental health. These interventions may be used in combination with pharmacological therapies and other non-pharmacological therapies to provide a comprehensive approach to ALD management.

Liver transplantation: In cases of advanced ALD that have progressed to liver failure, liver transplantation may be necessary. Liver transplantation involves replacing the damaged liver with a healthy liver from a donor. It is a major surgical procedure that requires long-term medical management and monitoring.

It is important to note that non-pharmacological therapies should be used in concurrence with pharmacological therapies to effectively manage ALD. Regular medical monitoring and follow-up care are also essential to prevent further liver damage and improve overall health (Siddiqi, Sajja, and Latt, 2020; Ayares et al., 2022; Nielsen, Askgaard, and Thiele, 2022).

19.6.3 Herbal Therapy

ALD is a form of liver injury caused by damage. Alcohol's complicated mechanism of liver injury includes alterations in the distribution of intestinal microbes, inflammation of the liver, the development of oxidative stress, and an imbalance in lipid metabolism. Natural substances provide a number of advantages over conventional treatments, such as glucocorticoids and PTX, including lower toxicity and more potential uses. Supplemental or alternative treatments that include hepato-protective agents, like silymarin, hesperidin, curcumin, etc., have shown promising results. However, there are obvious drawbacks to using natural compounds. The low bioavailability of most naturally occurring substances limits their clinical usefulness. Without standardized pharmaceutical technology, it is hard to determine the best drug form and dosage. This means the full extent of liver protection cannot be achieved. Due to a lack of research, the mechanisms of action of natural substances are still unknown, and most compounds have not been tested in double-blinded, placebo-controlled clinical trials to determine their efficacy. It is undeniable that natural chemicals hold great promise as potential ALD treatments. However, clinical trials are still required for systematic reviews in the field of ALD research. We anticipate this review will serve as a theoretical foundation for future investigations into the pathogenesis and progression mechanisms of ALD and the subsequent development of treatment drugs for the disease (Yan et al., 2021).

19.7 SUMMARY AND CONCLUSIONS

The diagnosis of fibrosis in liver disease is important for the prognosis, stratification for treatment, and monitoring of treatment efficacy. The increasing incidence and prevalence of NAFLD have driven the search for accurate non-invasive tools for treating liver fibrosis in this condition. Since there are deranged lipid profile and liver function tests in clinical cases of NAFLD, different laboratory tests are extremely useful in achieving a better understanding of diseases, and thereby allow the making of decisions for better management. Among others, aminotransferase assay is the most commonly used screening test, as well as an endpoint for the resolution of disease in NAFLD.

REFERENCES

Adams, L. A. *et al.* (2005). The histological course of nonalcoholic fatty liver disease: A longitudinal study of 103 patients with sequential liver biopsies, *Journal of Hepatology*, 42(1), pp. 132–138. doi: 10.1016/J.JHEP.2004.09.012.

Adams, L. A. and Lindor, K. D. (2007). Nonalcoholic fatty liver disease. *Annals of Epidemiology*, 17(11), pp. 863–869. doi: 10.1016/J.ANNEPIDEM.2007.05.013.

Adams, W. L. *et al.* (1993). Alcohol-Related Hospitalizations of Elderly People: Prevalence and Geographic Variation in the United States. *JAMA*, 270(10), pp. 1222–1225. doi: 10.1001/JAMA.1993.03510100072035.

Abdelmalek, M. F. *et al.* (2010). Increased fructose consumption is associated with fibrosis severity in patients with nonalcoholic fatty liver disease, *Hepatology (Baltimore, Md.)*, 51(6), pp. 1961–1971. doi: 10.1002/HEP.23535.

Argo, C. K. *et al.* (2009). Systematic review of risk factors for fibrosis progression in non-alcoholic steatohepatitis. *Journal of Hepatology*, 51(2), pp. 371–379. doi: 10.1016/J.JHEP.2009.03.019.

Ayares, G. *et al.* (2022). Current Medical Treatment for Alcohol-Associated Liver Disease. *Journal of Clinical and Experimental Hepatology*, 12(5), pp. 1333–1348. doi: 10.1016/J.JCEH.2022.02.001.

Anty, R. and Gual, P. (2019). Pathogenesis of non-alcoholic fatty liver disease. *Presse Medicale (Paris, France: 1983)*, 48(12), pp. 1468–1483.

Bambha, K. *et al.* (2012). Ethnicity and Nonalcoholic Fatty Liver Disease. *Hepatology (Baltimore, Md.)*, 55(3), p. 769. doi: 10.1002/HEP.24726.

Becker, U. *et al.* (1996). Prediction of risk of liver disease by alcohol intake, sex, and age: A prospective population study. *Hepatology*, 23(5), pp. 1025–1029. doi: 10.1053/jhep.1996.v23.pm0008621128.

Bellentani, S. *et al.* (1997). Drinking habits as cofactors of risk for alcohol induced liver damage. The Dionysos Study Group. *Gut*, 41(6). doi: 10.1136/GUT.41.6.845.

Boudreau, D. M. *et al.* (2009). Health care utilization and costs by metabolic syndrome risk factors. *Metabolic Syndrome and Related Disorders*, 7(4), pp. 305–313. doi: 10.1089/MET.2008.0070.

Cantó, C. and Auwerx, J. (2012). Targeting sirtuin 1 to improve metabolism: All you need is NAD$^+$? *Pharmacological Reviews*, 64(1), pp. 166–187.

Chalasani, N. *et al.* (2010). Genome-wide association study identifies variants associated with histologic features of nonalcoholic Fatty liver disease. *Gastroenterology*, 139(5). doi: 10.1053/J. GASTRO.2010.07.057.

Chalasani, N. et al. (2012). The diagnosis and management of non-alcoholic fatty liver disease: Practice Guideline by the American Association for the Study of Liver Diseases, American College of Gastroenterology, and the American Gastroenterological Association. *Hepatology*, 55(6), pp. 2005–2023. https://doi.org/10.1002/hep.25762.

Chen, W.L. et al. (2012). α-Lipoic acid regulates lipid metabolism through induction of sirtuin 1 (SIRT1) and activation of AMP-activated protein kinase. *Diabetologia*, 55, 1824–35.

Cornier, M. A. *et al.* (2008). The metabolic syndrome. *Endocrine Reviews*, 29(7), pp. 777–822. doi: 10.1210/ER.2008-0024.

Daly, A. K. *et al.* (2011). Genetic determinants of susceptibility and severity in nonalcoholic fatty liver disease. *Expert Review of Gastroenterology & Hepatology*, 5(2), pp. 253–263. doi: 10.1586/EGH.11.18.

Dam-Larsen, S. *et al.* (2009). Final results of a long-term, clinical follow-up in fatty liver patients. *Scandinavian Journal of Gastroenterology*, 44(10), pp. 1236–1243. doi: 10.1080/00365520903171284.

Deleuran, T. *et al.* (2012). Cirrhosis and mortality risks of biopsy-verified alcoholic pure steatosis and steatohepatitis: A nationwide registry-based study. *Alimentary Pharmacology & Therapeutics*, 35(11), pp. 1336–1342. doi: 10.1111/J.1365-2036.2012.05091.X.

Dixon, J. B., Bhathal, P. S. and O'Brien, P. E. (2001). Nonalcoholic fatty liver disease: Predictors of nonalcoholic steatohepatitis and liver fibrosis in the severely obese. *Gastroenterology*, 121(1), pp. 91–100. doi: 10.1053/gast.2001.25540.

Dodson, M et al. (2019). Modulating NRF2 in disease: Timing is everything. *Annual Review of Pharmacology and Toxicology*, 6(59), pp. 555–75.

Douds, A. C. *et al.* (2003). Ethnic differences in cirrhosis of the liver in a British city: Alcoholic cirrhosis in South Asian men. *Alcohol and Alcoholism (Oxford, Oxfordshire)*, 38(2), pp. 148–150. doi: 10.1093/ALCALC/AGG040.

Dunn, W. *et al.* (2012). The interaction of rs738409, obesity, and alcohol: A population-based autopsy study. *The American Journal of Gastroenterology*, 107(11), pp. 1668–1674. doi: 10.1038/AJG.2012.285.

Eguchi, Y. *et al.* (2012). Prevalence and associated metabolic factors of nonalcoholic fatty liver disease in the general population from 2009 to 2010 in Japan: A multicenter large retrospective study. *Journal of Gastroenterology*, 47(5), pp. 586–595. doi: 10.1007/S00535-012-0533-Z.

Ekstedt, M. *et al.* (2006). Long-term follow-up of patients with NAFLD and elevated liver enzymes. *Hepatology (Baltimore, Md.)*, 44(4), pp. 865–873. doi: 10.1002/HEP.21327.

Eslam, M., Valenti, L. and Romeo, S. (2018).Genetics and epigenetics of NAFLD and NASH: Clinical impact. *Journal of Hepatology*, 68(2), pp. 268–79.

Fan, J. G. *et al.* (2005). Prevalence of and risk factors for fatty liver in a general population of Shanghai, China. *Journal of Hepatology*, 43(3), pp. 508–514. doi: 10.1016/J.JHEP.2005.02.042.

Fan, J. G. (2013). Epidemiology of alcoholic and nonalcoholic fatty liver disease in China. *Journal of Gastroenterology and Hepatology*, 28(Suppl 1), pp. 11–17. doi: 10.1111/JGH.12036.

Fan, L. et al. (2021). miR-552-3p modulates transcriptional activities of FXR and LXR to ameliorate hepatic glycolipid metabolism disorder. *Journal of Hepatology*, 74(1), pp. 8–19.

Finucane, M. M. *et al.* (2011). National, regional, and global trends in body-mass index since 1980: Systematic analysis of health examination surveys and epidemiological studies with 960 country-years and 9·1 million participants. *Lancet (London, England)*, 377(9765), pp. 557–567. doi: 10.1016/S0140-6736(10)62037-5.

Friedman, S.L. et al. (2018) Mechanisms of NAFLD development and therapeutic strategies. *Nature Medicine*, 24(7), pp. 908–22.

Hamaguchi, M. *et al.* (2005). The metabolic syndrome as a predictor of nonalcoholic fatty liver disease. *Annals of Internal Medicine*, 143(10). doi: 10.7326/0003-4819-143-10-200511150-00009.

Hardy, T. and Mann, D.A. (2016). Epigenetics in liver disease: from biology to therapeutics. *Gut*, 65(11),1895–905.

Hatton, J. *et al.* (2009). Drinking patterns, dependency and life-time drinking history in alcohol-related liver disease. *Addiction (Abingdon, England)*, 104(4), pp. 587–592. doi: 10.1111/J.1360-0443.2008.02493.X.

Idalsoaga, F. *et al.* (2020). Non-alcoholic Fatty Liver Disease and Alcohol-Related Liver Disease: Two Intertwined Entities. *Frontiers in Medicine*, 7, p. 448. doi: 10.3389/FMED.2020.00448/BIBTEX.

Ikejima, K., Kon, K. and Yamashina, S. (2020). Nonalcoholic fatty liver disease and alcohol-related liver disease: From clinical aspects to pathophysiological insights. *Clinical and Molecular Hepatology*, 26(4), pp. 728–735. doi: 10.3350/CMH.2020.0202.

Jennison, E. et al. (2019). Diagnosis and management of non-alcoholic fatty liver disease. *Postgraduate Medical Journal*, 95(1124), pp. 314–322. https://doi.org/10.1136/postgradmedj-2018-136316.

Kawaguchi, T. *et al.* (2012). Genetic polymorphisms of the human PNPLA3 gene are strongly associated with severity of non-alcoholic fatty liver disease in Japanese, *PloS one*, 7(6). doi: 10.1371/JOURNAL.PONE.0038322.

Kerr, W. C., Fillmore, K. M. and Marvy, P. (2000). Beverage-specific alcohol consumption and cirrhosis mortality in a group of English-speaking beer-drinking countries. *Addiction (Abingdon, England)*, 95(3), pp. 339–346. doi: 10.1046/J.1360-0443.2000.9533394.X.

Kitamoto, T. *et al.* (2013). Genome-wide scan revealed that polymorphisms in the PNPLA3, SAMM50, and PARVB genes are associated with development and progression of nonalcoholic fatty liver disease in Japan. *Human Genetics*, 132(7), pp. 783–792. doi: 10.1007/S00439-013-1294-3.

Kojima, S. I. *et al.* (2003). Increase in the prevalence of fatty liver in Japan over the past 12 years: Analysis of clinical background. *Journal of Gastroenterology*, 38(10), pp. 954–961. doi: 10.1007/S00535-003-1178-8.

Kotronen, A. *et al.* (2010). Non-alcoholic and alcoholic fatty liver disease - Two diseases of affluence associated with the metabolic syndrome and type 2 Diabetes: The FIN-D2D survey. *BMC Public Health*, 10(1), pp. 1–7. doi: 10.1186/1471-2458-10-237/FIGURES/4.

Kraus, W. L. and Hottiger, M. O. (2013). PARP-1 and gene regulation: Progress and puzzles. *Molecular Aspects of Medicine*, 34(6), pp. 1109–1123.

Louvet, A. and Mathurin, P. (2015). Alcoholic liver disease: Mechanisms of injury and targeted treatment. *Nature Reviews Gastroenterology and Hepatology*, 12(4), pp. 231–242. https://doi.org/10.1038/nrgastro.2015.35.

Lazo, M. *et al.* (2013). Prevalence of nonalcoholic fatty liver disease in the United States: The Third National Health and Nutrition Examination Survey, 1988–1994. *American Journal of Epidemiology*, 178(1), pp. 38–45. doi: 10.1093/AJE/KWS448.

Longato, L. *et al.* (2012). Insulin resistance, ceramide accumulation, and endoplasmic reticulum stress in human chronic alcohol-related liver disease. *Oxidative Medicine and Cellular Longevity*, 2012. doi: 10.1155/2012/479348.

Maharjan, P. et al. (2016). Biochemical changes in non-alcoholic fatty liver disease (NAFLD): A study in nepalese population. *Annals of Clinical Chemistry and Laboratory Medicine*, 2(2), pp. 15–20.

Marchesini, G. et al. (2016). EASL-EASD-EASO Clinical Practice Guidelines for the management of non-alcoholic fatty liver disease. *Journal of Hepatology*, 64(6), pp. 1388–1402. https://doi.org/10.1016/j.jhep.2015.11.004.

Marchesini, G. *et al.* (2003). Nonalcoholic fatty liver, steatohepatitis, and the metabolic syndrome. *Hepatology*, 37(4), pp. 917–923. doi: 10.1053/jhep.2003.50161.

Marcos, M. *et al.* (2009). Tumor necrosis factor polymorphisms and alcoholic liver disease: A HuGE review and meta-analysis. *American Journal of Epidemiology*, 170(8), pp. 948–956. doi: 10.1093/AJE/KWP236.

Mathurin, P. *et al.* (2007). Fibrosis progression occurs in a subgroup of heavy drinkers with typical histological features. *Alimentary Pharmacology & Therapeutics*, 25(9), pp. 1047–1054. doi: 10.1111/J.1365-2036.2007.03302.X.

Meier, P. and Seitz, H. K. (2008). Age, alcohol metabolism and liver disease. *Current Opinion in Clinical Nutrition and Metabolic Care*, 11(1), pp. 21–26. doi: 10.1097/MCO.0B013E3282F30564.

Mohapatra, S. *et al.* (2010). Social cost of heavy drinking and alcohol dependence in high-income countries. *International Journal of Public Health*, 55(3), pp. 149–157. doi: 10.1007/S00038-009-0108-9.

Naveau, S. *et al.* (1997). Excess weight risk factor for alcoholic liver disease. *Hepatology*, 25(1), pp. 108–111. doi: 10.1002/hep.510250120.

Nielsen, A. S., Askgaard, G. and Thiele, M. (2022). Treatment of alcohol use disorder in patients with liver disease. *Current Opinion in Pharmacology*, 62, pp. 145–151. doi: 10.1016/J.COPH.2021.11.012.

Ouyang, X. *et al.* (2008). Fructose consumption as a risk factor for non-alcoholic fatty liver disease. *Journal of Hepatology*, 48(6), pp. 993–999. doi: 10.1016/J.JHEP.2008.02.011.

Pan, Y. et al. (2018). Inhibition of Rac1 ameliorates neuronal oxidative stress damage via reducing Bcl-2/Rac1 complex formation in mitochondria through PI3K/Akt/mTOR pathway. *Experimental Neurology*, 300, 149–166.

Papatheodoridi, M. and Cholongitas, E. (2019). Diagnosis of Non-alcoholic Fatty Liver Disease (NAFLD): Current concepts. *Current Pharmaceutical Design*, 24(38), pp. 4574–4586. https://doi.org/10.2174/1381612825666190117102111.

Pardhe, B.D. et al. (2018). Metabolic syndrome and biochemical changes among non-alcoholic fatty liver disease patients attending a tertiary care hospital of Nepal. *BMC Gastroenterology*, *18*, pp. 1–8.

Petrasek, J. et al. (2013). STING-IRF3 pathway links endoplasmic reticulum stress with hepatocyte apoptosis in early alcoholic liver disease. *Proceedings of the National Academy of Sciences*, 110(41), pp. 16544–16549.

Raynard, B. *et al.* (2002). Risk factors of fibrosis in alcohol-induced liver disease. *Hepatology (Baltimore, Md.)*, 35(3), pp. 635–638. doi: 10.1053/JHEP.2002.31782.

Rehm, J. *et al.* (2009). Global burden of disease and injury and economic cost attributable to alcohol use and alcohol-use disorders. *Lancet (London, England)*, 373(9682), pp. 2223–2233. doi: 10.1016/S0140-6736(09)60746-7.

Rehm, J., Samokhvalov, A. V. and Shield, K. D. (2013). Global burden of alcoholic liver diseases. *Journal of Hepatology*, 59(1), pp. 160–168. doi: 10.1016/J.JHEP.2013.03.007.

Romeo, S. *et al.* (2008). Genetic variation in PNPLA3 confers susceptibility to nonalcoholic fatty liver disease. *Nature Genetics*, 40(12), pp. 1461–1465. doi: 10.1038/NG.257.

Sattar, N., Forrest, E. and Preiss, D. (2014). Non-alcoholic fatty liver disease. *BMJ, 349*, p. 4596 (1–8).

Schwartz, J. M. and Reinus, J. F. (2012). Prevalence and natural history of alcoholic liver disease. *Clinics in Liver Disease*, 16(4), pp. 659–666. doi: 10.1016/J.CLD.2012.08.001.

Schwimmer, J. B. *et al.* (2006). Prevalence of fatty liver in children and adolescents. *Pediatrics*, 118(4), pp. 1388–1393. doi: 10.1542/PEDS.2006-1212.

Seitz, H. K. and Stickel, F. (2007). Alcoholic liver disease in the elderly. *Clinics in Geriatric Medicine*, 23(4), pp. 905–921. doi: 10.1016/J.CGER.2007.06.010.

Shen, L. *et al.* (2003). Prevalence of nonalcoholic fatty liver among administrative officers in Shanghai: An epidemiological survey. *World Journal of Gastroenterology*, 9(5), pp. 1106–1110. doi: 10.3748/WJG.V9.I5.1106.

Siddiqi, F. A., Sajja, K. C. and Latt, N. L. (2020). Current Management of Alcohol-Associated Liver Disease. *Gastroenterology & Hepatology*, 16(11), p. 561. Available at: https://www.ncbi.nlm.nih.gov/pmc/articles/PMC8132623/ (Accessed: 17 April 2023).

Sookoian, S. and Pirola, C. J. (2012). The genetic epidemiology of nonalcoholic fatty liver disease: Toward a personalized medicine. *Clinics in Liver Disease*, 16(3), pp. 467–485. doi: 10.1016/J.CLD.2012.05.011.

Spadaro, L. *et al.* (2008). Effects of n-3 polyunsaturated fatty acids in subjects with nonalcoholic fatty liver disease. *Digestive and Liver Disease*, 40(3), pp. 194–199. doi: 10.1016/J.DLD.2007.10.003.

Speliotes, E. K. *et al.* (2011). Genome-Wide Association Analysis Identifies Variants Associated with Nonalcoholic Fatty Liver Disease That Have Distinct Effects on Metabolic Traits. *PLOS Genetics*, 7(3), p. e1001324. doi: 10.1371/JOURNAL.PGEN.1001324.

Stewart, S. H. (2002). Racial and ethnic differences in alcohol-associated aspartate aminotransferase and gamma-glutamyltransferase elevation. *Archives of Internal Medicine*, 162(19), pp. 2236–2239. doi: 10.1001/ARCHINTE.162.19.2236.

Stickel, F. *et al.* (2011). Genetic variation in the PNPLA3 gene is associated with alcoholic liver injury in caucasians, *Hepatology (Baltimore, Md.)*, 53(1), pp. 86–95. doi: 10.1002/HEP.24017.

Stickel, F. and Hampe, J. (2012). Genetic determinants of alcoholic liver disease, *Gut*, 61(1), pp. 150–159. doi: 10.1136/GUTJNL-2011-301239.

Stranges, S. *et al.* (2004). Greater hepatic vulnerability after alcohol intake in African Americans compared with Caucasians: A population-based study. *Journal of the National Medical Association*, 96(9), p. 1185. Available at: /pmc/articles/PMC2568464/?report=abstract (Accessed: 4 May 2023).

Sullivan, S. (2010). Implications of Diet on Nonalcoholic Fatty Liver Disease. *Current Opinion in Gastroenterology*, 26(2), p. 160. doi: 10.1097/MOG.0B013E3283358A58.

Swain, M. et al. (2017). Biochemical profile of nonalcoholic fatty liver disease patients in eastern India with histopathological correlation. *Indian Journal of Clinical Biochemistry*, 32, pp. 306–314.

Tannapfel, A. *et al.* (2011). Histopathological diagnosis of non-alcoholic and alcoholic fatty liver disease. *Virchows Archiv : an International Journal of Pathology*, 458(5), pp. 511–523. doi: 10.1007/S00428-011-1066-1.

Tian, C. *et al.* (2010). Variant in PNPLA3 is associated with alcoholic liver disease. *Nature Genetics*, 42(1), pp. 21–23. doi: 10.1038/NG.488.

Torkadi PP, Apte IC and Bhute AK (2014). Biochemical evaluation of patients of alcoholic liver disease and non-alcoholic liver disease. *Indian J Clin Biochem*, 29(1), pp. 79–83.

Toshikuni, N., Tsutsumi, M. and Arisawa, T. (2014). Clinical differences between alcoholic liver disease and nonalcoholic fatty liver disease. *World Journal of Gastroenterology : WJG*, 20(26), p. 8393. doi: 10.3748/WJG.V20.I26.8393.

Trépo, E. *et al.* (2011). Common polymorphism in the PNPLA3/adiponutrin gene confers higher risk of cirrhosis and liver damage in alcoholic liver disease. *Journal of Hepatology*, 55(4), pp. 906–912. doi: 10.1016/J.JHEP.2011.01.028.

Williams, C. D. *et al.* (2011). Prevalence of nonalcoholic fatty liver disease and nonalcoholic steatohepatitis among a largely middle-aged population utilizing ultrasound and liver biopsy: A prospective study. *Gastroenterology*, 140(1), pp. 124–131. doi: 10.1053/J.GASTRO.2010.09.038.

Wilson, P. A. *et al.* (2006). Characterization of the human patatin-like phospholipase family. *Journal of Lipid Research*, 47(9), pp. 1940–1949. doi: 10.1194/JLR.M600185-JLR200.

Xu, M. J. et al. (2017). Targeting inflammation for the treatment of alcoholic liver disease. *Pharmacology & Therapeutics*, 180, 77–89.

Yan, J. *et al.* (2021). Natural Compounds: A Potential Treatment for Alcoholic Liver Disease?. *Frontiers in Pharmacology*, 12. doi: 10.3389/FPHAR.2021.694475.

Yang, A. L. *et al.* (2008). Epidemiology of Alcohol-Related Liver and Pancreatic Disease in the United States. *Archives of Internal Medicine*, 168(6), pp. 649–656. doi: 10.1001/ARCHINTE.168.6.649.

You, M. et al. (2017). Signal transduction mechanisms of alcoholic fatty liver disease: Emer ging role of lipin-1. *Current Molecular Pharmacology*, 10(3), pp. 226–236.

Younossi, Z. M. et al. (2016). Global epidemiology of nonalcoholic fatty liver disease—Meta-analytic assessment of prevalence, incidence, and outcomes. *Hepatology*, 64(1), pp. 73–84. https://doi.org/10.1002/hep.28431.

Zelber-Sagi, S. *et al.* (2007). Long term nutritional intake and the risk for non-alcoholic fatty liver disease (NAFLD): A population based study. *Journal of Hepatology*, 47(5), pp. 711–717. doi: 10.1016/J.JHEP.2007.06.020.

20 Common Pathogens Involved in Metabolic Diseases

Riya Patel, Santhana Kumar, Arun Soni, Sanjeev Acharya, and Niyati Acharya

20.1 INTRODUCTION

The biochemical procedures that enable individuals to develop, reproduce, heal injuries, and adapt to their surroundings are collectively referred to as metabolism. These mechanisms are hampered by metabolic abnormalities. The word "metabolism" refers to the multiple different chemical processes that the body goes through to prolong life and normal operation. Any aspect of metabolism can be harmed by conditions referred to as metabolic disorders (1).

When the metabolism process fails, the body either has too much or not enough of the necessary nutrients it needs to stay healthy; this is known as a metabolic disease. The mechanism of metabolism is intricate and entails a variety of tissues, organs, and biochemicals. The probability of something going wrong, resulting in a metabolic disease, is therefore very high (2).

Numerous pathogens have continued to thrive on humans and have increased into the trillions. This study's goal is to scientifically analyze and synthesize recent findings on the involvement of pathogens and processes in the progression and emergence of serious metabolic disorders (3).

In the human colon, there are up to 1,000 different kinds of bacteria that together code for over 3 million genes and may be harmful to health. Cytotoxins, immunotoxins, and genotoxins are only a few of the substances created by the microbiota that may be toxic for the host (4).

Here, the relationships among biochemical pathways, pathophysiology, and metabolic illnesses need to be explored in order to pave the way for future therapeutic developments. The main pathogenic agents that cause metabolic disease are cellular and acellular microbes, such as bacteria and viruses (5).

Metabolic diseases pose a huge global health challenge as their frequency is rising drastically (6). The number of people with metabolic diseases increases with age, affecting more than 40% of people in their sixties and seventies (7).

According to the information that is now available, metabolic syndrome can be said to affect 20–30% of adults worldwide. The proportion is even higher in particular regions and subgroups of society. Nonetheless, the incidence is lower in lower-income locations where populations are younger, but as these populations age and become more affluent, the proportion will increase (8).

Different risk factors have been associated with metabolic diseases. The two main risk factors are central obesity and insulin resistance. There are various other factors that are associated with metabolic diseases, like disorders related to genetics, deficiencies of certain hormones, consuming too much food, and a certain number of other factors (9).

Obesity, type 2 diabetes (T2DM), liver lipid problems, and metabolic disorders are all conditions that have been linked to food, physical activity, aging, and genetic alterations. However, there is now a lot of data to suggest that additional environmental variables may be responsible for the significant rise in the prevalence of these metabolic illnesses (10).

In the human body, the stomach has the widest variety of microbes. These microbes have developed a parasitic connection with their host over the course of long-term coevolution; they are essential for controlling the host's immune system generally, as well as the intestinal barrier, nutrition, metabolism, and gene expression (11).

Particularly with the advent of metabolic illnesses, the gut flora plays a critical role in preserving the equilibrium of human health.

The comorbid condition known as metabolic syndrome is linked to a number of illnesses that are lifestyle-related. In order to maintain a healthy lifestyle and a long life, managing metabolic diseases is crucial. This is because many conditions, including obesity, diabetes, cardiovascular disease, liver damage, and brain disorders, can lead to metabolic syndrome. Supporting a healthy gut flora, enhancing immune responses, and lowering chronic inflammation are essential for achieving this goal. A balanced diet and moderate exercise are also advised (12).

The main emphasis of the present research will be the conclusions drawn from the most significant studies looking at the involvement of molecules from the microbiome in metabolic disorders.

20.2 PATHOGENS INVOLVED IN METABOLIC DISEASES

20.2.1 What Are Pathogens?

Emerging pathogens are those that cause new illnesses, significantly raise the incidence of existing illnesses, spread an existing illness to a new area, or infect a new host. Human mucosal and epidermal surfaces are home to billions of commensal bacteria, and this ecosystem is crucial to the body's defense against infections, notably respiratory diseases (13).

The pathogens may be introduced more gradually by the establishment of newly permissive abiotic variables, such as climatic or atmospheric conditions, as in climate change, or other environmental factors.

Furthermore, mutation, hybridization, and horizontal gene transfer are other ways that pathogens might acquire new genes. The accessibility of whole-genome sequencing and the aggregation of genetic information have made it possible to take a population-phylogenetic relationship approach to the origin of virulence (14).

Pathogens are the microorganisms or agents that cause diseases in living organisms. They include bacteria, viruses, fungi, protozoa, and parasites. Pathogens can enter the body through various routes, such as the respiratory tract, the digestive tract, and the organs, leading to various symptoms and health problems (15).

Through direct contact with infected surfaces or items, or indirect contact with bodily fluids like blood, saliva, or mucus, pathogens can be transferred from one person to another. Some pathogens can also be transmitted by insects or other animals that act as vectors, such as mosquitoes that carry the malaria parasite.

20.2.2 Types of Pathogens

The category of illnesses referred to as "metabolic disorders", which interfere with the body's metabolism, has been linked to a variety of distinct pathogen types.

20.2.2.1 Bacteria

Many bacterial species have been linked to metabolic disorders. For instance, *Helicobacter pylori*, a bacteria responsible for chronic inflammation of the stomach lining, has been linked to an increased probability of developing metabolic syndrome, a combination of disorders that increases the risk of heart disease, stroke, and diabetes. *Escherichia coli* and *Lactobacillus* are two other bacteria that have been proven to have an impact on lipid and glucose metabolism (13).

20.2.2.2 Viruses

Metabolic illnesses have been linked to some viruses. For instance, obesity in both humans and animals has been linked to adenovirus-36 (AD-36), a virus that may infect both humans and animals. A higher risk of developing cardiovascular disease and metabolic syndrome has been associated with the pervasive cytomegalovirus (CMV), which can harm humans and cause viral disorders. Viruses are little pathogens that need a host cell to reproduce. They have the ability to spread a variety of illnesses, from the common cold to more serious ailments like HIV/AIDS and COVID-19 (16).

20.2.2.3 Fungi

Metabolic diseases have been linked to specific species of fungi. For instance, there is a higher chance of developing metabolic disorders and obesity when *Candida albicans*, a fungus that can infect individuals and cause diseases, is present. Multicellular organisms known as fungi have the potential to infect people, especially those with compromised immune systems. Examples of fungi infections include candidiasis, ringworm, and athlete's foot (17).

20.2.2.4 Parasites

There is evidence that some parasites cause metabolic disorders. *Toxoplasma gondii* infection, for example, has been linked to an increased risk of developing metabolic syndrome and insulin resistance. The term "parasite" refers to a creature that depends on another organism, known as the "host", for its existence. The health of people may be impacted by parasites such as tapeworms, lice, and malaria (18).

20.2.3 How Do Pathogens Spread?

Microorganisms called pathogens, including bacteria, viruses, fungus, and parasites, can infect people, animals, and plants and lead to disease. There are various ways they might spread, including the following.

Pathogens can be transmitted by immediate physical contact with an affected individual or animal. For instance, touching, kissing, or sexual contact can transfer contagious illnesses, including the flu, the common cold, and STDs.

Pathogens can also be transmitted through indirect contact with an infected person or object. This can involve handling infected objects, such as tissues or clothing, or touching contaminated surfaces, like a doorknob or tabletop. The common cold, the flu, and gastrointestinal disorders are among the illnesses that can be contracted through indirect contact.

Airborne transmission: When an infected person talks, coughs, or sneezes, droplets are usually generated that allow pathogens to travel through the air. Airborne infections have a short range and can spread to adjacent people. Measles, chickenpox, and tuberculosis are a few examples of illnesses that can spread via airborne transmission.

Waterborne transmission: Pathogens can spread through contaminated water, including lakes, rivers, and drinking water sources, in a process known as "waterborne transmission". Cholera, dysentery, and hepatitis A are a few diseases that can spread via waterborne transmission.

Foodborne transmission: Contaminated foods like meat, eggs, and dairy products can spread pathogens. *Salmonella*, *E. coli*, and *Listeria* are a few infections that can spread by foodborne transmission (19–21).

To prevent the spread of germs, it is important to practice good hygiene habits, which include frequent hand washing, covering coughs and sneezes, avoiding contact with sick individuals, and properly handling and cooking food.

Depending on the pathogen and illness in question, there are various ways in which pathogens linked to metabolic disorders can spread.

Diabetes: Inflammation in the pancreas brought on by pathogens like viruses and bacteria can harm insulin-producing cells and result in diabetes. These infections can be transmitted either directly, by coming into contact with bodily fluids like blood or saliva, or indirectly, by coming into contact with contaminated objects (22).

Obesity: Adenovirus-36 and other viruses have been linked to obesity in both people and animals. These pathogens can spread through tainted food and drink, as well as direct contact with infected human fluids (23).

Metabolic diseases: The risk of heart disease, stroke, and diabetes is increased by a group of conditions known as metabolic diseases. The development of metabolic syndrome may be influenced by pathogens, such as some types of bacteria, that produce persistent inflammation. These diseases can spread via direct or indirect contact with sick people, tainted food, and tainted water (24).

Several of the methods used to stop the spread of other types of infections can also be employed to stop the spread of pathogens that cause metabolic disorders. Pathogens can be stopped from spreading by following good hygiene habits like frequent hand washing and avoiding sick people. A balanced diet, regular exercise, and good overall health all help lower the risk of metabolic disorders.

20.2.4 Etiology of Pathogens That Affect Human Health

The ability of the pathogen to live and reproduce in various conditions, its capacity to elude the immune system, and the vulnerability of the host to infection are some of the elements that can have an impact on the genesis of diseases. Pathogens can spread through indirect contact, such as contact with contaminated objects or tainted food, or direct contact, such as through bodily fluids or skin-to-skin contact. Knowing the viruses' etiologies is a crucial first step in creating efficient preventative and treatment plans to safeguard human health (25).

Depending on the type of disease, different pathogens that affect human health have different etiologies.

Infections: Pathogens can produce infections, which can vary in severity from mild to severe and impact different regions of the body. Infections might manifest as fever, coughing, sneezing, exhaustion, and diarrhea.

Chronic diseases: By interfering with normal cellular function and causing chronic inflammation, certain infections, particularly those caused by viruses and bacteria, can contribute to the onset of chronic diseases like cancer and autoimmune disorders.

Allergies: Those who are allergic to certain microorganisms, such as mold or pollen, may experience allergic reactions. Sneezing, itching, hives, and swelling are some allergy signs and symptoms.

Foodborne illness: Foodborne illnesses are caused by pathogens that contaminate food and can range in severity from minor gastrointestinal discomfort to serious illness and even death.

Pandemics: Pandemics are widespread disease outbreaks that can result in high rates of illness and mortality. Pathogens that can produce pandemics include influenza viruses and coronaviruses.

It is crucial to prevent diseases from spreading in order to sustain healthy health. Practice excellent hygiene, such as frequently washing hands and covering coughs and sneezes; avoid contact with sick people; and get immunized against infectious diseases, as these are some methods for preventing the transmission of infections. Maintaining a healthy lifestyle that includes regular exercise, a balanced diet, and adequate sleep can also support an effective immune system that is better able to defend itself against illnesses (26–28).

20.2.5 Pathogens in Metabolic Diseases

In humans, the host and the gut bacteria have coevolved in a symbiotic relationship. With the defense the gut bacteria offer against viruses, they aid the host. Moreover, they help by protecting the gastrointestinal barrier's stability, promoting the production of nutrients, and producing molecules like short-chain fatty acids.

Metabolic diseases are a broad group of disorders that affect the body's metabolism and can lead to various health problems, including diabetes, obesity, and cardiovascular diseases. While the exact causes of metabolic diseases are not fully understood, several pathogens have been linked to these conditions.

Here are some examples:

Helicobacter pylori: This bacterium is known to cause chronic inflammation of the stomach lining, which can lead to ulcers and increase the risk of stomach cancer. According to certain studies, *H. pylori* infection has also been associated with the emergence of metabolic syndrome, a cluster of diseases that increases the risk of heart disease, stroke, and diabetes.

Adenovirus: Several studies have linked infection with adenovirus-36 (AD-36) to obesity in humans and animals. AD-36 is a type of virus that can infect both humans and animals and has been shown to promote fat accumulation and insulin resistance in an experimental study.

Cytomegalovirus: This virus frequently causes viral infections among individuals, and some research indicates that cytomegalovirus (CMV) infection may raise the chance of developing cardiovascular disease and metabolic disorders.

20.2.5.1 Gut Microbiota

The gut microbiota, which consists of trillions of microorganisms living in the intestinal tract, has also been implicated in metabolic diseases.

There are bacteria, archaea, and eukaryotes in the gut microbiota. The most prevalent gut microbes are bacteria, and the phyla Bacteroidetes, Firmicutes, and Actinobacteria are numerically dominant among them (29).

Several individual bacteria from these taxa have been linked to the emergence of metabolic disorders. Maintaining gut immunity and homeostasis requires a balanced bacterial population. "Dysbiosis" is the term for an imbalance in the gut microbiota, which has effects on metabolism (30).

Several lines of evidence show that changes in the gut microbiota are linked to the emergence of a variety of gastrointestinal tract diseases, such as colon cancer and IBD4, as well as a number of diseases associated with non-digestive systems. It has been demonstrated that the gut microbiota has a substantial impact on metabolic disorders (31).

Maintaining the host's physiological processes is crucially dependent on the gut bacteria. A number of metabolic illnesses can start as a result of a breakdown in the delicate host–microbiota contact equilibrium. Metabolites, which are microscopic compounds (1,500 Da) that serve as intermediates or by-products of microbial metabolism, allow the intestinal microbiota to communicate with the host. These molecules may originate from the bacteria themselves or may result from the metabolism of food or host-derived substrates (32).

The physiology and physiopathology of metabolic illnesses are significantly influenced by the compounds formed by the gut microbiota (33).

20.3 ROLE OF PATHOGENS IN METABOLIC DISEASES

The mechanisms by which pathogens can influence the emergence of metabolic disorders include the following.

Inflammation: Metabolic illnesses like metabolic syndrome and insulin resistance have been related to chronic inflammation in the body brought on by infection with particular microorganisms.

Alterations: Dysbiosis, which has been connected to metabolic illnesses like insulin resistance and obesity, is a condition in which pathogens in the gut upset the delicate balance of microorganisms.

Changes in metabolism: It has been demonstrated that several infections, like adenovirus-36, can affect glucose and lipid metabolism and promote fat formation, which can lead to the emergence of metabolic diseases.

Immune system dysfunction: An infection in the immune system can result in chronic low-grade inflammation, which has been related to metabolic disorders.

20.3.1 Metabolic Diseases

A class of disorders known as metabolic diseases manage the regular operation of numerous metabolic systems and have an impact on the body's capacity to turn food into energy. These diseases can be caused by a variety of factors, including genetic mutations, pathogens, deficiencies in specific enzymes or hormones, and environmental factors such as poor diet and physical inactivity (34).

Hyperglycemia, dyslipidemia, hypertension, obesity, and insulin resistance are only a few of the disease risk factors that are grouped together under the term "metabolic dysfunction". The risk of cardiovascular disorders such as acute myocardial infarction and stroke is dramatically increased by metabolic disturbances. Many different cell types, tissues, organs, inflammatory signaling cascades, and humoral components are involved in the etiology of metabolic diseases (35).

Type 2 diabetes (T2DM) and cardiovascular disease (CVD) are two of the most significant global public health issues. A poor diet, obesity, and being overweight all constitute significant risks factors for developing a variety of diseases (36).

Moreover, dietary fiber is well known for its positive metabolic effects because of its role in the lowering of cholesterol levels, enhanced control of blood glucose levels, and improved body weight regulation. Knowledge of the gut microbiota and its connection to the host's metabolic control has advanced significantly over the past few decades (37).

In the past 20 years, the occurrence of metabolic disorders has increased due to rising caloric intake and decreased levels of physical activity. Obesity, non-alcoholic fatty liver disease, and other pathological illnesses are clustered together as a category of disorders known as metabolic disorders.

When taken together, the risk of cardiovascular disease and death is considerably increased by diabetes, hypertension, gestational diabetes mellitus, low hyperinsulinemia, hepatic steatosis (NASH), hyperlipidemia, and insulin resistance (38).

3.2 What Causes Metabolic Diseases?

The process of metabolism is intricate and includes several biochemicals, tissues, and organs. Metabolic disorders interfere with the body's capacity to digest food and turn it into energy. Metabolic disorders can take many different forms, and the reasons for them can vary depending on the particular ailment. Therefore, the likelihood that something could go wrong and result in a metabolic illness is very high (39).

An increasing amount of research is demonstrating how fat accumulation has a pathogenic role in various organs. The various causes of metabolic syndrome interact with one another. Levels of exercise and diet are two variables that can be managed. Age and genes are two variables that cannot be altered (40).

Metabolic syndrome is primarily caused by a person's weight. Free fatty acid levels might rise as a result of fat cells, particularly those in the abdomen. Free fatty acids can increase the levels of several substances and hormones that impact how the body controls blood sugar levels. It is possible that the body is not getting enough insulin, a hormone that controls how much blood sugar muscles and organs absorb. This is caused by insulin resistance (41).

Moreover, immune system cells can encourage the body's extra fat cells to produce chemicals that exacerbate inflammation. Blood vessels may develop plaque, a waxy substance, as a result of this inflammation. Blood vessels may become blocked if plaque breaks off. Insulin resistance, high blood pressure, and disorders of the heart and blood vessels are all brought on by inflammation (42).

Some common causes of metabolic disorders include the following.

3.2.1 Genetics

In many different ways, genes can affect how metabolic systems work. Many metabolic disorders can be caused by genetic mutations that affect the body's ability to process certain nutrients. These genetic mutations can be inherited from one or both parents. For instance, a genetic mutation in people with Gaucher's disease causes the synthesis of the enzyme glucocerebrosidase, which breaks down lipids, to be restricted. This may result in a negative accumulation of body fat (43).

3.2.2 Hormonal Imbalance

Hormonal imbalances, such as those caused by thyroid disorders, can affect metabolism and lead to metabolic disorders. Over a woman's lifetime, the microbiota has a profound impact on the reproductive endocrine glands through interactions with estrogen, androgens, insulin, and other hormones. The investigation of the underlying mechanisms and potential causes of microbiota-hormone-mediated disease, as well as the development of fresh therapeutic and preventive approaches, should receive more attention (44).

3.2.3 Environmental Factors

Obesity, type 2 diabetes, hypertension, hyperlipidemia, and cardiovascular disease are among the modern health epidemics that result from a disrupted connection between the microbiota and the environment. Exposure to certain toxins or chemicals can disrupt metabolic processes and lead to metabolic disorders.

3.2.4 Sedentary Lifestyle

A lack of physical exercise is believed to cause the deaths of about 3.2 million people per year in the worldwide population of people under the age of 15, who account for about 31% of the population. A lack of physical activity can contribute to metabolic disorders by reducing muscle mass, slowing down metabolism, and promoting weight gain. It is commonly established that a lack of physical exercise – or, more specifically, physical inactivity – negatively impacts health. Responsible for 6% of worldwide mortality, physical inactivity is the fourth-highest risk factor for death (45).

The majority of physical activity-related instruction in clinical practice is focused on increasing physical activity levels, with less attention paid to reducing inactivity, even though inactivity poses a similar danger to one's health and increases the prevalence of numerous diseases (46).

3.2.5 Medications

Certain medications, such as corticosteroids and some antipsychotic drugs, can disrupt metabolic processes and lead to metabolic disorders. The major causes of death worldwide are cardiovascular diseases such as atherosclerosis, myocardial infarction, hypertension, cardiac hypertrophy, and heart failure, as well as metabolic diseases like diabetes, obesity, and non-alcoholic fatty liver disease. Cardiovascular and metabolic disorders (CVMDs) continue to have a high morbidity and mortality rate, despite major advancements in prevention and treatment over the past 20 years. Even though there is ample evidence that these medications are successful in treating CVMDs, major adverse effects could still occur (47).

3.2.6 Aging

As an organism ages, its cellular activity declines, and various tissues deteriorate systemically, impairing function and making the organism more susceptible to mortality. A growing body of research indicates that age-related illnesses and growing older are closely linked to an imbalance between energy supply and demand. Many therapies, including increased physical activity, calorie counting, and naturally occurring chemicals that target essential pathways for longevity, may be used to restore this imbalance. Metabolism diminishes with age, which can lead to type 2 diabetes and other metabolic problems such as insulin resistance (48).

3.2.7 Organ Dysfunction

Organs engaged in metabolism are susceptible to malfunction. Diabetes, for instance, can develop when the pancreas is unable to produce enough insulin to control blood glucose levels. Crosstalk aids in coordination and homeostasis maintenance, but acute or ongoing failure in one organ leads to the dysregulation of other organs. Several signal molecules, including cytokines and growth factors, whose excessive or incorrect release results in organ malfunction or disease, contribute to the dysregulation of metabolism (e.g., obesity, type 2 diabetes) (49).

3.2.8 Mitochondrial Dysfunction

The little energy-producing organelles found in cells are mitochondria. The efficiency with which mitochondria function and the amount of energy they can generate can be impacted by environmental events, mutations in the mitochondria or cell DNA, or both. Obesity, insulin resistance, atherogenic dyslipidemia (high triglycerides, low HDL cholesterol), and hypertension are all symptoms of metabolic syndrome. Recently, research has focused on the role that mitochondria play in the pathogenesis of metabolic conditions such as obesity, metabolic syndrome, and type 2 diabetes. The oxidative stress and systemic inflammation present in metabolic syndrome are a result of mitochondrial malfunction (50).

20.3.3 Major Diseases That Result from Metabolic Abnormalities

There are a number of diseases that arise as a result of metabolic disorders. Some of these include diabetes mellitus and hypertension, among others (Figure 20.1).

20.3.3.1 Diabetes and Other Metabolic Diseases

Elevated blood sugar levels brought on by issues with insulin generation or action are the hallmark of this illness. Diabetes, one of the illnesses with the fastest global growth rates, is predicted to affect 693 million individuals by 2045. The final common mechanism on which numerous metabolic abnormalities converge is hyperglycemia, which serves as the diagnostic criterion for a set of disorders collectively referred to as diabetes (51).

Diabetes is a condition that inhibits the body from effectively utilizing insulin to regulate blood sugar levels. The most prevalent kinds of diabetes include the following.

Type 1: The immune system accidentally targets pancreatic cells in type 1 diabetes (T1DM), which lowers the quantity of insulin generated. To control their blood sugar levels, people with type 1 diabetes need to take daily insulin prescriptions. Type 1 diabetes mellitus is hypothesized

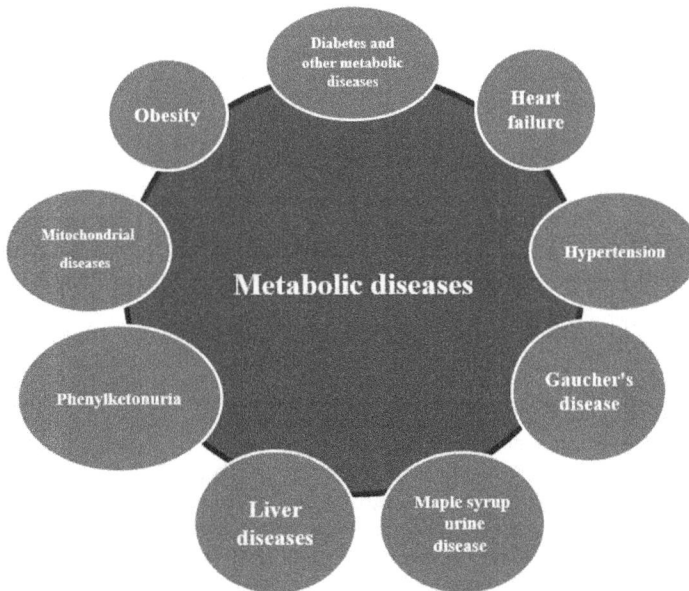

Figure 20.1 Metabolic problems come in a wide variety of forms due to the intricacy of the metabolism

to be caused by autoimmune processes that result in the death of beta cells that produce insulin in the pancreatic islets (52).

Type 2: Type 2 diabetes is a condition in which the body uses insulin incorrectly. It can appear at any age and can be brought on by specific lifestyle choices, such as an unhealthy diet. Many studies have shown that persistent low-grade inflammation and type 2 diabetes are both influenced by subclinical inflammation, which also raises the likelihood of insulin resistance and hyperglycemia, two hallmarks of metabolic syndrome (53).

Gestational diabetes: Some women experience this during pregnancy, and it typically goes away after delivery. But it could increase the risk of type 2 diabetes in the future. Gestational diabetes mellitus (GDM) is currently the most prevalent medical pregnancy complication, and young women are increasingly likely to suffer overt diabetes and undiagnosed hyperglycemia (54).

High blood glucose levels are the outcome of diabetes mellitus, a chronic metabolic condition that impairs the body's capacity to make or use insulin. Although diabetes mellitus is not caused by a single infection, other infectious agents have been associated with the onset or development of the condition. These agents include the following.

Coxsackievirus B: It is believed that this enterovirus results in type 1 diabetes by causing the body to assault the pancreatic cells that make its own insulin. The discovery that enteroviral components (VP1 capsid protein and/or RNA) are present in the blood, monocytes, gut mucosa, and pancreas, as well as circulating anti-enterovirus immunoglobulins (IgM, IgG, and IgA), is supported by epidemiological and clinical evidence. These findings are more frequently observed in patients with T1DM than in healthy individuals (55).

Cytomegalovirus (CMV): The common herpesvirus cytomegalovirus (CMV) has been linked to a higher incidence of type 2 diabetes, as well as a worsening of diabetic sequelae, such as retinopathy and nephropathy. Many viral infections have been linked to a higher risk of developing diabetes mellitus.

Rubella, mumps, Epstein–Barr, varicella zoster, and cytomegalovirus (CMV) are among the viruses that have been linked to type 1 diabetes. One of the most well-studied environmental causes of type 1 diabetes is enterovirus (56).

Helicobacter pylori: In addition to being recognized as causing peptic ulcers, the bacterium *Helicobacter pylori* has been connected to the emergence of insulin resistance and type 2 diabetes. Diabetes impairs the cellular and humoral immune systems' ability to operate, making a person more vulnerable to *H. pylori* infection.

Mycobacterium tuberculosis: This tuberculosis-causing bacterium has been connected to an elevated risk of type 2 diabetes because it generates persistent inflammation (57).

Candida albicans: *Candida albicans* is a yeast that is frequently found in the human gut and can make people sick if their immune systems are already compromised. Insulin resistance and the development of type 2 diabetes have both been linked to it. Diabetes mellitus (DM), a metabolic disorder, predisposes people to fungal infections, particularly those connected with *Candida* species, as a result of its immunosuppressive effects on the patient (58).

It is important to keep in mind that, while it is possible that these illnesses play a part in the development or progression of diabetes mellitus, the majority of cases of the condition are explained by a mix of hereditary, nutritional, and environmental factors.

Obesity: Around 20% of Western populations are affected by obesity, which is becoming a more significant health burden. Obese people are far more likely to develop type 2 diabetes, hypertension, coronary heart disease, stroke, fatty liver disease, dementia, obstructive sleep apnea, and many cancers.

Even though it is widely accepted that being overweight raises the risk of type 2 diabetes, dyslipidemia, fatty liver disease, chronic subclinical inflammation, hypertension, and cardiovascular disease, to create innovative approaches for the prevention and treatment of these conditions, identification and characterization of the molecular pathways underlying the connection between obesity and cardiometabolic diseases are essential (59).

The complex and multidimensional condition of obesity is impacted by a number of environmental, genetic, and lifestyle variables. Although there is no one particular pathogen that causes obesity, some infectious agents have been associated with the onset or development of the condition. They consist of the following.

Adenovirus-36 (AD-36): This virus has been found to promote obesity in animals and is related to obesity in people. There are many different causes of obesity, including biological factors. According to research, the human adenovirus subtype 36 (Adv36) is an adaptogenic agent that alters metabolism. The incidence of Adv36 and its clinical implications in humans have been the subject of a variety of studies (60).

Human herpesvirus-4 (HHV-4): The Epstein–Barr virus, also referred to as HHV-4 (EBV), has been linked to obesity in several studies, presumably as a result of its effects on insulin resistance.

Helicobacter pylori: In addition to being recognized as causing peptic ulcers, the bacterium *Helicobacter pylori* has been connected to the emergence of insulin resistance and obesity. Research on both animals and humans has demonstrated that the gut microbiota can control the host's energy homeostasis and, as a result, influence the development of obesity. Several studies have looked into the connection between *Helicobacter pylori* and obesity. According to certain research, those who had had *Helicobacter pylori* infections had higher BMIs than those who had not (61).

Gut microbiota: According to recent research, the development of obesity may be influenced by abnormalities in the gut microbiota, such as the overgrowth of particular bacterial species. The study of the gut microbiomes of obese people was motivated by the concept that the gut microbiota may play a significant environmental role in obesity. Numerous studies have linked obesity to the *Christensenellaceae* family, as well as the genera *Methanobacteriales*, *Lactobacillus*, *Bifidobacterium*, and *Akkermansia*. The variety of the gut flora is an important element of obesity as well (62).

It is crucial to remember that while these infections may contribute to the onset or progression of obesity, a combination of genetic, dietary, and environmental factors primarily contribute to the condition's development.

20.3.3.2 Heart Failure

Heart failure arises when the heart is unable to pump enough blood to meet the needs of the body. Heart failure is not caused by a single pathogen; however, some infectious agents have been associated with its onset or progression (Table 20.1). The complexity of heart failure is reflected in the diversity of classifications and categorizations that are now in use, which results in significant variation in reported estimates of the incidence of heart failure, hospitalizations, and mortality rates (63).

Pathogens linked to cardiac failure include some of the following.

Coxsackievirus B: This virus has been linked to myocarditis, a condition in which the heart muscle is inflamed and can eventually fail. An overlooked factor in heart failure is viruses. Furthermore, there are cardiovascular hazards associated with a number of viral illnesses. It is essential to comprehend the common and distinctive processes by which each virus impairs heart function in order to guide therapeutic strategies.

Chlamydia pneumoniae: This bacterium has been associated with the onset of atherosclerosis, an accumulation of plaque in the arteries that can result in heart failure.

Streptococcus pneumoniae: Due to its capacity to result in endocarditis, an inflammation of the inner lining of the heart, this bacterium has been linked to the emergence of heart failure.

It is crucial to remember that while these pathogens may contribute to the onset or progression of heart failure, the condition is usually brought on by a confluence of genetic, behavioral, and environmental variables. As a result, changing one's lifestyle and receiving medical care are frequently necessary for heart failure prevention and management (71).

Table 20.1 Pathogens involved in heart failure

Virus	Mechanism of cardiac damage	References
Coxsackievirus B	Lysing cardiomyocytes, interfering with their ability to function, and immune-mediated injury	(64)
Human Herpesvirus 6	Cardiovascular endothelial cell infection, immune system harm, and immunosuppression	(65)
Epstein–Barr Virus	Direct cardiomyocyte infection and direct lymphocytic infiltration into the heart	(66)
Cytomegalovirus	Cardiomyocyte, fibroblast, and endothelial cell infection; T-cell-mediated injury; activation of autoantibodies	(67)
Varicella-zoster Virus	Heart inflammation and disturbed electrical activity	(68)
Human Immunodeficiency Virus	Immune system damage, immunosuppression, cardiomyocyte infection, and an increased susceptibility to additional cardiotropic viruses	(69)
Influenza Virus	Immune-mediated damage, direct myocardial injury, and mainly unknown routes	(70)

20.3.3.3 *Pathogens Involved in Hypertension*

High blood pressure, commonly known as hypertension, is a complicated medical issue that is influenced by a variety of variables, such as heredity, way of life, and environmental factors. While there is no single disease that specifically causes hypertension, some infectious agents may play a role in the onset of the condition in some people, according to a study.

The following are examples of such agents.

Helicobacter pylori: This bacterium is typically found in the stomach and has been linked to a number of diseases, including gastric cancer and stomach ulcers. Several studies suggest that *H. pylori* infection may possibly contribute to the development of hypertension. One of the most prevalent chronic infections in the world, *Helicobacter pylori* infection causes a range of gastrointestinal and non-gastrointestinal symptoms. Among other factors, the etiology of metabolic syndrome has been connected to *Helicobacter pylori*. The most recent studies emphasizing a connection between *Helicobacter pylori* and metabolic syndrome caused by arterial hypertension and non-alcoholic fatty liver disease are emphasized in this review (72).

Chlamydia pneumoniae: Pneumonia and other respiratory illnesses can be brought on by this particular strain of bacterium. According to certain studies, *C. pneumoniae* may contribute to the onset of hypertension by inducing an inflammatory reaction in the blood vessels. One of the most common infectious agents in the world, according to serological research, it can cause a variety of clinical symptoms, such as flare-ups of chronic obstructive lung disease and chronic asthma. Serological correlations with coronary artery disease, strokes, transient cerebral ischemia, and asymptomatic carotid atherosclerosis have been shown by a number of studies (73).

Viruses: The herpes simplex virus (HSV) and the cytomegalovirus (CMV) have both been linked to hypertension. According to one idea, these viruses may promote blood vessel inflammation, which then results in hypertension.

20.3.3.4 *Pathogens Involved in Liver Diseases*

Hepatitis viruses: The two viruses most often linked to liver illness are the hepatitis B virus (HBV) and the hepatitis C virus (HCV). These viruses have the potential to inflame and harm the liver, which can result in diseases such as cirrhosis and liver cancer. The metabolism of lipids and glucose depends heavily on the liver. Many liver diseases, including chronic hepatitis, cirrhosis, and hepatocellular carcinoma, are brought on by chronic hepatitis B virus (HBV) or hepatitis C virus (HCV) infection. Due to the epidemic of type 2 diabetes mellitus (T2DM) and obesity, the prevalence of metabolic syndrome (MetS) is increasing (74).

Non-alcoholic fatty liver disease (NAFLD): NAFLD, which results in inflammation and liver damage, causes fat to accumulate in the liver. While the actual cause of NAFLD is uncertain, some evidence suggests that dysbiosis of the gut microbiota may play a role in the disease's development. More people are becoming aware of the significance of the human gut microbiota in non-alcoholic fatty liver disease (NAFLD). Long-term consumption of an unhealthy diet (such as one high in sugar or saturated fat) starts the dysbiosis of the gut microbiota, which in turn disrupts barrier function and immunological homeostasis. The components and metabolites produced by bacteria in the gut, or gut microbiota, are transported to the liver by the portal vein (75).

Parasites: In numerous parasitic illnesses, the liver plays a critical role. Infections with parasites, such as those brought on by liver flukes (such as *Opisthorchis viverrini*), can damage and inflame the liver over time, increasing the chance of developing liver cancer. The prevalence of morbidity and death from parasites in the liver has greatly increased globally due to their capacity to cause cancer, cirrhosis, liver failure, and recurrent cholangitis. Although the ideal immune response to exogenous germs is tolerance rather than immunization, it has recently been hypothesized that the liver provides a favorable immunological environment for parasites (76).

Bacteria: Changes in the microorganisms that reside in the gastrointestinal tract have an impact on the etiology and progression of many illnesses, including liver and gastrointestinal diseases. Infections with bacteria, such as those brought on by *Streptococcus sp.* and *Escherichia coli*, can result in liver abscesses, a condition in which pus-filled pockets develop in the liver tissue.

In addition to host–bacterial interactions, viable bacteria or microbial products influence healthy physiology and disease susceptibility, either locally via signaling to various intestinal mucosal cell populations or more distantly via such signalling to the liver and other organs (77).

20.3.3.5 *Pathogens Involved in Gaucher's Diseases*

Glucocerebrosidase deficiency results from mutations in the GBA gene, which is a rare genetic abnormality that causes Gaucher's disease (GCase). The lack of the lysosomal enzyme glucocerebrosidase causes glucosylceramide, the enzyme's substrate, to build up in lysosomal macrophages, resulting in the uncommon autosomal recessive genetic illness known as Gaucher's disease (78).

Some examples of pathogens that have been associated with Gaucher's diseases include the following.

Mycobacterium tuberculosis: According to one study, people with Gaucher's disease are more likely than the general population to contract tuberculosis (TB); the study posited that these people may be more prone to contracting TB since they lack GCase.

Helicobacter pylori: According to a different study, people with Gaucher's disease are more likely to have the bacterium *H. pylori*, which can result in stomach ulcers and other gastrointestinal issues. The build-up of glucocerebroside in the stomach lining may create an ideal environment for the growth and colonization of *H. pylori*.

Influenza virus: A patient with Gaucher's disease who experienced severe respiratory symptoms and was later identified as having an influenza A virus infection was the subject of a case report. The scientists hypothesized that the patient's lack of GCase may have increased the infection's severity.

20.3.3.6 *Pathogens Involved in Maple Syrup Urine Disorder*

Maple syrup urine disorder (MSUD) is a metabolic condition characterized by the presence of excessive levels of branch-chain amino acids (BCAAs) and their related branched-chain ketoacids (BCKAs) as a result of a flaw in the enzyme that breaks down these acids (79).

Enteroviruses: Viral infections with enteroviruses, such as coxsackievirus, were suspected to have caused metabolic decompensation in a number of recorded instances of MSUD. Although the precise method by which enteroviruses cause the symptoms of MSUD is not entirely understood, it is believed to involve an increase in BCAA breakdown.

20.4 PREVENTIVE MEASURES

When a metabolic disease's symptoms are evident, it is crucial to seek medical attention and treatment because prompt action can help manage the condition and prevent its consequences (Figure 20.2).

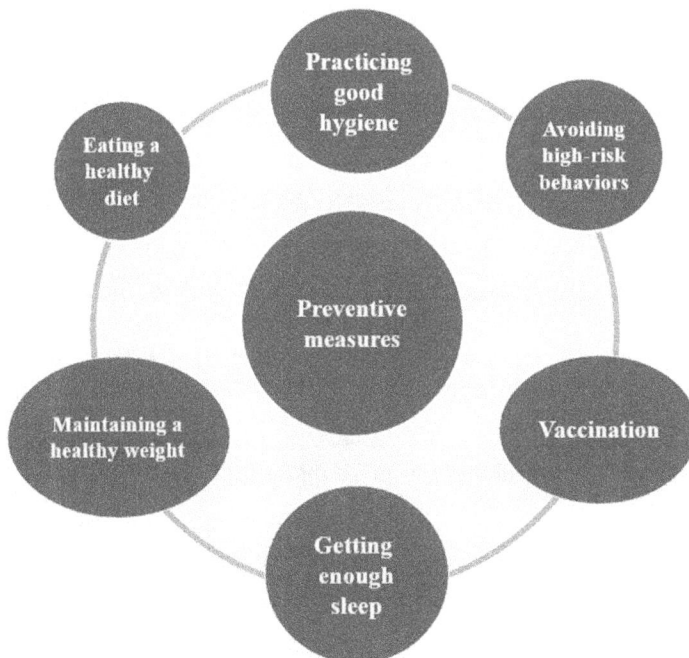

Figure 20.2 Preventive measure to reduce the incidence of metabolic disorders

20.5 CONCLUSIONS

Although some pathogens have been linked to metabolic disorders, it is important to note that the connection between infection and disease is complicated and not entirely understood. Metabolic illnesses can also be caused by many other variables, including genetics, nutrition, and lifestyle. Several articles outlining converging lines of evidence suggest that increased intestinal permeability and bacterial translocation are involved in the emergence of such metabolic diseases. The physiology and physiopathology of metabolic illnesses are significantly influenced by the metabolites produced by the gut microbiota and the focus of current research is experiencing shift from general public census data to more multiomics-based translational investigations and related findings.

REFERENCES

1. Alves A, Bassot A, Bulteau AL, Pirola L, Morio B. Glycine metabolism and its alterations in obesity and metabolic diseases. *Nutrients*. 2019;11(6):1356.

2. Ruiz-Ojeda FJ, Méndez-Gutiérrez A, Aguilera CM, Plaza-Díaz J. Extracellular matrix remodeling of adipose tissue in obesity and metabolic diseases. *Int. J. Mol. Sci.* 2019;20(19):4888.

3. Ding RX, Goh WR, Wu RN, Yue XQ, Luo X, Khine WW, Wu JR, Lee YK. Revisit gut microbiota and its impact on human health and disease. *J Food Drug Anal*. 2019;27(3):623–31.

4. Moran-Ramos S, López-Contreras BE, Canizales-Quinteros S. Gut microbiota in obesity and metabolic abnormalities: A matter of composition or functionality? *Arch Med Sci*. 2017;48(8):735–53.

5. Moos WH, Faller DV, Glavas IP, Harpp DN, Kamperi N, Kanara I, Kodukula K, Mavrakis AN, Pernokas J, Pernokas M, Pinkert CA. Pathogenic mitochondrial dysfunction and metabolic abnormalities. *Biochem. Pharmacol*. 2021;193:114809.

6. Agus A, Clément K, Sokol H. Gut microbiota-derived metabolites as central regulators in metabolic disorders. *Gut*. 2021;70(6):1174–82.

7. Cariou B, Byrne CD, Loomba R, Sanyal AJ. Nonalcoholic fatty liver disease as a metabolic disease in humans: A literature review. *Diabetes Obes. Metab*. 2021;23(5):1069–83.

8. Grundy SM. Metabolic syndrome pandemic.*Arterioscler Thromb. Vasc. Biol*. 2008;28(4):629–36.

9. Ferrara D, Montecucco F, Dallegri F, Carbone F. Impact of different ectopic fat depots on cardiovascular and metabolic diseases. *J. Cell. Physiol*. 2019;234(12):21630–41.

10. Heindel JJ, Blumberg B, Cave M, Machtinger R, Mantovani A, Mendez MA, Nadal A, Palanza P, Panzica G, Sargis R, Vandenberg LN. Metabolism disrupting chemicals and metabolic disorders. *Reprod. Toxicol*. 2017;68:3–3.

11. Liu R, Hong J, Xu X, Feng Q, Zhang D, Gu Y, Shi J, Zhao S, Liu W, Wang X, Xia H. Gut microbiome and serum metabolome alterations in obesity and after weight-loss intervention. *Nat. Med*. 2017;23(7):859–68.

12. Santa K, Kumazawa Y, Nagaoka I. Prevention of Metabolic Syndrome by Phytochemicals and Vitamin D. *Int. J. Mol. Sci*. 2023;24(3):2627.

13. Khan R, Petersen FC, Shekhar S. Commensal bacteria: An emerging player in defense against respiratory pathogens. *Front. Immunol*. 2019;10:1203.

14. Denamur E, Clermont O, Bonacorsi S, Gordon D. The population genetics of pathogenic Escherichia coli. *Nat. Rev. Microbiol*. 2021;19(1):37–54.

15. Gurung K, Wertheim B, Falcao Salles J. The microbiome of pest insects: It is not just bacteria. *Entomol. Exp. Appl.* 2019;167(3):156–70.

16. Sankaran N, Weiss RA. *Viruses: Impact on Science and Society. Encyclopedia of Virology* (Vol. 1, pp. 671–80). 4th Edition, Academic Press; 2021.

17. Köhler JR, Casadevall A, Perfect J. The spectrum of fungi that infects humans. *Cold Spring Harb. Perspect. Med.* 2015;5(1):a019273.

18. Haque R. Human intestinal parasites. *J. Health Popul. Nutr.* 2007;25(4):387–91.

19. Van Seventer JM, Hochberg NS. Principles of infectious diseases: transmission, diagnosis, prevention, and control. *Int. Encyclopedia Public Health.* 2017;22:22–39.

20. Richard M, Knauf S, Lawrence P, Mather AE, Munster VJ, Müller MA, Smith D, Kuiken T. Factors determining human-to-human transmissibility of zoonotic pathogens via contact. *COMICR.* 2017;22:7–12.

21. Stein RA, Chirilă M. Routes of transmission in the food chain. *Foodborne Pathog. Dis.* 2017 (pp. 65–103). Academic Press.

22. Sommer P, Sweeney G. Functional and mechanistic integration of infection and the metabolic syndrome. *Korean Diabetes J.* 2010;34(2):71–6.

23. Ponterio E, Gnessi L. Adenovirus 36 and obesity: An overview. *Viruses.* 2015;7(7):3719–40.

24. Troha K, Ayres JS. Metabolic adaptations to infections at the organismal level. *Mod. Trends Immunol.* 2020;41(2):113–25.

25. Rahman M, Sobur M, Islam M, Ievy S, Hossain M, El Zowalaty ME, Rahman AM, Ashour HM. Zoonotic diseases: Etiology, impact, and control. *Microorganisms.* 2020;8(9):1405.

26. Lindahl JF, Grace D. The consequences of human actions on risks for infectious diseases: A review. *Infect. Ecol. Epidemiology.* 2015;5(1):30048.

27. Griffiths EC, Pedersen AB, Fenton A, Petchey OL. The nature and consequences of coinfection in humans. *J. Infect.* 2011;63(3):200–6.

28. Galli SJ, Tsai M, Piliponsky AM. The development of allergic inflammation. *Nature.* 2008;454(7203):445–54.

29. Rinninella E, Raoul P, Cintoni M, Franceschi F, Miggiano GA, Gasbarrini A, Mele MC. What is the healthy gut microbiota composition? A changing ecosystem across age, environment, diet, and diseases. *Microorganisms.* 2019;7(1):14.

30. Myhrstad MC, Tunsjø H, Charnock C, Telle-Hansen VH. Dietary fiber, gut microbiota, and metabolic regulation—Current status in human randomized trials. *Nutrients.* 2020;12(3):859.

31. Ding RX, Goh WR, Wu RN, Yue XQ, Luo X, Khine WW, Wu JR, Lee YK. Revisit gut microbiota and its impact on human health and disease. *J. Food Drug Anal.* 2019;27(3):623–31.

32. Lamichhane S, Sen P, Dickens AM, Orešič M, Bertram HC. Gut metabolome meets microbiome: A methodological perspective to understand the relationship between host and microbe. *Methods.* 2018;149:3–12.

33. Agus A, Clément K, Sokol H. Gut microbiota-derived metabolites as central regulators in metabolic disorders. *Gut.* 2021;70(6):1174–82.

34. Blegvad C, Nybo Andersen AM, Groot J, Zachariae C, Barker J, Skov L. Clinical characteristics including cardiovascular and metabolic risk factors in adolescents with psoriasis. *J. Eur. Acad. Dermatol. Venereol.* 2020;34(7):1516–23.

35. Akbar N, Azzimato V, Choudhury RP, Aouadi M. Extracellular vesicles in metabolic disease. *Diabetologia.* 2019;62:2179–87.

36. Forouzanfar MH, Afshin A, Alexander LT, Anderson HR, Bhutta ZA, Biryukov S, Brauer M, Burnett R, Cercy K, Charlson FJ, Cohen AJ. Global, regional, and national comparative risk assessment of 79 behavioural, environmental and occupational, and metabolic risks or clusters of risks, 1990–2015: A systematic analysis for the Global Burden of Disease Study 2015. *Lancet.* 2016;388(10053):1659–724.

37. Makki K, Deehan EC, Walter J, Bäckhed F. The impact of dietary fiber on gut microbiota in host health and disease. *Cell Host Microbe.* 2018;23(6):705–15.

38. Diehl AM, Day C. Cause, pathogenesis, and treatment of nonalcoholic steatohepatitis. *N. Engl. J. Med.* 2017;377:2063–72.

39. Moszak M, Szulińska M, Bogdański P. You are what you eat—The relationship between diet, microbiota, and metabolic disorders—A review. *Nutrients.* 2020;12(4):1096.

40. Kitada M, Koya D. Autophagy in metabolic disease and ageing. *Nat. Rev. Endocrinol.* 2021;17(11):647–61.

41. Sharma BR, Kanneganti TD. NLRP3 inflammasome in cancer and metabolic diseases. *Nat. Immunol.* 2021;22(5):550–9.

42. Kawai T, Autieri MV, Scalia R. Adipose tissue inflammation and metabolic dysfunction in obesity. *Am. J. Physiol. Cell Physiol.* 2021;320(3):C375–91.

43. Nilsson PM, Tuomilehto J, Rydén L. The metabolic syndrome–what is it and how should it be managed? *Eur. J. Prev. Cardiol.* 2019;26(2_suppl):33–46.

44. Qi X, Yun C, Pang Y, Qiao J. The impact of the gut microbiota on the reproductive and metabolic endocrine system. *Gut Microbes.* 2021;13(1):1894070.

45. World Health Organization. *Global Recommendations on Physical Activity for Health.* World Health Organization; 2010.

46. Park JH, Moon JH, Kim HJ, Kong MH, Oh YH. Sedentary lifestyle: Overview of updated evidence of potential health risks. *Korean J. Fam. Med.* 2020; (6):365.

47. Feng X, Sureda A, Jafari S, Memariani Z, Tewari D, Annunziata G, Barrea L, Hassan ST, Šmejkal K, Malaník M, Sychrová A. Berberine in cardiovascular and metabolic diseases: from mechanisms to therapeutics. *Theranostics.* 2019;9(7):1923.

48. Amorim JA, Coppotelli G, Rolo AP, Palmeira CM, Ross JM, Sinclair DA. Mitochondrial and metabolic dysfunction in ageing and age-related diseases. *Nat. Rev. Endocrinol.* 2022;(4):243–58.

49. Armutcu F. Organ crosstalk: The potent roles of inflammation and fibrotic changes in the course of organ interactions. *Inflamm. Res.* 2019;68:825–39.

50. Prasun P. Mitochondrial dysfunction in metabolic syndrome. *Biochim. Biophys. Acta.* 2020;1866(10):165838.

51. Cole JB, Florez JC. Genetics of diabetes mellitus and diabetes complications. *Nat. Rev. Nephrol.* 2020;7:377–90.

52. Roep BO, Thomaidou S, van Tienhoven R, Zaldumbide A. Type 1 diabetes mellitus as a disease of the β-cell (do not blame the immune system?). *Nat. Rev. Endocrinol.* 2021 (3):150–61.

53. Oguntibeju OO. Type 2 diabetes mellitus, oxidative stress and inflammation: Examining the links. *Int. J. Physiol. Pathophysiol. Pharmacol.* 2019;11(3):45.

54. McIntyre HD, Catalano P, Zhang C, Desoye G, Mathiesen ER, Damm P. Gestational diabetes mellitus. *Nat. Rev. Dis. Primers.* 2019;5(1):47.

55. Nekoua MP, Alidjinou EK, Hober D. Persistent coxsackievirus B infection and pathogenesis of type 1 diabetes mellitus. *Nat. Rev. Endocrinol.*2022;18(8):503–16.

56. Hjelmesæth J, Müller F, Jenssen T, Rollag H, Sagedal S, Hartmann A. Is there a link between cytomegalovirus infection and new-onset posttransplantation diabetes mellitus? Potential mechanisms of virus induced β-cell damage. *Nephrol. Dial.* 2005;20(11):2311–5.

57. Nodoushan SA, Nabavi A. The interaction of Helicobacter pylori infection and type 2 diabetes mellitus. *Adv. Biomed. Res.* 2019;8:15 (1–16).

58. Rodrigues CF, Rodrigues ME, Henriques M. Candida sp. infections in patients with diabetes mellitus. *J. Clin. Med.* 2019;8(1):76.

59. Blüher M. Adipose tissue dysfunction contributes to obesity related metabolic diseases. *Best Pract. Res. Clin. Endocrinol. Metab.* 2013;27(2):163–77.

60. da Silva Fernandes J, Schuelter-Trevisol F, Cancelier AC, Goncalves e Silva HC, de Sousa DG, Atkinson RL, Trevisol DJ. Adenovirus 36 prevalence and association with human obesity: A systematic review. *Int. J. Obes.* 2021 (6):1342–56.

61. Baradaran A, Dehghanbanadaki H, Naderpour S, Pirkashani LM, Rajabi A, Rashti R, Riahifar S, Moradi Y. The association between Helicobacter pylori and obesity: A systematic review and meta-analysis of case–control studies. *Clin. Diab. Endocrinol.* 2021 (1):1–1.

62. Liu BN, Liu XT, Liang ZH, Wang JH. Gut microbiota in obesity. *World J. Gastroenterol.* 2021;27(25):3837.

63. Groenewegen A, Rutten FH, Mosterd A, Hoes AW. Epidemiology of heart failure. *Eur. J. Heart Failure.* 2020;22(8):1342–56.

64. Martens CR, Accornero F. Viruses in the heart: Direct and indirect routes to myocarditis and heart failure. *Viruses.* 2021;13(10):1924.

65. Murakami Y, Tanimoto K, Fujiwara H, An J, Suemori K, Ochi T, Hasegawa H, Yasukawa M. Human herpesvirus 6 infection impairs Toll-like receptor signaling. *Virol. J.* 2010;7(1):1–5.

66. Chimenti C, Russo A, Pieroni M, Calabrese F, Verardo R, Thiene G, Russo MA, Maseri A, Frustaci A. Intramyocyte detection of Epstein-Barr virus genome by laser capture microdissection in patients with inflammatory cardiomyopathy. *Circulation.* 2004;110(23):3534–9.

67. Magno Palmeira M, Umemura Ribeiro HY, Garcia Lira Y, Machado Jucá Neto FO, da Silva Rodrigues IA, Fernandes da Paz LN, Nascimento Pinheiro MD. Heart failure due to cytomegalovirus myocarditis in immunocompetent young adults: A case report. *BMC Res. Notes.* 2016;9:1–5.

68. Cersosimo A, Riccardi M, Amore L, Cimino G, Arabia G, Metra M, Vizzardi E. Varicella zoster virus and cardiovascular diseases. *Monaldi Arch. Chest Dis.* 2022. DOI: 10.4081/monaldi.2022.2414.

69. Bloomfield GS, Alenezi F, Barasa FA, Lumsden R, Mayosi BM, Velazquez EJ. Human immunodeficiency virus and heart failure in low-and middle-income countries. *JACC: Heart Failure.* 2015;3(8):579–90.

70. Kadoglou NP, Bracke F, Simmers T, Tsiodras S, Parissis J. Influenza infection and heart failure—Vaccination may change heart failure prognosis? *Heart Failure Rev.* 2017 329–36.

71. Martens CR, Accornero F. Viruses in the heart: Direct and indirect routes to myocarditis and heart failure. *Viruses.* 2021;13(10):1924.

72. Kountouras J, Papaefthymiou A, Polyzos SA, Deretzi G, Vardaka E, Soteriades ES, Tzitiridou-Chatzopoulou M, Gkolfakis P, Karafyllidou K, Doulberis M. Impact of Helicobacter pylori-related metabolic syndrome parameters on arterial hypertension. *Microorganisms.* 2021;(11):2351.

73. Cook PJ, Lip GY, Davies P, Beevers DG, Wise R, Honeybourne D. Chlamydia pneumoniae antibodies in severe essential hypertension. *Hypertension.* 1998;31(2):589–94.

74. Wang CC, Cheng PN, Kao JH. Systematic review: Chronic viral hepatitis and metabolic derangement. *AP&T.* 2020;51(2):216–30.

75. Ji Y, Yin Y, Li Z, Zhang W. Gut microbiota-derived components and metabolites in the progression of non-alcoholic fatty liver disease (NAFLD). *Nutrients.* 2019;11(8):1712.

76. Peters L, Burkert S, Grüner B. Parasites of the liver–epidemiology, diagnosis and clinical management in the European context. *J. Hepatol.* 2021;75(1):202–18.

77. Hendrikx T, Schnabl B. Indoles: Metabolites produced by intestinal bacteria capable of controlling liver disease manifestation. *J. Intern. Med.* 2019;286(1):32–40.

78. Nguyen Y, Stirnemann J, Belmatoug N. Gaucher disease: A review. *La Revue de Medecine Interne.* 2019;40(5):313–22.

79. Xu J, Jakher Y, Ahrens-Nicklas RC. Brain branched-chain amino acids in maple syrup urine disease: Implications for neurological disorders. *Int. J. Mol. Sci.* 2020;21(20):7490.

Index

For Product Safety Concerns and Information please contact our EU
representative GPSR@taylorandfrancis.com
Taylor & Francis Verlag GmbH, Kaufingerstraße 24, 80331 München, Germany